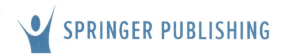

GET THE MOST FROM YOUR BOOK

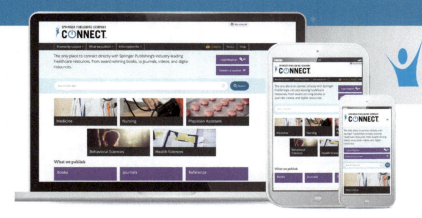

VOUCHER CODE:

7LVR6NBU

Online Access

Your print purchase of *The Handbook of Health Behavior Change,* Sixth Edition, includes **online access via Springer Publishing Connect**™ to increase accessibility, portability, and searchability.

Insert the code at http://connect.springerpub.com/content/book/978-0-8261-4265-8 or scan the QR code and insert the voucher code today!

Having trouble? Contact our customer service department at *cs@springerpub.com*

Instructor Resource Access for Adopters

Let us do some of the heavy lifting to create an engaging classroom experience with a variety of instructor resources included in most textbooks SUCH AS:

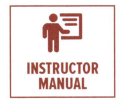
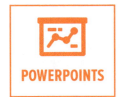
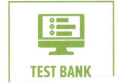

Visit **https://connect.springerpub.com/** and look for the **"Show Supplementary"** button [to see] what is available to instructors! First time using Springer Publishing Connect?

Email **textbook@springerpub.com** to create an account and start unlocking valuable resou[rces].

THE HANDBOOK OF HEALTH BEHAVIOR CHANGE

ANGIE L. CRADOCK, ScD, MPE, is a principal research scientist and deputy director at the Prevention Research Center on Nutrition and Physical Activity at the Harvard T.H. Chan School of Public Health in the Department of Social and Behavioral Sciences. Dr. Cradock's research focuses on the social, policy, and environmental factors associated with physical activity and nutrition.

KRISTINA H. LEWIS, MD, MPH, SM, is an internal medicine physician, board-certified in obesity medicine, whose clinical practice is in adult weight management. She is also an associate professor at the Wake Forest University School of Medicine at the Department of Epidemiology and Prevention, with a joint appointment at the Department of Implementation Science.

JUSTIN B. MOORE, PhD, MS, is a behavioral scientist who specializes in the design, implementation, and evaluation of behavioral interventions to promote healthy lifestyles in clinical and community settings. He is a professor and vice-chair for the Department of Implementation Science at the Wake Forest University School of Medicine, with joint appointments at the Department of Epidemiology and Prevention and the Department of Family and Community Medicine.

THE HANDBOOK OF HEALTH BEHAVIOR CHANGE

SIXTH EDITION

Angie L. Cradock, ScD, MPE
Kristina H. Lewis, MD, MPH, SM
Justin B. Moore, PhD, MS

Editors

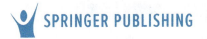

Copyright © 2025 Springer Publishing Company, LLC
All rights reserved.
First Springer Publishing edition: 978-0-8261-6780-4, 1998; subsequent editions, 2004; 2008; 2014; 2018

No part of this publication may be reproduced, stored in a retrieval system, or transmitted in any form or by any means, electronic, mechanical, photocopying, recording, or otherwise, without the prior permission of Springer Publishing Company, LLC, or authorization through payment of the appropriate fees to the Copyright Clearance Center, Inc., 222 Rosewood Drive, Danvers, MA 01923, 978-750-8400, fax 978-646-8600, info@copyright.com or at www.copyright.com.

Springer Publishing Company, LLC
902 Carnegie Center/Suite 140
Princeton, NJ 08540
www.springerpub.com
connect.springerpub.com

Acquisitions Editor: David D'Addona
Content Development Editor: Julia Curcio
Production Editor: Joseph Stubenrauch
Compositor: Amnet

ISBN: 978-0-8261-4264-1
e-book ISBN: 978-0-8261-4265-8
DOI: 10.1891/9780826142658

SUPPLEMENTS:

 A robust set of instructor resources designed to supplement this text is located at http://connect.springerpub.com/content/book/978-0-8261-4265-8. Qualifying instructors may request access by emailing textbook@springerpub.com.

Instructor Materials:
LMS Common Cartridge–All Instructor Resources ISBN: 978-0-8261-3744-9
Instructor Manual ISBN: 978-0-8261-4267-2
Instructor Test Bank ISBN: 978-0-8261-4268-9
Instructor PowerPoint Presentations ISBN: 978-0-8261-4266-5
Instructor Sample Syllabus ISBN: 978-0-8261-5239-8
Transition Guide: Fifth to Sixth Edition ISBN: 978-0-8261-5139-1

24 25 26 27 / 5 4 3 2 1

The author and the publisher of this Work have made every effort to use sources believed to be reliable to provide information that is accurate and compatible with the standards generally accepted at the time of publication. Because medical science is continually advancing, our knowledge base continues to expand. Therefore, as new information becomes available, changes in procedures become necessary. We recommend that the reader always consult current research and specific institutional policies before performing any clinical procedure or delivering any medication. The author and publisher shall not be liable for any special, consequential, or exemplary damages resulting, in whole or in part, from the readers' use of, or reliance on, the information contained in this book. The publisher has no responsibility for the persistence or accuracy of URLs for external or third-party Internet websites referred to in this publication and does not guarantee that any content on such websites is, or will remain, accurate or appropriate.

Library of Congress Cataloging-in-Publication Data
Names: Cradock, Angie L., editor. | Lewis, Kristina H., editor. |
  Moore, Justin B., editor.
Title: The handbook of health behavior change / Angie L. Cradock, Kristina
  H. Lewis, Justin B. Moore, editors.
Description: Sixth edition. | New York : Springer Publishing Company,
  [2025] | Includes bibliographical references and index.
Identifiers: LCCN 2024013926 (print) | LCCN 2024013927 (ebook) | ISBN
  9780826142641 (paperback) | ISBN 9780826142658 (ebook)
Subjects: MESH: Health Promotion | Health Behavior | Patient Compliance | Healthy Lifestyle
Classification: LCC RA776.9 (print) | LCC RA776.9 (ebook) | NLM WA 590 | DDC 613—dc23/eng/20240625
LC record available at https://lccn.loc.gov/2024013926
LC ebook record available at https://lccn.loc.gov/2024013927

Contact sales@springerpub.com to receive discount rates on bulk purchases.

Publisher's Note: **New and used products purchased from third-party sellers are not guaranteed for quality, authenticity, or access to any included digital components.**

Printed in the United States of America by Gasch Printing.

This edition is dedicated to the scientists, community members, and practitioners who work tirelessly to ensure that everyone can lead a healthy, fulfilling life regardless of their race, ethnicity, gender, socioeconomic status, or geography.

CONTENTS

Contributors   ix
Preface   xiii
Acknowledgments   xv
Instructor Resources   xvii

I. THEORIES, FRAMEWORKS, AND MEASURES RELEVANT TO HEALTH BEHAVIORS

1. How Policy, Society, and Economics Shape Health Behaviors   *1*
Vahé Heboyan and J. Dustin Tracy

2. Population Health, Social Ecology, and Community-Engaged Research   *21*
Scott D. Rhodes, Benjamin D. Smart, Ana D. Sucaldito, Amanda E. Tanner, and Enbal Shacham

3. Interventions With the Family System: Translating Theory Into Practice   *39*
Emily R. Hamburger, Lindsay S. Mayberry, and Sarah S. Jaser

4. Individual-Level Theories   *60*
Jay E. Maddock

5. Developmental and Cultural Influences on Behavior and Health   *82*
Crystal S. Lim and E. Thomaseo Burton

6. Measuring Health Behaviors at the Individual and Community Levels   *100*
Alexandra D. Monzon, Jessica S. Pierce, Lindsay A. Taliaferro, and Rachel M. Wasserman

II. PRIORITIZED BEHAVIORS FOR PRIMARY PREVENTION OF DISEASE

7. Dietary Behavior Change   *119*
Tracy E. Crane and Samantha Werts-Pelter

8. Physical Activity   *139*
Jylana L. Sheats, Sandra J. Winter, and Abby C. King

9. Tobacco, Alcohol, and Other Drugs   *164*
Oluwole Jegede, Joyce Rivera, Mark Jenkins, and Ayana Jordan

10. Vaccines   *192*
Abram L. Wagner

11. Sexual and Reproductive Health   *212*
Jewel Gausman, Kathryn Barker, Mahesh Karra, and Ana Langer

12. Behavior Change Approaches to Preventing Unintentional Injuries   *236*
David A. Sleet and Andrea C. Gielen

VIII CONTENTS

III. PRIORITIZED BEHAVIORS FOR SECONDARY PREVENTION

13. Screening for Cancer *253*
Kirsten Nguyen and Jennifer Richmond

14. Cardiovascular Disease: A Focus on Primary and Secondary Prevention *274*
Krupal Jay Hari, Yashashwi Pokharel, and Justin B. Moore

15. Diabetes Management Behaviors: The Key to Optimal Health and Quality of Life Outcomes *294*
Korey K. Hood and Ryan D. Tweet

16. Obesity *316*
Loneke T. Blackman Carr and Veronica R. Johnson

17. Mental and Behavioral Health *341*
Katherine Sanchez and Marisol Vargas Vilugron

IV. INTERVENING IN SETTINGS AND SYSTEMS TO MODIFY HEALTH BEHAVIORS

18. School Interventions to Support Health Behavior Change *357*
Rebekka M. Lee, Andria B. Eisman, and Steven L. Gortmaker

19. Chronic Disease Prevention in the Worksite *373*
Elizabeth Ablah, Mary T. Imboden, and Anna L. Zendell

20. Healthcare Provider and System Interventions Promoting Health Behavior Change *392*
Kristina H. Lewis

21. The Roles of the Built Environment in Supporting Health Behavior Change *413*
Angie L. Cradock

Index *437*

CONTRIBUTORS

Elizabeth Ablah, PhD, MPH, CPH, Professor, University of Kansas School of Medicine, Wichita, Kansas

Kathryn Barker, ScD, MPH, Assistant Adjunct Professor, Medicine, University of California, San Diego, San Diego, California

Loneke T. Blackman Carr, PhD, MA, RD, Assistant Professor, Department of Nutritional Sciences, University of Connecticut, Storrs, Connecticut

E. Thomaseo Burton, PhD, MPH, Clinical Psychologist, Children's Hospital of Philadelphia, Philadelphia, Pennsylvania

Angie L. Cradock, ScD, MPE, Principal Research Scientist and Deputy Director, Department of Social and Behavioral Sciences, T.H. Chan School of Public Health, Harvard University, Boston, Massachusetts

Tracy E. Crane, PhD, RDN, Associate Professor, College of Medicine, University of Miami and Sylvester Cancer Center, Miami, Florida

Andria B. Eisman, PhD, Associate Professor, Division of Kinesiology, Health, and Sport Studies, College of Education, Wayne State University, Detroit, Michigan

Jewel Gausman, ScD, MHS, Senior Research Associate, Women and Health Initiative, Department of Global Health and Population, T.H. Chan School of Public Health, Harvard University, Boston, Massachusetts

Andrea C. Gielen, ScM, ScD, FAAHB, Professor Emerita, Bloomberg School of Public Health, Johns Hopkins, Baltimore, Maryland

Steven L. Gortmaker, PhD, Professor, Department of Social and Behavioral Sciences, T.H. Chan School of Public Health, Harvard University, Boston, Massachusetts

Emily R. Hamburger, MEd, Graduate Research Assistant, University of Nebraska-Lincoln, Lincoln, Nebraska

Krupal Jay Hari, MD, Department of Cardiology, Internal Medicine, Wake Forest Medical Center, Winston-Salem, North Carolina

Vahé Heboyan, PhD, Associate Professor, Health Management, Economics, and Policy Department, Augusta University, Augusta, Georgia

Korey K. Hood, PhD, MS, Professor of Pediatrics, Endocrinology, Professor of Psychiatry and Behavioral Sciences, Child and Adolescent Psychology, Stanford University, Stanford, California

X CONTRIBUTORS

Mary T. Imboden, PhD, MS, Assistant Professor, George Fox University and Health Enhancement Research Organization, Newberg, Oregon

Sarah S. Jaser, PhD, William R. Long Director, Professor, Division of Pediatric Psychology, Vanderbilt University Medical Center, Nashville, Tennessee

Oluwole Jegede, MD, MPH, Assistant Professor, Yale School of Medicine, New Haven, Connecticut

Mark Jenkins CEO and Founder, Connecticut Harm Reduction Alliance, Hartford, Connecticut

Veronica R. Johnson, MD, Assistant Professor, Department of Medicine, Division of General Internal Medicine, Northwestern University Feinberg School of Medicine, Chicago, Illinois

Ayana Jordan, MD, PhD, Assistant Professor, Adjunct of Psychiatry, Yale School of Medicine, Affiliated Faculty, Yale Institute for Global Health, New Haven, Connecticut

Mahesh Karra, MSc, ScD, Assistant Professor, Global Development Policy, Frederick S. Pardee School of Global Studies, Boston University, Boston, Massachusetts

Abby C. King, PhD, David and Susan Heckerman Professor, Professor and Vice Chair for Academic Affairs, Department of Epidemiology and Population Health; Professor of Medicine, Stanford Prevention Research Center; Director, Stanford Healthy Aging Research and Technology Solutions, Palo Alto, California

Ana Langer, MD, Professor of the Practice of Public Health, Emerita, Department of Global Health and Population, T.H. Chan School of Public Health, Harvard University, Boston, Massachusetts

Rebekka M. Lee, ScD, Lecturer, Department of Social and Behavioral Sciences, T.H. Chan School of Public Health, Harvard University, Boston, Massachusetts

Kristina H. Lewis, MD, MPH, SM, Associate Professor, Department of Epidemiology and Prevention, School of Medicine, Wake Forest University, Winston-Salem, North Carolina

Crystal S. Lim, PhD, ABPP, Associate Professor and Chair, Department of Health Psychology, University of Missouri, Columbia, Missouri

Jay E. Maddock, PhD, Regents Professor, Texas A&M University, College Station, Texas

Lindsay S. Mayberry, PhD, Associate Professor, Vanderbilt University Medical Center, Nashville, Tennessee

Alexandra D. Monzon, PhD, Postdoctoral Research Fellow, Center for Healthcare Delivery Science, Nemours Children's Health, Orlando, Florida

Justin B. Moore, PhD, MS, Professor and Vice-Chair, Department of Implementation Science, School of Medicine, Wake Forest University, Winston-Salem, North Carolina

CONTRIBUTORS **XI**

Kirsten Nguyen, School of Medicine, Vanderbilt University, Nashville, Tennessee

Jessica S. Pierce, PhD, Psychologist and Research Scientist, Center for Healthcare Delivery Science, Nemours Children's Health, Orlando, Florida

Yashashwi Pokharel, MD, MSCR, Cardiology, Department of Internal Medicine, Atrium Health Wake Forest Baptist, School of Medicine, Wake Forest University, Winston-Salem, North Carolina

Scott D. Rhodes, PhD, MPH, Professor, Department of Social Sciences and Health Policy, School of Medicine, Wake Forest University, Winston-Salem, North Carolina

Jennifer Richmond, PhD, MSPH, Assistant Professor, Division of Public Health Sciences, Department of Social Sciences and Health Policy, School of Medicine, Wake Forest University, Winston-Salem, North Carolina

Joyce Rivera, ABD, MA, Founder, Chief Executive Officer, St. Ann's Corner of Harm Reduction, Bronx, New York

Katherine Sanchez, PhD, LCSW, Baylor Scott & White Research Institute, Dallas, Texas

Enbal Shacham, PhD, MPH, Professor, Department of Behavioral Science and Health Equity, St. Louis University, St. Louis, Missouri

Jylana L. Sheats, PhD, MPH, Clinical Associate Professor, Department of Social, Behavioral and Population Science, Tulane University School of Public Health and Tropical Medicine, New Orleans, Louisiana

David A. Sleet, PhD, FAAHB, Professor Emeritus, San Diego State University, San Diego, California; Senior Associate, Injury Prevention, Bizzell US and Bizzell Global LLC, New Carrollton, Maryland

Benjamin D. Smart, MD, MS, Department of Global Public Health, Karolinska Institutet, Stockholm, Sweden

Ana D. Sucaldito, PhD, Postdoctoral Research Fellow, Department of Social Sciences and Health Policy, School of Medicine, Wake Forest University, Winston-Salem, North Carolina

Lindsay A. Taliaferro, PhD, MPH, CHES, Assistant Professor, Department of Population Health Sciences, College of Medicine, University of Central Florida, Orlando, Florida

Amanda E. Tanner, PhD, MPH, Professor, Department of Public Health Education, University of North Carolina Greensboro, Greensboro, North Carolina

J. Dustin Tracy, PhD, Assistant Professor, Health Management, Economics, and Policy Department, Augusta University, Augusta, Georgia

Ryan D. Tweet, PsyD, Assistant Professor, Division of Endocrinology, Diabetes and Clinical Nutrition, Oregon Health & Science University School of Medicine, Portland, Oregon

Marisol Vargas Vilugron, LCSW, Baylor Scott & White Research Institute, Dallas, Texas

XII CONTRIBUTORS

Abram L. Wagner, PhD, MPH, Assistant Professor, Epidemiology, Assistant Professor of Global Health, Department of Epidemiology, School of Public Health, University of Michigan, Ann Arbor, Michigan

Rachel M. Wasserman, PhD, Psychologist and Assistant Research Scientist, Nemours Children's Health, Center for Healthcare Delivery Science, Orlando, Florida

Samantha Werts-Pelter, MPH, Research Program Administration Officer II, Department of Health Promotion Sciences, Mel and Enid Zuckerman College of Public Health, University of Arizona, Tucson, Arizona

Sandra J. Winter, PhD, MHA, Executive Director, Senior Coastsiders, Half Moon Bay, California

Anna L. Zendell, PhD, MSW, Program Director, School of Health and Natural Sciences, Bay Path University, Longmeadow, Massachusetts

PREFACE

CHALLENGES AND OPPORTUNITIES

In the United States and across the globe, the past 5 years have resulted in seismic shifts in the challenges to population health and well-being that future public health professionals must be prepared and equipped to address. This new edition of *The Handbook of Health Behavior Change* seeks to consider and explore these current and emerging public health challenges. This edition fits in the *Handbook*'s long-standing tradition of serving as a practical guide for graduate students on the key theories, methods, and strategies they will need to be effective in promoting health behavior changes in their communities and workplaces. As editors, we aimed for this edition to include behaviors and health topics of major interest, including those related to the leading causes of death and morbidity in the United States among adults and children, which have notably shifted over time. We sought to ensure that health and health equity were considered both in the discussion of health challenges and in the framing of effective strategies. This focus is essential to ensure the future workforce will be able to recognize the importance of equity considerations for health behavior change and apply an equity lens as they look at data, conduct research, or design programs to effect health behavior change in multiple settings.

In this sixth edition, we also sought to integrate several new features to facilitate a variety of learning and teaching styles and to ensure alignment with core public health competencies. Each chapter begins with learning objectives and focuses on providing multiple examples of the chapter content in practice through case studies and practical examples. Figures and tables provide content in varied formats to promote reader engagement and extend the text in ways that support understanding and visual identification of key issues and learnings. Chapter authors provide a summary of key points, and each chapter includes discussion questions to help guide students' deeper engagement with the content and provide a jumping-off point for classroom work, or with study groups. With these features, we hope this edition provides a practical road map for teaching the next generation of students about the key challenges and opportunities for health behavior change and insights into social and behavioral science-based approaches to disease prevention.

IN THIS TEXT

In this new edition, you will find the sections are reorganized to focus in four areas: The first section, "Theories, Frameworks, and Measures Relevant to Health Behaviors," considers and expands on the theories that draw from multiple disciplines and perspectives. The organization of this section's theory presentation begins with the broadest, economic, policy, and systems perspectives and moves down to the individual-level theories. This organization is intentional and may differ from the approach that is typical of behavior change texts, which commonly begin at the individual level and then zoom out to the environmental level. This section starts with a strong population health grounding in two new chapters that address the ways that policy can employ economics to shape health behaviors and population health and community theories of change. Chapter 1 explains how the choices individuals make often involve weighing the costs and benefits of their actions (or inaction), and how policies might be developed with this understanding in mind. Chapter 2 introduces concepts of population health, social ecology, community-engaged research, and health equity that permeate the remainder of the book. The middle of this section addresses family systems before outlining

XIV PREFACE

the most commonly used individual-level theories in behavior change research and practice. This section rounds out with a chapter focused on developmental and cultural influences on behavior and health (Chapter 5) and ends with guidance for measuring health behaviors at the individual and community levels (Chapter 6).

The second section, "Prioritized Behaviors for Primary Prevention of Disease," addresses behaviors and health topics of interest, including those related to the shifting landscape of the leading causes of death and morbidity in the United States among adults and children and priority public health concerns that were not considered in the prior editions. The sixth edition covers health-related behaviors that contribute to the leading chronic diseases in the U.S. population, including a chapter focused on dietary behavior change (Chapter 7), physical activity (Chapter 8), and tobacco, alcohol, and other drugs (Chapter 9). This section includes a new chapter on vaccines (Chapter 10). This new chapter as well as the two other new chapter topic areas, sexual and reproductive health (Chapter 11) and injury prevention (Chapter 12), help inform a new focus on these emerging public health concerns and provide students and instructors with resources to engage in productive discussions in these topic areas.

In the third section, "Prioritized Behaviors for Secondary Prevention," we continue to cover core areas of prevention that address chronic diseases, including cardiovascular disease, diabetes, and obesity, that now impact the majority of the U.S. population. Chapter 13 addresses secondary prevention behaviors, including screening for cancers, and Chapter 14 reviews the challenges facing those with cardiovascular disease, highlighting the evidence underscoring the essential role of aggressive risk factor management and behavioral–lifestyle modification for patients with this highly prevalent disease. In their examination of the challenges of managing diabetes (Chapter 15), the authors explore how to best manage the different types of diabetes and the barriers that prevent effective management in diverse patient populations. In Chapter 16, key concepts are discussed regarding the prevalence, diagnosis, and treatment of obesity, which continues to negatively impact the health of populations in developed and developing countries worldwide. This sixth edition also includes a new chapter (Chapter 17) on mental and behavioral health outcomes, with a particular focus on conditions commonly encountered in primary care and community settings—anxiety and depression.

Finally, the sixth edition concludes with the fourth section, "Intervening in Settings and Systems to Modify Health Behaviors," which covers setting-specific examples of interventions and strategies that focus on key settings for public health interventions. Readers will find updated content and discussion on settings including the schools where students learn (Chapter 18), as well as worksites (Chapter 19), including updates to new styles of work, such as remote work structures and how changes in work have influenced intervention practices. We close out this section with a chapter focused on healthcare providers and system interventions (Chapter 20), before heading into the community with a focus on the built environments that we live within (Chapter 21).

A robust set of instructor resources designed to supplement this text, including an instructor's manual, PowerPoints, test bank, and syllabus, can be accessed by qualified instructors at http://connect.springerpub.com/content/book/978-0-8261-4265-8. Qualifying instructors may request access by emailing textbook@springerpub.com.

As editors of this sixth edition, we recognize a long history since its initial publication in 1988 and its tenure as a practical guide for public health prevention and behavior change strategies for students. We trust that, in this updated edition, the content and topics of focus will continue to be practical and meaningful and engage a new generation of public health students, professionals, and leaders in seeking impactful actions in policy and practice to support and benefit the health of our population and promote greater health equity.

In health,

Angie L. Cradock
Kristina H. Lewis
Justin B. Moore

ACKNOWLEDGMENTS

Great thanks to:

- Marisa E. Hilliard, Kristin A. Riekert, Judith K. Ockene, and Lori Pbert, the editors of the fifth edition of *The Handbook of Health Behavior Change*, for providing a strong foundation for the sixth edition.

- The returning and new authors of the sixth edition, for sharing insights and knowledge with the public health professionals that will shape our future population health policy and practices.

- David D'Addona, Senior Editor, and Julia Curcio, Content Development Editor, at Springer Publishing, for keeping us focused on the tasks at hand while supporting us every step of the way.

Angie: Great thanks to my team at home, Kevin, Finn, and Caimin. I could not ask for a better crew.

Kristina: Thank you to my mother, JoAnn, for igniting my love of public health, and my father, Darrell, for sparking my scientific curiosity. I'm grateful for childhood days spent looking at green slime under a microscope and family dinnertime conversations about HIV prevention in Tanzania.

Justin: I would like to thank my wife, Theresa, and my dogs, Scarlett and Ginger, for reminding me that work–life balance is essential if I'm going to save the world . . . eventually.

INSTRUCTOR RESOURCES

 A robust set of instructor resources designed to supplement this text is located at http://connect.springerpub.com/content/book/978-0-8261-4265-8. Qualifying instructors may request access by emailing textbook@springerpub.com.

- LMS Common Cartridge–All Instructor Resources
- Instructor Manual
- Instructor Test Bank
- Instructor PowerPoint Presentations
- Instructor Sample Syllabus
- Transition Guide: Fifth to Sixth Edition

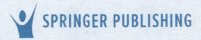

Visit http://connect.springerpub.com/content/book/978-0-8261-4265-8 and look for the "**Show Supplementary**" button on the **book homepage**.

PART I: THEORIES, FRAMEWORKS, AND MEASURES
RELEVANT TO HEALTH BEHAVIORS

CHAPTER 1

HOW POLICY, SOCIETY, AND ECONOMICS SHAPE HEALTH BEHAVIORS

VAHÉ HEBOYAN AND J. DUSTIN TRACY

LEARNING OBJECTIVES

- Identify how social determinants combined with individual behavior impact health.
- Understand how economic principles explain health behaviors.
- Recognize why markets may not work well when health is involved.
- Describe the various policy tools available to try to change health behaviors and which are likely to be effective in a particular circumstance.
- Understand the concept and use of economic analysis and economic evaluation techniques in shaping health policy and programming.
- Identify how communication regarding a policy might be as important as the policy itself.

INTRODUCTION

In the United States, there are large discrepancies in health based on race and sex. While life expectancy is a very tangible, observable measure of these inequities, similar discrepancies persist across many other health measures, including rates of obesity, high blood pressure (hypertension), diabetes, and cancer. While the COVID-19 epidemic exacerbated these differences, it also helped draw the public spotlight inequities that were previously the domain of researchers and policy makers. While some differences in health outcomes may be due to genetic and biological factors, race and sex are correlated with many other aspects that impact health in a variety of ways. Researchers and policy makers refer to the nonmedical factors that influence health outcomes as the social determinants of health (SDOH).

The World Health Organization (WHO) describes SDOH as ". . . the conditions in which people are born, grow, work, live, and age, and the wider set of forces and systems shaping the conditions of daily life. These forces and systems include economic policies and systems, development agendas, social norms, social policies and political systems" (WHO, 2023). The U.S. Centers for Disease Control and Prevention (CDC) organizes SDOH into five areas (**Figure 1.1**): (a) economic stability, (b) education access and quality, (c) health access and quality, (d) neighborhood and built environment, and (e) social community context (U.S. Department of Health and Human Services. Office of Disease Prevention and Health Promotion, 2023).

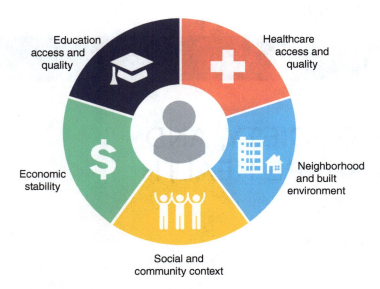

FIGURE 1.1 Social determinants of health.
Source: From U.S. Department of Health and Human Services. Office of Disease Prevention and Health Promotion. (2023). *Healthy people 2030: Social determinants of health.* Office of the Assistant Secretary for Health, Office of the Secretary, U.S. Department of Health and Human Services. https://health.gov/healthypeople/priority-areas/social-determinants-health.

As health behaviors do not occur in a vacuum, SDOH are important to behavior change. Behaviors take place in the context of and are shaped by the environment in which the person exhibits the behavior. Considering existing health disparities and the importance of social and environmental contributors to those disparities, one of the expressed goals of the CDC is to increase health equity, meaning decrease the differences we see among groups. The CDC pursues policies, programs, and interventions to reduce conditions we know lead to poorer health. While in an ideal world everyone would adopt and maintain healthy behaviors, there is a recognition that behavior change can be harder when SDOH create barriers to a healthy lifestyle. Therefore, policy or programmatic solutions that address these factors external to the individual may be necessary in some populations to better support equitable health outcomes. Economic inequality is one major determinant of health outcomes, and while it is beyond the CDC or the U.S. Department of Health and Human Services (HHS) to create economic stability they may be able to enact policies that decrease the impact that economic instability has on health. Healthy People 2030 is a data-driven campaign targeting objectives toward this goal. Healthy People 2030's website (health.gov/healthypeople) displays the leading health indicators and the disparities among them.

LIFE EXPECTANCY

As mentioned previously and shown in **Figure 1.2**, there are large differences in life expectancy across races in the United States. More specifically, an Asian American person could expect to live almost 14 years longer than a Native American or Alaskan Native in 2019 and over 18 years by 2021. One unusual trend in these data is that life expectancy is decreasing during the time frame examined. Historically, life expectancy had increased over time largely due to technological and knowledge progress we made in preventing diseases, improving treatment, and increasing quality of life. For example, a baby born in 2000 was expected to live more years than one born in 1990. Overall, about half the decrease in life expectancy during the period shown in the figure was due to increased deaths from COVID-19. As you can see, the impact varies substantially by race and ethnicity. In the years 2019 to 2021, Asian Americans had a larger decrease in life expectancy due to increases in cancer than due to COVID-19 (Arias et al., 2022).

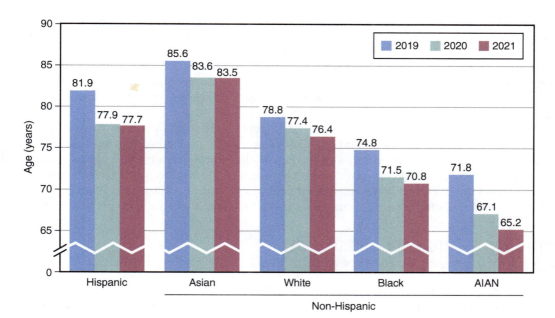

FIGURE 1.2 Life expectancy at birth, by Hispanic origin and race: United States, 2019 to 2021.
AIAN, American Indian or Alaskan Native.
Source: From Arias, E., Tejada-Vera, B., Kochanek, K. D., & Ahmad, F. B. (2022). *Provisional life expectancy estimates for 2021* (Vital Statistics Rapid Release. Report 23, Issue). https://stacks.cdc.gov/view/cdc/118999.

The CDC also estimates life expectancy by state and sex. These estimates can be accessed as an interactive map at www.cdc.gov/nchs/data-visualization/state-life-expectancy/index_2020.htm.

THE ROLES OF HEALTH POLICIES AND ECONOMICS IN INFLUENCING HEALTH

Health policies seek to improve population and individual health outcomes from the present state through disruption of the status quo. This is accomplished in many ways, including changing access and affordability of healthcare, adopting policies that promote preventive care (e.g., vaccinations and cancer screenings), regulating the quality of services provided by healthcare organizations and providers, addressing health disparities, and shaping more effective healthcare delivery methods. For example, the disparity in life expectancy across race and sex and the general decrease in life expectancy might inspire politicians and health agencies to consider policies that could reverse this trend. Policies aim to disrupt the status quo. Economics explains why the status quo exists.

There exist several road maps for behavioral targets that are thought to impact health and longevity, and thus could form a helpful guide for policy makers seeking to achieve this goal. *Healthy People 2030*, being one of these reports, made a detailed assessment of health in the United States and developed a 10-year plan to improve health. The assessment included many measures of health and components of health, as well as the factors that impact health. Based on the assessment, 359 core or measurable objectives were developed. One of these was to reduce the lung cancer death rate, explaining "[l]ung cancer is one of the most common and deadly cancers in the United States. Although lung cancer death rates have decreased in recent years, there are significant disparities by sex and race/ethnicity. Evidence shows that screening and interventions to prevent tobacco initiation and help people quit smoking can help lower the number of lung cancer deaths." In 2018, there were 34.8 lung

4 | • THEORIES, FRAMEWORKS, AND MEASURES RELEVANT TO HEALTH BEHAVIORS

cancer deaths per 100,000 people. A goal was set to try to reduce it to 25.1 deaths by 2030 through changing behaviors. The most recent data show that progress has been made on the goal; in 2021, there were only 31.7 deaths per 100,000. Healthy People 2030 also emphasized SDOH and therefore includes components to specifically address communities with high smoking rates or low rates of lung cancer screening. For example, Native Americans smoke at higher rate than other races, while Black Americans are screened for lung cancer at lower rates (Arrazola et al., 2023; Kunitomo et al., 2022).

Creation of health policy encompasses several steps, including a process for setting the goals of a policy, specifying the actual goals, developing the policy or programmatic interventions, and the actions to achieve those goals, and the processes to track progress toward achieving the goals. Lawmakers, government agencies at all levels, nonprofits, and even private companies might have policies related to health. Good policy will use data to understand the problem and will often use economics to analyze behavior and how it might be changed.

ECONOMIC PRINCIPLES IMPORTANT TO HEALTH POLICY DEVELOPMENT

Economics plays a vital role in shaping health policies and informing of their impact. *Economics* is a social science that studies how scarce resources, such as time, healthy foods, and medical care, are distributed and, often, asks if another allocation or distribution system would improve welfare and outcomes. Economics also studies how people (and firms run by people) make decisions, including how they use scarce resources, such as money, time, and inputs. Formally, economics is very mathematical and relies on equations and proofs in analysis. Economics also provides some fundamental concepts that provide insight into why the present situation exists and what policies are likely to be successful in improving health outcomes or other goals.

Before diving deeper into the types of economic analyses, it is important to distinguish between economics and related disciplines, such as finance and accounting. *Finance* is the science of money management and deals with the allocation of assets and liabilities over time under conditions of certainty and uncertainty. *Accounting* is the science of providing a framework to record, summarize, and report financial transactions to relevant organizations. Meanwhile, economics is the science of allocation of scarce resources to the best users. These resources not only include monetary resources, but also labor, land, production inputs, and time. Therefore, economic analysis goes beyond studying monetary decisions to include the broader set of resource allocation and decisions. In this chapter, we focus on intuition and outcomes. Like any discipline, economics has many very specific terms and jargon. To the degree possible, we avoid that jargon in favor of language understandable to a broader audience.

Although many factors influence health outcomes or a particular attribute of health, economics has powerful statistical tools and mathematical models to analyze and isolate the effect of individual determinants on health outcomes. Economists often analyze policy change, natural experiments, or cutoff rules to isolate casual effects of determinants of health. Economists have made many important contributions to our understanding of SDOH, such as the impact of neonatal nutrition (Lavy et al., 2016), neonatal air pollution (Currie & Neidell, 2005), air pollution on violence (Herrnstadt et al., 2021), and the relationship between education and health (Brunello et al., 2016), among many other areas.

Economics provides much insight into why SDOH differ among people. Raj Chetty and collaborators (2020) have made significant contributions to our understanding of the lack of intergenerational economic mobility. One is very likely to enjoy economic stability if one's parents enjoy it. Education and social networks play a large role in determining employment prospects and other economic opportunities. In a market economy, income and purchasing power are essential. Presumably, everyone would prefer to live in a location that is free of pollutants that adversely affect health, and therefore housing in these locations will be more expensive. Subsequently, individuals or families with lower income might not be able to afford to live in such locations. The same principles will hold for any scarce resource that increases health, be it a gym membership, quality food, or medical treatment. Employment in situations in which there are health risks generally pays more to compensate for these risks. People with more opportunities or who face fewer financial pressures will probably not take these jobs because even with extra pay it is not worth the risk. This might be compounded by the previous problem; housing near workplaces where there are risks might have similar risks (Badger et al., 2018).

CASE STUDY 1.1: THE OPPORTUNITY ATLAS

The Opportunity Atlas (www.opportunityatlas.org) is an interactive map based on research done by the U.S. Census Bureau, Brown University, and Harvard University. They used the Internal Revenue Service (IRS) and census data from 20 million Americans born between 1978 and 1983 to study how economic opportunity varies by neighborhood, race, sex, and parents' income. The authors of this chapter looked up the neighborhood immediately surrounding our university's main campus. It had very high economic opportunity, particularly in comparison with the surrounding areas. However, the advantage was driven by outcomes for females. There was also variation by parent income. What is notable is there are only data for White individuals. Out of privacy concerns, estimates are suppressed if they represent too few people. We also noticed the incarnation and teenage pregnancy rates were fairly high given the projected income of the area.

Making "The Best Choice"

Economists refer to the process of making the best choice as optimizing utility. We refer to the amount of money the person has to spend as a budget constraint. Given that a person's preferences for goods, equations that convert amounts of good to a utility number, and the current prices, there is mathematical process to determine which amount of each good they should get to have the highest utility possible. Economics offers a systematic way to understand which choice is the best for a person from that person's perspective. Given a certain amount of money to spend, the person will optimally spend that money to consume goods and services (hereafter referred to as simply goods) that provide the most benefits to them. This includes housing, food, clothing, entertainment, cell phones, computers, and so forth. Getting more of any one good means getting less of another good (e.g., if we have $100 to spend in a day, we might not have anything left on other goods or services if we spend all of it to take the family to a dinner). Sometimes, it means giving up a future good (e.g., if we spend more rather than save today, it means we will have less to spend in the future). Economics holds that people feel better off when consuming more than less and that greater variety in goods (to a point) is preferred. For example, people are better off spending some money on housing and some money on food rather than all on either, or eating a variety of foods than just one thing all the time. However, economics also allows for individual preferences; one person may like a luxurious house and inexpensive food, while another may like a simpler house and expensive food. Given the same budget, the best choices vary between the two. The choice that is best also depends on the set of prices for the available goods. If the prices of one good decrease, this generally means people will buy more of that good. Alternatively, if prices of a good increase, people will substitute away from it and buy other goods in place of it. These price changes might come from taxes or subsidies and are used by decision-makers in healthcare and public health to influence people's choices and behaviors, such as reduce sin behaviors (e.g., smoking or sugary beverages) and achieve healthcare and public health goals.

Markets

Economics considers people's efficiency at producing a particular good or service compared with efficiencies of others who they might trade with at producing the same good. Economists say that a person, a firm, or a country should produce the good or service in which it has a comparative advantage compared with the others. Resources are used (or allocated) more efficiently when individuals or firms specialize in the production of a particular good or service in which they are the best and trade for other goods or services that others are the best to provide. This is true even if someone else might be more efficient at it. The economic term for this is *specialization,* which implies that one becomes more efficient as they deepen their knowledge and practice in that task, and switching tasks may decrease efficiency. Economics also has insights on production and trade. In short, some places or people are better suited to produce a particular good or service by utilizing their comparative advantage. This leads to the modern economy where different agents in the economy produce certain products and services and trade for the rest. Instead of producing all goods we consume, individuals exchange our labor with employers for money and use it to buy all goods and services that we consume.

Trade, buying and selling of goods, occurs in *markets.* All markets have producers and consumers. In rare cases, one might be in both roles. Like the way consumers make the best choice given the circumstances, producers such as farmers, food processors, supermarket operators, or healthcare firms will produce a set of goods that will maximize their profits. The actions of producers and consumers jointly determine the price and quantity of the goods sold. Economists call this *market equilibrium.* Increasing demand for these goods, holding quantity supplied constant, increases price and increases quantity consumed (with other conditions remaining the same, known as "ceteris paribus" in economics; **Figure 1.3b**.) Meanwhile, decreasing demand while ceteris paribus has the opposite effect (**Figure 1.3a**). Similarly, increasing supply of goods decreases price and subsequently increases quantity consumed (**Figure 1.3c**) Decreasing supply has the opposite effect, ceteris paribus (**Figure 1.3d**) All will have spillover to other markets of complements and substitutes. As we will demonstrate later, these market concepts are directly related to health policy and behaviors in ways that might not be immediately apparent.

Relationships Between Goods

Economics also offers insight into how consumption of a good relates to consumption of another good. If the goods are *complements,* consumption of one increases the benefit of the other and vice versa. For example, a person might enjoy either workout clothing or a gym membership (without the other); however, combined, they are even more enjoyable. Another example might be that both surgery and physical therapy individually help to recover from an injury; however, in combination, the benefit of each (and subsequently the health outcome) is enhanced. If goods are *substitutes,* consumption of one decreases the benefit or need of the other. For example, on any given trip, it is likely that a person will use either public transport (which includes walking on both ends of the trip) or drive themselves. Similarly, generic and brand-name drugs are substitutes, and a higher price of the brand-name drugs implies that patients may choose a cheaper generic alternative, but never both. Related to substitutes are *inferior goods,* which are consumed less as people's budget increases, and people substitute away from them. For example, fast food can be viewed as an inferior good because as our incomes increase, we will start to substitute away from it toward better quality food. Understanding these relationships can be key to understanding policy and policy impact, because a policy that changes the price of one good (e.g., through taxation) will impact the consumption of other goods differently if the other good is complement than if it is a substitute.

Table 1.1 illustrates how the concepts of substitutes and complements might be leveraged by policy makers to improve health or facilitate healthful choices. Policies that impact the price of a good, either subsidies or taxes, directly on the good are likely to be the most effective at altering consumption but may not be an option in all cases. For example, if a goal is

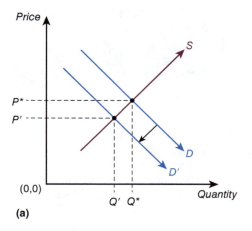 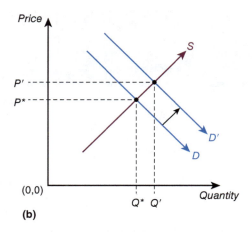

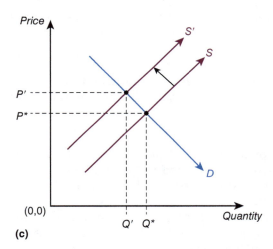 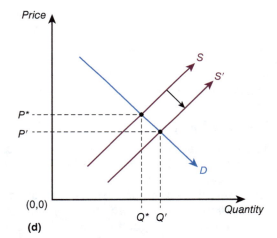

FIGURE 1.3 Supply and demand relationships and the impact of various shocks to the equilibrium.
Notes: Panel (a) illustrates the effect of demand decrease. For example, an information campaign that informed people about the negative health consequences of a particular product. Panel (b) illustrates the effect of demand increase, such as an information campaign that informed people about the positive health consequences of a particular product. Panel (c) illustrates the effect of supply decrease. A tax or other penalty on a product would be an example; this increases the price to the consumer. Panel (d) illustrates the effect of supply increase. A subsidy on a product would be an example; this decreases the price to the consumer.

to promote (or discourage) fruit consumption, imposing a subsidy (or tax) on fruits might be difficult due to several reasons, such as political will. However, policy targeting a substitute or a complement might also produce the desired result.

These fundamentals establish the ways in which policy operates. If policy makers want to decrease consumption of a particular good or service (e.g., junk food, cigarettes, etc.) that has a negative impact on health, they can attempt to decrease demand or supply of that good (or a complement). Alternatively, they could try to increase supply or demand of a substitute that does not have the same negative impact on health. If policy makers were trying to encourage or promote a behavior, the opposite would hold for each. In trying to determine which path to take, it would be helpful to consider what is most feasible and what is most likely to work. If

TABLE 1.1 Potential Policies to Increase Consumption of Fruits, That Is, Goods With Positive Health Impact

GOOD TARGET BY POLICY	RELATIONSHIP TO FRUIT	POLICY	EFFECTS AND MECHANISMS
Fruit	–	Subsidy	A subsidy on fruit would lower the price and increase its consumption. (See Figure 1.3d for a graphical account.)
Candy bars	Substitute	Tax	A tax on candy bars would lead people to buy less of them and choose other snacks in their place. Fruit consumption is expected to increase. (See Figure 1.3c for the effect on candy bars and Figure 1.3b for the effect on fruit.)
Yogurt	Complement	Subsidy	A subsidy on yogurt would lower the price and increase consumption of yogurt and things that go well with yogurt, for example, fruit. Fruit consumption is expected to increase. (See Figure 1.3d for the effect on yogurt and Figure 1.3b for the effect on fruit.)

there is already a plentiful supply of a good that promotes health, trying to increase the supply of it is unlikely to have the desired effect. A policy to increase demand might be more effective.

Market Failures

There are times when there are *market failures*. Economics has articulated the conditions that are likely to result in a well-functioning market. We encourage the curious reader to explore those conditions. In this chapter, we will constrain the discussion to only highlight a few reasons markets that impact health behaviors may fail.

Asymmetric information is the economic term when one party in the transaction is better informed about the good or service being exchanged in a way that they could exploit the privileged information to gain a competitive advantage over other party. For example, doctors have much better information about the likely benefit (or lack thereof) of medical treatments. An unscrupulous doctor could tell patients that a treatment has greater benefit than it actually does, and the patients would opt for treatments they would not opt for with accurate information, resulting in greater profit for the doctors. Another example relevant to health behaviors is health insurance. Here, the patient is often better informed about their own medical issues than the insurance company. This can lead to *adverse selection*, where people who are more likely to need medical care are more likely to buy insurance and/or select a plan with better coverage and benefits. This leads to an increased cost for the insurance company, which might in turn raise prices to accommodate higher risks. This process can cycle until no one can afford insurance. The Affordable Care Act (ACA) imposed a mandate to buy insurance to minimize the adverse selection.

Externality is the economic term for an impact to a third party that is not included in the price of a trade between a producer and a consumer. For example, prior to the Clean Air Act of 1970, steel producers used coal to smelt iron ore, and people downwind were left to deal with the pollution and health consequences due to air pollution. The price of the steel does not reflect the health consequences incurred by those downwind. This pollution is an externality. In contrast, as discussed earlier, an employer who is seeking labor in conditions where there is pollution will need to pay the worker more to compensate for unhealthy working conditions, or higher insurance premiums due to higher probability of sickness due to air pollution. The pollution experienced by the worker is not an externality to the transaction. The employer has an incentive to reduce pollution to avoid paying higher premiums to the workers. The same pollution can be an externality in one transaction and internalized in another. However, what is most important to note is the price does not fully reflect the impact of the pollution, so there is some externality. Externalities can also be positive. For example, when you get a flu shot, you benefit from a reduced likelihood of getting the flu, but the people around you also benefit because if you do not get the flu you cannot infect them. Externalities provide a clear case for policy intervention, commonly adding a tax (when they are negative) or subsidy (when they are positive), which adjusts the price to reflect the true costs or benefits to society.

Moral hazard takes place when one party engages in risky behavior where the consequences are borne by the others. For example, persons with health insurance might behave differently (e.g., engage in risky behaviors or avoid preventive care) when protected by an insurance from financial consequences. There are two types of moral hazard. The first type is *ex ante* and concerns behavior before an incident takes place. Being insured might cause some people to engage in more risky behaviors than they would have if were not insured, because the cost of treatment will be paid by the insurance. These behaviors might include dangerous activities such as sky diving, bungee jumping, smoking, or poor diet. However, uninsured individuals might be deterred from such activities because of the cost of medical care they might face. The fact that the person will still have the pain and suffering related to the illness or injury limits moral hazard. The second type is *ex post* and concerns behavior after an incident, where individuals might opt for more expensive treatment if the insurer is paying compared with the situation when they had to pay out of pocket. Some literature (e.g., Balafoutas et al., 2017) also examines what has been labeled *second-degree* moral hazard, which also involves asymmetric information. Here, a provider, knowing that the person has insurance, recommends more expensive treatment than is necessary, but the person might be unaware that there is a less expensive option with similar health outcome.

THE ECONOMIC RATIONALE FOR POLICY INTERVENTION

Having discussed the economic principles that help explain present health behaviors and outcomes, we now explore how health policies aim to disrupt that status quo to improve population and individual health outcomes. Policy makers have a broad array of tools they can employ to try to change health behaviors and outcomes. These include information campaigns, subsidies, taxes, limits or restrictions, mandates, and prohibitions. Information campaigns are the least restrictive to people's freedom of choice, and prohibitions are the most restrictive. Having identified an overly prevalent or undesired health outcome or behavior, a shrewd policy maker will employ economics to understand why the markets are producing that behavior or outcome, specifically if it is the result of one of the above-listed market failures. Identifying the reason for the failure indicates likely remedies.

Addressing Asymmetry of Information With Policy

Market failures caused by asymmetric information (described previously) provide a clear rationale for policy intervention. This assumes at least some of the consumers making unhealthy choices are doing so because they do not realize the choice is unhealthy and they might later regret the choice. Moreover, with good information, they would make the healthy choice. If people do not have adequate information, they cannot make the best choice for themselves and this might have a negative impact on their health or happiness. Through providing information, a policy helps the market function more efficiently. There is much long-established health policy we take for granted and probably do not even think of. For example, the U.S. Department of Agriculture (USDA) has for decades established rules about what can be sold as food and how it is labeled. These policies keep dangerous ingredients out of food, and they also prohibit fraud such as watering down milk or adding sawdust to bread—these seemingly egregious examples were once concerns for consumers before policy changes prohibited this behavior by companies. The USDA also dictates what can be called Grade A beef or how much an egg must weigh to be labeled "large." While these types of policies might seem trivial, this standardization of goods is essential to market efficiency. It allows the consumer to easily compare prices between stores, and forces suppliers to compete with each other.

Another type of policy to promote healthy choices is the requirement for certain types of information to be made available to potential consumers. Providing consumers with more information about what they are purchasing can help them understand the value of a good and its potential impact on their health. The USDA requires nutritional labels to be placed on packaged foods and beverages (www.fda.gov/food/food-labeling-nutrition/changes-nutrition-facts-label) in an attempt to provide consumers with information they might not know about the nutritional value of the item, so they might use that information to make healthier choices. A more recent example of information provision is the laws enacted by some cities and states that require that restaurant menus include how many calories items contain. Warning labels on cigarettes are also a form of information provision. Information campaigns might also be employed to have a similar effect.

Addressing Externalities With Policy

When markets fail to correctly price a good due to externalities associated with the good, this provides a clear rationale for policy to correct markets. An individual's decision to drink and drive has potential impacts on many people beyond them. Drinking and driving leads to the injuries and deaths of others, so there is strict policy to avoid severe outcomes. Smoking also imposes consequences on others. Before the mid-1990s, cigarette smoking was common in most restaurants and other public indoor places. A change occurred when California passed the first statewide ban on smoking in restaurants in 1995. Early bans were framed as protecting workers (waitstaff, etc.) from the harmful effects of secondhand smoke. However, many nonsmoking patrons also benefited. However, even when individuals' actions only harm themselves, this does not mean there is no cost to others. Smoking leads to multiple severe diseases such as cancer and cardiovascular complications. In the late 1990s, the federal and state governments sued tobacco companies to recover costs of medical care to smokers provided by publicly funded healthcare. Consuming unhealthy foods leads to obesity and associated diseases such as diabetes, which also burden publicly funded care and therefore this might be a reason for policy intervention. "Sin Taxes" (discussed later in this chapter) are often seen as trying to correct for externalities. A policy can also correct for positive externalities such as subsidizing health insurance and adopting policies that promote preventive care (e.g., vaccinations and cancer screenings).

Market Failures Specific to Healthcare and Potential Policy Remedies

Health insurance markets are particularly prone to failure. Failure can come in two directions; either only people who need much care buy insurance, or insurers can refuse to sell policies to people who through no fault of their own will have high costs. A policy that mandates an action can solve both. To address the first failure, the ACA imposed an individual mandate that was designed to ensure everyone bought insurance. To address the second, it forced insurers to sell to everyone and price only on the basis of age and smoking status. Another example of a mandate is mental health insurance laws, commonly known as mental health parity laws, which intend to improve access to needed treatment and to prevent discrimination in insurance coverage by requiring equal coverage for mental health treatment and treatment for other medical conditions (Harris et al., 2006; Heboyan et al., 2021; Li & Ma, 2020).

A policy maker might also believe many consumers place too much emphasis on the short-term outcomes and too little on the long-term outcomes (exhibit *present bias*). This too is a rationale for intervention. In the example of food, this means thinking too much about how good some less healthy food might taste compared with a healthier alternative, and not enough thinking of the long-term health risks, such as obesity, heart disease, cancer, and so forth. Policy makers might correct this with a tax on the less healthy food. Similarly, a subsidy on healthier food may help consumers make choices more aligned with what they would wish they had decided when experiencing consequence. We already noted a policy maker might impose a policy due to the externalities involved. This additional consideration gives further justification of the policy and might have implications for the size of the tax or subsidy. Similar logic may apply to other behaviors with negative public health consequences. Children and adolescents are often considered to lack the brain development to weigh long-term consequences or otherwise understand their choice. As such, there is often a policy to protect them (e.g., it is illegal to market cigarettes to minors).

Traditional health policies and tools for changing health behaviors and achieving targeted health outcomes have been in the form of incentives and disincentives (Cohen et al., 2016). For example, we impose insurance penalties in the form of extra monthly payments for those who are smokers, or increase the price of undesirable goods, such as sugary beverages and cigarettes, through taxation. Although many of these policies are effective, some of them are politically and socially controversial as they seem to infringe on liberty (e.g., taxation or prohibition of smoking at certain places), or raise ethical and moral issues as well as conflicts of interest (e.g., conscripting organs from dying patients, hence opening a market for human organs). As a result, such policies initiate political debates between libertarians and paternalists about the role of the government (Cohen et al., 2016). A classic example of such manifestation is the recent COVID-19 pandemic and the fierce debate surrounding vaccination mandates.

"Sin Taxes" as Policy Instruments to Change Unhealthy Behavior

A *sin tax* is an informal term for an excise tax placed on specific products or services that are deemed harmful to the individuals or the society, such as cigarettes, gambling, alcohol, sugary beverages, fast foods, and so forth. For example, tax on cigarettes or sugary beverages lowers the demand for these products by making them more expensive to purchase (**Figure 1.3c**). However, the true impact of the taxes will largely depend on the pass-through rate as producers may be willing and able to absorb some or all increased prices. Further, consumers may substitute expensive products for cheaper (or generic brand) alternatives, thus keeping consumption quantities the same.

Tobacco taxes, along with other tobacco control policies such as smoke-free laws, are major public policy instruments adopted by federal, state, and local governments to prevent or control tobacco use. It aims at raising tobacco prices to prohibitive levels, thus forcing smokers to quit or reduce smoking. The economic theory and existing applied research suggest that tobacco control policies (increased prices, tobacco-free ordinances, etc.) nudge smokers toward reducing or quitting smoking. Higher taxes lead to higher cigarette prices, which can bring shifts in the supply–demand equilibrium and can lower demand for cigarettes, ceteris paribus. Economic theory also suggests that heavy smokers and low-income individuals are price-sensitive, given the disproportionately higher share of their income is spent on cigarettes. Contrarily, heavy smokers are often thought to be price-insensitive due to nicotine-induced addiction (Chen et al., 2013). In the United States, federal excise tax on cigarettes increased from $0.24 per pack in 1995 to $1.01 in 2009, and the average state excise tax rose from $0.33 per pack to $1.20 over the same period (CDC, 2009). As of June 30, 2018, taxes range considerably from $0.17 per pack in Missouri to $4.35 in New York (CDC, 2018). The empirical literature points to the potency of taxes and smoke-free air (SFA) policies reducing smoking, steering smokers toward quitting, preventing smoking initiation, and improving a broad set of smoking outcomes (Chaloupka, 1991; Colman & Remler, 2008; Nesson, 2017; Peterson et al., 1992; Wamamili & Garrow, 2017).

Sugary beverages are among the major contributors to obesity and chronic diseases such as diabetes. Many states and cities have introduced sugary beverage taxes as a policy mechanism

12 I • THEORIES, FRAMEWORKS, AND MEASURES RELEVANT TO HEALTH BEHAVIORS

to nudge reduction of consumption and generate revenue to promote healthier lifestyle in their communities (Oddo et al., 2019). The city of Berkley was the first U.S. locality to introduce a sugary beverage tax in 2014, and several other municipalities and states around the United States followed suit. Flynn (2023) used data from the Youth Risk Behavior Surveillance System to study the impact of sugary beverage tax on health outcomes in Philadelphia, San Francisco, and Oakland. The results showed that higher taxes were associated with lower sugary beverage consumption in Philadelphia and reductions in average body mass index (BMI) in all three cities, although these improvements were concentrated among female and non-White respondents. White and colleagues (2023) found that sugary beverage taxes resulted in substantial decline in volume of sugary beverage consumption in Oakland, California, even 2 years after tax implementation. While a growing body of literature suggests that sugary beverage taxes are effective policy tools, several studies also suggest that the substitution of sweetened foods for sugary beverages due to increased taxes may effectively offset the decrease in sugary beverage consumption (Lozano-Rojas & Carlin, 2022).

It is important to note that many policies have trade-offs and negative consequences. In the case of the abovementioned examples, the opponents of tax increases argue that these taxes disproportionately affect low-income individuals since they must spend larger portion of their (already low) disposable income on these products. In turn, evidence suggests that individuals from lower socioeconomic status (SES) are more likely to be affected by unhealthy behaviors, such as consuming cigarettes or sugary beverages or not seeking medical care due in part to lack of financial resources. Thus, the opponents argue such taxes may exacerbate the already dire health of individuals of low SES.

INTERVENTIONS BASED ON BEHAVIORAL ECONOMICS

Behavioral economics, a subfield of economics, combines the elements of marketing, psychology, and social sciences to examine situations in which peoples' behavior deviates from what traditional economics describes as rational. It utilizes much more sophisticated tools to shape behavior to achieve desired policy targets. It allows the modeling and predicting of behaviors utilizing traditional economic analysis tools, but with more accurate assumptions about human behavior and rationality. Doing so, it addresses the two major problems associated with the incentives and disincentives approach. First, proposed policies may challenge cultural and normative views in society and become politically difficult to implement, such as raising taxes in conservative states. Second, proposed policies may backfire and result in unintended consequences (Cohen et al., 2016). A good example of the latter is the vaccination mandates during (and after) the COVID-19 pandemic, where in certain localities the population resented these mandates as infringement on their liberties. As a result, higher vaccination rates might have been achieved in the absence of such mandates or through use of other approaches, such as behavioral nudge or incentives, yielding desired results without challenging the normative and societal views.

Behavioral economic interventions evolved over the last decades as an alternative to politically or socially controversial policies. They nudge behavior change without imposing and without forbidding any options or significantly changing their economic incentives (Thaler & Sunstein, 2008, p. 6). Richard Thaler, who won the Nobel Prize in economics and coauthored the book *Nudge* (Thaler & Sunstein, 2008), advocated that nudges are less paternalistic than prohibitions, taxes or other penalties because they minimally limit people's freedom and ability to make their choices, while still being effective. Prohibitions are clearly the most restrictive and do not allow the choice at all or at least not legally. Taxes and penalties impose negative consequences if the consumer makes a choice contrary to what the policy makers desire. Nudges, in contrast, impose no penalty.

Nudge opens with a story about a cafeteria that decides, rather than having candy bars immediately in front of the cash register, to position fresh fruit there instead. In either arrangement, both the candy bars and fresh fruit are available in the cafeteria. However, by switching which is most easily accessed, the cafeteria can promote healthier behavior without limiting consumer choice.

Similarly, by changing the default, or what happens if someone does nothing, policy makers can also shift decisions. By changing from drivers needing to check a box to get an organ donor designation on their license, to needing to check a box to NOT get the designation, policy makers were able to get many more people to register as organ donors (Johnson & Goldstein, 2003). Thaler and Sunstein (2008) advocate that defaults can be employed in many situations, including enrollment in Medicare Part D plans. There, they argue the default should be the plan that minimizes the enrollees' out-of-pocket costs based on their current prescriptions. Buildings can also be designed so that the stairs are more convenient or visible than the elevators, and thus encourage people to take the stairs (Zimring et al., 2005).

Nudges might also employ social norms and remind people about what most people do or what they are expected to do. In traditional economics, how many other people choose some option should not affect another person's decision; if that other person was already making the best choice for them, it remains the best choice. However, behavioral economics has shown us that informing people about the choices of others can impact their own decisions. For example, providing information about how water and electric use compares with neighbors promotes people to conserve water and electricity (Allcott, 2011; Ferraro & Price, 2013). These examples are tangential to public health. However, a similar dynamic might exist in the healthcare exchange markets established by the ACA. The government regularly provides information about how many people bought health insurance through them and this might contribute to their increasing popularity.

Communication about health risk or an intervention program can also influence behavior. A message could emphasize the health gains from physical activity, or it could focus on the health risks of inactivity. Both communicate the same information: It is better for your health to be more active than less active. The difference is merely in framing, as the former is a gain framing, while the latter is a loss framing. Based on the assertion "losses loom greater than gains" (Kahneman & Tversky, 1979, p. 279), there have been many experiments that show that emphasizing losses can slightly increase the amount of effort exerted in a wide range of contexts (Ferraro & Tracy, 2022). The opposite seems to hold true in health contexts. Emphasizing health gains is generally more effective if the health gain is emphasized (Gallagher & Updegraff, 2011). It is also important that message be urgent enough to motivate reaction, but not be so alarming as to invoke fear or other negative reactions (Dillard & Shen, 2005).

Once a policy maker is considering policy to change present health behaviors and outcomes, there might be several options. The next section examines how the policy maker can compare those options and see if any are viable and which might be best or most efficient.

EVALUATION OF HEALTH POLICIES, PROGRAMS, AND INTERVENTIONS

Economic analyses are essential to the evaluation of the effectiveness or impact of health policies, programs, and interventions. For example, imagine that you are the director of a public health agency. As the director, you will be offered numerous policy and program alternatives to achieve the desired outcomes. However, due to budget constraints, only a subset of these policies and programs can be implemented at any given time. Therefore, before adopting policies and programs, it is critical to have a good understanding of and if and how effective these policies and programs are and how they compare with each other. Health economists employ various economic methods and tools, such as econometric models and economic evaluation techniques, to study policy and program effectiveness that might guide policy maker's or agency director's decision on policy and program selection and budget allocation.

Economic evaluations have become critical components of public health research and programming. These tools provide policy makers the economic cost associated with designing, delivering, or scaling up a particular program, intervention, or policy. Conducting an evaluation of each option enables decision-makers to better allocate scarce public health and healthcare resources. Economic evaluation is a comparative analysis of alternative courses of action in terms of both their costs and consequences. It identifies, measures, estimates values, and compares the costs (inputs) and consequences (outcomes) of the alternatives being considered. The costs and the consequences (outcomes) are the two essential characteristics of economic analyses to consider as they distinguish economic evaluations from other healthcare evaluations, such as efficacy or effectiveness evaluation, program evaluation, or outcome or cost description (Drummond et al., 2005). **Figure 1.4** provides a simple illustration of how economic evaluations aid in decision-making.

Economic evaluations allow us to better understand if the health procedure, service, or program is worth doing compared with other things we could do with these same resources. It helps us find answers to important healthcare and public health questions, such as if we are satisfied that the healthcare (public health) resources should be spent in this way rather than some other way, or if clinicians should check the blood pressure of each adult who walks into their offices, or if hospital administrators should purchase every piece of new diagnostic equipment. Economic evaluation provides us with criteria for deciding between alternative strategies that have different costs and/or consequences.

Information on the costs and effectiveness of alternative strategies to improve health outcomes can serve as an important policy tool to guide decision-making process on how to achieve public health and healthcare objectives. All economic evaluation techniques measure various types of costs in monetary units. However, they significantly differ in the ways they measure outcomes.

Economic costs associated with implementing programs, policies, and interventions are collected over their entire duration. These costs enable us to calculate the full economic cost of delivering each activity/intervention. These costs are classified into medical and nonmedical costs. Examples of medical costs include cost of organizing and operating the health centers, health sector costs incurred by the department of health, medical care costs paid by patients and their families to obtain care, or costs of medical supplies and drugs. Nonmedical costs are those associated with the intervention or the care, but not directly related to medical inputs and supplies. For example, a patient may have to spend money and time to come to a facility, and although it is related to receiving care it is not an input in the production of medical care. There are also indirect costs, which are the costs that were incurred due to the use of the medical program or intervention under consideration, such as loss of income due to taking time off to attend a medical appointment. Calculated economic costs serve as the basis for all three economic evaluation techniques described later. Based on the costs and outcomes, economists calculate cost to outcomes ratios, and incremental cost to outcome ratio. The former is defined as the "total cost" divided by the "total outcome," and the latter is defined as the "difference in cost" divided by the "difference in outcome" (e.g., effect of an additional dollar spent on a public health awareness campaign). While the average cost to outcome ratio informs us how much it costs to deliver a specific intervention per unit of outcome, the incremental ratio will inform us what is the extra cost of adopting one activity/intervention compared with another. These ratios also

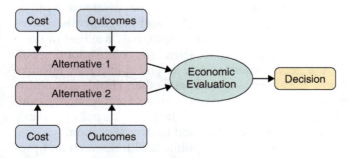

FIGURE 1.4 Economic evaluation and decision-making process.

enable us to rank activities/interventions. See Table 1.2 for an example of potential policies to decrease soda consumption. There are four main types of economic evaluations. Table 1.3 summarizes these economic evaluation methods, contrasting their similarities and differences.

Drummond et al. (2005) illustrate a cost-effectiveness analysis (CEA) with an example based on Hull et al. (1981), which conducted a CEA of strategies to treat deep vein thrombosis (DVT; Table 1.4). In this study, 516 patients with clinically suspected DVT were examined. Alternative methods of diagnosis (i.e., the alternatives to examine) were impedance

TABLE 1.2 Potential Policies to Decrease Consumption of Soda, That Is, Goods With Negative Health Impact			
GOOD TARGET BY POLICY	**RELATIONSHIP TO SODA**	**POLICY**	**EFFECTS AND MECHANISMS**
Soda	–	Tax	A tax on soda would increase the price and decrease its consumption. (See Figure 1.3c for a graphical account.)
Bottled water	Substitute	Subsidy	A subsidy on bottled water would lead people to buy more of it and choose fewer other beverages. Soda consumption is expected to decrease. (See Figure 1.3d for the effect on bottled water and Figure 1.3a for the effect on soda.)
Pizza	Complement	Tax	A tax on pizza would raise the price and decrease consumption of pizza and things that go well with pizza, for example, soda. Soda consumption is expected to decrease. (See Figure 1.3c for the effect on pizza and Figure 1.3a for the effect on soda.)

TABLE 1.3 Economic Evaluations and Their Characteristics		
EVALUATION TYPE	**COSTS CONSIDERED**	**OUTCOME MEASURES**
Cost minimization analysis	All present and future costs are measured from the perspective of analyses. These are calculated for each alternative.	All competing alternatives are measured by the same outcome, and all alternatives have the same outcome; for example, same number of people to be vaccinated.
Cost-effectiveness analysis	All present and future costs are measured from the perspective of analyses. These are calculated for each alternative.	All competing alternatives are measures in the same units and are comparable. They do not have the same outcome; for example, number of people vaccinated.
Cost utility analysis	All present and future costs are measured from the perspective of analyses. These are calculated for each alternative.	Health outcomes, such as number of life years gained due to successful treatment, are transformed into QALY to capture both mortality and morbidity. It can be used to compare interventions targeting various outcomes.
Cost-benefit analysis	All present and future costs are measured from the perspective of analyses. These are calculated for each alternative.	All outcomes are transformed into a monetary unit using various economic valuation techniques. It can be used to compare dissimilar projects.

QALY, quality-adjusted life years.

TABLE 1.4 Cost-Effectiveness Analysis of Alternative Strategies for Deep Vein Thrombosis

ALTERNATIVE	COSTS (U.S. DOLLARS)	OUTCOME (NUMBER OF CORRECT DIAGNOSIS)	COST TO OUTCOME RATIO (U.S. DOLLARS PER CORRECT DIAGNOSIS)
IPG (alone)	321,488	142	2,264
IPG plus outpatient venography if IPG is negative	603,552	201	3,003
Increment (alternative 2 over alternative 1)	282,064	59	4,781

IPG, impedance plethysmography.
Source: From Drummond, M., Sculpher, M., Torrance, G., O'Brien, B., & Stoddart, G. (2005). *Methods for the economic evaluation of health care programmes* (3rd ed.). Oxford University Press.

plethysmography (IPG) alone and IPG plus outpatient venography if IPG is negative. The authors used the correctly identified cases by the tests as the effectiveness or outcome measure. The results indicate that IPG alone is more cost-effective than its alternative ($2,264 vs. $3,003) and therefore is more preferred from an economic point of view. In this example, the second alternative is simply first intervention plus an additional test. Therefore, in such circumstances, it is also important to evaluate the incremental cost-effectiveness ratio, which is equal to $4,781 per correct diagnosis when an additional test is used. It informs the decision-maker that to achieve an additional 59 correct diagnosis, we will need to pay this amount per each.

In contrast to CEA, *cost utility analysis* (CUA) expresses outcomes as the number of life years adjusted for change in the quality of life due to said programs, polices, or interventions. It combines morbidity and mortality into a single measure. CUA is preferred when quality of life is an important outcome. Many diseases do not create any significant reduction in life years but may affect patients' physical, emotional, and social function or morbidity. As illustrated in **Figure 1.5,** person A did not receive an intervention (e.g., a novel treatment or healthier life choices) and therefore has fewer quality-adjusted life years (QALYs) compared with person B, who has received the intervention. Letters A and B on the diagram represent lifetime utility for persons A and B. More specifically, utility gained by person A is represented by the blue area, while utility gained due to intervention by person B is represented by blue plus tan-shaded areas. Area B is larger and the difference corresponds to the impact of the intervention, ceteris paribus.

The most common outcome measure used in CUA is the QALY. However, other alternatives exist as well, such as health-adjusted person-years (HAPY), health-adjusted life expectancy (HALE), quality-adjusted life expectancy (QALE), disability-adjusted life years (DALYs), and years of healthy life (YHL). Like CEA, CUA uses cost per outcome ratios (e.g., U.S. dollars per QALY or U.S. dollar per DALY) and incremental ratio to compare alternatives.

Shaw and colleagues (2021) used a decision analysis model to conduct a comparative CUA of postoperative discharge pathways following posterior spinal fusion for scoliosis in nonambulatory cerebral palsy patients. In this study, the authors compared the traditional discharge (TD) approach with the novel accelerated discharge (AD) pathway. The results, summarized in **Table 1.5,** indicate that AD is an economically preferred approach since it costs less per one unit of outcome than the alternative.

Cost-benefit analysis (CBA) is used to compare very dissimilar projects, where CEA or CUA would be impractical. Alternatives are compared using the cost to benefit ratio or the benefit to cost ratio. The latter is very popular with stakeholders and is an equivalent to the return-on-investment (ROI) measure. Heboyan and colleagues (2023) estimated the ROI of a COVID-19 vaccination incentivization campaign in Augusta, Georgia. The results of their study showed that not only vaccination intervention protected population health, but it also resulted in significant healthcare benefits and an ROI of over 100.

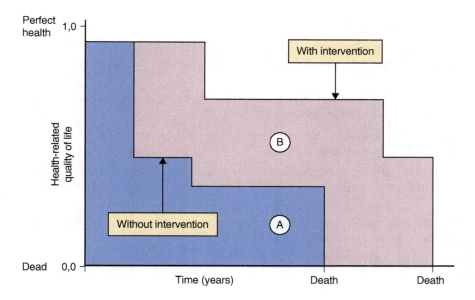

FIGURE 1.5 Quality-adjusted life years (QALY) gained from an intervention, program, or policy.
Source: Image courtesy of Jmarchn.

TABLE 1.5 Comparative Effectiveness of Accelerated and Traditional Discharge Pathway Following Posterior Spinal Fusion			
ALTERNATIVE STRATEGY	COST (U.S. DOLLARS)	EFFECTIVENESS (LIFE YEARS)	CUA RATIO (U.S. DOLLARS/LIFE YEARS)
Accelerated discharge	67,069	15.38	4,361
Traditional discharge	81,312	15.37	5,290

CUA, cost utility analysis.
Source: From Shaw, K. A., Heboyan, V., Fletcher, N. D., & Murphy, J. S. (2021). Comparative cost-utility analysis of postoperative discharge pathways following posterior spinal fusion for scoliosis in non-ambulatory cerebral palsy patients. *Spine Deform, 9*(6), 1659–1667. https://doi.org/10.1007/s43390-021-00362-y.

CONCLUSION

Health policies are a set of decisions, interventions, and actions that are undertaken within the society to disrupt the status quo by shifting resources and/or mandating certain actions to improve the underlying public health and healthcare outcomes (Heboyan et al., 2021). A good policy is guided by sound understanding of economic fundamentals to identify, conceptualize, and remedy the problem. Evidence-based policy will use data and other evidence to guide policy. Interventions that are effective in achieving desired results can be kept, expanded, and replicated, while those that are ineffective can be altered or canceled. Economic analysis and evaluations play a critical role in shaping our understanding of the effectiveness of policies, programs, and interventions designed to achieve desired healthcare and public health goals. Those curious about this field of study are encouraged to incorporate learning opportunities on economics concepts and topics into their courses of study. We firmly believe that economics knowledge will be an invaluable addition to one's skill set, especially those with ambitions to seek leadership opportunities within healthcare and public health.

SUMMARY KEY POINTS

- Economic stability, education access and quality, health access and quality, neighborhood and built environment, and social community context are important to health outcomes.
- Economic principles such as trading off costs and benefits to make the best of a situation can explain many health-related behaviors.
- Externalities, asymmetric information, and budget constraints can undermine how well markets for health-related goods function.
- Because agents respond to incentives, policies such as subsidies and taxes or other penalties can be utilized to encourage or discourage consumption of health-related goods.
- Social norms and political feasibility are essential considerations in proposing a change in the status quo. In such situations, decision-makers and advocates should consider behavioral nudge as a more viable alternative.
- Economists use various analytic and evaluation methods, and the choice of the specific approach depends on the objectives of the analysis and the context of policy, program, and intervention.
- Communication regarding a policy might be as important as the policy itself.

DISCUSSION QUESTIONS

1. Describe one trade-off you make and how it impacts your health.
2. Describe one exchange you make that has an externality. What is the externality? Is it positive or negative? Who is the third party that bears the externality?
3. Describe a public health problem and how you would use a behavioral nudge to improve it.
4. Review the map here: www.cdc.gov/nchs/data-visualization/state-life-expectancy/index_2020.htm. Looking at this map, how does your home state compare to the neighboring states or other states in the United States?
5. Revisit The Opportunity Atlas (http://www.opportunityatlas.org). If you were born in the United States, zoom in or use the search function to find the neighborhood where you were born. Alternatively, find the neighborhood in which you presently live or study. What are the overall economic opportunities in that neighborhood? How much does projected salary vary by race, gender, and parent income in that neighborhood? How do the opportunities and variation within them compare to the surrounding neighborhoods? You may also want to look at other places you have lived or perhaps where you attend school now. Are the data for those neighborhoods consistent with your experience of them? Think about the school systems in those areas. Do they help explain the variation or lack thereof? What other characteristics and institutions might offer some explanation?

A robust set of instructor resources designed to supplement this text is located at http://connect.springerpub.com/content/book/978-0-8261-4265-8. Qualifying instructors may request access by emailing textbook@springerpub.com.

REFERENCES

Allcott, H. (2011). Social norms and energy conservation. *Journal of Public Economics*, *95*(9), 1082–1095. https://doi.org/10.1016/j.jpubeco.2011.03.003

Arias, E., Tejada-Vera, B., Kochanek, K. D., & Ahmad, F. B. (2022). *Provisional life expectancy estimates for 2021* (Vital Statistics Rapid Release. Report 23, Issue). https://stacks.cdc.gov/view/cdc/118999

Arrazola, R. A., Griffin, T., Lunsford, N. B., Kittner, D., Bammeke, P., Courtney-Long, E. A., & Armour, B. S. (2023). US cigarette smoking disparities by race and ethnicity–keep going and going! *Preventing Chronic Disease*, *20*, E45. https://doi.org/10.5888/pcd20.220375

Badger, E., Miller, C. C., Pearce, A., & Quealy, K. (2018). Extensive data shows punishing reach of racism for Black boys. *The New York Times*. https://www.nytimes.com/interactive/2018/03/19/upshot/race-class-white-and-black-men.html

Balafoutas, L., Kerschbamer, R., & Sutter, M. (2017). Second-degree moral hazard in a real-world credence goods market. *The Economic Journal*, *127*(599), 1–18. https://doi.org/10.1111/ecoj.12260

Brunello, G., Fort, M., Schneeweis, N., & Winter-Ebmer, R. (2016). The causal effect of education on health: What is the role of health behaviors? *Health Economics*, *25*(3), 314–336. https://doi.org/10.1002/hec.3141

Centers for Disease Control and Prevention. (2009). Federal and state cigarette excise taxes–United States, 1995–2009. *Morbidity and Mortality Weekly Report (MMWR)*, *58*(19), 524–527.

Centers for Disease Control and Prevention. (2018). *State Tobacco Activities Tracking and Evaluation (STATE) system*. http://www.cdc.gov/statesystem/

Chaloupka, F. (1991). Rational addictive behavior and cigarette smoking. *Journal of Political Economy*, *99*(4), 722–742. https://doi.org/10.1086/261776

Chen, C. M., Chang, K. L., & Lin, L. (2013). Re-examining the price sensitivity of demand for cigarettes with quantile regression. *Addictive Behaviors*, *38*(12), 2801–2804. https://doi.org/10.1016/j.addbeh.2013.07.003

Chetty, R., Friedman, J. N., Saez, E., Turner, N., & Yagan, D. (2020). Income segregation and intergenerational mobility across colleges in the United States*. *The Quarterly Journal of Economics*, *135*(3), 1567–1633.

Cohen, I. G., Lynch, H. F., & Robertson, C. T. (2016). *Nudging health: Health law and behavioral economics*. Johns Hopkins University Press.

Colman, G. J., & Remler, D. K. (2008). Vertical equity consequences of very high cigarette tax increases: If the poor are the ones smoking, how could cigarette tax increases be progressive? *Journal of Policy Analysis and Management*, *27*(2), 376–400. https://doi.org/doi:10.1002/pam.20329

Currie, J., & Neidell, M. (2005). Air pollution and infant health: What can we learn from California's recent experience? *The Quarterly Journal of Economics*, *120*(3), 1003–1030. http://www.jstor.org/stable/25098761

Dillard, J. P., & Shen, L. (2005). On the nature of reactance and its role in persuasive health communication. *Communication Monographs*, *72*(2), 144–168. https://doi.org/10.1080/03637750500111815

Drummond, M., Sculpher, M., Torrance, G., O'Brien, B., & Stoddart, G. (2005). *Methods for the economic evaluation of health care programmes* (3rd ed.). Oxford University Press.

Ferraro, P. J., & Price, M. K. (2013). Using nonpecuniary strategies to influence behavior: Evidence from a large-scale field experiment. *The Review of Economics and Statistics*, *95*(1), 64–73. https://doi.org/10.1162/REST_a_00344

Ferraro, P. J., & Tracy, J. D. (2022). A reassessment of the potential for loss-framed incentive contracts to increase productivity: A meta-analysis and a real-effort experiment. *Experimental Economics*, *25*(5), 1441–1466. https://doi.org/10.1007/s10683-022-09754-x

Flynn, J. (2023). Do sugar-sweetened beverage taxes improve public health for high school aged adolescents? *Health Economics*, *32*(1), 47–64. https://doi.org/10.1002/hec.4609

Gallagher, K. M., & Updegraff, J. A. (2011). Health message framing effects on attitudes, intentions, and behavior: A meta-analytic review. *Annals of Behavioral Medicine*, *43*(1), 101–116. https://doi.org/10.1007/s12160-011-9308-7

Harris, K. M., Carpenter, C., & Bao, Y. (2006). The effects of state parity laws on the use of mental health care. *Medical Care*, *44*(6), 499–505. https://doi.org/10.1097/01.mlr.0000215813.16211.00

Heboyan, V., Allen, K., & Merchen, L. (2023). *Investing in public health: Cost-benefit analysis of VaxUp! Augusta COVID-19 vaccination initiative*. Georgia Public Health Assocuation Anual Meeting, Jekyll Island, GA.

Heboyan, V., Douglas, M. D., McGregor, B., & Benevides, T. W. (2021). Impact of mental health insurance legislation on mental health treatment in a longitudinal sample of adolescents. *Medical Care*, *59*(10), 939–946. https://doi.org/10.1097/mlr.0000000000001619

Herrnstadt, E., Heyes, A., Muehlegger, E., & Saberian, S. (2021). Air pollution and criminal activity: Microgeographic evidence from Chicago. *American Economic Journal: Applied Economics*, *13*(4), 70–100. https://doi.org/10.1257/app.20190091

Hull, R., Hirsh, J., Sackett, D. L., & Stoddart, G. (1981). Cost effectiveness of clinical diagnosis, venography, and noninvasive testing in patients with symptomatic deep-vein thrombosis. *New England Journal of Medicine, 304*(26), 1561–1567. https://doi.org/10.1056/nejm198106253042602

Johnson, E. J., & Goldstein, D. (2003). Do defaults save lives? *Science, 302*(5649), 1338–1339. https://doi.org/doi:10.1126/science.1091721

Kahneman, D., & Tversky, A. (1979). Prospect theory: An analysis of decision under risk. *Econometrica, 47*(2), 263–291. https://doi.org/10.2307/1914185

Kunitomo, Y., Bade, B., Gunderson, C. G., Akgün, K. M., Brackett, A., Tanoue, L., & Bastian, L. A. (2022). Evidence of racial disparities in the lung cancer screening process: A systematic review and meta-analysis. *Journal of General Internal Medicine, 37*(14), 3731–3738. https://doi.org/10.1007/s11606-022-07613-2

Lavy, V., Schlosser, A., & Shany, A. (2016). *Out of Africa: Human capital consequences of in utero conditions* (working paper; w21894). National Bureau of Economic Research.

Li, X., & Ma, J. (2020). Does mental health parity encourage mental health utilization among children and adolescents? Evidence from the 2008 Mental Health Parity and Addiction Equity Act (MHPAEA). *Journal of Behavioral Health Services & Research, 47*(1), 38–53. https://doi.org/10.1007/s11414-019-09660-w

Lozano-Rojas, F., & Carlin, P. (2022). The effect of soda taxes beyond beverages in Philadelphia. *Health Economics, 31*(11), 2381–2410. https://doi.org/10.1002/hec.4586

Nesson, E. (2017). Heterogeneity in smokers' responses to tobacco control policies. *Health Economics, 26*(2), 206–225. https://doi.org/10.1002/hec.3289

Oddo, V. M., Krieger, J., Knox, M., Saelens, B. E., Chan, N., Walkinshaw, L. P., Podrabsky, M., & Jones-Smith, J. C. (2019). Perceptions of the possible health and economic impacts of Seattle's sugary beverage tax. *BMC Public Health, 19*(1), 910. https://doi.org/10.1186/s12889-019-7133-2

Peterson, D. E., Zeger, S. L., Remington, P. L., & Anderson, H. A. (1992). The effect of state cigarette tax increases on cigarette sales, 1955 to 1988. *American Journal of Public Health, 82*(1), 94–96.

Shaw, K. A., Heboyan, V., Fletcher, N. D., & Murphy, J. S. (2021). Comparative cost-utility analysis of postoperative discharge pathways following posterior spinal fusion for scoliosis in non-ambulatory cerebral palsy patients. *Spine Deformity, 9*(6), 1659–1667. https://doi.org/10.1007/s43390-021-00362-y

Thaler, R. H., & Sunstein, C. R. (2008). *Nudge: Improving decisions about health, wealth, and happiness*. Yale University Press.

U.S. Department of Health and Human Services. Office of Disease Prevention and Health Promotion. (2023). *Healthy people 2030: Social determinants of health*. Office of the Assistant Secretary for Health, Office of the Secretary, U.S. Department of Health and Human Services. https://health.gov/healthypeople/priority-areas/social-determinants-health

Wamamili, B. M., & Garrow, A. P. (2017). Have higher cigarette taxes in the United States discouraged smoking? A review of data from 1999–2013. *Tobacco Prevention & Cessation, 3*, 15. https://doi.org/10.18332/tpc/70561

White, J. S., Basu, S., Kaplan, S., Madsen, K. A., Villas-Boas, S. B., & Schillinger, D. (2023). Evaluation of the sugar-sweetened beverage tax in Oakland, United States, 2015–2019: A quasi-experimental and cost-effectiveness study. *PLoS Medicine, 20*(4), e1004212. https://doi.org/10.1371/journal.pmed.1004212

World Health Organization. (2023). *Social determinants of health*. https://www.who.int/health-topics/social-determinants-of-health#tab=tab_1

Zimring, C., Joseph, A., Nicoll, G. L., & Tsepas, S. (2005). Influences of building design and site design on physical activity: Research and intervention opportunities. *American Journal of Preventive Medicine, 28*(Suppl. 2), 186–193. https://doi.org/10.1016/j.amepre.2004.10.025

CHAPTER 2

POPULATION HEALTH, SOCIAL ECOLOGY, AND COMMUNITY-ENGAGED RESEARCH

SCOTT D. RHODES, BENJAMIN D. SMART, ANA D. SUCALDITO, AMANDA E. TANNER, AND ENBAL SHACHAM

LEARNING OBJECTIVES

- Provide a brief introduction to population health and the history leading up to modern epidemiology and public health.
- Identify and describe the key characteristics of socioecological models.
- Define and understand the rationale for community-based participatory research (CBPR).
- Outline the ENGAGED for CHANGE process as a strategy to develop multilevel health behavior change interventions.
- Describe the use of the empowerment theory-based community forum as a dissemination method and a strategy to identify the next steps for community change.

FOUNDATIONS OF POPULATION HEALTH, EPIDEMIOLOGY, AND COMMUNITY-BASED BEHAVIOR CHANGE

Population health is a concept within public health that focuses on understanding health outcomes of a specific population. It replaces the individual with the community or population as the primary focus (National Academies of Sciences, Engineering, and Medicine, 2023). While a precise definition of population is not widely agreed upon, most definitions of population health emphasize the importance of examining social and structural determinants of health, in addition to biomedical factors, as well as describing health outcome disparities between groups (Kindig, 2015). An important concept closely linked to population health is epidemiology, a descriptive science concerned with studying the occurrence, spread, and control of health and disease states and the determinants within a population (Mausner & Kramer, 1985).

Epidemiology contains valuable tools for investigating, measuring, and tracking disease, which are critical to describing health trends over time within populations and among population subgroups. By specifically defining the population and explicitly measuring health and disease markers, those concerned with improving population health can identify priorities and develop strategies to move closer to their goals by addressing social and structural determinants of health. Modern epidemiology is marked by three major eras (Susser & Susser, 1996)—sanitary statistics, germ theory, and chronic disease epidemiology. This first era of sanitary statistics dates to the early 19th century when "miasma" was the prevailing paradigm used to describe the cause and spread of disease. At that time, it was thought that diseases were caused by foul emanations from "air, water, and places." This era left its mark in the lexicon with words like *malaria*, which means *bad* (mal) *air* (aria; Young, 2004).

In the latter part of the 19th century, however, "contagionists" challenged the concept of miasma. They believed that diseases were caused by organisms passed from individual to individual. French chemist Louis Pasteur (1822–1895) proposed the germ theory of disease, suggesting that microorganisms were the cause of disease. The contagionists eventually prevailed, as careful experimentation and observation identified more and more bacteria (germs) that apparently caused tuberculosis, diphtheria, cholera, and other diseases previously believed to be linked to the worst miasmas (Karamanou et al., 2012). To illustrate, cholera was a major global challenge faced in the 19th century, with frequent large-scale epidemics in European cities. John Snow, an English physician widely considered to be the founder of modern epidemiology, conducted pioneering investigations on cholera epidemics in England. In 1854, he demonstrated that contaminated water was the main source of cholera epidemics. His investigation of a cholera epidemic in London led to his conclusion that contaminated water from the Broad Street water pump was the source of the disease, and consequently the removal of the handle led to cessation of the epidemic (Tulchinsky, 2018).

In 1876, German scientist Robert Koch (1843–1910) demonstrated the procedures for linking a specific microbe to a specific disease by identifying the cause of anthrax, and in 1884 Koch and Friedrich Loeffler (1852–1915) established the criteria for confirming a relationship between a causative microbe and a disease. This approach, known as "Koch's postulates," remains a gold standard for confirming the causative agents of most infectious diseases (Karamanou et al., 2012). Thus, the germ theory and the modern concept of disease transmission emerged during the late 19th and first half of the 20th century (Ewald, 2004). The germ theory led to a number of critical advances, including the development of vaccines and antibiotics (Young, 2004). Because of these advances, death rates from infectious diseases fell substantially in the United States, and overall life expectancy increased by the middle of the 20th century. In 1900, the average life expectancy at birth was 48 years for women and 46 years for men, but by 1950 it had increased to 71 and 66 years, respectively. In 2022, life expectancy estimates rose to 80 for women and 75 for men (Arias et al., 2023).

By the second half of the 20th century, disease patterns in higher income countries were increasingly characterized by chronic, noninfectious diseases, which harkened the beginning of a third period: the era of chronic disease epidemiology (Susser & Susser, 1996). Chronic diseases are also referred to as noncommunicable diseases (NCDs). To date, this era has focused on using advances in epidemiology and biostatistics to identify and understand risk factors for diseases. A risk factor is a variable that has been shown statistically to be positively associated with a negative health outcome. The power of identifying risk factors is that it leads us one step closer to discovering true causality, and it also provides focus areas for population and public health and medical interventions.

Most of the current global burden of diseases is attributed to NCDs, due to improvements worldwide in public health, medicine, and living conditions. NCDs surpassed injuries and the so-called "Group I diseases" (e.g., communicable, maternal, neonatal, and nutritional diseases) as the leading global cause of disability-adjusted life years in the mid-2000s (GBD 2015 Disease and Injury Incidence and Prevalence Collaborators, 2016). Currently, heart disease, cancer, accidents, and stroke are among the leading causes of death in the United States, accounting for more than two-thirds of all deaths (National Center for Health Statistics, 2016). New infectious diseases, such as COVID-19, have emerged, and others such as HIV infection continue to profoundly affect the health of vulnerable populations. These infections have also negatively impacted the management of chronic diseases and complicate their medical care further. Ample evidence suggests that many causes of premature morbidity and mortality can be prevented or at least delayed through behavior change (Mokdad et al., 2004). Therefore, adherence to preventive health behaviors is key to promoting health and prolonging life (Breslow & Enstrom, 1980).

Early attempts to understand and influence the prevention, development, and/or maintenance of disease included the development of several models of *individual* behavior change, such as the health belief model (Rosenstock, 1974), the theory of planned behavior (Ajzen & Fishbein, 1980), and the transtheoretical model (Prochaska & DiClemente, 1983), which emphasize changes in behavior and cognition to promote health. Most health promotion interventions based on these models focus on the individual as the unit of change and attempt to modify an individual's behavior. The individual approach to behavior change, which typically focuses on those at increased risk, may have reduced impact as this approach often neglects the complex influences influencing behavior (Mayer et al., 2008). In addition, insufficient attention has been given to the communities where people live, work, and play, and how these environments affect behavior (Cashman et al., 2008). For example, knowledge of healthcare resources and access to healthcare can influence uptake of and adherence to biomedical innovations, such as preexposure prophylaxis (PrEP), postexposure prophylaxis (PEP), and antiretroviral therapy (ART) to prevent HIV and reduce HIV-related morbidity and mortality. However, knowledge of resources and access to healthcare are not always sufficient; other social and structural determinants of health, also sometimes referred to as the "social drivers of health" (Mann-Jackson et al., 2022), play profound roles in HIV prevention and care. For example, there is growing recognition that populations at increased HIV risk may need access to educational opportunities, jobs with fair wages and insurance, positive supportive relationships, transportation resources, and legal pathways to immigration, as examples (Mann-Jackson et al., 2018, 2022; Painter et al., 2019; Smart et al., 2020).

To date, we have seen that rigorously designed and theoretically informed behavior change interventions that focus solely on the individual often provide only modest changes in health behavior, and often these interventions have not consistently translated into lasting behavior change or had a population-level impact (Glasgow et al., 2004). A criticism of some of these interventions is that they often are not tailored to address the multilevel contexts that influence behaviors (Mann-Jackson et al., 2021; Sprague & Simon, 2021).

The primary purpose of this chapter is to provide an overview of several approaches that support the consideration of multilevel factors involved in influencing behaviors. We describe socioecological models, community-based participatory research (CBPR), and the development of multilevel interventions and dissemination of study findings using approaches that are aligned with CBPR. To place this chapter into a more applied context, we incorporate the ongoing HIV epidemic in the United States as examples throughout.

SOCIOECOLOGICAL MODELS

The word *ecology*, which has its origins in the biological sciences, is concerned with the interrelations between organisms and their environment (Bronfenbrenner, 1992). Many other disciplines, such as psychology, sociology, and public health, have adapted ecological models to define frameworks for how people interact with their physical, social, and cultural environments (Stokols, 1996). Within the realm of health behavior research and practice, socioecological models provide a framework for the development of multilevel interventions that can systematically address mechanisms of change at various levels of an individual's environment. Socioecological models can be viewed, in part, as a reaction to the limited explanatory power of earlier behavioral and cognitive models of behavior change that primarily focused on the *individual* as the unit of analysis and did not produce a profound or sustained change in behavior when targeted in interventions (Stokols, 1996). The innovation of the socioecological models is their consideration of both internal and external influences on health and behavior that range from biological to global levels, as well as the interaction among these factors (Mayer et al., 2008).

Characteristics of Socioecological Models

At the very core of socioecological models is the concept that behavior has multiple levels of influences, often including individual (e.g., biological and psychological), interpersonal (e.g., social and cultural), institutional, community, and societal (e.g., culture, structures, and policies) factors. Socioecological models can provide a comprehensive framework to identify, understand, and intervene on the multiple influences on health behaviors. Essentially, socioecological models can be used to develop comprehensive intervention approaches that systematically address mechanisms of change at various levels of influence. Socioecological models are often visualized as nested circles, with the smallest circle being the individual and the largest circle being societal-level factors (**Figure 2.1**). This emphasizes the interconnectedness of health-driving factors.

Socioecological models have several key characteristics worth noting. First, these models help tease out the multiple factors that influence a particular behavior or constellation of behaviors at multiple levels, such as the individual, interpersonal, institutional, community, and societal levels (Bronfenbrenner, 1992; Stokols, 1996). To illustrate, preventing HIV historically was viewed as an individual's personal responsibility. At the beginning of the HIV epidemic, there was a predominate focus on the need for gay, bisexual, queer, and other men who have sex with men (GBQMSM) to correctly and consistently use condoms and limit their number of

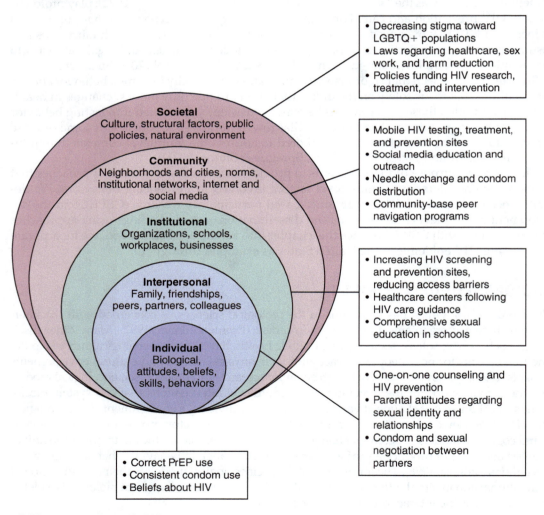

PrEP, pre-exposure prophylaxis

FIGURE 2.1 Adapted version of a socioecological model with examples from HIV prevention in the United States.
PrEP, pre-exposure prophylaxis.

sexual partners to reduce the risk of HIV transmission. Risk behavior was viewed solely as a personal choice, where the individual decided whether or not to use a condom. Hence, there was a proliferation of individual-level interventions designed to increase consistent condom use behaviors (Gamarel et al., 2022). However, while individual-level HIV prevention and care interventions can increase protective behaviors and reduce risk, their reach tends to be limited and they do not acknowledge the complexities of and multiple influences on behavior. Instead, a person's physical and social situation—essentially a person's entire environment—profoundly affects their behavior well beyond their personal attributes. Researchers, clinicians, practitioners, health educators, and so forth now recognize that solutions to the HIV epidemic must come from addressing the problem on multiple levels by considering the complex multiple levels of influence that coalesce to affect behaviors and HIV risk (Dibble et al., 2022).

Another characteristic of socioecological models is the recognition of the complex nature of human environments. For example, descriptions of environments are not limited to their objective (actual) physical and social attributes, but can also be extended to their subjective (perceived) qualities. For example, the perception of low availability to quality HIV care or a lack of providers who do not provide culturally congruent services may negatively influence decisions to access care, whether these perceptions are accurate or not. In addition, independent components of an environment can be combined into composite relationships (Stokols, 1996).

The third characteristic is that, similar to the way environments can be described in terms of their complexity, participants in those environments are affected by and can be studied at a number of levels, ranging from the individual to small groups, to larger organizations, to populations (Bronfenbrenner, 1992; Stokols, 1996). Rather than focusing exclusively on the individual or the population, socioecological models recognize that coordinated efforts and methodologies are necessary to understand phenomena and effectively intervene on their antecedents and the factors that influence these phenomena. Using the HIV epidemic as an example, some of the changes needed to end the HIV epidemic include individual-level behavior changes such as using condoms and/or taking PrEP, PEP, or ART consistently as prescribed; however, structural changes are also critical (Bono et al., 2023; Phillips et al., 2021; Raifman et al., 2023; Rimmler et al., 2022). For example, there may be need for clinics to be open at different hours to be more accessible to populations carrying disproportionate burdens of HIV; clinic spaces that are welcoming to sexual and gender minorities, as well as people of different ages; providers who are trained in respectfully working with vulnerable populations such as LGBTQ+ persons; and better public transportation to ensure community members have access to services. There may also be a need for changes around access to healthcare resources, like health insurance. Of course, these are only a few of the multilevel structural factors that may affect the HIV epidemic, and it is important to acknowledge that different factors may affect subgroups differently. Thus, contexts are critical, and there may be different contexts that should be explored, understood, and intervened on. Different countries have different contexts that influence HIV risk, and within countries there may be different contexts by region. The HIV epidemic in the U.S South, for example, is different from the epidemic in other regions. Stigma related to sexual orientation, gender identity, and sexual behaviors, as well as stigma related to HIV, have been noted to be particularly strong in the South (Sullivan et al., 2021). Thus, efforts to reduce HIV risk in this region may benefit from a stronger focus on stigma and its many forms and impact.

Furthermore, although beyond the scope of this chapter, the impact of climate change and disaster response is also an important factor in the environment. Studies coming out of drought-ridden countries in Africa suggest that lack of employment opportunities increases both sex work and HIV (Lieber et al., 2021; Logie et al., 2021). In the United States, the COVID-19 pandemic led to canceled appointments and routine management of HIV. For example, those living with or at risk of HIV were isolated, and testing for HIV and sexually transmitted infections (STIs) was limited (Rhodes et al., 2021).

The fourth characteristic of socioecological models focuses on the fact that there are elements of an individual's environment that can either facilitate or impede health behaviors. In other words, an individual's ability to independently make "good" choices can be influenced

26 | • THEORIES, FRAMEWORKS, AND MEASURES RELEVANT TO HEALTH BEHAVIORS

by the social and environmental contexts in which they live, work, and play (Stokols, 1996). For example, PrEP is now an effective prophylaxis to prevent HIV, yet many of those at risk do not take PrEP for a variety of reasons related to social and environmental contexts. Early on, for example, there was stigma against PrEP use; users were thought to be "promiscuous" (Fields et al., 2021). Furthermore, PrEP remains difficult to access; one must perceive that they are at risk for HIV infection, one must see a provider, have periodic lab tests, and be able to afford PrEP and the associated costs. These examples underscore the profound impact that context can have on the opportunities people have and the choices they make. Another example within HIV prevention is the use of syringe services programs and other harm reduction initiatives to reduce the transmission of HIV among persons who inject drugs. The availability of these types of programs and initiatives, which have been shown to reduce the transmission of HIV (Fernandes et al., 2017), depends on government policies, political will, community perceptions, and of course funding. Ultimately, although choices are considered to be made at the individual level, the environment often dictates the options that are available.

The fifth characteristic of socioecological models recognizes that even within a given environmental context, individual behavioral responses will vary (Stokols, 1996). Understanding individual responses can help create more tailored interventions that may be most beneficial to specific subgroups. For example, recent research suggests that linking PrEP use to other priorities, such as medically supervised gender-affirming hormone therapy, among some transgender women can reduce misconceptions about PrEP use, increase access to PrEP, and increase its uptake among this population. However, not all transgender women receive or wish to receive gender-affirming hormone therapy (Rhodes et al., 2024). Therefore, socioecological models can incorporate individual-level differences in combination with contextual factors to identify the most promising strategies for a given subgroup.

Finally, the socioecological framework acknowledges the dynamic nature of behavior. Environments do not remain constant, and behavioral choices must be made and acted on in the context of a continually changing environment. Thus, flexibility and adaptability must be built into any multilevel model of behavior change.

A MULTILEVEL STRATEGY FOR HIV PREVENTION

CASE STUDY 2.1: HOLA

As described, there is a need for multilevel interventions that move beyond individual-level behavior change to reduce risks and promote health. Here, we describe *HOLA*, an intervention that was developed in Spanish by a CBPR partnership in North Carolina in response to a need for culturally congruent, effective multilevel interventions to reduce the disproportionate effects of HIV and other STIs among Latinx GBQMSM, and transgender women (Rhodes, Alonzo, et al., 2020; Rhodes et al., 2013; Sun et al., 2015; Tanner et al., 2014). *HOLA* harnesses natural helping through the deliberate selection, careful training, and ongoing support of Latinx GBQMSM and transgender women who serve as community-based peer navigators. These navigators, known as *navegantes* (navigators), are chosen because they are natural helpers. They are informal, lay community leaders whom other community members naturally turn for advice, emotional support, and tangible aid. They share similar backgrounds and demographic characteristics of the community of focus: Latinx GBQMSM and transgender women.

Through *HOLA* training, *navegantes* become sources of reliable information about HIV, risk, protection, and other resources within their social networks. *Navegantes* work within their existing social networks of Latinx GBQMSM and transgender women, promoting behavior change through fulfilling multiple roles: health advisors, opinion leaders, and community advocates. As health advisors, *navegantes* raise awareness of HIV and local

(continued)

2 • POPULATION HEALTH, SOCIAL ECOLOGY, AND COMMUNITY-ENGAGED RESEARCH

CASE STUDY 2.1: HOLA (*continued*)

prevention and care services and help social network members access services. For example, a social network member may hesitate to seek HIV testing because they do not trust the provider to maintain their confidentiality, or fear they may be stigmatized for their sexual orientation, gender identity, and/or assumed immigration status. Thus, the *navegante* describes the testing process and how providers are required to maintain confidentiality. As opinion leaders, *navegantes* reframe health-compromising and bolster positive community norms and expectations about testing and use of PrEP and HIV care services. *Navegantes* are taught the concept of reciprocal determinism from the social cognitive theory (Bandura, 1986) to illustrate how attitudes and behaviors are influenced by and influence one's environment (e.g., community). For example, some Latinx GBQMSM and transgender women may think that providers only offer PrEP to those who are "promiscuous" (perceived negatively; Rhodes, Alonzo, et al., 2020); thus, *navegantes* provide medically accurate information about PrEP and how providers view it as an important HIV prevention tool to encourage use and also congratulate and affirm PrEP users for overcoming fear to discuss PrEP with their providers. They promote changes within communities regarding how PrEP is perceived, for example, and serve as role models for others within their networks and communities. Further, some Latinx GBQMSM and transgender women may think that they are being treated as experimental subjects without their consent when seeking care in the United States, and *navegantes* may help them process through these perceptions and improve their understanding about medicine, PrEP, and so forth. Third, as community advocates, *navegantes* elevate the voices of Latinx GBQMSM and transgender women to providers. *Navegantes* participate in tours of local HIV service providers. Tours provide *navegantes* direct experiences with accessing prevention and care services that will not only help them support their social network members in using services but also build relationships with providers to facilitate communication and advocacy. For example, *navegantes* may advocate for off-site testing events, longer clinic hours, and alternatives to making appointments. We have seen health departments change policies around documentation requirements based on *navegante* mobilization and advocacy. Thus, all in all, *navegantes* work at multiple levels, including the individual, community, and structural levels, to address the influences of HIV prevention and care (Rhodes, Alonzo, et al., 2017, 2020; Rhodes, Alonzo, Mann, Freeman, et al., 2015).

While the implementation of a multilevel intervention based on socioecological models can be seen as complex, individuals must have a supportive environment that supports behavior change and healthier lifestyles to make effective and sustained changes (Eng et al., 2009). Awareness and use of multilevel models in addressing HIV, as well as other diseases, have begun to erode the long-held beliefs that education is the only element necessary to make the "right choices" and that failure to make the right choices is a failure to take personal responsibility. Socioecological models do not obviate the role of education in promoting healthy changes, but instead underscore the need for creating an environment that makes the healthier choices feasible and sustainable by addressing multiple levels of influence.

COMMUNITY-BASED PARTICIPATORY RESEARCH

Research aimed at addressing the multilevel social and structural determinants of health, eliminating health disparities, and promoting health equity can benefit from meaningful community engagement and authentic community partnership as integral processes throughout the entire research process. Traditional outside experts (e.g., academic researchers, clinicians, and public health practitioners) may have limited understanding and appreciation of how social, cultural, political, and economic contexts and individuals interact within communities

(Cashman et al., 2008; Rhodes et al., 2014). Thus, understanding and intervening on the complex behavioral, contextual, and environmental factors that influence health and well-being within communities benefit from multiple perspectives, insights, and experiences. The outside expert or community outsider (e.g., academic researcher) can work best with community members, who themselves are experts. CBPR, a form of community engagement, has emerged as an approach to intervention development, implementation, and evaluation in public health and medicine (Rhodes, 2014).

In the past few decades, CBPR has gained recognition as an often-effective approach to addressing persistent public health disparities because the approach may produce more informed understandings of health phenomena and thus more effective interventions (Rhodes, 2014; Wallerstein & Minkler, 2002).

The National Institutes of Health (NIH) Office of Behavioral and Social Sciences Research (OBSSR) describes CBPR as:

> an applied collaborative approach that enables community residents to more actively participate in the full spectrum of research (from conception – design – conduct – analysis – interpretation – conclusions – communication of results) with a goal of influencing change in community health, systems, programs or policies.

Whereas traditional research assumes the academic researcher is in the best position to set the research agenda for a community or population (Israel et al., 1998, 2005), CBPR unites community members, other relevant shareholders (e.g., representatives from community organizations), and academic researchers to actively participate in the research.

Note that the term *stakeholder* has been commonly used as an encompassing term for partners, collaborators, and shareholders; however, it groups all parties into one term, despite different constituencies, roles, levels of engagement, and perhaps most importantly power. It also has a negative connotation for some tribal and Indigenous communities. Thus, the term is being used less, and in fact the U.S. Centers for Disease Control and Prevention (CDC) recommends replacing it with other more respectful and specific terms, such as *contributors, funders, consultants, coalition members, working partners, community affected,* or *interested groups* (www.cdc.gov/healthcommunication/Preferred_Terms.html).

CBPR builds bridges among community members, those who serve communities through service delivery and practice, and academic researchers. Incorporating the experiences of community members, who are experts in their lived experiences and their community's needs, priorities, and assets, and the experiences of representatives from community organizations with sound science can promote the reduction of health disparities and achieve health equity through deeper and more informed understandings of health-related phenomena and the identification of actions (e.g., interventions, programs, policies, and system changes) that are more relevant; culturally congruent; and likely to be effective, sustained, if warranted, and scalable (Clinical and Translational Science Awards Consortium Community Engagement Key Function Committee Task Force on the Principles of Community Engagement, 2011; Committee to Review the Clinical and Translational Science Awards Program at the National Center for Advancing Translational Sciences & Institute of Medicine, 2013; Kost et al., 2017; Rhodes, 2014; Rhodes, Mann-Jackson, et al., 2017; Rhodes et al., 2018).

Similarly, study designs, including those used to evaluate actions, that are informed by multiple perspectives may be more authentic to the community and to the ways that community members convene, interact, and act. Thus, interventions, for example, may be more innovative; recruitment benchmarks, including enrollment and retention rates, may be higher; measurement may be more precise; data collection may be more acceptable, complete, and meaningful; analysis and interpretation of findings may be more accurate; and sustainability and meaningful dissemination of findings may be more likely (Rhodes, 2014; Rhodes, Mann-Jackson, et al., 2017, 2020; Rhodes et al., 2018). Furthermore, by working *with* rather than merely *in* communities, partners applying community-engaged research approaches like

CBPR may strengthen a community's overall capacity to problem-solve through participation in the research process.

CBPR continues to gain prominence in public health research due to its ongoing documented contributions to community and population health. For example, the CDC established the Prevention Research Centers Program in more than 30 schools of public health and medicine to support the use of CBPR through collaborations of academic institutions and community partners in conducting research in underserved communities. The Institute of Medicine (IOM) identified CBPR as one of the eight essential content areas for emerging public health professionals (IOM, 2003). Since that time, more than a dozen institutes at the NIH have released funding opportunity announcements dedicated to CBPR. Along with these initiatives, experts in CBPR have developed guidelines and further refined methods to support this research approach (Clinical and Translational Science Awards Consortium Community Engagement Key Function Committee Task Force on the Principles of Community Engagement, 2011; Committee to Review the Clinical and Translational Science Awards Program at the National Center for Advancing Translational Sciences & Institute of Medicine, 2013; Israel et al., 2013; Rhodes, 2014) in an effort to better implement and evaluate the impact of CBPR.

Using Community-Based Participatory Research to Develop Interventions Through ENGAGED for CHANGE

It is well-established that interventions designed to improve health are more likely to be effective, replicated, and sustained when they are developed though blending the perspectives of diverse shareholders including community members, those most closely affected by a health issue; service providers and practitioners from health departments/clinics and other community organizations, who have expansive experiences based in service delivery; and academic researchers with expertise in science and theory and ready access to the scientific literature (Rhodes, 2014; Wallerstein & Duran, 2010). However, while the theory behind CBPR is well-established, there remains a need for sound methods and strategies that align with the approach. ENGAGED for CHANGE is one such strategy that provides a framework for developing an intervention to meet the needs and priorities, while building on the assets of a community, to positively affect health and well-being. Each letter of ENGAGED for CHANGE signifies one step within the process (Table 2.1; Rhodes, Mann, et al., 2017; Rhodes, Mann-Jackson, et al., 2017; Rhodes et al., in press).

The first step in the process involves *expanding the partnership*. CBPR partnerships often lack sufficient representation of key community or academic partners. Partnerships may not always have the expertise, connections, or other resources that are needed to move a project forward. Thus, it may be necessary to expand representation of shareholders whose expertise is needed. Of course, the expansion of representation is not easy. It can take months to identify potential members, build trust, and increase understanding of the rationale for CBPR partnerships and the relevant processes, history, and goals.

The second step is *establishing an intervention team*, which is a small working group, tasked with overseeing the entire intervention development process. The team works collaboratively with the CBPR partnership, providing updates and brainstorming solutions to challenges faced. This team must have broad and diverse representation of community members, organization representatives, and academic researchers; its work cannot be done in isolation and requires thorough involvement of members representing all partner types.

The third step includes the *gathering of literature and extant data*. This next step allows the intervention team and partnership to build on what is known about community needs, priorities, and assets. These may include community assessments that are regularly conducted by public health departments, hospitals, and local foundations; epidemiological and disparity reports from state and national agencies; data collected and synthesized by community-based organizations used in their own service delivery and grant proposals; and other sources,

THEORIES, FRAMEWORKS, AND MEASURES RELEVANT TO HEALTH BEHAVIORS

	STEP	OBJECTIVE
TABLE 2.1 Steps in ENGAGED for CHANGE		
E	1. Expand the partnership.	To ensure that necessary key partners and perspectives are not missing from the partnership
N	2. iNtervention team is established.	To assign responsibility for moving the intervention development process forward to a small team representing the partnership and its diversity
G	3. Gather existing literature and data.	To build on what is already known in terms of epidemiological data; existing local, regional, national, and global data; and so forth
A	4. Assess community needs, priorities, and assets.	To ensure that community needs, priorities, and assets are blended with existing data
G	5. Generate and refine intervention priorities.	To begin the process of focusing intervention goals based on community needs, priorities, and assets
E	6. Evaluate and incorporate appropriate and meaningful theory.	To apply theory when appropriate and ensure the intervention is informed by theory
D	7. Design an intervention conceptual or logic model.	To describe the logic of the intervention (what is expected to happen)
for		
C	8. Create objectives and craft activities and materials.	To develop and refine intervention objectives and all necessary activities and materials, ensuring activities and materials are clearly linked to objectives
H	9. Hone and pretest all activities and materials.	To ensure activities and materials make sense for those for whom they are designed
A	10. Administer intervention pilot test.	To ensure intervention components fit together coherently
N	11. Note the process of implementation during the pilot test.	To document challenges, problems, weaknesses, and successes identified through the pilot test
G	12. Gather feedback from the pilot and those who conducted and participated in the pilot.	To include all perspectives in the intervention editing step
E	13. Edit the intervention based on feedback.	To refine the intervention based on lessons learned from the pilot

including those from traditional academic research efforts (e.g., peer-reviewed publications). A partnership approach to this step is important because different members will be aware of and have access to different types of existing literature and data depending on their different roles (e.g., organization representatives and academics), and gathering information from a broad range of sources helps to have a more complete picture of the current community landscape and inequities.

Because not all necessary literature and data may be readily available, the partnership must also *assess the needs, priorities, and assets of communities* themselves. This may be accomplished using qualitative and quantitative methods. It is important to note that a key hallmark of CBPR is the movement from knowledge generation to action (Israel et al., 1998). Thus, data collection should focus on answering questions not already answered and collecting data critical to moving toward action.

Based on existing data and data uncovered by the previous step, the intervention team *generates priorities*, presents them to the entire CBPR partnership, and iteratively refines intervention priorities based on feedback. This step helps focus intervention goals based on needs, priorities, and assets. This step also leads to the next: *evaluating and incorporating appropriate and meaningful theory*. Discussions of theory enable partners to understand processes of change, at whatever level, from a systematic perspective, and identify where and how theory fits into their lived experiences. Understanding theory and integrating it with community member perspectives on their own lived experiences is critical to making informed decisions about interventions.

The seventh step in the ENGAGED for CHANGE process is the *design of an intervention conceptual or logic model*. A conceptual or logic model enables partnership members to visually depict and see the logic in their thinking, discuss their assumptions, and engage in a process of blending perspectives, insights, and experiences with theory while keeping an eye on outcomes. During these discussions, community members may describe their real-world experiences and perspectives on health within contexts and evaluate what might and might not work to reach expected outcomes. Representatives from community organizations may provide insights based on their rich experience in service provision, and academic researchers may synthesize the literature and provide expertise in health behavior theory and health promotion. During development of the logic model, new variables may be identified for measurement, including mediating and moderating variables and outcomes.

The eighth step includes the *creation of objectives and crafting activities and materials* that align with these objectives. Intervention team members collaboratively draft objectives and craft activities and materials. In this step, the team develops a general outline for the intervention, including goals, objectives, key messages, and theoretical underpinnings. Intervention activities are then outlined, refined, and developed. Relevant culturally congruent materials are also developed at this stage. This process is iterative, with multiple opportunities for the intervention team and partnership members to provide feedback.

Partnership members, even those who represent the community, become more alike others within the partnership (including organization representatives and academic researchers) and can become "out of touch" with their community peers. Thus, it is critical to *hone and pretest intervention activities and materials* with community members outside of the partnership who may be naive to the research and the partnership.

Next, *administering a pilot test of the intervention* can be essential to analyzing activities and materials for attention, comprehension, personal relevance, credibility, and acceptability by those for whom the activities and materials are developed. Questions include the following: (a) Do activities and materials motivate and sustain the audience's attention and interest? (b) Are activities and materials perceived as they were intended? (c) Is there anything offensive in them? (d) Does the audience recognize and identify with the activities and materials?

It is important to learn as much as one can from the pilot test, and thus it is important to *note the process of its implementation*. Details may identify where the intervention is vague, unclear, or confusing. Instructions may need to be refined, for example. Furthermore, *gathering feedback from the pilot* and those involved through quantitative and qualitative methods can be critical to making necessary tweaks.

Finally, the last step is to *edit and revise the intervention based on feedback*. This may be an iterative process, with the intervention team revisiting previous steps of the ENGAGED for CHANGE model. This process is crucial to ensure that the most promising intervention—based on the unique needs of the community and sound science—is used and evaluated. After all, the goal is to develop an intervention that has the highest potential for success.

CASE STUDY 2.2: APPALACHIAN ACCESS PROJECT

The ENGAGED for CHANGE strategy has been used by the North Carolina Community-Academic Partnership, a long-standing CBPR partnership (Rhodes, 2014; Rhodes et al., in press), to develop an intervention known as the *Appalachian Access Project* (Rhodes et al., in press). Because GBQMSM, transgender, and nonbinary persons in Appalachia are at an increased risk for HIV, STIs, hepatitis C virus (HCV) infection, and mpox (formerly known as monkeypox) infection, and are less likely to use prevention and care services, the partnership applied each step of ENGAGED for CHANGE to systematically develop the intervention to increase use of HIV, STI, HCV, and mpox prevention and care services.

Through the use of ENGAGED for CHANGE, the *Appalachian Access Project* intervention is able to meet the needs and priorities of underserved and minoritized communities in rural Appalachia through community-based peer navigation and mobile health (mHealth). It contains five modules to train GBQMSM, transgender, and nonbinary persons to serve as navigators (known as "community health leaders") within their social networks. The modules are designed to increase awareness of HIV, STIs, HCV, and mpox, and their prevention and care; provide guidance on how to promote use of services, including PrEP, syringe services, and medically supervised gender-affirming hormone therapy; improve understanding of social and structural determinants of health; increase ability to effectively communicate and apply social support strategies in person and through mHealth social media; and work with systems to reduce multilevel barriers to prevention and care. While the testing of the intervention is ongoing, the systematic process provided by ENGAGED for CHANGE ensured that the intervention was based on the experiences, perspectives, and strengths of all partners, thus meeting the needs and priorities of communities and ensuring that the intervention has the greatest potential to be efficacious. If the intervention is efficacious, it will be an important tool in our efforts to reduce health disparities in parts of the United States and within communities that are severely underserved.

Dissemination Through Use of the Empowerment Theory-Based Community Forum

The translation of findings into action is a hallmark of CBPR (Israel et al., 1998; Rhodes, 2014). Through community-engaged dissemination, multilevel changes can be identified and promoted. The empowerment theory-based community forum is a highly collaborative process that translates findings into the next steps, including practice, research, intervention, and policy priorities and recommendations, through a process that brings together community members, multisectoral partners (including organization representatives), and academic researchers to do just that (Rhodes, Alonzo, Mann, Sun, et al., 2015; Rhodes et al., 2011).

The process includes convening partnership members, organization representatives, and academic researchers to review and discuss study findings. Study findings could be from any type of study observational or longitudinal (e.g., intervention). As a group, attendees respond to four empowerment theory-based trigger questions that move from concrete ("What do you see in these findings?" "In what ways do these findings make/not make sense to you?") to action ("What can be done?" "What can we do?"; Figure 2.2). Based on the latter two triggers, attendees brainstorm potential strategies that are displayed on newsprint. Next, using a nominal group process (Rhodes, Alonzo, Mann, Sun, et al., 2015; Rhodes, Song, et al., 2015; Rhodes et al., 2011), attendees define practice, research, intervention, and policy priorities for the next steps based on two criteria, *importance* and *feasibility* (Green et al., 1999), to ensure priorities have potential to address health inequities, decrease health disparities, and are realistic.

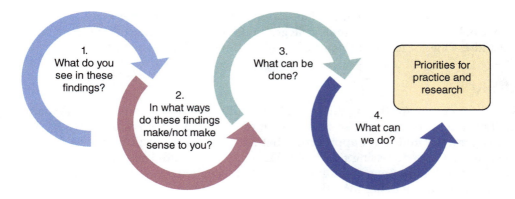

FIGURE 2.2 Triggers used in the empowerment theory-based community forum.

Subsequently, attendees then divide into small groups based on the defined priorities, their own interests, and where they think they might have influence. For example, representatives from law enforcement may choose to join a small group that is focused on intimate partner violence and HIV. Each small group defines the next steps and determines responsibility. They develop recommendations for carrying out identified priorities. They then reconvene to the larger group to present their next steps or action plans. Action plans may include a timeline laying out the next steps, as well as a list of additional individuals and organizations that might be key to engaging. The forum may also identify additional priorities for future research and intervention development, including policy-level interventions. A final report of findings and practice, research, intervention, and policy priorities and recommendations can be developed and distributed to attendees and others for whom the findings could be relevant (e.g., local- and state-level health department representatives and representatives from sectors that did not attend).

This community forum approach was used to translate findings into action in a study of HIV disparities among GBQMSM. Subsequent actions that were led by forum attendees were (a) redirection of state prevention funds to develop GBQMSM safe spaces for facilitated community dialogue around intimacy, norms and perceptions, and HIV risk; (b) a statewide conference to develop advocacy skills among formal and informal GBQMSM community leaders; (c) novel ways to support persons living with HIV; (d) creative uses of social media to make community-level change; and (e) new research partnerships, one of which went on to explore the impact of immigration policy on healthcare use among Latine persons (Rhodes et al., 2011, 2014).

In a non–HIV-related project that was designed to explore barriers to healthcare access and utilization and identify potentially effective intervention strategies to increase access among members of the Korean community in North Carolina, the empowerment theory-based community forum was used to move focus group and in-depth interview findings into action. The actions that were identified through the forum process included the development of (a) low-literacy materials to educate members of the Korean community about how to access local healthcare services, (b) a lay health advisor program to support navigation of service access and utilization, (c) church-based health programming, and (d) provider education to reduce misconceptions about Korean community needs (Rhodes, Song, et al., 2015).

Underlying the empowerment theory-based community forum is the idea that addressing the social and structural determinants of health requires changes at multiple levels as well as coordinated efforts across sectors. Academic researchers cannot do it alone, and community members cannot do it alone. Working together, community members, organizational representatives, and academic researchers can learn from one another and develop more informed understanding of health phenomena. At the same time, however, each partner can translate findings to change the factors within their realms of influence, at whatever level. Through participation in an empowerment theory-based community forum, nontraditional partners (e.g., nonprofit organizations, public libraries, community colleges, and HIV service organizations) have come together to address the social determinants of health of transgender populations.

CONCLUSION

No single solution exists for the significant public health challenges we face. Furthermore, health equities and disparities are seen across different populations and population subgroups. Thus, targeted multilevel approaches that harness socioecological models and use CBPR are promising for addressing the challenges we face in health promotion and disease prevention. For health improvement at the population level, there must be dramatic shifts at multiple levels that make it easier for individuals to be healthy. Unraveling the multiple contexts that contribute to health requires a comprehensive and coordinated effort across several levels by individuals, communities, researchers, policy makers, and government agencies.

SUMMARY KEY POINTS

- Population health focuses on understanding the health outcomes of a specific population.
- Epidemiology contains valuable tools for investigating, measuring, and tracking disease, which are critical to describing health trends over time within populations and among population subgroups.
- Within the realm of health behavior research and practice, socioecological models provide a framework for the development of multilevel interventions that can systematically address mechanisms of change at various levels of an individual's environment.
- Research aimed at addressing the multilevel social and structural determinants of health, eliminating health disparities, and promoting health equity can benefit from meaningful community engagement and authentic community partnership as integral processes throughout the entire research process.

DISCUSSION QUESTIONS

1. Consider the concept of "population health." What "population" do you identify being a member of? Do you consider yourself part of more than one population?
2. What health concerns do you consider relevant to your population(s)?
3. Do you feel that there are resources in your community to serve your population(s) health concerns? How could they be improved?
4. How would the ENGAGED for CHANGE strategy interact in your population? Would you expect this intervention to serve your community well?
5. What social determinants affect the health of your population? Have you encountered any barrier to receiving care?

A robust set of instructor resources designed to supplement this text is located at http://connect.springerpub.com/content/book/978-0-8261-4265-8. Qualifying instructors may request access by emailing textbook@springerpub.com.

REFERENCES

Ajzen, I., & Fishbein, M. (1980). *Understanding attitudes and predicting social behavior*. Prentice Hall.

Arias, E., Kochanek, K. D., Xu, J., & Tejada-Vera, B. (2023). *Provisional life expectancy estimates for 2022. Vital Statistics Rapid Release*. https://www.cdc.gov/nchs/data/vsrr/vsrr031.pdf

Bandura, A. (1986). *Social foundations of thought and action: A social cognitive theory*. Prentice-Hall.

Bono, R. S., Pan, Z., Dahman, B., Deng, Y., & Kimmel, A. D. (2023). Urban-rural disparities in geographic accessibility to care for people living with HIV. *AIDS Care, 35*(12), 1844–1851. https://doi.org/10.1080/09540121.2022.2141186

Breslow, L., & Enstrom, J. E. (1980). Persistence of health habits and their relationship to mortality. *Preventive Medicine, 9*(4), 469–483. https://doi.org/10.1016/0091-7435(80)90042-0

Bronfenbrenner, U. (1992). Ecological systems theory. In R. Vasta (Ed.), *Six theories of child development: Revised formulations and current issues* (pp. 187–249). Jessica Kingsley Publishers.

Cashman, S. B., Adeky, S., Allen, A. J., Corburn, J., Israel, B. A., Montaño, J., Rafelito, A, Rhodes, S. D., Swanston, S., Wallerstein, N., & Eng, E. (2008). The power and the promise: Working with communities to analyze data, interpret findings, and get to outcomes. *American Journal of Public Health, 98*(8), 1407–1417. https://doi.org/10.2105/AJPH.2007.113571

Clinical and Translational Science Awards Consortium Community Engagement Key Function Committee Task Force on the Principles of Community Engagement. (2011). *Principles of community engagement* (2nd ed.). Washington Department of Health and Human Services.

Committee to Review the Clinical and Translational Science Awards Program at the National Center for Advancing Translational Sciences, & Institute of Medicine. (2013). *The CTSA program at NIH: Opportunities for advancing clinical and translational research*. https://doi.org/10.17226/18323

Dibble, K. E., Murray, S. M., Wiginton, J. M., Maksut, J. L., Lyons, C. E., Aggarwal, R., Augustinavicius, J. L., Al-Tayyib, A., Sey, E. K., Ma, Y., Flynn, C., German, D., Higgins, E., Anderson, B. J., Menza, T. W., Orellana, E. R., Flynn, A. B., Wermuth, P. P., Kienzle, J., . . . Baral, S. D. (2022). Associations between HIV testing and multilevel stigmas among gay men and other men who have sex with men in nine urban centers across the United States. *BMC Health Services Research, 22*(1), 1179. https://doi.org/10.1186/s12913-022-08572-4

Eng, E., Rhodes, S. D., & Parker, E. A. (2009). Natural helper models to enhance a community's health and competence. In R. J. DiClemente, R. A. Crosby, & M. C. Kegler (Eds.), *Emerging theories in health promotion practice and research* (Vol. 2, pp. 303–330). Jossey-Bass.

Ewald, P. W. (2004). Evolution of virulence. *Infectious Disease Clinics of North America, 18*(1), 1–15. https://doi.org/10.1016/s0891-5520(03)00099-0

Fernandes, R. M., Cary, M., Duarte, G., Jesus, G., Alarcão, J., Torre, C., Costa, S., Costa, J., & Carneiro, A. V. (2017). Effectiveness of needle and syringe programmes in people who inject drugs—An overview of systematic reviews. *BMC Public Health, 17*(1), 309. https://doi.org/10.1186/s12889-017-4210-2

Fields, E. L., Thornton, N., Long, A., Morgan, A., Uzzi, M., Sanders, R. A., & Jennings, J. M. (2021). Young black MSM's exposures to and discussions about PrEP while navigating geosocial networking apps. *Journal of LGBT Youth, 18*(1), 23–39. https://doi.org/10.1080/19361653.2019.1700205

Gamarel, K. E., King, W. M., & Operario, D. (2022). Behavioral and social interventions to promote optimal HIV prevention and care continua outcomes in the United States. *Current Opinion in HIV and AIDS, 17*(2), 65–71. https://doi.org/10.1097/coh.0000000000000717

GBD 2015 Disease and Injury Incidence and Prevalence Collaborators. (2016). Global, regional, and national incidence, prevalence, and years lived with disability for 310 diseases and injuries, 1990–2015: A systematic analysis for the Global Burden of Disease Study 2015. *The Lancet, 388*(10053), 1545–1602. https://doi.org/10.1016/s0140-6736(16)31678-6

Glasgow, R. E., Klesges, L. M., Dzewaltowski, D. A., Bull, S. S., & Estabrooks, P. (2004). The future of health behavior change research: What is needed to improve translation of research into health promotion practice? *Annals of Behavioral Medicine, 27*(1), 3–12. https://doi.org/10.1207/s15324796abm2701_2

Green, L. W., Krueter, M., & Krueter, M. W. (1999). *Health promotion planning: An educational and environmental approach* (3rd ed.). Mayfield Publications. https://doi.org/10.1016/j.amepre.2006.12.006

Institute of Medicine. (2003). *The future of the public's health in the 21st century*. National Academy Press.

Israel, B. A., Eng, E., Schulz, J. A., &Parker, E. A. (Eds.). (2013). *Methods in community-based participatory research for health*. Jossey-Bass.

Israel, B. A., Parker, E. A., Rowe, Z., Salvatore, A., Minkler, M., López, J., Butz, A., Mosley, A., Coates, L., Lambert, G., Potito, P. A., Brenner, B., Rivera, M., Romero, H., Thompson, B., Coronado, G., & Halstead, S. (2005). Community-based participatory research: Lessons learned from the Centers for Children's Environmental Health and Disease Prevention Research. *Environ Health Perspect,113*(10), 1463-1471. https://doi.org/10.1289/ehp.7675.

36 I • THEORIES, FRAMEWORKS, AND MEASURES RELEVANT TO HEALTH BEHAVIORS

Israel, B. A., Schulz, A. J., Parker, E. A., & Becker, A. B. (1998). Review of community-based research: Assessing partnership approaches to improve public health. *Annu Rev Public Health, 19*, 173–202. https://doi.org/10.1146/annurev.publhealth.19.1.173

Karamanou, M., Panayiotakopoulos, G., Tsoucalas, G., Kousoulis, A. A., & Androutsos, G. (2012). From miasmas to germs: A historical approach to theories of infectious disease transmission. *Le Infezioni in Medicina, 20*(1), 58–62.

Kindig, D. (2015). What are we talking about when we talk about population health? *Health Affairs*. https://doi.org/10.1377/forefront.20150406.046151

Kost, R. G., Leinberger-Jabari, A., Evering, T. H., Holt, P. R., Neville-Williams, M., Vasquez, K. S., Coller, B. S., & Tobin, J. N. (2017). Helping basic scientists engage with community partners to enrich and accelerate translational research. *Academic Medicine, 92*(3), 374–379. https://doi .org/10.1097/acm.0000000000001200

Lieber, M., Chin-Hong, P., Whittle, H. J., Hogg, R., & Weiser, S. D. (2021). The synergistic relationship between climate change and the HIV/AIDS epidemic: A conceptual framework. *AIDS and Behavior, 25*(7), 2266–2277. https://doi.org/10.1007/s10461-020-03155-y

Logie, C. H., Toccalino, D., Reed, A. C., Malama, K., Newman, P. A., Weiser, S., Harris, O., Berry, I., & Adedimeji, A. (2021). Exploring linkages between climate change and sexual health: A scoping review protocol. *BMJ Open, 11*(10), e054720. https://doi.org/10.1136/bmjopen-2021-054720

Mann-Jackson, L., Alonzo, J., Garcia, M., Trent, S., Bell, J., Horridge, D. N., & Rhodes, S. D. (2021). Using community-based participatory research to address STI/HIV disparities and social determinants of health among young GBMSM and transgender women of colour in North Carolina, USA. *Health and Social Care in the Community, 29*(5), e192–e203. https://doi.org/10.1111 /hsc.13268

Mann-Jackson, L., Ravindran, S., Perez, A., & Linton, J. M. (2022). Navigating immigration policy and promoting health equity: Practical strategies for clinicians. *Journal of Hospital Medicine, 17*(3), 220–224. https://doi.org/10.1002/jhm.12792

Mann-Jackson, L., Song, E. Y., Tanner, A. E., Alonzo, J., Linton, J. M., & Rhodes, S. D. (2018). The health impact of experiences of discrimination, violence, and immigration enforcement among Latino men in a new settlement state. *American Journal of Men's Health, 12*(6), 1937–1947. https://doi .org/10.1177/1557988318785091

Mausner, J. S., & Kramer, S. (1985). *Epidemiology: An introductory text*. W. B. Saunders Company.

Mayer, K., Pizer, H. F., & Venkatesh, K. K. (2008). The social ecology of HIV/AIDS. *Medical Clinics of North America, 92*(6), 1363–1375, x. https://doi.org/10.1016/j.mcna.2008.06.003

Mokdad, A. H., Marks, J. S., Stroup, D. F., & Gerberding, J. L. (2004). Actual causes of death in the United States, 2000. *JAMA, 291*(10), 1238–1245. https://doi.org/10.1001/jama.291.10.1238

National Academies of Sciences, Engineering, and Medicine. (2023). *Population health in challenging times: Insights from key domains: Proceedings of a workshop*. https://www.nationalacademies.org /our-work/population-health-in-challenging-times-insights-from-key-domains-a-workshop

National Center for Health Statistics (2016). *Health, United States, 2015: With special feature on racial and ethnic health disparities*. https://pubmed.ncbi.nlm.nih.gov/27308685/

Painter, T. M., Song, E. Y., Mullins, M. M., Mann-Jackson, L., Alonzo, J., Reboussin, B. A., & Rhodes, S. D. (2019). Social support and other factors associated with HIV testing by Hispanic/Latino gay, bisexual, and other men who have sex with men in the U.S. South. *AIDS and Behavior, 23*(Suppl. 3), 251–265. https://doi.org/10.1007/s10461-019-02540-6

Phillips, G., McCuskey, D., Ruprecht, M. M., Curry, C. W., & Felt, D. (2021). Structural interventions for HIV prevention and care among US men who have sex with men: A systematic review of evidence, gaps, and future priorities. *AIDS and Behavior, 25*(9), 2907–2919. https://doi.org/10.1007/s10461 -021-03167-2

Prochaska, J. O., & DiClemente, C. C. (1983). Stages and processes of self-change of smoking: Toward an integrative model of change. *Journal of Consulting and Clinical Psychology, 51*(3), 390–395. https:// doi.org/10.1037/0022-006x.51.3.390

Raifman, J., Cheng, D. M., Skinner, A., Hatzenbuehler, M. L., Mayer, K. H., & Stein, M. D. (2023). State same-sex marriage policies and pre-exposure prophylaxis implementation among men who have sex with men in the United States. *Journal of the International AIDS Society, 26*(11), e26180. https:// doi.org/10.1002/jia2.26180

Rhodes, S. D. (2014). Authentic engagement and community-based participatory research for public health and medicine. In S. D. Rhodes (Ed.), *Innovations in HIV prevention research and practice through community engagement* (pp. 1–10). Springer Publishing Company.

Rhodes, S. D., Alonzo, J., Mann, L., Freeman, A., Sun, C. J., Garcia, M., & Painter, T. M. (2015). Enhancement of a locally developed HIV prevention intervention for Hispanic/Latino MSM: A partnership of community-based organizations, a university, and the Centers for Disease Control and Prevention. *AIDS Education and Prevention, 27*(4), 312–332. https://doi.org/10.1521 /aeap.2015.27.4.312

Rhodes, S. D., Alonzo, J., Mann, L., Song, E., Tanner, A. E., Arellano, J. E., Rodriguez-Celedon, R., Garcia, M., Freeman, A., Reboussin, B. A., & Painter, T. M. (2017). Small-group randomized controlled trial to increase condom use and HIV testing among Hispanic/Latino gay, bisexual, and other men who have sex with men. *American Journal of Public Health, 107*(6), 969–976. https://doi.org/10.2105/AJPH.2017.303814

Rhodes, S. D., Alonzo, J., Mann, L., Sun, C. J., Simán, F. M., Abraham, C., & Garcia, M. (2015). Using photovoice, Latina transgender women identify priorities in a new immigrant-destination state. *International Journal of Transgenderism, 16*(2), 80–96. https://doi.org/10.1080/15532739.2015.1075928

Rhodes, S. D., Alonzo, J., Mann-Jackson, L., Aviles, L. R., Tanner, A. E., Galindo, C. A., Bessler, P. A., Courtenay-Quirk, C., Garcia, M., Sucaldito, A. D., Smart, B. D, Goldenberg, T., & Reboussin, B. A. (2024). Preexposure prophylaxis uptake among Spanish-Speaking transgender women: A randomized controlled trial in North and South Carolina, 2019–2022. *American Journal of Public Health, 114*(1), 68–78. https://doi.org/10.2105/ajph.2023.307444

Rhodes, S. D., Alonzo, J., Mann-Jackson, L., Song, E. Y., Tanner, A. E., Garcia, M., Smart, B. D., Baker, L. S., Eng, E., & Reboussin, B. A. (2020). A peer navigation intervention to prevent HIV among mixed immigrant status Latinx GBMSM and transgender women in the United States: Outcomes, perspectives and implications for PrEP uptake. *Health Education Research, 35*(3), 165–178. https://doi.org/10.1093/her/cyaa010

Rhodes, S. D., Daniel, J., Alonzo, J., Duck, S., Garcia, M., Downs, M., Hergenrather, K. C., Alegría-Ortega, J., Miller, C., Allen, A. B., Gilbert, P. A., & Marsiglia, F. F. (2013). A systematic community-based participatory approach to refining an evidence-based community-level intervention: The HOLA intervention for Latino men who have sex with men. *Health Promotion Practice, 14*(4), 607–616. https://doi.org/10.1177/1524839912462391

Rhodes, S. D., Hergenrather, K. C., Vissman, A. T., Stowers, J., Davis, A. B., Hannah, A., Alonzo, J., & Marsiglia, F. F. (2011). Boys must be men, and men must have sex with women: A qualitative CBPR study to explore sexual risk among African American, Latino, and white gay men and MSM. *American Journal of Men's Health, 5*(2), 140–151. https://doi.org/10.1177/1557988310366298

Rhodes, S. D., Mann, L., Alonzo, J., Downs, M., Abraham, C., Miller, C., Stowers, J., Ramsey, B., Simán, F. M., Song, E., Vissman, A. T., Eng, E., & Reboussin, B. A. (2014). CBPR to prevent HIV within ethnic, sexual, and gender minority communities: Successes with long-term sustainability. In S. D. Rhodes (Ed.), *Innovations in HIV prevention research and practice through community engagement* (pp. 135–160). Springer Publishing Company.

Rhodes, S. D., Mann, L., Siman, F. M., Alonzo, J., Vissman, A. T., Nall, J., & Tanner, A. E. (2017). ENGAGED for CHANGE: An innovative community-based participatory research strategy to intervention development. In N. Wallerstein, B. Duran, J. Oetzel, & M. Minkler (Eds.), *Community-based participatory research for health* (3rd ed.) (pp. 189-206). Jossey-Bass.

Rhodes, S. D., Mann-Jackson, L., Alonzo, J., Bell, J. C., Tanner, A. E., Martinez, O., Simán, F. M., Oh, T. S., Smart, B. D., Felizzola, J., & Brooks, R. A. (2020). The health and well-being of Latinx sexual and gender minorities in the USA: A call to action. In A. D. Martinez & S. D. Rhodes (Eds.), *New and emerging issues in Latinx health* (pp. 217–236). Springer Publishing Company.

Rhodes, S. D., Mann-Jackson, L., Alonzo, J., Garcia, M., Tanner, A. E., Smart, B. D., Horridge, D. N., Van Dam, C. N., & Wilkin, A. M. (2021). A rapid qualitative assessment of the impact of the COVID-19 pandemic on a racially/ethnically diverse sample of gay, bisexual, and other men who have sex with men living with HIV in the US South. *AIDS and Behavior, 25*(1), 58–67. https://doi.org/10.1007/s10461-020-03014-w

Rhodes, S. D., Mann-Jackson, L., Alonzo, J., Siman, F. M., Vissman, A. T., Nall, J., Abraham, C., Aronson, R. E., & Tanner, A. E. (2017). ENGAGED for CHANGE: A community-engaged process for developing interventions to reduce health disparities. *AIDS Education and Prevention, 29*(6), 491–502. https://doi.org/10.1521/aeap.2017.29.6.491

Rhodes, S. D., Song, E., Nam, S., Choi, S. J., & Choi, S. (2015). Identifying and intervening on barriers to healthcare access among members of a small Korean community in the southern USA. *Patient Educ Couns, 98*(4), 484–491. https://doi.org/10.1016/j.pec.2015.01.001

Rhodes, S. D., Tanner, A. E., Alonzo, J., Mann-Jackson, L., Chaffin, J. W., Garcia, M., . . . Kline, D. M. (in press). Using ENGAGED for CHANGE to develop a multicultural intervention to reduce disparities among sexual and gender minorities in Appalachia. *Progress in Community Health Partnerships: Research, Education, and Action*. https://preprint.press.jhu.edu/pchp/preprints/using-engaged-change-develop-multicultural-intervention-reduce-disparities-among-sexual

Rhodes, S. D., Tanner, A. E., Mann-Jackson, L., Alonzo, A., Siman, F. M., Song, E. Y., Bell, J., Irby, M. B., Vissman, A. T., & Aronson, R. E. (2018). Promoting community and population health in public health and medicine: A stepwise guide to initiating and conducting community-engaged research. *Journal of Health Disparities Research and Practice, 11*(3), 16–31.

Rimmler, S., Golin, C., Coleman, J., Welgus, H., Shaughnessy, S., Taraskiewicz, L., Lightfoot, A. F., Randolph, S. D., & Riggins, L. (2022). Structural barriers to HIV prevention and services:

Perspectives of African American women in low-income communities. *Health Education and Behavior, 49*(6), 1022–1032. https://doi.org/10.1177/10901981221109138

Rosenstock, I. M. (1974). Historical origins of the health belief model. *Health Education Monographs, 2*(4), 328–335.

Smart, B. D., Mann-Jackson, L., Alonzo, J., Tanner, A. E., Garcia, M., Refugio Aviles, L., & Rhodes, S. D. (2020). Transgender women of color in the U.S. South: A qualitative study of social determinants of health and healthcare perspectives. *International Journal of Transgender Health, 23*(1–2), 164–177. https://doi.org/10.1080/26895269.2020.1848691

Sprague, C., & Simon, S. E. (2021). Ending HIV in the USA: Integrating social determinants of health. *The Lancet, 398*(10302), 742–743. https://doi.org/10.1016/s0140-6736(21)01236-8

Stokols, D. (1996). Translating social ecological theory into guidelines for community health promotion. *American Journal of Health Promotion, 10*(4), 282–298. https://doi.org/10.4278/0890-1171-10.4.282

Sullivan, P. S., Satcher Johnson, A., Pembleton, E. S., Stephenson, R., Justice, A. C., Althoff, K. N., Bradley, H., Castel, A. D., Oster, A. M., Rosenberg, E. S., Mayer, K. H., & Beyrer, C. (2021). Epidemiology of HIV in the USA: Epidemic burden, inequities, contexts, and responses. *The Lancet, 397*(10279), 1095–1106. https://doi.org/10.1016/s0140-6736(21)00395-0

Sun, C. J., Garcia, M., Mann, L., Alonzo, J., Eng, E., & Rhodes, S. D. (2015). Latino sexual and gender identity minorities promoting sexual health within their social networks: Process evaluation findings from a lay health advisor intervention. *Health Promotion Practice, 16*(3), 329–337. https://doi.org/10.1177/1524839914559777

Susser, M., & Susser, E. (1996). Choosing a future for epidemiology: I. Eras and paradigms. *American Journal of Public Health, 86*(5), 668–673. https://doi.org/10.2105/ajph.86.5.668

Tanner, A. E., Reboussin, B. A., Mann, L., Ma, A., Song, E., Alonzo, J., & Rhodes, S. D. (2014). Factors influencing healthcare access perceptions and care-seeking behaviors of Latino sexual minority men and transgender individuals: HOLA intervention baseline findings. *Journal of Health Care for the Poor and Underserved, 25*(4), 1679–1697. https://doi.org/ 10.1353/hpu.2014.0156

Tulchinsky, T. H. (2018). John Snow, Cholera, the Broad Street Pump; waterborne diseases then and now. In *Case studies in public health* (pp. 77–99). Elsevier Press.

Wallerstein, N., & Duran, B. (2010). Community-based participatory research contributions to intervention research: The intersection of science and practice to improve health equity. *American Journal of Public Health, 100*(Suppl. 1), S40–S46. https://doi.org/10.2105/ajph.2009.184036

Wallerstein, N., & Minkler, M. (Eds.). (2002). *Community-based participatory research for health.* Wiley.

Young, T. K. (2004). *Population health, concepts, and methods* (2nd ed.). Oxford University Press.

CHAPTER 3

INTERVENTIONS WITH THE FAMILY SYSTEM: TRANSLATING THEORY INTO PRACTICE

EMILY R. HAMBURGER, LINDSAY S. MAYBERRY, AND SARAH S. JASER

LEARNING OBJECTIVES

- Differentiate "family support" from "social support" in relation to health behavior.
- Identify and differentiate between the three levels of measurement and intervention in family interventions.
- Describe overarching theories underlying health behavior change interventions within the family system for pediatric and adult populations.
- Describe the potential benefits of technology applications to family interventions for health behavior.
- Identify the benefits of community engagement for family-based interventions to promote health equity.

INTRODUCTION

For most people, families help define "health" and "illness" and shape expectations and tolerances for certain health outcomes for themselves and others (e.g., obesity; Weihs et al., 2002). The family is also the context in which daily health behaviors occur (Grey et al., 2015; Weihs et al., 2002). Families share routines (e.g., mealtimes, bedtimes) and rituals (e.g., holiday celebrations, vacations, religious observations) that shape health behaviors, such as dietary choices and type and frequency of physical activity (Crespo et al., 2013). Other health behaviors can be shaped by family norms and values, such as smoking or other drug use, and the prioritization of healthcare access or adherence to prescribed medication can be influenced by family values, religion, or competing family priorities. Family roles and responsibilities, such as childcare, caring for siblings, meal preparation, working long hours or engaging in after-school activities, and caregiving for an older adult or disabled family member, can interfere with or support health behaviors and health behavior change. In response to these realities of daily life and to research demonstrating the strong role of the family in health behavior, researchers have sought to promote health behavior change by intervening with the family system. As with many other areas of research and clinical work, recent years have seen an increase in utilization of digital delivery modalities for interventions with the family system, which have improved access and convenience for many populations. Additionally, there has been growing attention to the role of culture and community in family system interventions for health behavior change.

40   I • THEORIES, FRAMEWORKS, AND MEASURES RELEVANT TO HEALTH BEHAVIORS

In this chapter, we define terms that shape research and interventions with the family system and describe two overarching theories supporting the notion of interventions with the family system. Next, we describe specific theories and frameworks that have been applied to develop and/or evaluate interventions with the family system. For each framework, we provide illustrative exemplars of interventions applying the theory or framework to promote health behavior change, drawing from a wide variety of behaviors and target populations, including children, adolescents, and adults (Table 3.1). Our approach reflects a theoretical overview with examples, rather than a comprehensive review of family interventions for changing health behavior. As a result, many effective family interventions may not be discussed. Finally, we offer critiques of the existing literature and directions for future research to further inform and shape interventions within the family system for health behavior, including recommendations to promote health equity.

Defining the Family System

When considering the family as a setting for and/or target for intervention, a definition of family must be narrow enough to be useful in intervention but broad enough to include all the significant actors and accommodate the multiple forms that families take in modern society (Weihs et al., 2002). In this context, *family* has been defined as "a group of intimates with strong emotional bonds (identification, attachment, loyalty, reciprocity, and solidarity) and with a history and a future as a group" (Weihs et al., 2002, p. 8). This definition sets family support apart from social support based on three core assumptions: (a) these relationships persist over time, (b) they are emotionally intense and play a critical role in development, and (c) they involve high levels of intimacy in everyday life and require coordination of roles to meet daily demands. Each of these unique aspects of family also informs how and why family members influence health behavior more than other people involved in the life of an individual.

The "family system" has two theoretical and definitional underpinnings. The first comes from the social-ecological theory (Bronfenbrenner, 1992), which describes the individual as embedded within and influenced by multiple systems, ranging from the microsystems, which represent the groups (e.g., family) and institutions (e.g., school, church) that immediately and directly affect the individual, to the macrosystem, which includes attitudes and cultural norms in which the individual and their microsystems are embedded (Figure 3.1). An ecological understanding of the family system may explain how this microsystem affects each individual member and how the family may be affected by larger systems (e.g., politics, healthcare policy, cultural shifts). For example, public benefit programs providing food assistance (e.g., the Supplemental Nutrition Assistance Program) allow families to make healthier food choices, as cheaper foods are often higher in calories and lower in nutritional value; or if a community builds new walking trails, the family might be more likely to go on walks or bike rides, resulting in increased physical activity in the individual. Interventions applying an ecological theory understanding of the family system seek to improve an individual's ability or motivation to make or sustain a health behavior by focusing on the unidirectional effect of the family system on the individual—in other words, changing the microsystem in which the intervention participant is expected to perform a behavior to increase the likelihood of successful behavior change.

The second comes from family systems theory (Whitchurch & Constantine, 1993), which considers the family as a unit of interest and a target for behavior change. The systems theory states that all systems (including living organisms, business organizations, governments, and the family) are shaped by the same key principles. These include the following:

- *Interdependence and mutual influence:* Each of the components in a system is interdependent because their actions influence, and are influenced by, the behaviors of all other components in the system (Broderick, 1990; Whitchurch & Constantine, 1993). The components can be individual family members or subsystems (e.g., parents, siblings). Interdependence and mutual influence are characteristics that

TABLE 3.1 Intervention Examples by Level of Intervention

	INTERVENTION PARTICIPANT(S)	ROLE OF FAMILY MEMBER(S)	RELEVANT BEHAVIOR CHANGE TARGETS	LEVEL OF OUTCOMES MEASURED	RELEVANT THEORETICAL MODELS	EXAMPLE INTERVENTIONS
Family-focused	Person with condition	Family issues addressed, no participation in intervention	Individual health behaviors	Individual	Self- and family management framework (Grey et al., 2015)	The initial coping skills training intervention (Grey et al., 2000), later adapted to be family-based by including parents (Grey et al., 2009)
Family-based	Person with condition and one or more family members, or family member only	Family issues addressed, family member participates in intervention	Individual and dyadic health behaviors	Individual and/or dyadic	Actor–partner interdependence model (Cook & Kenny, 2005)	Behavioral weight loss plus home environment modification (Gorin et al., 2013); secondhand smoke exposure prevention (Borrelli et al., 2016); communication and coping (Jaser et al., 2019)
Family-level	All family members	Family issues addressed, all members participate in intervention	Family-level behaviors (e.g., routines, cohesion)	Individual and/or family	Common fate model (Kenny & La Voie, 1985), developmental model of self- and social regulation (Wiebe et al., 2018)	La Familia and GROW (Barkin et al., 2012; Po'e et al., 2013); WebMAP2 (Palermo et al., 2016, 2018); Family/Friends Activation to Motivate Self-Care (Mayberry, El-Rifai et al., 2022)

GROW, Growing Right Onto Wellness.

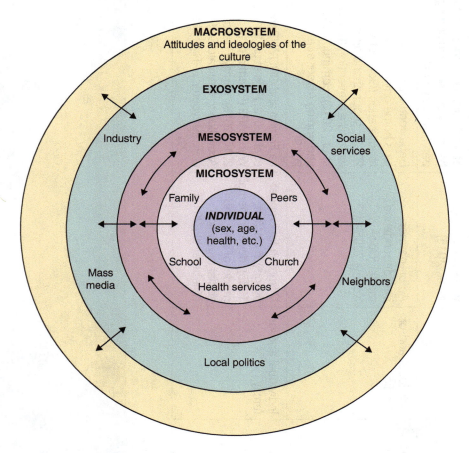

FIGURE 3.1 Bronfenbrenner's ecological theory.
Source: From Prout, T. A., Wadkins, M. J., & Kufferath-Lin, T. (2022). *Essential interviewing and counseling skills: An integrated approach to practice.* Springer Publishing Company.

help define the boundaries of a system; the individuals included in a "family" may be defined as those who are interdependent and exert mutual influence on the other members.

- *Nonsummativity:* Nonsummativity is the assumption that the whole is greater than the sum of its parts; this accounts for emergent properties, which are characteristics or processes that only exist and are observable at the group level (e.g., cohesion, communication patterns). These group-level emergent properties exert influence on the individuals, just as the individuals shape and inform the group-level properties through feedback. An individual may find it difficult to change their behavior in the family context but easy in other contexts, indicating a group-level property may be exerting influence. However, if the individual makes the behavior change in the family context, they may change that group-level property by doing so.
- *Feedback:* According to the systems theory, change occurs in a cyclical pattern (Whitchurch & Constantine, 1993). As one actor performs a behavior, the consequences and reactions of the system to that behavior in turn influence the future behaviors of the actor. The feedback can reinforce the new behavior (e.g., one family member starts smoking, and another smokes with them; one family member begins walking at night, and others walk with them) or dampen

it (e.g., one family member plans healthier meals, the other family members refuse to eat it with them). Interventions applying the family systems theory ideally work with the entire family, or a subsystem within the family system (e.g., the couple or parent–child dyad), and target relationships, family processes (e.g., communication, problem-solving, parenting), or emergent properties of the family (e.g., family cohesion, hostility) to increase the likelihood of successful behavior change. However, engaging multiple members of a family can prove logistically challenging and sometimes harmful to the individual if family members are unwilling to participate or engage in harmful ways. Thus, some interventions using the family systems theory seek to address feedback from the family system without requiring the participation of multiple members (e.g., Shaffer et al., 2022).

Levels of Intervention

The term *family-based* is used most often to describe family interventions for behavior change. As seen in Table 3.1, this definition means the intervention occurs "within the family," in the same way that community-based interventions occur within a community setting. Family-based often means the target patient and at least one other family member must be involved in the intervention. In contrast, family-oriented or family-focused interventions involve a single individual but have content that addresses family issues. For example, a nurse discussing with a patient how they should ask their family to accommodate their medication regimen may be conducting a family-oriented/family-focused intervention, but this intervention would not be considered family-based unless a family member was present and participating in the discussion. A family-based intervention may also include an intervention with a parent who seeks to change a health behavior in the child. For instance, the communication and coping intervention (Jaser et al., 2019) targeted depressive symptoms and parenting practices for mothers of adolescents with type 1 diabetes (T1D) with the intent of improving adolescents' diabetes management. This approach could be conceptualized as family-based because this intervention targets a family process (i.e., parenting practices) to influence an outcome (i.e., diabetes management) in another family member. In contrast, family-level interventions that include all members of the family system are the gold standard from a family systems perspective (Whitchurch & Constantine, 1993), but are often difficult to achieve. Family-level interventions often aim to change a family-level process (e.g., family routines) or emergent property (e.g., family communication), and in turn influence individual health behaviors.

Analogously, the outcomes and targeted mechanisms for these interventions occur and are measured on the individual, dyadic, and family levels (see Table 3.1). Individual-level mechanisms targeted by interventions may include the degree to which the individual is supported by their family to perform a health behavior (perceived support) or things family members have done to make the behavior possible or easier (received instrumental support). Dyadic-level mechanisms may include relationship quality. For example, a weight loss intervention for couples may succeed in changing behavior only to the degree that it improves relationship quality while encouraging the behavior. Family-level mechanisms might include family cohesion or family values about a behavior or expectations of a health outcome. Each of the theories described in this chapter suggests targeted mechanisms at the individual, dyadic, and/or family level, and likewise suggests analyses at different levels. Decisions about the level an intervention will target, measure, and analyze depend on the theoretical frameworks used and the health behaviors targeted, but also on practical considerations such as sample size (e.g., family-level analyses require far more participants than individual-level analyses), resources (e.g., costs, space, access to families vs. individuals), and acceptability of engaging more than one family member among the target population (e.g., culture, norms, and availability of family members).

Analyzing outcomes at the dyadic and family levels requires theoretical and analytic models to frame an individual's health behaviors and outcomes as a function of variables attributable to the individual *and* variables attributable to member(s) of the family or on the family level (Table 3.2). Commonly used statistical procedures assume *independent observations*—that each individual observation is not systematically correlated with any other. The family systems theory assumes *interdependent observations*—that family members' observations will be more similar to one another than to other observations (Kenny & Cook, 1999). Models and frameworks may suggest interdependence but analyze outcomes at the individual level; only a few require analysis at the dyadic or family level.

THEORIES AND EXEMPLAR INTERVENTIONS

Social-Ecological Theory

The following examples are supported by the tenets of the social-ecological theory (Bronfenbrenner, 1992). As described in greater depth earlier, the social-ecological perspective views the individual as existing within and influenced by multiple levels of systems, both proximal and distal. Each of the following frameworks and interventions seeks to alter the effects of the family microsystem on the individual in order to influence health behaviors.

SELF- AND FAMILY MANAGEMENT FRAMEWORK

Grey and colleagues (2015) have presented the self- and family management framework for use with chronic conditions. As the name suggests, this framework combines aspects of both self-management and family management models and builds on more general stress adaptation models. Self-management has been described in several ways, but definitions typically include the dynamic, interactive tasks that an individual engages in to manage a chronic illness and incorporate them into their daily life (Grey et al., 2015). Family management, then, refers to the processes that a family engages in to integrate the treatment and needs of the person with the condition into their family's day-to-day routine. For many, self-management and family management overlap and interact, and this relationship may change over the course of the individual's life. This is particularly true for children, adolescents, and young adults. Young children may depend entirely on their parents to provide and organize their healthcare, while older adolescents may manage their condition almost completely independently. As a child matures, families often begin sharing healthcare responsibilities and transitioning to more independent management.

The self- and family management framework includes facilitators and barriers, processes, proximal outcomes, and distal outcomes. In this framework, facilitators and barriers are similar to risk and protective factors and comprised preexisting elements in an individual or family's life that positively or negatively affect how they are able to engage with the management process. Facilitators and barriers identified in this model include personal/lifestyle factors, health status, resources, environment, and healthcare system factors. These factors are proposed to impact the process of health management, which includes the broad categories of focusing on illness needs, activating resources, and living with the condition. The extent to which the individual or family is able to successfully navigate these tasks influences *proximal outcomes* (including behaviors, cognitions, biomarkers, and symptom management) as well as *distal outcomes* (health status; individual and family outcomes, such as quality of life; and healthcare, including access and unitization).

TABLE 3.2 Theory and Case Study Summary

THEORY OR FRAMEWORK	KEY CONCEPTS	EXEMPLAR INTERVENTION	CROSS-CULTURAL CONSIDERATIONS
Social-ecological theory (Bronfenbrenner, 1986, 1992)	• The individual is embedded within and influenced by *multiple systems.* • Systems range from *microsystems* (groups, family, institutions), which influence the individual directly, to *macrosystems* (attitudes, cultural norms), which impact microsystems and individuals.		• Culture is captured within the macrosystem. • The individual and family are impacted by broader systems, which may either promote or diminish health disparities. • Interventions may wish to utilize the strengths of the individual/family's systems and address areas of negative impact.
Self- and family management framework (Grey et al., 2015)	• *Facilitators and barriers* include personal/lifestyle factors, resources, and healthcare system factors. • Facilitators and barriers impact *health management processes*, including focusing on illness needs, activating resources, and living with the condition. • Navigation of these processes influences *proximal outcomes* (e.g., behaviors, biomarkers, symptom management) and *distal outcomes* (e.g., health status, quality of life, healthcare utilization).	• Coping skills training (Grey et al., 2000): – Targeted processes such as social problem-solving, conflict resolution, and stress management – Diabetes self-efficacy, and parental guidance and control over diabetes management and child depressive symptoms included as proximal outcomes – Glycemic measures, diabetes-related quality of life, and family functioning included as distal outcomes	• Facilitators and barriers will vary among individuals, cultures, and communities. • Interventions should consider the factors most salient to each population. • Proximal and distal outcomes may highlight disparities to prioritize in future interventions.
Parent and family factors framework (Palermo & Chambers, 2005)	• *Multiple levels* of family variables. • *Individual parenting variables* are embedded within the context of *parent–child dyadic variables*, which are in turn embedded within the *family environment.* • Emphasis is on *developmental factors* such as age and developmental status.	• WEbMAP2 (Palermo et al., 2016): – Targeted individual parenting practices – Concurrently addressed dyadic variables by targeting quality of communication and parent–child interactions – Reward systems created to influence family environment	• Cultural values and norms around parenting and family relationships should be considered when designing and implementing interventions. • Expectations regarding what is developmentally appropriate may differ across cultures and communities.

(continued)

TABLE 3.2 Theory and Case Study Summary (*continued*)

THEORY OR FRAMEWORK	KEY CONCEPTS	EXEMPLAR INTERVENTION	CROSS-CULTURAL CONSIDERATIONS
Therapeutic triangle in healthcare (Doherty & Baird, 1983)	• *Family members* play a role in patient–provider interactions. • *Patient–provider interactions* can be *supported or undermined* by family. • Provider recommendations can be aligned or misaligned with the *strengths and abilities* of the family.	• mHealth+CarePartners (Piette et al., 2015): – Collected information and provided feedback to patients via phone – Caregivers received emails with support suggestions – Providers received fax messages in the event of worsening symptoms	• Systems-level intervention may provide an opportunity to aid providers in aligning with the strengths of the patient and the family.
Family systems theory (Whitchurch & Constantine, 1993)	• *Interdependence*: Actions of each component in a system mutually influence all other components of the system. • *Nonsummativity*: Emergent properties exist and are observable only at the group level. • *Feedback*: Behaviors of one actor elicit consequences and reactions within a system that influence future behaviors of the actor in a cyclical pattern. • It seeks to alter *dyadic and family-level processes*.		• Involving the community as well as the family acknowledges the interdependence between the two groups. • Cultural strengths may be considered an emergent property arising at a family and community level. • The feedback that behaviors elicit will vary among differing populations and cultures.
Family system–illness model (Rolland, 1999)	• *Psychosocial types of illness and disability* are considered. • Key *family systems variables* include family vulnerabilities, strengths, coping skills, and culture. • *Development over time* includes phases such as crisis, chronic, long-haul, and terminal phases.	• Behavioral family systems therapy for diabetes (BFST-D; Wysocki et al., 2008): – Communication and problem-solving skills included as family system variables – Targeted adolescence, a stage of life where conflict and diabetes outcomes typically worsen	• Perceptions of chronic and acute illness and disability vary widely between populations. • Expectations for family involvement across time may also be impacted by cultural norms.

THEORY OR FRAMEWORK	KEY CONCEPTS	EXEMPLAR INTERVENTION	CROSS-CULTURAL CONSIDERATIONS
Actor–partner interdependence model (Cook & Kenny, 2005)	• the model assumes an individual actor's outcome is determined by their *own predictors* as well as that of *meaningful others.* • it includes *two actor paths* (the individual's behavior predicts their own outcome) and *two partner paths* (the individual's behavior predicts their partner's outcome). • it posits that an *individual's success* with health behavior change will be impacted by their *partner's ability* to make the same changes.	• OurRelationship (Doss et al., 2013): – Includes opportunities for joint meetings in addition to individual – Targets the individual's behavior, including behavior that elicits maladaptive responses from their partner – Assumes that an individual's behavior changes will be impacted by their partner's behavior changes	• The role of various members of the family will differ across cultures. • Care should be taken to ensure that target behaviors are culturally informed. • Identities and cultures may vary between the actor and partner of a single dyad.
Common fate model (Kenny & La Voie, 1985)	• *Emergent properties* influence actors in the group. • Actors shape the group and emergent properties through *feedback.* • It seeks to alter outcomes in all *family members.* • Engaging and monitoring all family members are difficult and *resource-intensive.*	• Salud Con La Familia (Barkin et al., 2012): – Routines around meals and nutrition, physical activity, and media use included as emergent properties – Family routines shaped by individual family members' behavior	• Broader cultural norms will impact the emergent properties of the family. • Resources and strengths within the community or population should be considered to reduce family and interventionist burden.
Developmental model of self- and social regulation (Berg et al., 2017; Weibe et al., 2018)	• *Self-regulation* includes emotions, cognitions, and behaviors. • *Social regulation* includes disclosures to others, requesting that they be involved, asking for helpful involvement, and managing harmful involvement. • Both types of regulation impact each other, as well as *diabetes-related outcomes.*	• FAMS (Mayberry, Berg, et al., 2021; Mayberry, El-Rifai et al., 2022): – Supports target individual in regulating important others across multiple relationships (social regulation) – Goal setting and monitoring (self-regulation) aid in identifying when and how to activate social support	• Appropriate self and social regulation will be different across contexts, populations, cultures, and roles. • These factors will also impact what type of support is feasible and acceptable in relationships.

FAMS, Family/Friend Activation to Motivate Self-Care.

CASE STUDY 3.1: COPING SKILLS TRAINING FOR YOUTH WITH TYPE 1 DIABETES

Grey and colleagues (2000) developed a coping skills training (CST) intervention for youth with T1D to improve glycemic outcomes. The initial CST intervention consisted of group sessions with adolescents (age 12–20), in which the interventionists used role-playing and discussion to teach coping skills, such as social problem-solving and conflict resolution, including strategies to communicate better with parents (Grey et al., 2000). In this way, the intervention was family-focused, as parents were not directly included. In the next phase of their work, children with T1D between the ages of 8 and 12 were randomly assigned to either a CST or a general education (GE) group along with their parents (Grey et al., 2009). By involving parents in the intervention along with the adolescents, the intervention shifted from being family-focused to family-based. Children in the CST group met for six, 90-minute sessions in groups of two to five. Parents met concurrently and reunited with their children at the end of the session for discussion. The CST intervention utilized the process-level components of the self- and family-management framework to impact proximal and distal outcomes. Processes targeted included social problem-solving, conflict resolution, and stress management, all of which integrated diabetes management into the family's larger social environment. Researchers measured several cognitive proximal outcomes, such as diabetes self-efficacy and child-reported depressive symptoms, as well as the behavioral proximal outcome of parental guidance and control over diabetes management. Glycemic outcomes (such as HbA1c), diabetes-related quality of life, and family functioning represent distal outcomes.

Although the researchers' primary hypotheses—that children in the CST group would demonstrate greater improvements in glycemic outcomes, quality of life, depressive symptoms, self-efficacy, and family functioning—were not supported, families in both groups did see benefits in quality of life, reduction of depressive symptoms, decreased issues with coping, reduced parental guidance and control regarding diabetes management, and increased diabetes self-efficacy. Unmeasured factors, such as the social support anecdotally reported in both groups, may have impacted the children's glycemic outcomes and psychosocial adjustment, resulting in improved outcomes for both groups. Because family-based interventions target more proximal outcomes (e.g., communication), it may be more difficult to observe significant changes in more distal factors, such as glycemic outcomes or quality of life.

PARENT AND FAMILY FACTORS FRAMEWORK

The parent and family factors framework, proposed by Palermo and Chambers (2005), is an extension and application of the socioecological framework that has been applied in health behavior change interventions. The authors sought to address gaps in the chronic pain literature, noting that the existing theoretical frameworks for understanding pediatric chronic pain lacked a comprehensive conceptualization of parent and family factors and did not provide an adequate context for understanding these effects. Their integrative model embeds individual parenting variables within the context of parent–child dyadic variables, which are further situated within the overall family environment. As such, this framework suggests family assessment at multiple levels to fully understand how each level of variables functions within the broader family context and the reciprocal effects of family factors on children's pain and functional outcomes. Additionally, this framework highlights the need to position these relationships within the developmental context, considering factors such as age and developmental status. Working within this framework, interventions target specific parent or family factors to improve children's pain and functional outcomes. For example, by teaching parents to reinforce and reward children's school attendance and exercise, rather than offering solicitous responses (e.g., paying attention to pain symptoms, allowing the child to avoid normal activities), children may be more likely to engage in those desired health behaviors and ultimately have better outcomes.

CASE STUDY 3.2: WEBMAP2

An example of an intervention based on the parent and family factors framework is WebMAP2, a family-based cognitive behavioral therapy (CBT) intervention delivered via the internet, which was developed by Palermo and colleagues (2016). A randomized controlled trial compared WebMAP2 with an internet pain education intervention in a sample of adolescents with chronic pain (Palermo et al., 2016). WebMAP2 involved weekly 30-minute sessions for both parent and child with homework assignments over 8 weeks. The parent modules aimed to improve parenting practices and the quality of communication and interactions with their child, in line with the parent and family factors framework. The intervention also focused on creating reward systems to reinforce the child's participation in their regular daily activities, even during pain episodes. Parents and children completed assessments regarding pain intensity and daily activity limitations due to pain prior to and posttreatment. Compared with the internet-delivered pain education control group, consisting of modules with publicly available information, the CBT intervention group experienced statistically significant reductions in daily activity limitations, as well as improvements in sleep quality and parent response (but not pain intensity) over 6 months, indicating the efficacy of the intervention (Palermo et al., 2016). This intervention was adapted and tested in a pilot study with adolescents with sickle cell disease and their parents; researchers found a high degree of family engagement, and participants reported that they found the intervention to be useful, interesting, and easy to use (Palermo et al., 2018).

THERAPEUTIC TRIANGLE IN HEALTHCARE

Doherty and Baird (1983) developed a relational model for the role of family members in patient–provider interactions that connects the patient, family, and healthcare provider in the management of a chronic condition. According to this model, interactions between the patient and the provider can be supported or undermined by the family, and the provider can make recommendations aligned or misaligned with the strengths or abilities of the family. Acknowledging all parties in the triangle and coordinating their efforts toward the same behavior change goals, therefore, is thought to result in better care and better management of chronic conditions.

CASE STUDY 3.3: mHEALTH+CAREPARTNERS

In line with the therapeutic triangle model, the mHealth+CarePartner intervention uses mobile health (mHealth) technology to enhance communication about and support for self-management among patients with heart failure (Piette et al., 2015). The technologies used included automated interactive voice response (IVR) calls to patients with heart failure, faxes to healthcare providers, and emails to out-of-home informal caregivers called "CarePartners." Participants were randomly assigned to mHealth or mHealth+CarePartners. The mHealth group received IVR calls weekly for 12 months, which inquired about overall health, heart failure symptoms, and self-management behaviors, and provided feedback tailored to their response. Participants' providers received an automated fax when the participant reported worsening of shortness of breath or a significant weight increase. The mHealth+CarePartners group received the same components, but an adult caregiver who lived outside the participant's home also received weekly emails providing a report based on the participants' IVR call responses, with suggestions for ways the CarePartner could monitor and support the patient. CarePartners also received guidance about how to communicate in a positive way, while avoiding conflict with the participant

(continued)

50 | • THEORIES, FRAMEWORKS, AND MEASURES RELEVANT TO HEALTH BEHAVIORS

CASE STUDY 3.3: mHEALTH+CAREPARTNERS (*continued*)

and any in-home caregivers present. This trial evaluated the linkage of patients with their care providers against a completed therapeutic triangle, also incorporated the patients' families. As compared with the mHealth group, the mHealth+CarePartners group showed improved medication adherence at 6- and 12-month assessments, and increased family communication about heart failure at 6 months, providing support to the therapeutic triangle as an effective method to promote chronic disease self-management. This intervention is also being evaluated among patients with type 2 diabetes and depression.

Family Systems Theory

The following frameworks and interventions build upon the key principles of the family systems theory: interdependence, nonsummativity, and feedback. These examples seek to alter dyadic- and family-level processes, such as communication and problem-solving, in order to effect change in the individual's health behaviors.

THE FAMILY SYSTEMS–ILLNESS MODEL

The family systems–illness (FSI) model (Rolland, 1999) was developed as a strengths-based framework for the provision of psychoeducation, assessment, and intervention for families coping with illness and disability. The FSI model addresses three dimensions: (a) the psychosocial types of illness and disability, (b) key family systems variables (e.g., family vulnerabilities, strengths, coping skills, belief systems, culture), and (c) development over time. A unique attribute of the FSI model is that it can be used with a variety of health conditions by including attributes of the illness as one dimension of the model. Important illness characteristics considered in the FSI model include onset (acute vs. gradual), course (progressive vs. constant vs. relapsing), outcome (nonfatal vs. possible shortened life span vs. fatal), level and kind of disability, and level of uncertainty. In addition to being adaptive enough to accommodate multiple health conditions, another advantage to using the FSI model is attention to the time dimension of chronic illnesses. Rolland (1999) was one of the first to integrate different phases over the course of an illness into a theoretical model, including the crisis phase, the chronic long-haul phase, and the terminal phase, and to acknowledge that families need different forms of support and have different strengths and weaknesses at each of these phases.

The FSI model is transactional, as each element of the model influences the others reciprocally, and each is influenced by the characteristics of the larger systems in which the family system is embedded. Thus, the FSI model attends to interactions between the phase of the illness and the family life cycle (i.e., family formation, parenting young children, launching children, later life) and the developmental phases of each individual family member. At different phases of the illness, certain family processes and characteristics vary in importance. The impact of the illness on family functioning and the ability of the family to manage the illness are functions of the *goodness of fit* between illness characteristics and family and individual development (Rolland, 1999).

The behavioral family systems therapy (BFST) intervention is an example of an intervention based on the FSI model. The BFST was developed to improve parent–adolescent conflict by teaching family problem-solving and family communication skills and addressing extreme beliefs with cognitive restructuring and acknowledging and addressing problems with family structure that interfere with problem-solving and communication (Robin & Foster, 1989). Wysocki and colleagues tested a BFST intervention in families of adolescents with T1D to address the shift in the family life cycle (from raising a young child to raising an adolescent). Adolescence can be one of the most challenging times for families managing T1D; during this time, parents often find themselves torn between allowing the child to develop autonomy and self-efficacy and wanting to monitor diabetes management. Failure to ensure the adolescent follows treatment recommendations can lead to medical complications, but the consequences of preventing successful differentiation during adolescence can create intrafamilial conflict and impair the development of self-efficacy critical for the adolescent to manage the illness long term (Harris et al., 2008).

CASE STUDY 3.4: BFST-D

The BFST intervention was adapted to be more diabetes-specific (BFST-D) by including training on behavioral contracting related to diabetes management, education on using blood glucose data to make diabetes management decisions, targeting diabetes-related problems, and parent simulation of diabetes (parents engaged in multiple daily blood glucose checks and injections of saline on the same schedule as the child for 1 week; Wysocki et al., 2006). Families of adolescents who were not meeting glycemic targets were randomized to either the BFST-D intervention (n = 36, 12 sessions over 6 months), an educational support group (n = 36, 12 meetings over 6 months), or standard care (n = 32). Families in the BFST-D group demonstrated changes in parent–child communication (measured objectively), with a decrease in negative communication in adolescents and their mothers, an increase in positive communication in mothers, and an improvement in problem-solving skills that were sustained over 18 months (Wysocki et al., 2008). There were no significant changes in fathers' communication between groups over time. Further, adolescents with higher HbA1c at baseline showed greater improvements in adherence relative to the other treatment groups (Wysocki et al., 2006). Thus, the BFST-D intervention used the FSI model to promote behavior change to improve diabetes-related outcomes in a time when family life cycle phases, individual development, and illness demands often result in conflict and worsening diabetes outcomes.

ACTOR–PARTNER INTERDEPENDENCE MODEL

The actor–partner interdependence model (APIM; Cook & Kenny, 2005) accommodates and quantifies the assumption of interdependence at the level of the dyad. The interdependence assumption in the APIM is that an individual actor's outcome is determined by that actor's own predictor(s) (e.g., characteristics, behaviors) and that of meaningful others (e.g., partner, parent); therefore, the APIM includes two actor paths and two partner paths. The actor paths are the predictive pathways between each individual's health behavior and their own health outcome, whereas the partner paths are the predictive pathways between each individual's health behavior and their *partner's* health outcome (Cook & Kenny, 2005). The core assumptions of the APIM inform any intervention that includes both partners with the same condition, as well as those that target partners' psychological well-being in an attempt to improve the patient's health behavior or outcome. These interventions include partners based on the assumption that an individual's success with health behavior change will be facilitated (or made more difficult) by their partner's ability to make the same changes.

Gorin and colleagues (2013) incorporated the components of the APIM into a randomized controlled trial of a home environment-focused weight loss program for adults and members of their household. In their trial, dyads were randomized either to a standard behavioral weight loss (BWL) program or behavioral weight loss plus home environment modifications (BWL+H). For the BWL group, only the target participants received treatment, whereas both participants and their partners received treatment in the BWL+H group. Both groups met weekly for 6 months, followed by biweekly meetings for the next 12 months. All participants were placed on a standardized diet; given information and resources about diet and physical activity; and instructed on behavioral skills such as problem-solving, cognitive restructuring, goal setting, and stimulus control. Additionally, the BWL+H group was provided with a number of supplementary modifications for their home environment (e.g., exercise equipment, subscriptions to healthy eating and exercise magazines, and serving-size appropriate dishes).

52 I • THEORIES, FRAMEWORKS, AND MEASURES RELEVANT TO HEALTH BEHAVIORS

At 6 months, partners' participation in exercise significantly increased for the BWL+H group, whereas the BWL group showed significant decreases. BWL+H participants lost significantly more weight than those in the BWL group at 6 months, and partners in the BWL+H condition lost more weight than those in the BWL condition at 6 months and 18 months (Gorin et al., 2013).

This intervention offers support for the APIM in the contexts of physical activity and diet by demonstrating that individuals are more successful at implementing behavior changes together with a partner than when attempted alone, and partners are also likely to benefit from such interventions.

Notably, interventions using the APIM for physical activity and diet have found behavior change outcomes are moderated by important factors such as age, gender, and relationship type. For instance, the BWL+H intervention was more beneficial for women participants than men (although there was no gender effect among partners; Gorin et al., 2013). In addition, a recent review on the inclusion of family members in weight loss interventions found that the relationship between partners is important to consider; including spouses may be beneficial, but adolescents achieved greater weight loss when family members were not included (McLean et al., 2003).

CASE STUDY 3.5: OURRELATIONSHIP

The APIM framework lends itself well to couples' interventions that target behavior at an individual level to improve relationship functioning, as these interventions act upon outcome variables via both actor and partner pathways. One such intervention, OurRelationship, has adapted the components of the integrative behavioral couple therapy for web-based delivery (Doss et al., 2013). This 6-week, 8- to 10-hour program is largely completed by each member of the dyad individually, with opportunities for the couple to have virtual, joint meetings with a coach.

The OurRelationship intervention seeks to disrupt the polarization process, in which the members of the dyad elicit maladaptive reactions in their partner (often inadvertently) and react to their partner with problematic behaviors. The program prompts users to examine how differences, external stress, hidden emotions, and patterns of communication contribute to relationship dysfunction. Recommendations tailored to the user's previous responses are provided to help identify ways that they and their partner might alter their behavior. Finally, the couple is guided by either the program or coach as they take turns sharing the insights they have gathered and potential solutions they have developed over the course of the intervention.

The utilization of individually delivered content provides flexibility in scheduling and pace and allows each party the time and privacy to reflect on the concepts presented. This format allows for individuals to participate in the program even if their partner does not. Greater levels of distress were reported by individuals whose partners did not enroll in the intervention, emphasizing the importance of providing an option for individuals to participate on their own (Barton et al., 2020).

While OurRelationship does not specifically target health outcomes, randomized trials demonstrated improvements in perceived health and health behaviors, including alcohol use, insomnia, and exercise. The effect sizes for these improvements were larger for the subset of individuals who initially reported difficulties in these domains at baseline than for the entire sample, with medium and small effect sizes, respectively (Doss & Hatch, 2022).

COMMON FATE MODEL

The common fate model (CFM; Kenny & La Voie, 1985) accommodates and quantifies the assumptions of interdependence and *nonsummativity,* and therefore allows for measurement and analysis at the individual, dyadic, and group levels. Nonsummativity assumes the whole is greater than the sum of its parts; this accounts for emergent properties (i.e., characteristics or processes that only exist and are observable at the group level). Further, these emergent properties exert influence on the actors within that group, just as the actors shape and inform the group-level properties through feedback. Examples of emergent properties affecting health behavior change include family routines and rituals around food and meal preparation. CFM provides information on how group-level properties affect individual actors (Galovan et al., 2017). CFM informs interventions seeking to affect health behaviors and outcomes in all family members. Such interventions are rare, as it is difficult and resource-intensive to engage all family members in an intervention and to measure outcomes in all family members.

CASE STUDY 3.6: SALUD CON LA FAMILIA

The Salud Con La Familia (Health With the Family) program by Barkin and colleagues (2012) is an example of an intervention based on CFM. Families of Latin American, preschool-age children were randomized to a behavioral intervention or a school readiness program. The intervention was culturally tailored to be relevant to Latin American families and consisted of weekly 90-minute sessions, delivered over 12 weeks, aimed at improving health behaviors in the family, including better nutrition, increased physical activity, and decreased media use. Children whose families participated in the program experienced a significant reduction in body mass index (BMI) over 3 months, as compared with those in the school readiness program. In this study, researchers intervened with the parents to change family practices to reduce children's BMI.

Another example of the CFM model is Buller and colleagues' (2021) social media campaign, *Health Chat*, which targeted mothers' permissiveness around their daughters' use of indoor tanning with the goal of reducing both mothers' and daughters' indoor tanning. In this yearlong campaign, mothers in the intervention group were added to a private Facebook group and received posts covering topics such as communication with teens about indoor tanning, alternatives, associated risks, and social norms around indoor tanning. The results of this study indicated that mothers in the intervention group engaged in more communication with daughters regarding indoor tanning and had lower intentions to indoor-tan themselves, as well as decreased permissiveness for indoor tanning (parental permission is typically required for minors). However, no differences in actual indoor tanning were reported (Buller et al., 2021).

Developmental Model of Self- and Social Regulation

Berg, Wiebe, and colleagues developed the developmental model of self- and social regulation of diabetes management (Berg et al., 2017), which focuses on the dual processes required to manage diabetes successfully across the life span. This model, depicted in **Figure 3.2**, postulates that outcomes of diabetes management are a function of self-regulation (emotions, cognitions, behaviors) and social regulation (disclosing needs to others, requesting their involvement, asking for helpful involvement, and managing harmful involvement). Moreover, one's self-regulation capacity can influence their ability to regulate important others toward outcomes. As people age, they become increasingly responsible for both self-regulation and regulating others (e.g., parents, friends, romantic partners, coworkers) toward successful disease management. Parent–child coordination throughout childhood transitions to involve others as children age into adulthood. This framework reflects the key principle of *feedback* from the family systems theory, but rather than suggesting interventions with the system to improve feedback this framework focuses on developing the skills of adults to manage/regulate feedback across diverse relationships.

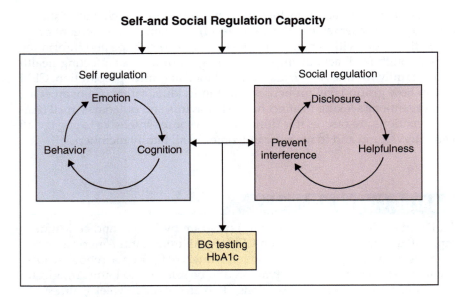

FIGURE 3.2 Self-Disclosure and Social Regulation model.
BG, blood glucose; HbA1c, hemoglobin A1c.

The Family/Friend Activation to Motivate Self-Care (FAMS) intervention applies this understanding of family systems theory and feedback by focusing on building skills of the person with diabetes to regulate important others, across multiple relationships. FAMS is a mobile phone-delivered intervention using phone coaching and text messaging that has been evaluated among adults with type 2 diabetes (Mayberry, Berg et al., 2021) and adapted for emerging adults (ages 18–24) with T1D (Mayberry et al., under review). FAMS focuses on goal setting and monitoring—reflecting the self-regulation component of this framework—and building skills to identify and ask for helpful involvement toward their goals, and minimize, manage, or redirect harmful involvement related to their goals—reflecting the social regulation component of this framework. FAMS also includes the option to enroll a support person to receive text messages tailored to the goals set by the person with diabetes, and therefore can activate an existing helpful individual to provide additional support. In addition to improved self-efficacy and self-care behaviors, FAMS has demonstrated improvements in helpful family/friend involvement and reductions in harmful family/friend involvement through intervening with the person with diabetes (Mayberry, Berg et al., 2021). Moreover, improvements in hemoglobin A1c (HbA1c) were mediated by improvements in family/friend involvement over time (Roddy et al., 2022), supporting the developmental model of self- and social regulation.

CONCLUSION

In this chapter, we noted the characteristics differentiating "family support" from "social support" in relation to health behavior. Further, we have identified the three levels of measurement and intervention in family interventions (individual, dyadic, and family). We describe the two overarching theories—the social-ecological theory and the family systems theory—underlying interventions with the family system, and we identified examples of frameworks for health behavior change within each. We discussed interventions that exemplified a key tenet of the theory or framework, but the study authors may not have characterized the intervention using the associated framework. In a previous edition, we highlighted limitations such as barriers to dissemination and scalability and a lack of diversity among participants. However, digitally delivered interventions have improved access for many populations, and recent publications have included more diverse samples as well as culturally tailored interventions.

In the remaining section, we will describe future directions, including the potential benefits of technology applications to family interventions for health behavior.

Future Directions

Majority of family-based interventions in pediatric populations are conducted with mothers (Phares et al., 2005). Strikingly, in a systematic review of 213 obesity prevention and treatment trials targeting children and adolescents, only 6% of parent participants were fathers (Morgan et al., 2017). Thus, researchers must find novel strategies to engage fathers and other caregivers in family interventions. Similarly, although children of single parents are often at higher risk for poor outcomes than children from two-parent families, single parents are harder to engage in research studies (Brown et al., 2008). Given the increased financial burden on single-parent families, strategies for increasing engagement in this population may dovetail with strategies to increase engagement in lower income populations. Interventions among adults are increasingly recognizing the importance of family members who live separately from the target participants, which is an important advancement in the field's understanding of family (Mayberry, Berg et al., 2021).

An additional challenge is disseminating effective family-based interventions to real-world settings. Many of the interventions described here are time- and resource-intensive, and research is needed to find ways to disseminate these approaches into low-resource settings. For example, a smoking cessation intervention for parents of children with asthma found improvements in secondhand smoke exposure and asthma morbidity in children after two brief home visits and four 15-minute phone calls (Borrelli et al., 2016).

The next generation of family-based interventions can take a page from the personalized medicine field, in which there is greater tailoring of protocols. By examining moderators of interventions, we can determine *for whom* they are most effective (Kraemer et al., 2002). For example, analyses of treatment moderators for the pediatric pain intervention described earlier (WebMAP2) indicated that younger adolescents (age 11–14) and those whose parents experienced lower levels of distress demonstrated greater response to the CBT program (Murray et al., 2020). Recently, there have been efforts to develop and advance typological approaches to understanding the family for adults with chronic conditions (e.g., Bouldin et al., 2019). These studies have sought to identify types of family interactions around disease management or health and explore associations with health behaviors and outcomes. Across these three studies, the same number of types has emerged, and the types share similarities across studies; there is a more collaborative type, a more distant type, an avoidant or unobligated type, and a more conflicted or combative type. The types are associated with behavioral and psychosocial outcomes and predict mortality risk. This area of research is rapidly emerging and holds promise for revolutionizing how we think about designing and delivering family interventions. Typologies can be applied to inform tailoring of intervention components/content and to evaluate differential effects. As the science on family typologies advances, we may be able to predict outcomes by type and better match interventions to type to maximize benefits.

Finally, we expect to see an increased use of technology in family-based interventions as mHealth approaches can overcome some of the limitations described earlier (Shaffer et al., 2022). Delivering interventions digitally makes it more feasible to include family members who live apart from the patient, even if they live hundreds of miles away, and to provide ongoing support for behavior change or self-management, such as the mHealth+CarePartners intervention and the FAMS intervention (described earlier). These approaches may also increase the racial/ethnic and sociodemographic diversity of study samples by minimizing demands (e.g., travel to intervention sessions) on participating families.

Technology also creates opportunities to disseminate effective family-based programs more widely. For example, the intervention for pediatric pain by Palermo and colleagues (described earlier) is an effective web-based family intervention, and the intervention for mothers of teens aimed at reducing indoor tanning was delivered via Facebook posts (Buller et al., 2021). Further, the use of telehealth (e.g., Skype) to deliver interventions that have established efficacy may reduce the burden for families and improve accessibility to specialized providers, particularly those living in rural areas (Harris et al., 2015). Finally, technology presents opportunities for automated tailoring of intervention components or content to consistently individualize protocols based on patient and family needs (Head et al., 2013).

In addressing health disparities, community engagement is critical to ensure input from populations that have been historically underrepresented in research, to ensure that the intervention addresses outcomes that are meaningful to them, and to identify potential barriers/facilitators to their participation (Holzer et al., 2014). Community engagement in research exists on a continuum, ranging from brief surveys, to conducting community engagement studios or focus groups, to including community members as collaborators and integral members of the research team (Boyer et al., 2018). In digital interventions, this often occurs through user-centered design processes that engage end users of the intervention in elicitation research, followed by iterative feedback on intervention prototypes (Lyon & Koerner, 2016). The development stage of interventions is particularly important for community involvement in order to facilitate recruitment and enrollment into trials, effectiveness, and sustainability.

SUMMARY KEY POINTS

- Family need not be strictly limited to immediate biological family members; family can be defined as a group of individuals with emotionally intense and highly intimate relationships that persist over time, impact development, and require coordination of roles to meet daily demands.

- The three levels of family intervention include family-focused, in which family issues are addressed with the individual with the condition to target individual health behaviors; family-based, in which the person with the condition and family member(s) participate in the intervention to target individual and dyadic health behaviors; and family-level, in which all family members participate in the intervention to target family-level behaviors.

- Interventions based on the social-ecological theory address the impact of the family microsystem on the individual in order to influence health behaviors.

- Interventions based on the family systems theory target dyadic and family processes to impact an individual's health behaviors and are shaped by the key principles of interdependence, nonsummativity, and feedback.

- Future interventions have the opportunity to include a wider range of family members, incorporate family typology to tailor protocols, utilize technology to improve access, and adopt community-based participatory research practices.

DISCUSSION QUESTIONS

1. To what extent does the definition of family presented in this chapter fit with how you define family?

2. What factors impact how you might choose which level of intervention to use with a particular population?

3. What barriers to engagement would you like to see future interventions address?

4. How might you incorporate technology into existing interventions?

5. Using the theories and frameworks presented in this chapter, in what ways can healthcare providers promote family involvement in health behavior change?

A robust set of instructor resources designed to supplement this text is located at http://connect.springerpub.com/content/book/978-0-8261-4265-8. Qualifying instructors may request access by emailing textbook@springerpub.com.

REFERENCES

Barkin, S. L., Gesell, S. B., Po'e, E. K., Escarfuller, J., & Tempesti, T. (2012). Culturally tailored, family-centered, behavioral obesity intervention for Latino-American preschool-aged children. *Journal of Pediatrics, 130*(3), 445–456. https://doi.org/10.1542/peds.2011-3762

Barton, A. W., Hatch, S. G., & Doss, B. D. (2020). If you host it online, who will (and will not) come? Individual and partner enrollment in a web-based intervention for distressed couples. *Prevention Science, 21*, 830–840. https://doi.org/10.1007/s11121-020-01121-7

Berg, C. A., Butner, J., Wiebe, D. J., Lansing, A. H., Osborn, P., King, P. S., Palmer, D. L., & Butler, J. M. (2017). Developmental model of parent-child coordination for self-regulation across childhood and into emerging adulthood: Type 1 diabetes management as an example. *Developmental Review, 46*, 1–26. https://doi.org/10.1016/j.dr.2017.09.001

Borrelli, B., McQuaid, E. L., Tooley, E. M., Busch, A. M., Hammond, S. K., Becker, B., & Dunsiger, S. (2016). Motivating parents of kids with asthma to quit smoking: The effect of the teachable moment and increasing intervention intensity using a longitudinal randomized trial design. *Addiction, 111*(9), 1646–1655. https://doi.org/ 10.1111/add.13389

Bouldin, E. D., Aikens, J. E., Piette, J. D., & Trivedi, R. B. (2019). Relationship and communication characteristics associated with agreement between heart failure patients and their Carepartners on patient depressive symptoms. *Aging & Mental Health, 23*(9), 1122–1129. https://doi.org/10.1080/13607863.2018.1481923

Boyer, A. P., Fair, A. M., Joosten, Y. A., Dolor, R. J., Williams, N. A., Sherden, L., Stallings, S., Smoot, D. T., & Wilkins, C. H. (2018). A multilevel approach to stakeholder engagement in the formulation of a clinical data research network. *Medical Care, 56* Suppl 10 Suppl 1(10 Suppl. 1), S22–S26. https://doi.org/10.1097/MLR.0000000000000778

Broderick, C. B. (1990). Family process theory. In J. Sprey (Ed.), *Fashioning family theory* (pp.171–206). Sage.

Bronfenbrenner, U. (1986). Recent Advances in Research on the Ecology of Human Development. In R. K. Silbereisen, K. Eyferth, & G. Rudinger (Eds.), *Development as action in context*. Springer, Berlin, Heidelberg. https://doi.org/10.1007/978-3-662-02475-1_15

Bronfenbrenner, U. (1992). Ecological systems theory. In R. Vasta (Ed.), *Six theories of child development: Revised formulations and current issues* (pp. 187–249). Jessica Kingsley Publishers.

Brown, R. T., Wiener, L., Kupst, M. J., Brennan, T., Behrman, R., Compas, B. E., Elkin, T. D., Fairclough, D. L., Friebert, S., Katz, E., Kazak, A. E., Madan-Swain, A., Mansfield, N., Mullins, L. L., Noll, R., Patenaude, A. F., Phipps, S., Sahler, O. J., Sourkes, B., & Zeltzer, L. (2008). Single parents of children with chronic illness: An understudied phenomenon. *Journal of Pediatric Psychology, 33*(4) 408–421. https://doi.org/10.1093/jpepsy/jsm079

Buller, D. B., Pagoto, S., Baker, K., Walkosz, B. J., Hillhouse, J., Henry, K. L., Berteletti, J., & Bibeau, J. (2021). Results of a social media campaign to prevent indoor tanning by teens: A randomized controlled trial. *Preventive Medicine Reports, 22*, 101382. https://doi.org/10.1016/j.pmedr.2021.101382

Cook, W. L., & Kenny, D. A. (2005). The actor–partner interdependence model: A model of bidirectional effects in developmental studies. *International Journal of Behavioral Development, 29*(2), 101–109. https://doi.org/10.1080/01650250444000405

Crespo, C., Santos, S., Canavarro, M. C., Kielpikowski, M., Pryor, J., & Feres-Carneiro, T. (2013). Family routines and rituals in the context of chronic conditions: A review. *International Journal of Psychology, 48*(5), 729–746. https://doi.org/10.1080/00207594.2013.806811

Doherty, W. J., & Baird, M. A. (1983). *Family therapy and family medicine: Toward the primary care of families*. Guilford Press.

Doss, B. D., Benson, L. A., Georgia, E. J., & Christensen, A. (2013). Translation of Integrative Behavioral Couple Therapy to a web-based intervention. *Family Process, 52*(1), 139–153. https://doi.org/10.1111/famp.12020

Doss, B. D., & Hatch, S. G. (2022). Harnessing technology to provide online couple interventions. *Current Opinion in Psychology, 43*, 114–118. https://doi.org/10.1016/j.copsyc.2021.06.014

Galovan, A. M., Holmes, E. K., & Proulx, C. M. (2017). Theoretical and methodological issues in relationship research: Considering the common fate model. *Journal of Social and Personal Relationships, 34*(1), 44–68. https://doi.org/10.1177/0265407515621179

Gorin, A. A., Raynor, H. A., Fava, J., Maguire, K., Robichaud, E., Trautvetter, J., Crane, M., & Wing, R. R. (2013). Randomized controlled trial of a comprehensive home environment-focused weight-loss program for adults. *Health Psychology, 32*(2), 128–137. https://doi.org/10.1037/a0026959

Grey, M., Boland, E. A., Davidson, M., Li, J., & Tamborlane, W. V. (2000). Coping skills training for youth with diabetes mellitus has long-lasting effects on metabolic control and quality of life. *The Journal of Pediatrics, 137*(1), 107–113. https://doi.org/10.1067/mpd.2000.106568

Grey, M., Schulman-Green, D., Knafl, K., & Reynolds, N. R. (2015). A revised self-and family management framework. *Nursing Outlook, 63*(2), 162–170. https://doi.org/10.1016/j.outlook.2014.10.003

Grey, M., Whittemore, R., Jaser, S., Ambrosino, J., Lindemann, E., Liberti, L., Northrup, V., & Dziura, J. (2009). Effects of coping skills training in school-age children with type 1 diabetes. *Research in Nursing & Health, 32*(4), 405–418. https://doi.org/10.1002/nur.20336

Harris, M. A., Antal, H., Oelbaum, R., Buckloh, L. M., White, N. H., & Wysocki, T. (2008). Good intentions gone awry: Assessing parental "miscarried helping" in diabetes. *Families, Systems, & Health, 26*(4), 393–403. https://doi.org/10.1037/a0014232

Harris, M. A., Freeman, K. A., & Duke, D. C. (2015). Seeing is believing: Using Skype to improve diabetes outcomes in youth. *Diabetes Care, 38*(8), 1427–1434. https://doi.org/10.2337/dc14-2469

Head, K. J., Noar, S. M., Iannarino, N. T., & Harrington, N. G. (2013). Efficacy of text messaging-based interventions for health promotion: A meta-analysis. *Social Science & Medicine, 97*, 41–48. https://doi.org/10.1016/j.socscimed.2013.08.003

Holzer, J. K., Ellis, L., & Merritt, M. W. (2014). Why we need community engagement in medical research. *Journal of Investigative Medicine: The Official Publication of the American Federation for Clinical Research, 62*(6), 851–855. https://doi.org/10.1097/JIM.0000000000000097

Jaser, S. S., Hamburger, E. R., Pagoto, S., Williams, R., Meyn, A., Jones, A. C., & Simmons, J. H. (2019). Communication and coping intervention for mothers of adolescents with type 1 diabetes: Rationale and trial design. *Contemporary Clinical Trials, 85*, 105844. https://doi.org/10.1016/j.cct.2019.105844

Kenny, D. A., & Cook, W. (1999). Partner effects in relationship research: Conceptual issues, analytic difficulties, and illustrations. *Personal Relationships, 6*(4), 433–448. https://doi.org/10.1111/j.1475-6811.1999.tb00202.x

Kenny, D. A., & La Voie, L. (1985). Separating individual and group effects. *Journal of Personality and Social Psychology, 48*(2), 339–348. https://doi.org/10.1037/0022-3514.48.2.339

Kraemer, H. C., Wilson, T., Fairburn, C. G., & Agras, W. S. (2002). Mediators and moderators of treatment effects in randomized clinical trials. *Archives of General Psychiatry, 59*(10), 877–883. https://doi.org/10.1001/archpsyc.59.10.877

Lyon, A. R., & Koerner, K. (2016). User-centered design for psychosocial intervention development and implementation. *Clinical Psychology: Science and Practice, 23*(2), 180–200. https://doi.org/10.1111/cpsp.12154

Mayberry, L. S., Berg, C. A., Greevy, R. A., Nelson, L. A., Bergner, E. M., Wallston, K. A., Harper, K. J., & Elasy, T. A. (2021). Mixed-methods randomized evaluation of FAMS: A mobile phone-delivered intervention to improve family/friend involvement in adults' type 2 diabetes self-care. *Annals of Behavioral Medicine, 55*(2), 165–178. https://doi.org/10.1093/abm/kaaa041

Mayberry, L. S., El-Rifai, M., Nelson, L. A., Parks, M., Greevy, R. A., Jr, LeStourgeon, L., Molli, S., Bergner, E., Spieker, A., Aikens, J. E., & Wolever, R. Q. (2022). Rationale, design, and recruitment outcomes for the Family/Friend Activation to Motivate Self-care (FAMS) 2.0 randomized controlled trial among adults with type 2 diabetes and their support persons. *Contemporary Clinical Trials, 122*, 106956. https://doi.org/10.1016/j.cct.2022.106956

Mayberry, L. S., Wiebe, D. J., Parks, M., Campbell, M. S., Beam, A. B., & Berg, C. A. (2024). Acceptability and feasibility of FAMS-T1D mHealth intervention to optimize self- and social regulation for emerging adults with type 1 diabetes. *Pilot and Feasibility Studies, 10*(1), 68. https://doi.org/10.1186/s40814-024-01497-1

Mayberry, L. S., Wiebe, D. J., Parks, M., Campbell, M. S., Beam, A. B., & Berg, C. A. (2024). Acceptability and feasibility of FAMS-T1D mHealth intervention to optimize social regulation for emerging adults with type 1 diabetes.

McLean, N., Griffin, S., Toney, K., & Hardeman, W. (2003). Family involvement in weight control, weight maintenance and weight-loss interventions: A systematic review of randomised trials. *International Journal of Obesity and Related Metabolic Disorders, 27*(9), 987–1005. https://doi.org/10.1038/sj.ijo.0802383

Morgan, P. J., Young, M. D., Lloyd, A. B., Wang, M. L., Eather, N., Miller, A., Murtagh, E. M., Barnes, A. T., & Pagoto, S. L. (2017). Involvement of fathers in pediatric obesity treatment and prevention trials: A systematic review. *Pediatrics, 139*(2), e20162635. https://doi.org/10.1542/peds.2016-263

Murray, C. B., de la Vega, R., Loren, D. M., & Palermo, T. M. (2020). Moderators of internet-delivered cognitive-behavioral therapy for adolescents with chronic pain: who benefits from treatment at long-term follow-up?. *The Journal of Pain, 21*(5–6), 603–615. https://doi.org/10.1016/j.jpain.2019.10.001

Palermo, T. M., & Chambers, C. T. (2005). Parent and family factors in pediatric chronic pain and disability: An integrative approach. *Pain, 119*(1–3), 1–4. https://doi.org/10.1016/j.pain.2005.10.027

Palermo, T. M., Dudeney, J., Santanelli, J. P., Carletti, A., & Zempsky, W. T. (2018). Feasibility and acceptability of internet-delivered cognitive behavioral therapy for chronic pain in adolescents with sickle cell disease and their parents. *Journal of Pediatric Hematology/Oncology, 40*(2), 122–127. https://doi.org/10.1097/MPH.0000000000001018

Palermo, T. M., Law, E. F., Fales, J., Bromberg, M. H., Jessen-Fiddick, T., & Tai, G. (2016). Internet-delivered cognitive-behavioral treatment for adolescents with chronic pain and their parents: A randomized controlled multicenter trial. *Pain, 157*(1), 174–185. https://doi.org/10.1097/j.pain.0000000000000348

Phares, V., Lopez, E., Fields, S., Kamboukos, D., & Duhig, A. M. (2005). Are fathers involved in pediatric psychology research and treatment? *Journal of Pediatric Psychology, 30*(8), 631–643. https://doi.org/10.1093/jpepsy/jsi050

Piette, J. D., Striplin, D., Marinec, N., Chen, J., Trivedi, R. B., Aron, D. C., Fisher, L., & Aikens, J. E. (2015). A mobile health intervention supporting heart failure patients and their informal caregivers: A randomized comparative effectiveness trial. *Journal of Medical Internet Research, 17*(6), e142. https://doi.org/10.2196/jmir.4550

Po'e, E. K., Heerman, W. J., Mistry, R. S., & Barkin, S. L. (2013). Growing Right Onto Wellness (GROW): A family-centered, community-based obesity prevention randomized controlled trial for preschool child-parent pairs. *Contemporary Clinical Trials, 36*(2), 436–449. https://doi.org/10.1016/j.cct.2013.08.013

Robin, A. L., & Foster, S. L. (1989). *Negotiating parent-adolescent conflict: A behavioral family systems approach*. Guilford Press.

Roddy, M. K., Nelson, L. A., Greevy, R. A., & Mayberry, L. S. (2022). Changes in family involvement occasioned by FAMS mobile health intervention mediate changes in glycemic control over 12 months. *Journal of Behavioral Medicine, 45*(1), 28–37. https://doi.org/10.1007/s10865-021-00250-w.

Rolland, J. S. (1999). Parental illness and disability: A family systems framework. *Journal of Family Therapy, 21*(3), 242–266. https://doi.org/10.1111/1467-6427.00118

Shaffer, K. M., Mayberry, L. S., Salivar, E. G., Doss, B. D., Lewis, A. M., & Canter, K. (2022). Dyadic digital health interventions: Their rationale and implementation. *Procedia Computer Science, 206*, 183–194. https://doi.org/10.1016/j.procs.2022.09.097

Weihs, K., Fisher, L., & Baird M. A. (2002). Families, health and behavior. *Families, Systems, & Health, 20*(1), 7–46. https://doi.org/10.1037/h0089481

Whitchurch, G. G., & Constantine, L. C. (1993). Systems theory. In P. G. Boss, W. J. Doherty, R. LaRossa, W. R. Schumm, & S. K. Steimnetz (Eds.), *Sourcebook of family theories and methods: A contextual approach* (pp. 325–352). Plenum Press.

Wiebe, D. J., Berg, C. A., Mello, D., & Kelly, C. S. (2018). Self- and Social-Regulation in Type 1 Diabetes Management During Late Adolescence and Emerging Adulthood. *Current Diabetes Reports, 18*(5), 23. https://doi.org/10.1007/s11892-018-0995-3

Wysocki, T., Harris, M. A., Buckloh, L. M., Mertlich, D., Lochrie, A. S., Taylor, A., Sadler, M., Mauras, N., & White, N. H. (2006). Effects of behavioral family systems therapy for diabetes on adolescents' family relationships, treatment adherence, and metabolic control. *Journal of Pediatric Psychology, 31*(9), 928–938. https://doi.org/10.1093/jpepsy/jsj098

Wysocki, T., Harris, M. A., Buckloh, L. M., Mertlich, D., Lochrie, A. S., Taylor, A., Sadler, M., & White, N. H. (2008). Randomized, controlled trial of behavioral family systems therapy for diabetes: Maintenance and generalization of effects on parent-adolescent communication. *Behavior therapy, 39*(1), 33–46. https://doi.org/10.1016/j.beth.2007.04.001

CHAPTER 4

INDIVIDUAL-LEVEL THEORIES

JAY E. MADDOCK

LEARNING OBJECTIVES

- Discuss the major components and applications of commonly used individual theories, including the social cognitive theory (SCT), the health belief model (HBM), the theory of planned behavior (TPB), the transtheoretical model (TTM), and the relapse prevention (RP) model.
- Describe how individual theories of health behavior change are used to guide both correlational and intervention-based research and the prominent role that these theories have played in health behavior research over more than five decades.
- Describe how individual theories have been applied to technology-enabled interventions and present opportunities for innovative approaches to theory development in this area.
- Describe how individual theories address health equity and ensure positive health behavior change for all.
- Apply knowledge of behavioral theories to develop interventions.

INTRODUCTION

While built, natural, political, and social environments play an important role in determining health outcomes, individual health behaviors are still essential in improving population health. Various behaviors affect human health, including substance abuse, unsafe sexual practices, injury prevention, physical activity, and others. The success of effective preventive and treatment regimens depends on individuals' willingness to undertake and maintain required behaviors. Given low rates of screening, immunization, and adherence to prescribed medical regimens (Finney Rutten et al., 2021; Lombardo et al., 2022) nor preventive health behaviors (Lee et al., 2022; Piercy et al., 2018), it is not surprising that behavioral scientists have devoted extensive effort to explain and predict individuals' health-related decisions. This effort has resulted in the development and widespread application of numerous individual-level behavior change theories.

Despite the increasing use of the socioecological model, multilevel frameworks, and theories that account for broader influences on health behavior, individual-level theories remain widely used in the research literature (Noar & Mehrotra, 2011; Painter et al., 2008). These theories focus on cognitive variables such as attitudes, beliefs, expectations, and their influencing factors. They are "rational" in assuming that individuals wish to maximize positive health outcomes. Guidelines for intervention development and evaluation have reiterated the importance of a solid theoretical base (Sniehotta et al., 2015; Winter et al., 2016).

The ongoing popularity of individual theories can be seen in recent trends. First, 20th-century theories are being applied in new ways in the 21st century as health behavior interventions are increasingly delivered digitally (Cliffe et al., 2021). Second, a globally connected world and new communication channels allow researchers and practitioners to apply individual theories in populations and settings far from those in which they were developed. As lessons learned from this work are shared, we gain insight into how culture and setting affect the generalizability of these theories (King, 2015). Third, the use of individual theories has extended well beyond the traditional health behaviors for which most were initially developed to study phenomena as diverse as antimicrobial stewardship (Heid et al., 2016), safety behaviors among Boko Haram victims in Nigeria (Tade & Nwanosike, 2016), and older adults' driving behavior (Kowalski et al., 2014).

The appeal of individual theories lies in their potentially powerful applications to health behavior research and practice. For instance, they can form a blueprint for intervention development and evaluation by helping identify the critical determinants of health behavior to influence and measure. Theories can also be used to predict future health actions, and more generally to help us sift through the complexity of human health-related behavior. Mitigating the potential value of these theories is the reality of unclear evidence about whether the explicit use of theories in intervention development enhances intervention efficacy. However, evidence is emerging that interventions based on theory are more efficacious (Murimi et al., 2017). Also, the utility and aptness of each theory for a given health behavior, population, or setting may differ. In addition, the considerable overlap in constructs or components across theories with varying terminology may make the existing menu of theories "overwhelming" to researchers and practitioners (Noar & Zimmerman, 2005).

The overall goal of this chapter is to offer a snapshot of five commonly used individual health behavior theories: the health belief model (HBM), social cognitive theory (SCT), theory of planned behavior (TPB), transtheoretical model (TTM) and relapse prevention (RP) model. A summary of the origins and primary components is provided for each. We also describe their empirical application and the results of meta-analyses or reviews that lend insight into their value. A meta-analysis is a study of studies where an overall effect between the studies is calculated. Where applicable, we note the critical attention that a theory has received, including significant limitations or recommendations for future directions. In addition, we provide an overview of the growing application of individual theories to internet-based (eHealth) and mobile (mHealth) interventions and address health equity in diverse populations. We discuss the overlap among theories and practical dimensions for comparing individual theories. The chapter concludes by discussing recent observations on health behavior theory research.

THE HEALTH BELIEF MODEL

The HBM was developed in the early 1950s by social psychologists at the U.S. Public Health Service (Rosenstock, 1974) to understand "the widespread failure of people to accept disease preventives or screening tests for the early detection of asymptomatic disease" (p. 328). The HBM was later applied to patients' symptom responses and adherence to prescribed medical regimens (Becker, 1974).

The essential components of the HBM are derived from a well-established body of psychological and behavioral theory. The HBM emphasizes personal beliefs and hypothesizes that behavior depends primarily on two variables: (a) the value placed by an individual on a particular goal and (b) the individual's estimate of the likelihood that a given action will achieve that goal (Maiman & Becker, 1974). In the context of health-related behavior, these variables were conceptualized as (a) the desire to avoid illness (or, if ill, to get well) and (b) the belief that a specific health action will prevent (or ameliorate) illness (i.e., the individual's estimate of the threat of illness and of the likelihood of being able, through personal action, to reduce that threat).

Specifically, the HBM consists of the following constructs (**Figure 4.1**): *perceived susceptibility,* or how likely someone believes they are to contract a condition; *perceived severity,* or feelings concerning the seriousness of contracting an illness (or of leaving it untreated)—while low perceptions of seriousness might provide insufficient motivation for behavior, very high perceived severity might inhibit action; *perceived benefits,* or beliefs regarding the effectiveness of the various actions available to reduce disease threat; *perceived barriers,* or the potential negative aspects of a particular health action that may reduce the chance of undertaking the recommended behavior; and *cues to action,* or stimuli to trigger the decision-making process.

According to the HBM, demographic, personal, social, and structural factors have the potential to influence health behaviors. However, these variables are believed to work through their effects on the individual's health motivations and subjective perceptions rather than functioning as direct causes of health action (Becker et al., 1974).

The HBM is well-represented in published research. Evidence supports the HBM's ability to account for substantial variance in undertaking preventive health actions, seeking diagnoses, and following prescribed medical advice. Recent reviews have found the HBM effective for various behaviors, including colorectal cancer screening, mammography, and COVID-19 preventive behaviors (Ritchie et al., 2021; Zewdie et al., 2022).

Additional examples of HBM application across various preventive behaviors continue to proliferate. These include condom use (Amevor & Tarkang, 2022), vaccination (Suess et al., 2022), and adherence to antihypertensive medication (Yang et al., 2016). Although the HBM is often used to explain behavior, it has also served as a blueprint for intervention design. Jones et al. (2014) conducted a systematic review of 18 HBM-based interventions targeted at improving adherence to a medical regimen. *Perceived benefits* and *perceived susceptibility* were

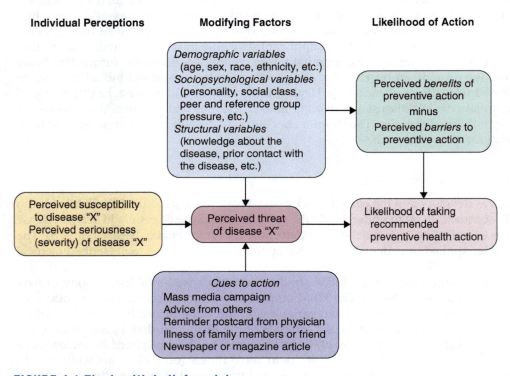

FIGURE 4.1 The health belief model.
Source: From the National Institute of Neurological Disorders and Stroke. National Institutes of Health. Bethesda, MD 20892.

included in virtually all studies; a *cue to action* was the model element least often addressed. About three-quarters of reviewed studies reported a statistically significant effect of the intervention on improving adherence. However, the likelihood of intervention success was independent of which HBM constructs were addressed. The authors argue that standardized tools are needed to measure HBM constructs, which could be adapted for given behaviors and diseases, to facilitate comparison across studies.

The HBM also has been criticized because it can only account for as much of the variance in individuals' health-related behaviors as can be explained by their attitudes and beliefs. It is clear that other forces influence health actions; for example, (a) some behaviors (e.g., cigarette smoking and brushing teeth) have a substantial habitual component, obviating any ongoing psychosocial decision-making process; (b) many health-related behaviors are undertaken for what are non–health-related reasons (e.g., stopping smoking to attain social approval); and (c) socioeconomic or environmental factors may prevent the individual from undertaking a preferred course of action (e.g., living in a city with high levels of air pollution). The model is based on the premise that "health" is a highly valued concern or goal for most individuals and that "cues to action" are widely prevalent; where these conditions are not satisfied, the model may not be helpful in or relevant to predicting behavior. This model appears most relevant for one-time preventive behaviors like vaccines and screening rather than daily lifestyle behaviors.

SOCIAL COGNITIVE THEORY

The central feature of SCT is the reciprocal nature of influences that produce behavior. Personal factors, existing behaviors, and the social and physical environments interact and, as a result, shape the new behavior. In SCT, several vital concepts explain and predict behavior based on how individuals learn: incentives, outcome expectations, and efficacy expectations. According to Bandura (1986), a person with given beliefs, information, attitudes, and needs functioning in given social and physical environments will engage in a behavior with a consequent outcome. In this way, behavior change and maintenance are primarily a function of (a) expectations about the outcomes resulting from engaging in behavior and (b) expectations about one's ability to engage in or execute the behavior. Thus, "outcome expectations" consist of beliefs about whether given behaviors will lead to given outcomes, whereas "efficacy expectations" consist of beliefs about how capable one is of performing the behavior that leads to those outcomes. The two constructs are linked in predicting, for example, exercise behavior (Young et al., 2014) and self-management of diabetes (Ghoreishi et al., 2019).

Both outcome and efficacy expectations reflect a person's beliefs about capabilities and the connections between behavior and outcome. These perceptions, then, and not necessarily "true" capabilities, influence behavior. In addition, it is essential to understand that the concept of self-efficacy relates to beliefs about capabilities of performing specific behaviors in particular situations (Marks et al., 2005); self-efficacy does not refer to a personality characteristic or a global trait that operates independently of contextual factors (Bandura, 1986). An individual's efficacy expectations will vary greatly depending on the particular task and context that confronts them.

Bandura (2002) argued that perceived self-efficacy influences all aspects of behavior, including the acquisition of new behaviors (e.g., a young adult learning how to use a particular contraceptive device), inhibition of existing behaviors (e.g., decreasing or stopping cigarette smoking), and disinhibition of behaviors (e.g., resuming sexual activity after myocardial infarction). Individuals with low self-efficacy for a particular task may ruminate about their deficiencies rather than thinking about accomplishing or attending to the task at hand; this impedes the successful performance of the task. Self-efficacy also affects the amount of effort a person will expend on a task and the degree of persistence in the face of obstacles. Finally, self-efficacy affects people's emotional reactions, such as anxiety and distress.

Efficacy expectations derive from four primary sources (Bandura, 1986). The first, termed *performance accomplishments*, refers to learning through personal experience, where one achieves mastery over a difficult task, which increases self-efficacy. Performance accomplishments attained through personal experience are the most potent source of efficacy expectations.

The second source is *vicarious experience*, which refers to learning that occurs through observation of events or other people, or models. To increase an observer's self-efficacy, it is crucial that the model is viewed as having overcome difficulties through determined effort rather than with ease and that the model is similar to the observer concerning other characteristics (e.g., age, gender).

"Verbal persuasion," or encouragement, constitutes the third source of efficacy expectations. Finally, one's "physiological state" provides information that can influence efficacy expectations. For example, people who experience sweaty palms and a racing heartbeat before they are about to give a talk find that their self-efficacy plummets; to someone just beginning an exercise program, fatigue and mild aches and pains may be mistakenly interpreted as a sign that they should not be physically active.

The behavior change techniques used in popular commercially available activity monitors are commonly based on SCT's goal-setting, self-monitoring, and feedback elements (Lyons et al., 2014).

CASE STUDY 4.1: HIP HOP HEALS

The "Hip Hop HEALS (Healthy Eating And Living in Schools)," a school-based intervention to improve children's food choices, provides an example of how SCT constructs are typically operationalized in program design (Williams et al., 2016). The program consisted of three 1-hour hip hop assembly style classes. In this program, children were given an opportunity for *performance accomplishments (mastery)* via a calorie balance video game, obtained *vicarious experience* in adopting healthy eating patterns via characters in animated cartoons and comic books, and received *verbal persuasion* in the form of encouragement from facilitators. Results showed a significant decreased purchased calories and unhealthy foods that lasted for at least 12 days after the intervention.

Other recent interventions demonstrate SCT's versatility; for example, SCT is the most frequently used theory informing the design of electronic games for children with diabetes.

SCT has been most often applied to explaining or promoting lifestyle behaviors. In a review and meta-analysis of SCT-based diet and physical activity interventions for adult cancer survivors, Stacey and colleagues found a significant pooled intervention effect on physical activity and that most studies were successful in changing at least one aspect of nutrition-related behavior (Stacey et al., 2015). However, in a caveat frequently found in reviews and meta-analyses of studies based on a given theory, the authors noted that SCT constructs were seldom well-described in the reviewed studies and rarely measured or tested. Recently, SCT has been extended to additional, emerging lifestyle behaviors, including vaping cessation (Berg et al., 2021) and spending time in nature (Maddock et al., 2022).

In a meta-analysis of observational studies of physical activity, 31% of the overall variance in outcomes was explained by SCT constructs (Young et al., 2014). They also found that self-efficacy and goals were more consistently associated with physical activity than outcome expectations or social–environmental factors. They point out that while self-efficacy is the SCT construct with the largest body of evidence supporting its links with behavior, goal setting via self-regulation appears to have similarly strong effects on behavior.

THEORY OF PLANNED BEHAVIOR

The prediction of behavioral intentions, as the direct antecedent to the behavior itself, is at the heart of Ajzen's TPB (Ajzen, 2011) and its predecessor, the theory of reasoned action (TRA; Ajzen & Fishbein, 1980). Predictors of behavioral intention, according to these models, are (1) an individual's *attitudes* toward the behavior, which are influenced, in turn, by their beliefs about the (a) likelihood and (b) desirability of outcomes resulting from the behavior; and (2) the *subjective norm* toward that behavior as perceived by the individual, determined by (a) what an individual perceives as the expectations of significant others about the behavior, as well as (b) how motivated a person is to comply with the beliefs of these significant others. The relative influence of these two components—attitude and subjective norms—on intention depends on the nature of the behavioral goal. For some behaviors, the attitudinal component will be the significant determinant of intention. In contrast, for others, the more the individual believes that significant others are in favor of the behavior, the stronger their intention to perform it will be. A refinement of the model by its creator was the addition of "descriptive norms" as part of the "normative beliefs" component (Ajzen, 2011). "Descriptive norms" are what a person perceives as others' actual *performance* of a particular behavior (such as the perceived extent to which peers practice safer sex), not just others' *views* of the behavior.

TPB expands on the TRA by including a component representing the perceived degree of control the person has over the behavior, a concept similar to Bandura's construct of self-efficacy (Ajzen, 2011). These control beliefs consider the presence and strength of personal and external factors that influence the behavior, such as having a workable plan, skills, social support, knowledge, time, money, willpower, and opportunity. By accounting for control perceptions, TPB increases its relevance to many health-related behaviors over which people have incomplete volitional control, such as following nutrition guidelines.

TPB posits that a solid intention to perform the behavior should result when attitudes and subjective norms are favorable and perceived control is high. These predictors do not solely explain the ultimate execution of the behavior, as actual control also plays an important part. According to the model (**Figure 4.2**), perceived behavioral control (PBC) can serve as a proxy for actual control over a behavior, and as such it may contribute to predicting actual behavior. In other words, successful behavior performance will result if individuals have the intention and sufficient control over the internal and external factors that influence such performance.

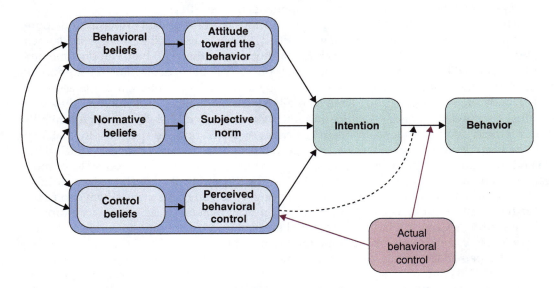

FIGURE 4.2 The theory of planned behavior.
Source: From Ajzen, I. (2013). Theory of planned behavior. https://people.umass.edu/aizen/pubs/REA.pdf. Copyright 2006 Icek Ajzen. Reprinted with permission.

Detailed guides are available to help researchers develop measures for each of the key TPB constructs and design TPB-based behavioral interventions, for example, selecting the specific theory components to attempt to influence a given behavior and population (Ajzen, 2013). TPB has been used extensively in health research and applied to various health-related behaviors (e.g., condom use, malaria prophylaxis, physical activity, and cancer screening).

TPB has been widely used in research, with over 4,200 papers listed in the Web of Science by April 2020 across a variety of disciplines (Bosnjak et al., 2020). McEachan and colleagues (2011) performed a random-effects meta-analysis of 206 prospective studies of health behaviors using TPB. Their analysis controlled for the effects of past behavior on future behavior and assessed how behavioral type (e.g., health-promoting vs. health risk), sample characteristics, and methodological factors (e.g., length of follow-up) moderated the ability of TPB to predict future behavior. The results of this analysis indicated that TPB explained 19% of the variance in behavior and 44% of the variance in intention across studies. Past behavior added 11% variance to the prediction of behavior and 5% to behavioral intention. In this analysis, TPB more successfully predicted behaviors related to diet and physical activity than risk detection, safer sex, and abstinence from drugs. Behaviors in the shorter term were better predicted than behaviors in the longer term, and self-report behavior measures were better predicted than objective measures. Notably, attitudes remained a strong predictor of intentions after controlling for past behavior, which, according to the authors, strengthens the case for trying to target attitudes as part of interventions.

The author of TPB has responded to recurrent criticisms of this model (Ajzen, 2011). For example, Ajzen notes that the model has been said to ignore the affective component of decision-making and to rely on a "rational-actor" approach to behavioral choices. He argues that both emotion and irrationality can be subsumed in the behavioral, normative, and control "beliefs" components of TPB, as these beliefs are not always formed rationally or accurately and are subject to influence by emotional state. Ajzen also describes attempts made by researchers to improve the predictive validity of the TPB by adding components. For instance, when predicting genetic testing behaviors, Wolff and colleagues (2011) added "anticipated affective outcomes" to the model's "behavioral beliefs" component; Kor and Mullan (2011) added "perceived autonomy support" to the prediction of sleep-hygiene behaviors. Ajzen cautions that for model parsimony, any new predictors proposed for addition to the model should meet strict criteria, for example, having a causal relationship with intention and action and conceptual independence from other components (Ajzen, 2011).

The debate over the utility of TPB continues. A more recent round of criticism and countercriticism was sparked by a commentary entitled "Time to Retire the Theory of Planned Behavior" (Sniehotta et al., 2014), in which the authors assert that TPB has well-documented limitations and that two aspects of the conceptual core of TPB, in particular, are not supported: the notion that the attitude–behavior association is mediated by intention, and the assertion that TPB constructs as a group fully mediate all external influences on behavior. They also assert that the model is better at explaining intention than actual behavior, which limits its utility in practice. Ajzen responds to these criticisms by reiterating the specific way that TPB should be used, including an extensive and specific formative research process (which Sniehotta and colleagues describe in a rebuttal as being so burdensome as to be impossible for most researchers) and argues that any other way of using the theory is not a fair test (Ajzen, 2015).

Questions about its overall value notwithstanding, Ajzen suggests several ways to refine TPB further. First, additional work might focus on how beliefs are activated according to mood and setting (Ajzen, 2011). Other potential areas of inquiry are past behavior and habit formation's role in determining behavioral intention and how stable "background factors"—for example, personality traits or demographic characteristics—might affect the relative importance of TPB components (Ajzen, 2011). Howland et al. (2016) report on an innovative extension of TPB to a dyadic level in assessing interpersonal influences on physical activity intentions and behaviors. In this study, a partner's PBC predicted a person's intentions to be physically active over and above their own PBC and other model predictors. The authors suggest that such a dyadic framework might extend to other individual theories. Several recent papers have examined further refinements to TPB, including examining the effect of group identification, affective and cognitive attitudes, and reexamining subjective norms (Canova & Manganelli, 2020; Willis et al., 2020).

TRANSTHEORETICAL MODEL

The TTM (Prochaska & Velicer, 1997), known more familiarly as the "stages of change" model, is one of the most prominent in health behavior research. TTM focuses on *behavior change,* unlike models like TPB that could be used equally to explain ongoing behaviors (Noar et al., 2008). Prochaska and colleagues developed TTM in the 1970s to identify the common elements of leading theories of psychotherapy and behavior change. In subsequent empirical work, the authors observed that smokers used different processes of change at different points in their attempts to quit, leading to the formulation of the "stage" aspect of TTM in which behavior change is viewed not as an event but as a six-stage process.

These stages, which represent a continuum and through which movement may take place backward as well as forward, are defined as the following (Prochaska & Velicer, 1997): *precontemplation,* where people are not considering a health behavior change in the near future (usually operationalized as 6 months); *contemplation,* where people are intending to change in the next 6 months and need to be motivated to do so; *preparation,* in which people intend to take action in the immediate future and need the skills to do so; *action,* where people are making a specific behavior change and can be supported by intervention strategies and guidelines; *maintenance,* where a new behavior becomes habitual and requires less ongoing effort, but where relapse prevention is still important; and the final stage, *termination,* which occurs when a behavior is permanently ingrained and may only be applicable to cessation behaviors.

Ten *processes of change,* or activities that people use to progress through the stages, are specified by TTM. Examples are counterconditioning (substituting healthy for less healthy behaviors), stimulus control (removing cues for unhealthy habits), and contingency management (e.g., a reward system). Other TTM constructs include *decisional balance* (an individual's perceived pros and cons of changing), *self-efficacy* (as per SCT), and *temptation* (the intensity of urges to engage in a specific behavior when in challenging situations). According to TTM, an intervention will be more effective if it is "stage-matched"—using the processes and principles of change appropriate for a given stage and health behavior. Thus, one way to test the validity of TTM is to do a "match–mismatch" experiment to assess whether stage matching enhances the intervention's effectiveness. At least one such study of a smoking cessation intervention found that participants in the "matched" condition made more significant forward movement in stages (Dijkstra et al., 2006). However, another found no advantage for the stage-matched condition (Aveyard et al., 2009). A meta-analysis of 33 matched and nonmatched interventions for physical activity found that they improved behavior, but that efficacy was not mediated by stage of change but by the other TTM constructs including self-efficacy and the processes of change (Romain et al., 2018).

Much of the early empirical work with TTM has been with smoking cessation—the health behavior that gave rise to the theory—but it has since been applied to a wide range of other health-related behaviors. For example, a 2008 meta-analysis examined 48 health behaviors studied using TTM principles in 120 data sets (Hall & Rossi, 2008). This meta-analysis found consistent support across behaviors for Prochaska's so-called "strong and weak principles of change," which state that for an individual to move from *precontemplation* to *action,* they need to experience approximately one standard deviation (*SD*) increase in their perceived "pros" of changing and about one-half *SD* decrease in the "cons" of changing.

Several reviews and meta-analyses have examined TTM-based interventions across various behaviors: smoking cessation (Cahill et al., 2010), physical activity (Kleis et al., 2021), medication adherence (Imeri et al., 2022), patients with chronic disease (Hashemzadeh et al., 2019), and diet and physical activity for weight loss (Tuah et al., 2011). Across reviews, authors noted the inconsistent and often incomplete application of the model and other methodological weaknesses, making it difficult to draw conclusive results about the value of TTM for behavior change interventions (Cahill et al., 2010). Based on a review of 35 trials, Cahill and colleagues (2010) concluded that stage-based, self-help interventions for smoking cessation are no more effective than non–stage-based equivalents. Tuah et al. (2011) found that TTM-based interventions for weight loss have a "limited" impact in the short term, with no strong evidence for sustained weight loss.

Despite—or perhaps because of—its popularity and the appealing prospect of stage-matched interventions having the potential to produce "unprecedented impacts on entire at-risk populations" (Prochaska & Velicer, 1997), TTM has inspired several critical articles describing what is viewed as the model's shortcomings. Indeed, one observer commented that TTM has not just fame but "notoriety" (Brug et al., 2005). Another note that the model seems better accepted among practitioners than researchers (Munro et al., 2007). Examples of articles critical of TTM are those of Sutton (2001) and West (2005). For example, some argue that there is only weak empirical evidence for the efficacy of stage-based interventions, the existence of discrete stages of behavior change, and the sequencing of readiness stages. Others have pointed to the arbitrary length of stages and the use of staging algorithms that lack validity, reliability, and consistency across studies; the difficulty of applying the model to complex behaviors like physical activity or dietary change; and a lack of evidence that moving people forward in stages ultimately results in behavior change or other health-related outcomes. Munro et al. (2007) also noted that stage-tailored interventions might be resource-intensive and inappropriate when rapid behavior change is desired.

It has also been noted that TTM tends to be selectively operationalized (Brug et al., 2005), resulting in an alternative explanation for nonsignificant findings. Ideas for improving how TTM is applied include increased precision of methods of staging individuals and expanding stage-transition strategies to include constructs from other theories/models (Brug et al., 2005). Better documentation of the fidelity of TTM application to interventions has also been suggested to deepen understanding of how—and whether—the model helps foster behavior change (Salmela et al., 2008). However, an informal review of the recent literature suggests that such documentation of fidelity of the application of theory in the intervention remains absent mainly from published reports of TTM-based interventions. It is important to note that this shortcoming is not unique to TTM but is shared across theories.

RELAPSE PREVENTION MODEL

RP is a cognitive behavioral model developed over three decades ago to help people change addictive behaviors and anticipate and cope with relapse (Hendershot et al., 2011; Marlatt & George, 1984). Rooted in SCT, the RP model (**Figure 4.3**) has been highly influential in practice, with the ability to self-regulate playing a vital role in an individual's vulnerability to relapse (Bandura, 1986). In fact, *relapse prevention* has become a generic term describing interventions that build coping skills for dealing with situations that place individuals at high risk of relapse (Marlatt, & George, 1984). Unlike the other theories and models discussed in this chapter, RP does not address initial behavior change, but instead deals with the ubiquitous challenge of maintaining the change over the long term. A significant contribution of this model is its elaboration of relapse not as a failure or end state but rather as a transitional process that may or may not lead to previous levels of the undesired behavior. Moreover, RP provides individuals with skills and strategies to prevent a single, temporary lapse from becoming a more protracted relapse (Marlatt & George, 1984).

The RP model recognizes two primary categories of factors that trigger or contribute to relapse: *immediate determinants* of relapse and *covert antecedents* (Hendershot et al., 2011). Among the *immediate determinants* are *high-risk situations*, which pose a threat to a person's sense of control over the behavior (including negative emotional states like depression, interpersonal conflict, social pressure, and external cues to engage in the behavior); *coping* (i.e.,

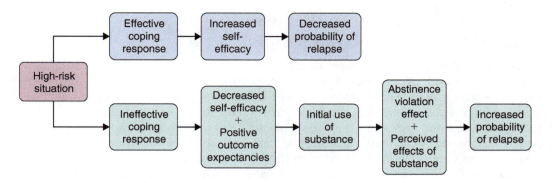

FIGURE 4.3 The relapse prevention model.
Source: From Marlatt, G. A., & Gordon, J. R. (Eds.). (1985). *Relapse prevention: Maintenance strategies in the treatment of addictive behaviors*. Guilford Press.

how the person responds to those situations; individuals who have mastered effective coping strategies are less likely to experience relapse, and success in coping also leads to greater self-efficacy to do so in the future); *outcome expectancies* for the behavior (most relevant are positive expectations; e.g., relapse is more likely if a person believes that the behavior will help with short-term stress reduction); and the *abstinence violation effect* (where a person who has an initial lapse feels guilt, a lack of control, and other negative emotions, which in turn make full-blown relapse more likely).

A second category of factors (Hendershot et al., 2011) consists of the broader and more subtle *covert antecedents* to relapse. These can be thought of as lifestyle factors that influence the extent to which a person is confronted with high-risk situations. A successful "lifestyle balance" of obligations and pleasurable activities is essential for managing overall stress levels that can foster high-risk situations for relapse. The RP model specifies cognitive and behavioral intervention strategies to deal with both immediate determinants of relapse, such as skills development and cognitive restructuring, and also encourages people to achieve a healthier, more balanced lifestyle to address relapse's covert antecedents. Notably, a reformulated "dynamic" version of the RP model now recognizes both "tonic" (stable personal characteristics) and "phasic" (situational or transient) influences on relapse, which interact in complex ways to determine the likelihood of relapse (see Hendershot et al., 2011, for a detailed discussion of this reformulated model).

Most empirical applications of the RP model have been to alcohol use and smoking (Hendershot et al., 2011), with an occasional application to a nonaddictive behavior such as physical activity (e.g., Stetson et al., 2005). The efficacy of the RP model has been examined in systematic reviews, meta-analyses, and randomized controlled trials (RCTs), as well as in studies of specific model components such as self-efficacy and negative affect (Hendershot et al., 2011). It has been noted that while the overall clinical effectiveness of the RP model has received some empirical support, "the diffuse application of RP approaches tends to complicate efforts to define RP-based treatments and evaluate their overall efficacy" (Hendershot et al., 2011, p. 2).

The RP model and its application to practice continue to evolve. For example, mindfulness-based RP refers to adding mindfulness techniques to the cognitive behavioral principles used in RP, with demonstrated promise in empirical studies (Witkiewitz et al., 2014). Other promising directions for this model (Hendershot et al., 2011) include using nonlinear statistical approaches to examine the complex interactions proposed by the reformulated model, exploring genetic influences on relapse and relapse prevention, teasing out the mechanisms of effects in efficacious RP-based interventions, and use of functional MRI to explore the neural correlates of relapse.

APPLYING HEALTH BEHAVIOR THEORIES TO TECHNOLOGY-ENABLED INTERVENTIONS

While individual theories have changed little over the years, they are being applied in new ways as intervention delivery methods keep pace with societal communication and information exchange changes. For example, the last decade has dramatically increased theory-informed interventions delivered via the internet (eHealth) or mobile devices (mHealth). mHealth includes short messaging services (SMS or text messages) and apps on internet-enabled smartphones, which may incorporate cameras, global positioning systems, and physiological sensors into intervention design (Bull & Ezeanochie, 2016). Social media interventions delivered via a variety of platforms are also rapidly increasing. A simple tabulation in 2015 and 2016 revealed that approximately one-quarter of the behavioral intervention studies published in *Health Education & Behavior* incorporated technology-enabled components. By 2019, a special section called *Apps, Social Media and Health* was published in the same journal. Digital interventions have the potential to provide health behavior change support to a larger and more diverse audience than could be reached in traditional ways, given their low marginal costs and the fact that mobile phone use is now widespread across socioeconomic and demographic groups, with approximately 82% of North Americans and 67% of adults globally having access to a smartphone as of 2021 (Bull & Ezeanochie, 2016; Laricchia, 2024). Evidence is accumulating regarding the efficacy of many digital health behavior change interventions across diverse populations and behaviors (Hou et al., 2014).

The degree to which classic health behavior theories have been integrated into technology-enabled health interventions is the subject of several articles and reviews. For example, Winter and colleagues reviewed 240 technology-enabled interventions for cardiovascular disease prevention and treatment published between 2010 and 2015. About half referenced a behavioral theory or model—most commonly SCT, TTM, or TPB (Winter et al., 2016). Riley et al. (2011) reviewed mHealth interventions in smoking, weight loss, adherence, and disease management. Most smoking and weight loss studies invoked theory; here, SCT was most frequently cited. A systematic review of 33 social media interventions in low- and middle-income countries found that only eight used a theoretical framework (Seiler et al., 2022).

In contrast, virtually no studies in this review targeting adherence or disease management cited a theoretical basis. Even simple reminder interventions for adherence could be more potent by addressing theory-informed mechanisms of behavior change (Riley et al., 2011). Bull and Ezeanochie (2016) found that only one-tenth of electronically delivered interventions tested in RCTs between 2005 and 2014 included a reference to theory in their design, implementation, or analysis descriptions. In a review of 38 internet-based interventions published between 2005 and 2015, Hou and colleagues (2014) found that most cited SCT or TTM. Conversely, a systematic review of social media interventions for vaccine hesitancy found that 60% were theory-based and most of these employed the HBM (Li et al., 2022).

CASE STUDY 4.2: THE NA MIKIMIKI PROJECT

The Na Mikimiki Project is an example of a technology-enabled, theoretically based physical activity intervention for ethnically diverse new mothers in a multiethnic population in Hawaii. The project focused on self-regulatory behavioral skills, self-efficacy, and social support. Based on extensive formative research, the intervention compared a phone and technology-based intervention with a traditional paper-based intervention (Albright et al., 2005, 2009). Mobile telephone counseling was provided with an average of 17 health educator lead calls, in addition to website and email-based resources, including stroller-friendly walking paths, newsletters, and skill building tips (Albright et al., 2012). Self-reported physical activity significantly increased in the technology-enabled group compared with the paper-based group (Albright et al., 2014).

Overall, the use of theory in technology-enabled interventions varies widely by intervention type and behavior of focus. Where theory is cited, it tends to be the same behavior change theories popular in nondigital interventions. SCT is widely used and has ready application to digital interventions' self-monitoring, individualized feedback, and goal-setting components. Reviews typically focus on research-tested interventions; the use of theory may be markedly less common in commercially available apps for behavior change, and researchers have called for increased collaboration between health behavior change experts and commercial app developers (Hingle et al., 2019). As with nonelectronic interventions, there is general agreement that behavior change theory is helpful for technology-enabled interventions, but there is also mixed empirical evidence. For example, in a review of text messaging interventions on a range of health topics, the authors found that those that were theory-based did not have significantly different outcomes than those that were not (Head et al., 2013).

Other researchers have identified limitations to applying individual theories to the new interventions currently being developed, especially mHealth interventions. For example, they differ from traditional programs because they can incorporate frequent interaction with participants, up to multiple times per day, in the same context that health behaviors occur, such as at home or during social events. Further, real-time inputs from participants—including self-reported symptoms, behavior, and information on the current context—can be used to individualize interventions (Riley et al., 2011). Indeed, the degree of tailoring and personalization of text messaging-based health promotion interventions is thought to be positively associated with intervention efficacy (Head et al., 2013).

Martín and colleagues wrote: "SCT and other related theories were developed primarily to explain differences between individuals, but explanatory theories of within-person behavioral variability are increasingly needed to support new technology-driven interventions that can adapt over time for each person" (Martín et al., 2014). Ideally, then, health behavior theories used in these interventions would be able to accommodate a high level of interactivity and adaptivity. However, traditional behavior change theories and models are generally linear and static (Riley et al., 2011). As an initial step to improving the fit of these theories to the more intensive, interactive interventions that are enabled by today's technology, Riley and colleagues developed a "dynamic computational model" of SCT based on a "control systems fluid analogy" derived from engineering principles, which enables precise predictions of an individual's behavior at a specific time based on specific changes in theory components (Riley et al., 2016).

There are many innovative strategies for melding technology with theory to develop effective and appealing interventions for behavior change. Examples include virtual reality (VR), alternate-world reality gaming, and virtual coaches (Winter et al., 2016). One potentially powerful complement to traditional behavior change theories that can be incorporated into VR and gaming applications are "story immersion"—an embedded narrative where participants feel part of the story (Georgieva & Georgiev, 2019). For example, a participant who takes on the part of a protagonist undergoing a behavior change in a vividly rendered world may be influenced by theoretical constructs like social norms and vicarious experiences woven into the story's narrative. Finally, health communication and dissemination theories might inform mHealth interventions to maximize user engagement and the cost-efficient scalability of technology-enabled interventions (Bull & Ezeanochie, 2016).

Although technological advances provide exciting opportunities for health behavior scientists and practitioners, Winter et al. (2016) offer two notes of caution. First, they point out that while technology development is rapid, funding cycles for research could be faster, potentially leaving investigators in a permanent state of catching up. Second, having more options for intervention delivery means more "whiches" to consider when applying behavioral theory: "Which behavioral techniques delivered through which technology channels should be used for which targeted behaviors and outcomes and for which population segments?" (p. 611).

COMPARING MULTIPLE THEORIES OF BEHAVIOR CHANGE

Although presented here as distinct, the behavioral theories discussed in this chapter share many common elements; for instance, beliefs, self-efficacy, and social influences are all found across theories, although they may go by different names. While the original developers of these theories focused on particular types of health behaviors (e.g., HBM for single-action preventive behaviors like screening; TTM for addictive behavior, smoking), in practice, all have been applied to a wide range of health-related behaviors. Noar and Zimmerman (2005) summarize the constructs common to HBM, TPB, SCT, and TTM, showing how a given concept is labeled and described within each theory. Network analysis by Gainforth et al. (2015) provides empirical support for most behavior change theories' close relationships and common origins. A comparison of similar constructs across the theories presented in this chapter is displayed in Table 4.1.

Differences in individual theories are also easy to spot: for example, TRA/TPB is concerned with behavioral intention as the outcome; other theories attempt to predict actual behavior. Some theories, like TTM, are stage-based and describe processes and predictors of stage movement en route to behavior change; others are continuous and describe how predictors work together to influence the likelihood of action (Head & Noar, 2014). Theories may be developed to predict, design behavior change strategies, or both (Head & Noar, 2014). However, the studies reviewed in this chapter suggest that this distinction is lost mainly in the "real world" of theory application. Theories also differ in the extent to which they prescribe how to operationalize and measure theoretical constructs. As noted by Young et al. (2014), there is a vast variation in how elements of SCT are operationalized. In comparison, the developers of TPB provide specific, modifiable items to measure theory constructs.

TABLE 4.1 Comparison of Similar Constructs Across Theories (With Smoking Cessation as an Example)

CONSTRUCT	HEALTH BELIEF MODEL	SOCIAL COGNITIVE THEORY	THEORY OF PLANNED BEHAVIOR	TRANSTHE-ORETICAL MODEL	RELAPSE PREVENTION MODEL
Attitudes toward a behavior	Benefits, barriers "If I quit smoking, I will be stressed out."	Outcome expectations, expectancies "If I smoke it will reduce my stress."	Attitudes "A cigarette calms me down when I am stressed."	Pros, cons "Smoking cigarettes relieves tension."	Positive outcome expectancies "If I don't smoke, I will feel better."
Ability to perform a behavior	Self-efficacy How confident are you that you will not smoke when you are out with friends?	Perceived behavioral control "I can choose whether I smoke or not when I'm out with friends."	Self-efficacy "How confident are you that you will not smoke when you are out with friends?"	Self-efficacy, temptation How tempted are you to smoke when you are out with friends?	Coping, self-efficacy "How confident are you that you will not smoke when you are out with friends?"

(continued)

TABLE 4.1 Comparison of Similar Constructs Across Theories (With Smoking Cessation as an Example) *(continued)*

CONSTRUCT	HEALTH BELIEF MODEL	SOCIAL COGNITIVE THEORY	THEORY OF PLANNED BEHAVIOR	TRANSTHE-ORETICAL MODEL	RELAPSE PREVENTION MODEL
Social norms	–	Social support *"I have someone I can talk to about quitting smoking."*	Normative beliefs and motivation to comply *"My best friend thinks I should smoke."* *"With regards to smoking, I want to do what my best friend thinks I should."*	–	–
Intentions	–	Self-control, self-regulation *"I am good at resisting temptation."*	Intentions *"I intend to stop smoking."*	Stage of change *"Are you planning to quit smoking in the next 6 months?"*	Rationalization, apparently irrelevant decisions *"It's just one cigarette."*

Many of the reviews cited in this chapter have noted the tendency for study authors to cite multiple theories as influences on intervention design. The overlap among popular individual theories can confuse practitioners and applied researchers trying to decide which option is best for a given application (Gainforth et al., 2015). Often, their choice will be based on what is familiar or commonly used in a given field. Some research has suggested that multiple-theory interventions may be less effective than their single-theory counterparts (Prestwich et al., 2014), although the reasons for this need to be clarified.

Noar and Zimmerman (2005) describe two broad directions the field could take to address theory overlap. The first is to focus on integrations of similar theories. Well-supported constructs from single theories are combined, tested across various behaviors, and refined as needed. According to Head and Noar (2014), the first significant attempt at such a unified theory was made in 1991 due to a workshop by developers of significant theories. The resulting integrated behavioral model, however, was seldom used subsequently. Over a decade later, this model was refined further by Fishbein and Ajzen, who recast it as the "Reasoned Action Approach" (RAA; Head & Noar, 2014). Only some empirical published studies have applied the RAA under that name, illustrating that the uptake of theoretical innovations into practice is slow and uncertain. Another example of an attempt to make a composite, or "best of," theory is Ryan's (2009) integrated theory of health behavior change, which blends concepts from multiple theories, selecting components based on the strength of empirical evidence for their efficacy. De Vries (2017) also proposes potential ways to examine and utilize integrated theoretical models using the I-change model as an example. The second broad direction is for researchers to emphasize head-to-head comparisons of theories, a point that we will return to in the following section. While such comparisons are still uncommon, several examples can be found in the literature (Montanaro & Bryan, 2014; Murphy et al., 2014).

FUTURE DIRECTIONS IN INDIVIDUAL THEORY DEVELOPMENT

Judging from the extensive application of individual-level theories to current health behavior research—especially the handful of popular theories described in this chapter—their value and utility would appear widely accepted. However, the link between theory use and intervention effectiveness appears weak, as suggested by a rigorous meta-analysis of nearly 200 physical activity and healthy eating interventions (Prestwich et al., 2014). Using a theory coding scheme to assess the use of theory to develop and evaluate interventions, these investigators found that very few reviewed studies used theory extensively. No meaningful associations were found between intervention effectiveness and type of theory use (e.g., linking behavior change techniques to a particular theoretical construct) or an "overall theory score" representing the extent of theory use. However, a meta-analysis of 204 experimental studies found that interventions designed to change attitudes, social norms, and self-efficacy led to medium effect size changes in intention and small to medium effect size changes in behavior (Sheeran et al., 2016). Other commentators have repeatedly called attention to shortcomings in health behavior theory development, particularly in the realm of theory testing and theory refinement.

Ideally, the field of health behavior theory would be dynamic, with ongoing development and modifications as new empirical evidence emerges (Munro et al., 2007; Noar & Head, 2014). Instead, some researchers refer to some popular theories as having a scientifically unhealthy "immortality" (Sniehotta et al., 2015); that is, they are never improved upon or retired. This stagnation may be due to a lack of rigorous testing and subsequent theory modification that would genuinely move the field forward (Head & Noar, 2014; Noar & Mehrotra, 2011; Weinstein, 2007). Although it is beyond the scope of this chapter to describe these critiques in detail, several issues will be highlighted here, and the reader is referred to more nuanced discussions in the cited works.

The first is how theories have traditionally been evaluated. The most common approach to theory testing is correlational, that is, the "which theory explains the most variance in a particular behavior" approach. However, whether data are cross-sectional or longitudinal, associations between cognitive variables and health behaviors are inflated because the relationships are likely bidirectional. Thus, any observed cognition/behavior association may be explained by the effect of the behavior on how one thinks about that behavior. This may be particularly true in the case of ongoing or habitual behaviors (Painter et al., 2008; Weinstein, 2007). For example, a person who has experienced the benefits of regular physical activity is likely to have a more favorable attitudes toward exercise. In other words, correlational approaches assess whether given theory-based constructs are associated with a particular health behavior when the actual question of interest is whether changes in theory-based constructs lead to changes in health behavior (Noar & Mehrotra, 2011; Sniehotta et al., 2015). Another criticism of the "correlational" approach is that it offers little precision or insight into the criteria required for empirical data to support a given theory; for example, what does it mean if some, but not all, hypothesized relationships among theoretical constructs are supported by the data in a given study (Hagger, 2015)?

Sniehotta and colleagues argue that the individual-level theory remains relevant despite these issues, as scholars from multiple disciplines seek innovative strategies to motivate behavior change to improve population health and quality of life. As part of this process, insightful, in-depth theories that help us understand how this can be accomplished will remain in demand. It is, therefore, incumbent on health behavior scientists to improve methods of theory development "in a way that mirrors recent improvements in methods for the development, reporting, and evaluation of interventions" (Sniehotta et al., 2015, p. 186).

Head and Noar (2014) note the tension between the generalizability of a theory and its accuracy and utility in a given domain. The former is often of interest to theory developers and the latter to those applying the theory (Head & Noar, 2014). They advocate for "living," behavior-specific versions of general theories that would incorporate knowledge gained from empirical work on that behavior and result in adding or removing theoretical constructs as indicated. A behavior-specific theory could inform the design of future interventions and be a more helpful version of a general theory (Noar & Head, 2014).

Noar and Mehrotra (2011) have proposed a "multimethodological theory-testing" framework to increase the rigor of theory testing and ultimately enhance the value of theory to practice. According to the authors, any single theory-testing approach has inherent limitations. For example, while theory-based interventions appear to support that theory if they are proven effective, in cases where the control condition consists of minimal intervention or none at all, the specific role of the theory in intervention efficacy remains to be determined. An alternative approach using sequential, complementary methodological tools have been suggested to test a theory. These tools include randomized lab experiments, randomized field experiments of theory-based interventions and mechanisms analysis, and meta-analysis of both lab and field experiments. Brewer and Gilkey (2012) propose "competitive hypothesis testing" as another means of increasing the value of theory testing. In this approach, researchers identify specific components of two theories that give rise to competing predictions about the relationships among particular variables; empirical data are then used to determine which theory better supports the hypotheses. Noar and Zimmerman (2005) suggest eight crucial research questions for direct comparisons of theories; for example, "Are certain theories or elements of theories better predictors of one-time behaviors as opposed to behaviors that must be maintained over time?"

A second, broader issue regarding individual-level theories of behavior change is that they typically downplay the importance of both the "biological underpinnings and consequences" of behavior and the social context in which it occurs (Institute of Medicine Committee on Health and Behavior: Research, Practice, and Policy, 2001). Most of the theories discussed in this chapter incorporate interpersonal influences on attitudes, beliefs, or other antecedents of behavior; such variables are likely to be influenced indirectly by one's environment (e.g., workplace restrictions on smoking may factor into one's "pros and cons" of smoking cessation as per the TTM; living in an high-crime area may impede self-efficacy for daily physical activity).

However, Glass and McAtee (2006) wrote that "much of public health continues to treat behaviors such as diet, smoking, violence, drug use, and sex work as if they were voluntary decisions, without regard to social constraints, inducements, or pressures" (p. 1652). A major limitation of individual theories is that they do not adequately account for the social determinants of health. The social determinants of health including poverty, housing, built environment, and education have been shown to be important underlying indicators of health behavior (Braveman & Gottlieb, 2014). Individual theories focus on rational action and do not account for limitation in a person's immediate environment. Food deserts and unwalkable communities can limit the ability of someone to change their behavior no matter how strong their intention is. With a limited food budget, providing inexpensive, calorically-dense food might be a more rational decision than eating more expensive fruits and vegetables. Individual theory-based interventions may be more effective when paired with the social-ecological approach focusing on social, organizational community, and policy issues, as well as individual motivations and skills.

Finally, applying individual theories to multiple health behavior change merits attention. Health behaviors tend to cluster and share common determinants at individual, interpersonal, and environmental levels (Klein et al., 2016). None of the individual-level theories in this chapter explicitly consider changing multiple health behaviors simultaneously (Noar et al., 2008). Noar et al. (2008) suggest three possible approaches to using theory as it relates to multiple behaviors, each with differing implications for theory-based interventions: (a) a *"behavior change principles" approach,* wherein common principles of health behavior change can be taught to individuals, who can apply them to multiple health behaviors; (b) a *global health/behavior category approach,* which suggests using broader categories such as weight control or management of a particular illness to organize and appeal to the motives for change regarding a variety of health behaviors; and (c) a *multiple behavioral approaches,* which involves intervening on multiple behaviors that may cluster together, like alcohol use and smoking. Empirical testing could reveal which of these theoretical approaches is optimal for given behaviors or circumstances. Klein et al. (2016) describe various approaches: "repurposing" evidence-based interventions from one related behavior to another—finally, a careful descriptive study of how multiple health behaviors cluster is also warranted.

THEORIES, FRAMEWORKS, AND MEASURES RELEVANT TO HEALTH BEHAVIORS

Other related questions that merit future exploration have to do with sequencing—that is, is it best to address multiple behaviors simultaneously or sequentially? Is there a logical hierarchy to changing behaviors (such as "gateway behaviors") and a maximum number of behaviors to target for change (Geller et al., 2017)? Finally, which individual-level theories can be applied most effectively to research and evaluate interventions focusing on multiple health behavior changes?

CONCLUSION

Individual health behavior change theories have influenced research and interventions for over five decades. Nevertheless, many questions about their optimal use and validity still need to be answered. With the increase in social-ecological approaches, it is essential for individual-based theories to address the larger social determinant of health in promoting health equity across populations. Taking theory testing and development in new directions—including, but not limited to, those mentioned in this chapter—may help ensure the relevance of individual-level theories in an era where a solid evidence base and multilevel, multidisciplinary, and multibehavior approaches are viewed as critical to addressing today's most prominent public health challenges.

SUMMARY KEY POINTS

- Despite an increased use of models such as the social-ecological model that include broader domains of influence, individual theories are still widely used.
- Many of the key concepts including beliefs, self-efficacy, and social influences are found across theories.
- eHealth and mHealth theory-based interventions are becoming more widespread.
- Health equity and the social determinants of health need to be considered across all theory-based interventions.
- Further testing and refinement should be conducted across all theories.

DISCUSSION QUESTIONS

1. Think of your participation in preventive screenings for your own health (yearly physicals, vaccines, blood tests, sexually transmitted infection [STI] testing, etc.). How do you decide which preventive screenings to have, if any? How do you decide what preventive care is important to you? What messages did you receive to have these beliefs?

2. Consider your perceived self-efficacy in terms of your own healthcare and, if applicable, the care of your family. Has your perceived self-efficacy always been the same, or has it increased or decreased at different times in your life? What factors influence how you feel about your self-efficacy?

3. How do you feel about the relationship between individual-level theories and social determinants of health? Can they be compatible with a worldview that is focused on equity? Why or why not?

4. Have you ever used eHealth or mHealth resources for your own health or the health of your family? Examples include remote monitoring apps; apps that track steps, nutrition, menstrual cycle, and activity; and apps that provide support for mental health, medication, or smoking cessation. If you have used one or more of these apps, how did you feel it influenced your behavior? Were there any downsides? If you have not used any of these apps, would you be willing to in the future? If so, what benefits would you expect? If not, what are your concerns?

5. What changes do you feel could be made to select (or all) individual-level theories of health to make them more current and user-friendly?

A robust set of instructor resources designed to supplement this text is located at http://connect.springerpub.com/content/book/978-0-8261-4265-8. Qualifying instructors may request access by emailing textbook@springerpub.com.

REFERENCES

Ajzen, I. (2011). The theory of planned behaviour: Reactions and reflections. *Psychology & Health*, 26(9), 1113–1127. https://doi.org/10.1080/08870446.2011.613995

Ajzen, I. (2013). *Theory of planned behavior*. https://people.umass.edu/aizen/pubs/REA.pdf

Ajzen, I. (2015). The theory of planned behaviour is alive and well, and not ready to retire: A commentary on Sniehotta, Presseau, and Araujo-Soares. *Health Psychology Review*, 9(2), 131–137. https://doi.org/10.1080/17437199.2014.883474

Ajzen, I., & Fishbein, M. (1980). *Understanding attitudes and predicting social behavior*. Prentice-Hall.

Albright, C. L., Maddock, J. E., & Nigg, C. R. (2005). Physical activity before pregnancy and following childbirth in a multiethnic sample of healthy women in Hawaii. *Women & Health*, 42(3), 95–110. https://doi.org/10.1300/j013v42n03_06

Albright, C. L., Maddock, J. E., & Nigg, C. R. (2009). Increasing physical activity in postpartum multiethnic women in Hawaii: Results from a pilot study. *BMC Womens Health*, 9, 4. https://doi.org/10.1186/1472-6874-9-4

Albright, C. L., Steffen, A. D., Novotny, R., Nigg, C. R., Wilkens, L. R., Saiki, K., Yamada, P., Hedemark, B., Maddock, J. E., Dunn, A. L., & Brown, W. J. (2012). Baseline results from Hawaii's Nā Mikimiki Project: A physical activity intervention tailored to multiethnic postpartum women. *Women & Health*, 52(3), 265–291. https://doi.org/10.1080/03630242.2012.662935

Albright, C. L., Steffen, A. D., Wilkens, L. R., White, K. K., Novotny, R., Nigg, C. R., Saiki, K., & Brown, W. J. (2014). Effectiveness of a 12-month randomized clinical trial to increase physical activity in multiethnic postpartum women: Results from Hawaii's Nā Mikimiki project. *Preventive Medicine*, 69, 214–223. https://doi.org/10.1016/j.ypmed.2014.09.019

Amevor, E., & Tarkang, E. (2022). Determinants of female condom use among female tertiary students in the Hohoe municipality of Ghana using the health belief model. *African Health Sciences*, 22(1), 1–10. https://doi.org/10.4314/ahs.v22i1.2

Aveyard, P., Massey, L., Parsons, A., Manaseki, S., & Griffin, C. (2009). The effect of transtheoretical model based interventions on smoking cessation. *Social Science & Medicine*, 68(3), 397–403. https://doi.org/10.1016/j.socscimed.2008.10.036

Bandura, A. (1986). *Social foundations of thought and action: A social cognitive thory*. Prentice-Hall.

Bandura, A. (2002). Social cognitive theory in cultural context. *Applied Psychology*, 51(2), 269–290. https://doi.org/10.1111/1464-0597.00092

Becker, M. H. (1974). The health belief model and sick role behavior. *Health Education Monographs*, 2, 409–419.

Becker, M. H., Drachman, R. H., & Kirscht, J. P. (1974). A field experiment to evaluate various outcomes of continuity of physician care. *American Journal of Public Health*, 64(11), 1062–1070. https://doi.org/10.2105/ajph.64.11.1062

Berg, C. J., Krishnan, N., Graham, A. L., & Abroms, L. C. (2021). A synthesis of the literature to inform vaping cessation interventions for young adults. *Addictive Behaviors*, 119, 106898. https://doi.org/10.1016/j.addbeh.2021.106898

Bosnjak, M., Ajzen, I., & Schmidt, P. (2020). The theory of planned behavior: Selected recent advances and applications. *Europe's Journal of Psychology*, 16(3), 352–356. https://doi.org/10.5964/ejop.v16i3.3107

Braveman, P., & Gottlieb, L. (2014). The social determinants of health: It's time to consider the causes of the causes. *Public Health Reports (Washington, D.C: 1974)*, 129 (Suppl. 2), 19–31. https://doi.org/10.1177/00333549141291S206

Brewer, N. T., & Gilkey, M. B. (2012). Comparing theories of health behavior using data from longitudinal studies: A comment on Gerend and Shepherd. *Annals of Behavioral Medicine*, 44(2), 147–148. https://doi.org/10.1007/s12160-012-9396-z

Brug, J., Conner, M., Harre, N., Kremers, S., McKellar, S., & Whitelaw, S. (2005). The transtheoretical model and stages of change: A critique: Observations by five commentators on the paper by Adams, J. and White, M. (2004) why don't stage-based activity promotion interventions work? *Health Education Research*, 20(2), 244–258. https://doi.org/10.1093/her/cyh005

Bull, S., & Ezeanochie, N. (2016). From foucault to freire through Facebook: Toward an integrated theory of mHealth. *Health Education & Behaviour*, 43(4), 399–411. https://doi.org/10.1177/1090198115605310

Cahill, K., Lancaster, T., & Green, N. (2010). Stage-based interventions for smoking cessation. *Cochrane Database of Systematic Reviews*, (11), CD004492. https://doi.org/10.1002/14651858.CD004492.pub4

Canova, L., & Manganelli, A. M. (2020). Energy-saving behaviours in workplaces: Application of an extended model of the theory of planned behaviour. *Europe's Journal of Psychology, 16*(3), 384–400. https://doi.org/10.5964/ejop.v16i3.1893

Cliffe, B., Tingley, J., Greenhalgh, I., & Stallard, P. (2021). mHealth interventions for self-harm: Scoping Review. *Journal of Medical Internet Research, 23*(4), e25140. https://doi.org/10.2196/25140

de Vries, H. (2017). An integrated approach for understanding health behavior: The I-change model as an example. *Psychology and Behavioral Science International Journal, 2*(2), Article 555585. https://doi.org/10.19080/pbsij.2.2

Dijkstra, A., Conijn, B., & De Vries, H. (2006). A match-mismatch test of a stage model of behaviour change in tobacco smoking. *Addiction (Abingdon, England), 101*(7), 1035–1043. https://doi.org/10.1111/j.1360-0443.2006.01419.x

Finney Rutten, L. J., Zhu, X., Leppin, A. L., Ridgeway, J. L., Swift, M. D., Griffin, J. M., St Sauver, J. L.,Virk, A., & Jacobson, R. M. (2021). Evidence-based strategies for clinical organizations to adress COVID-19 vaccine hesitancy. *Mayo Clinic Proceedings, 96*(3), 699–707. https://doi.org/10.1016/j.mayocp.2020.12.024

Gainforth, H. L., West, R., & Michie, S. (2015). Assessing connections between behavior change theories using network analysis. *Annals of Behavioral Medicine, 49*(5), 754–761. https://doi.org/10.1007/s12160-015-9710-7

Geller, K., Lippke, S., & Nigg, C. R. (2017). Future directions of multiple behavior change research. *Journal of Behavioral Medicine, 40*(1), 194–202. https://doi.org/10.1007/s10865-016-9809-8

Georgieva, I., & Georgiev, G. V. (2019). Reconstructing personal stories in virtual reality as a mechanism to recover the self. *International Journal of Environmental Research and Public Health, 17*(1), 26. https://doi.org/10.3390/ijerph17010026

Ghoreishi, M. S., Vahedian-Shahroodi, M., Jafari, A., & Tehranid, H. (2019). Self-care behaviors in patients with type 2 diabetes: Education intervention based on social cognitive theory. *Diabetes & Metabolic Syndrome, 13*(3), 2049–2056. https://doi.org/10.1016/j.dsx.2019.04.045

Glass, T. A., & McAtee, M. J. (2006). Behavioral science at the crossroads in public health: Extending horizons, envisioning the future. *Social Science & Medicine, 62*(7), 1650–1671. https://doi.org/10.1016/j.socscimed.2005.08.044

Hagger, M. S. (2015). Retired or not, the theory of planned behaviour will always be with us. *Health Psychology Review, 9*(2), 125–130. https://doi.org/10.1080/17437199.2015.1034470

Hall, K. L., & Rossi, J. S. (2008). Meta-analytic examination of the strong and weak principles across 48 health behaviors. *Preventive Medicine, 46*(3), 266–274. https://doi.org/10.1016/j.ypmed.2007.11.006

Hashemzadeh, M., Rahimi, A., Zare-Farashbandi, F., Alavi-Naeini, A. M., & Daei, A. (2019). Transtheoretical model of health behavioral change: A systematic review. *Iranian Journal of Nursing and Midwifery Research, 24*(2), 83–90. https://doi.org/10.4103/ijnmr.IJNMR_94_17

Head, K. J., & Noar, S. M. (2014). Facilitating progress in health behaviour theory development and modification: The reasoned action approach as a case study. *Health Psychology Review, 8*(1), 34–52. https://doi.org/10.1080/17437199.2013.778165

Head, K. J., Noar, S. M., Iannarino, N. T., & Grant Harrington, N. (2013). Efficacy of text messaging-based interventions for health promotion: A meta-analysis. *Social Science & Medicine, 97*, 41–48. https://doi.org/10.1016/j.socscimed.2013.08.003

Heid, C., Knobloch, M. J., Schulz, L. T., & Safdar, N. (2016). Use of the health belief model to study patient perceptions of antimicrobial stewardship in the acute care setting. *Infection Control & Hospital Epidemiology, 37*(5), 576–582. https://doi.org/10.1017/ice.2015.342

Hendershot, C. S., Witkiewitz, K., George, W. H., & Marlatt, G. A. (2011). Relapse prevention for addictive behaviors. *Substance Abuse Treatment, Prevention, and Policy, 6*(1), 17. https://doi.org/10.1186/1747-597X-6-17

Hingle, M., Patrick, H., Sacher, P. M., & Sweet, C. C. (2019). The intersection of behavioral science and digital health: The case for academic–industry partnerships. *Health Education & Behavior, 46*(1), 5–9. https://doi.org/10.1177/1090198118788600

Hou, S. I., Charlery, S. A., & Roberson, K. (2014). Systematic literature review of Internet interventions across health behaviors. *Health Psychology and Behavioral Medicine, 2*(1), 455–481. https://doi.org/10.1080/21642850.2014.895368

Howland, M., Farrell, A. K., Simpson, J. A., Rothman, A. J., Burns, R. J., Fillo, J., & Wlaschin, J. (2016). Relational effects on physical activity: A dyadic approach to the theory of planned behavior. *Health Psychology*. https://doi.org/10.1037/hea0000334

Imeri, H., Toth, J., Arnold, A., & Barnard, M. (2022). Use of the transtheoretical model in medication adherence: A systematic review. *Research in Social & Administrative Pharmacy: RSAP, 18*(5), 2778–2785. https://doi.org/10.1016/j.sapharm.2021.07.008

Institute of Medicine Committee on Health and Behavior: Research, Practice, and Policy. (2001). *Health and Behavior: The Interplay of Biological, Behavioral, and Social Influences*. National Academic Press.

Jones, C. J., Smith, H., & Llewellyn, C. (2014). Evaluating the effectiveness of health belief model interventions in improving adherence: A systematic review. *Health Psychology Review, 8*(3), 253–269. https://doi.org/10.1080/17437199.2013.802623

King, A. C. (2015). Theory's role in shaping behavioral health research for population health. *International Journal of Behavioral Nutrition and Physical Activity, 12,* 146. https://doi.org/10.1186/s12966-015-0307-0

Klein, W. M. P., Grenen, E. G., O'Connell, M., Blanch-Hartigan, D., Chou, W.-Y. S., Hall, K. L., Taber, J. M., & Vogel, A. L. (2016). Integrating knowledge across domains to advance the science of health behavior: Overcoming challenges and facilitating success. *Translational Behavioral Medicine, 7*(1), 98–105. https://doi.org/10.1007/s13142-016-0433-5

Kleis, R. R., Hoch, M. C., Hogg-Graham, R., & Hoch, J. M. (2021). The effectiveness of the transtheoretical model to improve physical activity in healthy adults: A systematic review. *Journal of Physical Activity & Health, 18*(1), 94–108. https://doi.org/10.1123/jpah.2020-0334

Kor, K., & Mullan, B. A. (2011). Sleep hygiene behaviours: An application of the theory of planned behaviour and the investigation of perceived autonomy support, past behaviour and response inhibition. *Psychology & Health, 26*(9), 1208–1224. https://doi.org/10.1080/08870446.2010.551210

Kowalski, K., Jeznach, A., & Tuokko, H. A. (2014). Stages of driving behavior change within the transtheoretical Model (TM). *Journal of Safety Research, 50,* 17–25. https://doi.org/10.1016/j.jsr.2014.01.002

Laricchia, F. (2024). Global smartphone penetration rate as share of the population from 2016 to 2023. Statista. https://www.statista.com/statistics/203734/global-smartphone-penetration-per-capita-since-2005/

Lee, S. H., Moore, L. V., Park, S., Harris, D. M., & Blanck, H. M. (2022). Adults meeting fruit and vegetable intake recommendations—United States, 2019. *MMWR. Morbidity and Mortality Weekly Report, 71*(1), 1–9. https://doi.org/10.15585/mmwr.mm7101a1

Li, L., Wood, C. E., & Kostkova, P. (2022). Vaccine hesitancy and behavior change theory-based social-media interventions: A systematic review. *Translational Behavioral Medicine, 12*(2), 243–272. https://doi.org/10.1093/tbm/ibab148

Lombardo, L., Ferguson, C., George, A., Villarosa, A. R., Villarosa, B. J., Kong, A. C., Wynne, R., & Salamonson, Y. (2022). Interventions to promote oral care regimen adherence in the critical care setting: A systematic review. *Australian Critical Care, 35*(5), 583–594. https://doi.org/10.1016/j.aucc.2021.08.010

Lyons, E. J., Lewis, Z. H., Mayrsohn, B. G., & Rowland, J. L. (2014). Behavior change techniques implemented in electronic lifestyle activity monitors: A systematic content analysis. *Journal of Medical Internet Research, 16*(8), e192. https://doi.org/10.2196/jmir.3469

Maddock, J. E., Suess, C., Bratman, G. N., Smock, C., Kellstedt, D., Gustat, J., Perry, C. K., & Kaczynski, A. T. (2022). Development and validation of self-efficacy and intention measures for spending time in nature. *BMC Psychology, 10*(1), 51. https://doi.org/10.1186/s40359-022-00764-1

Maiman, L. A., & Becker, M. H. (1974). The health belief model: Origins and correlates in psychological theory. *Health Education Monographs, 2,* 336–353. https://doi.org/10.1177/109019817400200404

Marks, R., Allegrante, J. P., & Lorig, K. (2005). A review and synthesis of research evidence for self-efficacy-enhancing interventions for reducing chronic disability: Implications for health education practice (Part II). *Health Promotion Practice, 6*(2), 148–156. https://doi.org/10.1177/1524839904266792

Marlatt, G. A., & George, W. H. (1984). Relapse prevention: Introduction and overview of the model. *British Journal of Addiction, 79*(3), 261–273. https://doi.org/10.1111/j.1360-0443.1984.tb00274.x

Martín, C. A., Rivera, D. E., Riley, W. T., Hekler, E. B., Buman, M. P., Adams, M. A., & King, A. C. (2014, 4–6 June). A dynamical systems model of Social Cognitive Theory. Paper presented at the 2014 American Control Conference. Portland, OR.

McEachan, R. R. C., Conner, M., Taylor, N. J., & Lawton, R. J. (2011). Prospective prediction of health-related behaviours with the theory of planned behaviour: A meta-analysis. *Health Psychology Review, 5*(2), 97–144. https://doi.org/10.1080/17437199.2010.521684

Montanaro, E. A., & Bryan, A. D. (2014). Comparing theory-based condom interventions: Health belief model versus theory of planned behavior. *Health Psychology, 33*(10), 1251–1260. https://doi.org/10.1037/a0033969

Munro, S., Lewin, S., Swart, T., & Volmink, J. (2007). A review of health behaviour theories: How useful are these for developing interventions to promote long-term medication adherence for TB and HIV/AIDS? *BMC Public Health, 7,* 104. https://doi.org/10.1186/1471-2458-7-104

Murimi, M. W., Kanyi, M., Mupfudze, T., Amin, M. R., Mbogori, T., & Aldubayan, K. (2017). Factors influencing efficacy of nutrition education interventions: A systematic review. *Journal of Nutrition Education and Behavior, 49*(2), 142–165.e1. https://doi.org/10.1016/j.jneb.2016.09.003

80 I • THEORIES, FRAMEWORKS, AND MEASURES RELEVANT TO HEALTH BEHAVIORS

Murphy, C. C., Vernon, S. W., Diamond, P. M., & Tiro, J. A. (2014). Competitive testing of health behavior theories: How do benefits, barriers, subjective norm, and intention influence mammography behavior? *Annals of Behavioral Medicine, 47*(1), 120–129. https://doi.org/10.1007/s12160-013-9528-0

Noar, S. M., Chabot, M., & Zimmerman, R. S. (2008). Applying health behavior theory to multiple behavior change: Considerations and approaches. *Preventive Medicine, 46*(3), 275–280. https://doi.org/10.1016/j.ypmed.2007.08.001

Noar, S. M., & Head, K. J. (2014). Mind the gap: Bringing our theories in line with the empirical data—A response to commentaries. *Health Psychololy Review, 8*(1), 65–69. https://doi.org/10.1080/17437199.2013.855593

Noar, S. M., & Mehrotra, P. (2011). Toward a new methodological paradigm for testing theories of health behavior and health behavior change. *Patient Education and Counseling, 82*(3), 468–474. https://doi.org/10.1016/j.pec.2010.11.016

Noar, S. M., & Zimmerman, R. S. (2005). Health behavior theory and cumulative knowledge regarding health behaviors: Are we moving in the right direction? *Health Education Research, 20*(3), 275–290. https://doi.org/10.1093/her/cyg113

Painter, J. E., Borba, C. P., Hynes, M., Mays, D., & Glanz, K. (2008). The use of theory in health behavior research from 2000 to 2005: A systematic review. *Annals of Behavioral Medicine: A Publication of the Society of Behavioral Medicine, 35*(3), 358–362. https://doi.org/10.1007/s12160-008-9042-y

Piercy, K. L., Troiano, R. P., Ballard, R. M., Carlson, S. A., Fulton, J. E., Galuska, D. A., George, S. M., & Olson, R. D. (2018). The physical activity guidelines for Americans. *JAMA, 320*(19), 2020–2028. https://doi.org/10.1001/jama.2018.14854

Prestwich, A., Sniehotta, F. F., Whittington, C., Dombrowski, S. U., Rogers, L., & Michie, S. (2014). Does theory influence the effectiveness of health behavior interventions? Meta-analysis. *Health Psychology, 33*(5), 465–474. https://doi.org/10.1037/a0032853

Prochaska, J. O., & Velicer, W. F. (1997). The transtheoretical model of health behavior change. *American Journal of Health Promotion, 12*(1), 38–48. https://doi.org/10.4278/0890-1171-12.1.38

Riley, W. T., Martin, C. A., Rivera, D. E., Hekler, E. B., Adams, M. A., Buman, M. P., Pavel, M., & King, A. C. (2016). Development of a dynamic computational model of social cognitive theory. *Translational Behavioral Medicine, 6*(4), 483–495. https://doi.org/10.1007/s13142-015-0356-6

Riley, W. T., Rivera, D. E., Atienza, A. A., Nilsen, W., Allison, S. M., & Mermelstein, R. (2011). Health behavior models in the age of mobile interventions: Are our theories up to the task? *Translational Behavioral Medicine, 1*(1), 53–71. https://doi.org/10.1007/s13142-011-0021-7

Ritchie, D., Van den Broucke, S., & Van Hal, G. (2021). The health belief model and theory of planned behavior applied to mammography screening: A systematic review and meta-analysis. *Public Health Nursing (Boston, Mass.), 38*(3), 482–492. https://doi.org/10.1111/phn.12842

Romain, A. J., Bortolon, C., Gourlan, M., Carayol, M., Decker, E., Lareyre, O., Ninot, G., Boiché, J., & Bernard, P. (2018). Matched or nonmatched interventions based on the transtheoretical model to promote physical activity. A meta-analysis of randomized controlled trials. *Journal of Sport and Health Science, 7*(1), 50–57. https://doi.org/10.1016/j.jshs.2016.10.007

Rosenstock, I. M. (1974). Historical origins of the health belief model. *Health Education Monographs, 2*(4), 328–335.

Ryan, P. (2009). Integrated theory of health behavior change: Background and intervention development. *Clinical Nurse Specialist, 23*(3), 161–170. https://doi.org/10.1097/NUR.0b013e3181a42373

Salmela, S., Poskiparta, M., Kasila, K., Vähäsarja, K., & Vanhala, M. (2008). Transtheoretical model-based dietary interventions in primary care: A review of the evidence in diabetes. *Health Education Research, 24*(2), 237. https://doi.org/10.1093/her/cyn015

Seiler, J., Libby, T. E., Jackson, E., Lingappa, J. R., & Evans, W. D. (2022). Social media-based interventions for health behavior change in low- and middle-income countries: Systematic review. *Journal of Medical Internet Research, 24*(4):e31889. https://doi.org/10.2196/31889

Sheeran, P., Maki, A., Montanaro, E., Avishai-Yitshak, A., Bryan, A., Klein, W. M., Miles, E., & Rothman, A. J. (2016). The impact of changing attitudes, norms, and self-efficacy on health-related intentions and behavior: A meta-analysis. *Health Psychology, 35*(11), 1178–1188. https://doi.org/10.1037/hea0000387

Sniehotta, F. F., Presseau, J., & Araujo-Soares, V. (2014). Time to retire the theory of planned behaviour. *Health Psychology Review, 8*(1), 1–7. https://doi.org/10.1080/17437199.2013.869710

Sniehotta, F. F., Presseau, J., & Araujo-Soares, V. (2015). On the development, evaluation and evolution of health behaviour theory. *Health Psychology Review, 9*(2), 176–189. https://doi.org/10.1080/17437199.2015.1022902

Stacey, F. G., James, E. L., Chapman, K., Courneya, K. S., & Lubans, D. R. (2015). A systematic review and meta-analysis of social cognitive theory-based physical activity and/or nutrition behavior change interventions for cancer survivors. *Journal of Cancer Survivorship: Research and Practice, 9*(2), 305–338. https://doi.org/10.1007/s11764-014-0413-z

Stetson, B. A., Beacham, A. O., Frommelt, S. J., Boutelle, K. N., Cole, J. D., Ziegler, C. H., & Looney, S. W. (2005). Exercise slips in high-risk situations and activity patterns in long-term exercisers: An application of the relapse prevention model. *Annals of Behavioral Medicine, 30*(1), 25–35. https://doi.org/10.1207/s15324796abm3001_4

Suess, C., Maddock, J., Dogru, T., Mody, M., & Lee, S. (2022). Using the health belief model to examine travelers' willingness to vaccinate and support for vaccination requirements prior to travel. *Tourism Management, 88*, 104405. https://doi.org/10.1016/j.tourman.2021.104405

Sutton, S. (2001). Back to the drawing board? A review of applications of the transtheoretical model to substance use. *Addiction, 96*(1), 175–186. https://doi.org/10.1046/j.1360-0443.2001.96117513.x

Tade, O., & Nwanosike, P. C. (2016). 'Nobody is sure of tomorrow'—Using the health belief model to explain safety behaviours among Boko Haram victims in Kano, Nigeria. *International Review of Victimology, 22*(3), 339–355. https://doi.org/10.1177/0269758016634184

Tuah, N. A., Amiel, C., Qureshi, S., Car, J., Kaur, B., & Majeed, A. (2011). Transtheoretical model for dietary and physical exercise modification in weight loss management for overweight and obese adults. *Cochrane Database of Systematic Reviews,* (10), CD008066. https://doi.org/10.1002/14651858.CD008066.pub2

Weinstein, N. D. (2007). Misleading tests of health behavior theories. *Annals of Behavioral Medicine: A Publication of the Society of Behavioral Medicine, 33*(1), 1–10. https://doi.org/10.1207/s15324796abm3301_1

West, R. (2005). Time for a change: Putting the transtheoretical (stages of change) model to rest. *Addiction (Abingdon, England), 100*(8), 1036–1039. https://doi.org/10.1111/j.1360-0443.2005.01139.x

Williams, O., DeSorbo, A., Sawyer, V., Apakama, D., Shaffer, M., Gerin, W., & Noble, J. (2016). Hip hop heals: Pilot study of a culturally targeted calorie label intervention to improve food purchases of children. *Health Education & Behavior, 43*(1), 68–75. https://doi.org/10.1177/1090198115596733

Willis, L., Lee, E., Reynolds, K. J., & Klik, K. A. (2020). The theory of planned behavior and the social identity approach: A new look at group processes and social norms in the context of student binge drinking. *Europe's Journal of Psychology, 16*(3), 357–383. https://doi.org/10.5964/ejop.v16i3.1900

Winter, S. J., Sheats, J. L., & King, A. C. (2016). The use of behavior change techniques and theory in technologies for cardiovascular disease prevention and treatment in adults: A comprehensive review. *Progress in Cardiovascular Diseases, 58*(6), 605–612. https://doi.org/10.1016/j.pcad.2016.02.005

Witkiewitz, K., Warner, K., Sully, B., Barricks, A., Stauffer, C., Thompson, B. L., & Luoma, J. B. (2014). Randomized trial comparing mindfulness-based relapse prevention with relapse prevention for women offenders at a residential addiction treatment center. *Substance Use & Misuse, 49*(5), 536–546. https://doi.org/10.3109/10826084.2013.856922

Wolff, K., Nordin, K., Brun, W., Berglund, G., & Kvale, G. (2011). Affective and cognitive attitudes, uncertainty avoidance and intention to obtain genetic testing: An extension of the theory of planned behaviour. *Psychology & Health, 26*(9), 1143–1155. https://doi.org/10.1080/08870441003763253

Yang, S., He, C., Zhang, X., Sun, K., Wu, S., Sun, X., & Li, Y. (2016). Determinants of antihypertensive adherence among patients in Beijing: Application of the health belief model. *Patient Educucation and Counseling, 99*(11), 1894–1900. https://doi.org/10.1016/j.pec.2016.06.014

Young, M. D., Plotnikoff, R. C., Collins, C. E., Callister, R., & Morgan, P. J. (2014). Social cognitive theory and physical activity: A systematic review and meta-analysis. *Obesity Reviews, 15*(12), 983–995. https://doi.org/10.1111/obr.12225

Zewdie, A., Mose, A., Sahle, T., Bedewi, J., Gashu, M., Kebede, N., & Yimer, A. (2022). The health belief model's ability to predict COVID-19 preventive behavior: A systematic review. *SAGE Open Medicine, 10*, 20503121221113668. https://doi.org/10.1177/20503121221113668

CHAPTER 5

DEVELOPMENTAL AND CULTURAL INFLUENCES ON BEHAVIOR AND HEALTH

CRYSTAL S. LIM AND E. THOMASEO BURTON

LEARNING OBJECTIVES

- Recognize theories of development related to health and strategies of health behavior change.
- Understand the importance of racial, ethnic, and gender identity development.
- Describe social determinants of health (SDOH) and provide examples.
- Identify examples of developmentally and culturally tailored health behavior change strategies.

INTRODUCTION

Health outcomes are often contingent on health behavior changes. For example, diagnosis of type 2 diabetes may indicate a need for dietary and exercise changes. Change may also entail a new regimen, such as monitoring blood sugar or taking medication. Supporting and encouraging health behavior change is a complex process. There is increasing recognition that a variety of factors play a role in supporting and implementing health behavior change strategies. Two such factors, developmental influences and cultural influences, will be the focus of this chapter. Although developmental and cultural influences will be discussed separately, it is important to recognize how the intersectionality, or interactions, between developmental and cultural factors can also impact engagement in a variety of health behaviors and effective change strategies.

CASE STUDY 5.1: PSYCHOLOGICAL DEVELOPMENT IN EMERGING ADULTHOOD

Madeline is a 20-year-old non-Hispanic White female. She is currently a sophomore in college and is attending a private university. Madeline is presenting for an outpatient psychological evaluation due to attention-related concerns. Madeline reports she first noticed attention issues impacting her functioning when she started college about 1.5 years ago. Her academic functioning has also been impacted. She was an A student in high school, but in college she has been earning Bs and Cs. She indicates that she has had a hard time adjusting to the style of teaching used in college compared with what she was used to in high school. Specifically, she described her high school courses being hands-on and experiential, while her college courses are primarily lecture-based. In college, Madeline has noticed she has trouble remaining seated for long periods of time during classes, gets

(continued)

CASE STUDY 5.1: PSYCHOLOGICAL DEVELOPMENT IN EMERGING ADULTHOOD (*continued*)

distracted easily (such as by her cell phone), and procrastinates on tasks she does not like or feels may require much mental effort. Madeline also reports issues with socializing, such as problems engaging in social relationships, interrupting others in conversation, and talking excessively.

Madeline also indicates symptoms of anxiety that first appeared when she started college. Madeline reports anxiety related to meeting new people and when taking tests. She also reports significant issues related to her sleep as she often stays up until the early morning hours engaging in various social media apps on her cell phone and playing video games. This results in her waking up late and missing many of her classes, having trouble paying attention, or feeling tired throughout the day.

At the start of college, Madeline began drinking alcohol, primarily in social settings. She reports drinking one to two times a week and having about six alcoholic drinks each time. She and her referring primary care provider are wondering if she may have attention deficit hyperactivity disorder (ADHD).

DEVELOPMENTAL INFLUENCES ON BEHAVIOR AND HEALTH

Broadly speaking, development represents functioning in a variety of domains, often thought to be associated with someone's age. Many dimensions of development are thought to impact behavior, health, and functioning, such as physical, biological, cognitive, social, emotional, psychological, gender identity, sexual identity, relational, and career/occupational domains. Development in many dimensions is thought to occur in successive and organized ways, such as gross motor skills in young children beginning as sitting up and then progressing to crawling, standing up, and then walking. In fact, many stage theories of development have been formulated, from Sigmund Freud's psychosexual stages to Erikson's psychosocial stages. Most widely recognized and empirically supported developmental theories explain one or more domains of development in a sequential order and provide expectations regarding timelines for normal or abnormal courses of functioning, often referred to as developmental milestones (Sheldrick et al., 2019). For young children, individual developmental milestones are considered indicators of developmental status that help identify children who may need early intervention services due to developmental delays (Sheldrick et al., 2019). Table 5.1 highlights the domains of typical development in early childhood, middle childhood, adolescents, emerging adulthood, and older adulthood. Developmental transitions, such as moving from adolescence to adulthood, are critical periods in a person's life when there are numerous changes in multiple domains of functioning, which may impact physical and mental health and engagement in specific health behaviors (Barkham et al., 2019). For example, adolescence has been recognized as a period of increased risk of medication nonadherence in youth with chronic medical conditions (Shih & Cohen, 2020).

Bioecological Theory

Urie Bronfenbrenner is considered the father of the ecological theory of development, which proposes there are interactions between a person and intersecting aspects of their environment. This theory was later expanded by Bronfenbrenner and others to the bioecological theory, where there are reciprocal interactions occurring between the person and the external environment that influence development (Education, 2019). Thus, interactions with the environment are important at specific times of development. Figure 5.1 demonstrates the bioecological model of human development. For example, language development occurs in a stepwise fashion, such as speaking one word, two words, and then multiple word sentences, but if an infant is not exposed to speech and language during this critical period of language development, their speech and language will be delayed.

TABLE 5.1 Developmental Considerations

	EARLY CHILDHOOD (0–5 YEARS)	MIDDLE CHILDHOOD (6–12 YEARS)	ADOLESCENCE (12–18 YEARS)	EMERGING ADULTHOOD (18–25 YEARS)	OLDER ADULTHOOD (65+ YEARS)
Physical					
Motor skills	Gradual development of gross (e.g., walking) and fine (e.g., pinching) motor skills	Improvements in motor coordination and control	Fully developed		Decline in muscle and bone strength decline; decreased flexibility
Sensory	Touch, hearing, taste, and smell fully developed	Vision fully developed			Declines in all five sensory systems
Sleep	Less sleep needed with age (e.g., time in REM sleep decreases)	About 10 hours of sleep needed	About 8–10 hours of sleep needed; sleep deprivation common	Continue to need about 8–10 hours of sleep	Need less sleep, but sleep difficulties more common
Cognitive					
Brain development	Dramatic development, especially rapid growth in frontal lobe; gradual development and increases in language skills	Continued growth throughout areas of the brain	Continued frontal lobe development	New growth and continued development in frontal lobe	Loss of brain weight and neurons
Thought processes	Development of mental representations; egocentric views	Thoughts become more logical, flexible, and organized	Systematic and logical thinking; increase in abstract ideas	Ability to question and evaluate information; greater internalization of morality	Memory recall difficulties
Socioemotional					
Peer relationships	Obtains ability to play and share with friends; frequently changing friends	Friends usually same gender; personal qualities and trust with peers become more important	Peers are major focus; increase in unsupervised peer activities	Romantic relationships become more physically and emotionally intimate	Number of friends decreases; peers are similar to self

	EARLY CHILDHOOD (0–5 YEARS)	MIDDLE CHILDHOOD (6–12 YEARS)	ADOLESCENCE (12–18 YEARS)	EMERGING ADULTHOOD (18–25 YEARS)	OLDER ADULTHOOD (65+ YEARS)
Socioemotional					
Self-esteem	Gradual increases in self-consciousness and self-awareness	Views of self determined by appearance, possessions, and activities	Changes in body image and increase in body dissatisfaction	Identity exploration	Multifaceted self-concept; response to sense of mortality important
Gender	Gender-specific stereotypes become more rigid	Understand differences between boys and girls; increased gender flexibility, but also increased identity to gendered traits	Continued development of gender identity	Integration of biological, psychological, and social aspects of gender; gender identity becomes stable	
Examples of Behavioral Interventions Based on Developmental Stage					
Targeted health behavior	Immunizations	Weight management	Reducing risk of HIV/STI	Vaping cessation	Improving memory
Developmentally tailored health behavior change intervention examples	Social norms approach intervention to address parental antivaccine conspiracy beliefs (e.g., parents given feedback about their own antivaccine beliefs, their estimation of other parents' antivaccine beliefs, and actual data about other parents' antivaccine beliefs; Cookson et al., 2021)	Family-focused individual and group intervention delivered via telehealth based on cognitive behavioral theory and child weight theory focusing on behavioral, nutrition, and physical activity (Davis et al., 2019)	Mother–daughter HIV/STI prevention program addressing individual, social, and structural factors of HIV/STI risk in South Africa (Donenberg et al., 2021)	Text messaging intervention providing social support and cognitive and behavioral coping skills training (Graham et al., 2021)	Assistive technology training interventions (reminder apps, voice recorder; Scullin et al., 2022)

STI, sexually transmitted infections.

86 I • THEORIES, FRAMEWORKS, AND MEASURES RELEVANT TO HEALTH BEHAVIORS

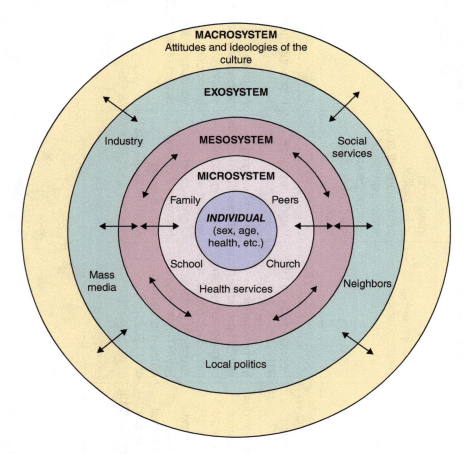

FIGURE 5.1 Bioecological model of human development.
Source: From Prout, T. A., Wadkins, M. J., & Kufferath-Lin, T. (2022). *Essential interviewing and counseling skills: An integrated approach to practice.* Springer Publishing Company.

Roles of Interactive Media Use in Development

Around the world, the use of technology, digital media, and social media is becoming more pervasive than ever before. In fact, the term *digital natives* was coined to describe children who were born and raised in a digital- and media-saturated world (Prensky, 2001). The ubiquitous presence of television, video games, personal computers and laptops, smartphones, tablets, and other mobile devices has had a profound effect on familial interactions, educational practices, and social development (Beyens et al., 2022; Ihmeideh & Alkhawaldeh, 2017). Moreover, the constant availability of social media content is linked to a number of behavioral and health outcomes, such as depression, anxiety, disordered eating, impaired sleep quality, and less engagement in physical activity (Keles et al., 2020; Shannon et al., 2022).

Considering that media use habits form early in life (Paudel et al., 2017), there is growing attention to how problematic interactions with media can influence development. Important considerations include how much time youth spend with media, the type of content consumed, and the degree to which media disrupts health-related activities such as social interaction, sleep, and physical activity (The U.S. Surgeon General's Advisory, 2023). Several professional organizations, including the World Health Organization (WHO) and the American Psychological Association (APA), have issued guidelines on restriction, regulation, and oversight of media use for children and adolescents (Association, 2023; WHO, 2019).

Despite the numerous developmental consequences linked to media use, there are certainly benefits of interactive technology. Social media can provide community, connection, and enhanced access for youth who may be otherwise isolated or marginalized (Charmaraman et al., 2022). For example, mobile health (mHealth) applications hold strong promise for facilitating efficient and equitable delivery and uptake of health behavior change information (Marcolino et al., 2018; WHO, 2011).

Identity Development

Identity development is a critical task of adolescence and emerging adulthood in which individuals grapple with the question "Who am I?" This process of defining oneself is complex and multifaceted (Erikson, 1968). Aspects of identity, which are influenced by familial, societal, and cultural factors, are coexisting, intersecting, and interactive, and can be more or less salient depending on context (Branje, 2022). This section focuses on two fundamental aspects of identity influenced by sociocultural context, racial identity and gender identity. The focus on race/ethnicity and gender does not imply that all individuals define themselves by these domains, nor does it suggest that individuals cannot or do not perceive themselves in a variety of other ways or that these types of identity development are occurring independently of each other.

RACIAL AND ETHNIC IDENTITY DEVELOPMENT

Race is a social construct that has no basis in science or genetics. Rather, the notion of race was established to divide people into superior and inferior groups based on arbitrary characteristics such as skin color. Nevertheless, the concept of race has been used to uphold systems of power, privilege, and oppression. Initial theories of racial identity development emerged during the civil rights movement to investigate how Black individuals understood their Black identities in the context of these aforementioned systems and have now expanded to examine how individuals from multiple racial/ethnic backgrounds (e.g., White, Asian, Hispanic) define themselves internally and are perceived externally in terms of social, political, and cultural factors (Moffitt & Rogers, 2022).

Developmental models of racial identity are important tools in understanding how racism-related stressors influence mental and physical health outcomes (Neblett et al., 2012). Scholars in the fields of sociology and psychology have attempted to identify patterns or stages that every individual goes through when recognizing their racial/ethnic identity. In reality, however, the process is different for each individual. While an exhaustive overview of the numerous models of racial/ethnic identity is beyond the scope of this chapter, **Figure 5.2** illustrates how racial/ethnic identity development is influenced by personal family, community, political, and social factors, and how at different stages an individual may be more vulnerable to deleterious health effects of racism.

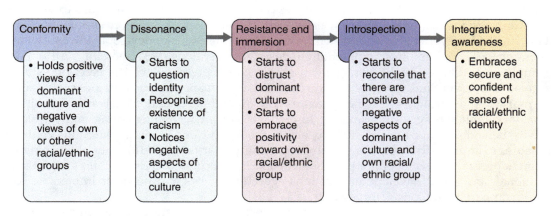

FIGURE 5.2 Model of racial/ethnic identity development.
Source: Adapted from Sue, D. W., & Sue, D. (1999). *Counseling the culturally different: Theory and practice.* John Wiley & Sons Inc.

GENDER IDENTITY DEVELOPMENT

Recently, there has been increased focus on gender identity development and how it influences health and engagement in health behaviors. *Gender identity* has been defined as a person's sense of themselves as male, female, both, or neither (Hines, 2020). Concepts specific to gender identity development can be traced to early theories of child development, with tenets tied to Lawrence Kohlberg's Theory of Gender Role Development first proposed in the 1960s. Kohlberg's theory primarily focused on stages of gender role development, where children first develop knowledge of gender stereotypes (e.g., girls wear dresses and have long hair, boys wear pants and have short hair), then begin to recognize their own gender identity and can label their gender (I am a girl, I am a boy), and gender constancy, the stage where children learn their gender will not change over time or if they engage in nongender-conforming activities (Hines, 2020). More recent theorists and researchers have called into question this theory given its cisgender-focused perspective (i.e., gender identity is consistent with biological sex) and the current expanding sociocultural conceptualizations of fluid gender identities and acceptance of transgender and nonconforming gender identities (Martinez, 2020). In addition, there is increased recognition that gender identity development involves numerous influences, primarily biological systems (hormones, timing of hormone exposure, etc.), socialization, and cognitive conceptualization, which all interact with each other over time (Hines, 2020). Mousavi and colleagues (2019) conducted qualitative interviews with girls and their parents to describe the role of socialization in gender identity development in the Middle East. They found that gender socialization occurred in the context of family (e.g., relationship with parents), relationships with both same-sex peers and the opposite sex, and society (i.e., sociocultural context). These methods of socialization impacted sexual self-expression, which then led to the achievement of a stabilized gender identity (Mousavi et al., 2019). Although this study occurred in the Middle East, it highlights the important interaction between culture through socialization and gender identify development, which is applicable to cultures throughout the world. Gender identity is widely recognized as influencing health-related attitudes and behaviors, which contribute to health and disease processes (Nielsen et al., 2021).

Examples of Developmentally Focused Health Behavior Change Strategies

There are numerous examples of health behavior change strategies and interventions that take into account developmental factors. In young children, parents or caregivers are often targeted in prevention and treatment strategies due to the role they play in regard to seeking out healthcare for their children, as well as their influence on the home environment (Lim et al., 2018). However, it is also important to consider dimensions of development, as well as parenting skills and abilities, in parenting-focused interventions (Bejarano et al., 2019). For example, in pediatric weight management programs for preschoolers, the parenting skills targeted in interventions typically include child behavior management strategies such as using praise and ignoring for specific behaviors (i.e., differential attention), rewarding healthy behaviors, limit setting, using time-out to manage tantrums, shaping eating and physical activity behaviors, exposures to introduce new foods, and implementing stimulus control measures to improve food choices and physical activity (Stark et al., 2018). Thus, weight management programs developed for preschoolers take into account the young child's cognitive, emotional, and social development, such as egocentric views and need for immediate rewards compared with long-term rewards.

However, in pediatric weight management interventions targeting adolescents and their caregivers, parent–child communication, behavioral contracts, and problem-solving are targeted skills caregivers and youth learn to implement together (Biggs et al., 2023). These programs are designed to target increases in systematic and logical thinking, which are characteristic of adolescence. Parental involvement is typically limited in interventions targeting adolescents to facilitate increased independence and self-efficacy regarding health behavior change strategies.

The recent global COVID-19 pandemic is an example of when developmental factors, represented by age, played a role in engagement in health prevention strategies. During the early months of the pandemic in the United States, age was found to be an important factor related to engagement in virus mitigation behaviors, such as wearing a mask (Hutchins et al., 2020). Specifically, adults 60 years or older reported engaging in more COVID-19 mitigation behaviors, including mask use, compared with adults 18 to 29 years of age (Hutchins et al., 2020). This disparity may have been associated with older adults being at increased risk of death from the virus compared with younger adults, but this difference in mitigation behaviors also led to increased incidence of confirmed cases in the young adult age group during this period of time. Young adults in the United States were also more hesitant to get COVID-19-specific vaccines compared with older U.S. adults (Szilagyi, Shah et al., 2021). Perceptions of disease risk and developmental differences in the perceptions of recommended prevention strategies are important to consider when introducing health prevention strategies and behaviors from a public health perspective.

CASE STUDY 5.2: PSYCHOLOGICAL DEVELOPMENT AND ADHD

Returning to Madeline, her case highlights the importance of developmental transitions in the context of physical and mental health, as well as health behavior change strategies. During the evaluation for ADHD, she indicated symptoms related to inattention were present in her childhood, but given the structure of her elementary, middle, and high school educational settings (i.e., experientially focused) and support from her parents and teachers, she was able to compensate in a variety of ways, such as by sitting in the front of her classes and by making lists to help her remember to complete tasks. However, after transitioning to a less structured setting that used different teaching strategies and with academic topics of increased difficulty in the college setting, it became difficult for her to compensate for her symptoms of inattention. Madeline's poor academic performance when starting college also contributed to her increased symptoms of anxiety. These symptoms of anxiety led to her drinking alcohol as a way to self-medicate and to help her feel more comfortable in social settings. Her use of her cell phone before bedtime made it more difficult to sleep and also increased her anxiety symptoms. Effectively treating her ADHD symptoms (via medications, evidence-based therapy) would substantially improve both her academic and psychological functioning, both of which could lead to reduced alcohol consumption.

The following recommendations were provided to Madeline to address her symptoms and improve her functioning: discuss if medication would be appropriate to treat symptoms of ADHD with her primary care medical provider; contact the Office of Disability Services at her university to determine academic accommodations that may be available; begin receiving counseling services through her university's student counseling center (general support groups and evidence-based psychological treatments focused on anxiety symptoms may especially be helpful); limit use of cell phone, especially social media and games, before bedtime; utilize other sleep hygiene techniques; and reduce engagement in binge drinking to help improve cognitive functioning and increase overall health.

CULTURAL INFLUENCES ON HEALTH AND BEHAVIOR

While there is a growing acknowledgment of the role of culture in human health and behavior, there is no singular definition of culture (Alesina & Giuliano, 2015). **Table 5.2** presents some key definitions. Despite the varied interpretations of culture, there is certainly considerable overlap among these definitions. It is clear that culture influences beliefs, behaviors, and response patterns. However, the concepts of health and behavior are cultural in and of themselves, as culture frames and shapes diverse perceptions of experiences. For example, interpretation of physical or mental symptoms, beliefs about what constitutes a disease, and attitudes about acceptable treatments and interventions are all influenced by culture (Brottman et al., 2020; Shahin et al., 2019). Taken together, cultural health beliefs influence how individuals and groups conceptualize health and how they define health problems. Furthermore, culture influences public health researchers and policy makers who develop health change interventions, as well as healthcare practitioners who implement these interventions. The concept of culture appears in many terms related to health and behavior change (**Table 5.3**).

TABLE 5.2 Key Definitions of Culture

DEFINITION	SOURCE
A way of life of a relatively large group of people; the generally accepted behaviors, beliefs, norms, values, attitudes, meanings, and concepts that influence individual and group	Hofstede (1997)
What is learned, shared, transmitted intergenerationally, and reflected in a group's values, beliefs, norms, behaviors, communication, and social roles	Rosal et al. (2014)
The sum total of integrated learned behavior patterns that are characteristic of the members of a society rather than the result of biological inheritance	Hoebel and Frost (1976)
A shared meaning and information system that allows a group to meet basic survival needs	Matsumoto (2007)

TABLE 5.3 Cultural Terms Related to Health and Behavior Change

TERM	DEFINITION	EXAMPLE
Cultural acceptability	Extent to which a treatment or intervention is relevant and engaging to members of a cultural group	A food insecurity intervention that serves a population of Muslim Americans does not include pork or pork products in its meal deliveries.
Cultural humility	Appreciation of the complexity of cultural differences and awareness that one will never be fully competent about the ever-changing nature of others' experiences; cultural humility is a lifelong commitment to self-evaluation, self-critique, and learning from others	Medical students volunteering at a health clinic in Haiti attend weekly seminars to examine their own biases and engage in ongoing learning about the roles of history, politics, and culture on the health of their patients.

(continued)

TABLE 5.3 Cultural Terms Related to Health and Behavior Change (*continued*)		
TERM	DEFINITION	EXAMPLE
Cultural responsiveness	Approach to health that is respectful of and relevant to the beliefs, practices, values, and linguistic needs of individuals and groups from diverse backgrounds and experiences	A community health center provides visit summaries and patient instructions in patients' preferred language.
Cultural sensitivity	Knowledge, awareness, and appreciation of norms, practices, and beliefs associated with other cultures and others' cultural identities	A research assistant conducting focus groups on dental hygiene practices always asks participants how they would like to be addressed before beginning the interview.

Health Equity

The pursuit of health equity, in which all people have a fair and just opportunity to attain their highest level of health, is contingent on appreciation of the role of culture (CDC, 2022c). More specifically, equitable health outcomes for all requires a culturally humble approach that acknowledges diverse beliefs, practices, and experiences. The health equity framework highlights the importance of systems-level change to acknowledge current and past injustices, address social and economic barriers to health and healthcare, and eliminate health disparities.

Health disparities refer to avoidable and unjust inequities in the quality of health, access to healthcare, and health outcomes experienced by groups based on sociodemographic characteristics like race/ethnicity, socioeconomic status, or environmental characteristics (Braveman, 2006). Many factors contribute to health disparities, including environmental conditions that affect where people are born, live, learn, work, and play. These factors, collectively known as the social determinants of health (SDOH), have a major impact on individuals' health, well-being, and quality of life (Gómez et al., 2021). The five broad domains of SDOH are illustrated in **Figure 5.3**. As can be seen in the scenarios presented, SDOH are often by-products of historical and contemporary racist and discriminatory policies.

Global Health Issues

As the world population surpasses eight billion, we must prioritize improving health and achieving health equity for all people, with an emphasis on populations made vulnerable due to systematic socioeconomic disadvantage. The most populous countries on Earth, China and India, are home to well over one billion people each. The tremendous cultural diversity within and between these countries highlights the vast differences in people's environments, resources, and social statuses. Nevertheless, health threats such as infectious diseases, pollution, and climate change affect everyone, regardless of economic factors. Similarly, political events such as war influence the collective experience of a population, although some are more susceptible to ill effects than others.

Scholars have noted that addressing health at a global level requires much more than financial resources (Garrett, 2007; Mantena et al., 2020). The billions of philanthropic dollars that are funneled into global health spending too often fail to consider contextual, developmental, and cultural factors that make unique health systems unique. Global health issues require comprehensive solutions that address cultural, political, social, infrastructural, educational, and technological factors (Koplan et al., 2009). Of course, such an expansive approach does require considerable investment of resources. In addition to striving for just and equitable health outcomes worldwide, the financial returns on investing in global health are

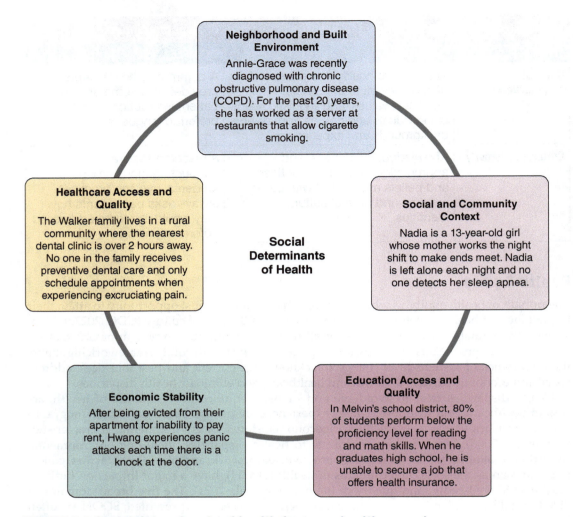

FIGURE 5.3 Social determinants of health framework with examples.
Source: Adapted from Healthy People 2030, U.S. Department of Health and Human Services, Office of Disease Prevention and Health Promotion. (n.d.). Social determinants of health. *Healthy People 2030*. U.S. Department of Health and Human Services. https://health.gov/healthypeople/objectives-and-data/social-determinants-health

impressive—reductions in morbidity and mortality are associated with economic growth in low- and middle-income countries (Jamison et al., 2013).

The 1946 Constitution of the WHO defined *health* as "a state of complete physical, mental, and social well-being." This suggests that addressing global health must transcend traditional medical clinics and requires efforts and perspectives beyond healthcare practitioners.

CASE STUDY 5.3: CULTURAL HUMILITY

Fatima is a graduate student studying public health in the United States. Fatima identifies as nonbinary and uses they/them pronouns. They are enrolled in a study abroad program and will spend a semester supporting the implementation of a mental and sexual health intervention for pregnant women in Liberia (Callands et al., 2023). In preparation for their trip, Fatima learns that between 1989 and 2003, Liberia endured a civil war that resulted in more than 150,000 deaths, as well as innumerable human rights violations such as torture and sexual violence (Vinck & Pham, 2013). These traumatic exposures

(continued)

CASE STUDY 5.3: CULTURAL HUMILITY (*continued*)

continue to affect physical, mental, and sexual health of many Liberians. Fatima discovers that Liberia's healthcare infrastructure is still recovering from the war, and the COVID-19 pandemic further stressed the already vulnerable healthcare system.

Fatima majored in psychology during college and is familiar with some evidence-based mental health treatments that were introduced in a psychopathology course. They are eager to apply their knowledge and even took an online course in trauma-focused cognitive behavioral therapy in the weeks leading up to their departure for Liberia. Fatima is relieved to know that English is the official language of Liberia but is shocked upon landing at the airport outside of Monrovia to hear a dialect of Liberian English that is not familiar.

Over the first several days, Fatima is oriented to their new surroundings. They learn more about the history of Liberia, including the conflict between Indigenous Africans and formerly enslaved African Americans and Afro-Caribbeans. Fatima also learns that during the civil war, girls and women frequently endured emotional, physical, and sexual abuse, including forced marriage, pregnancy, and childbirth. During a lecture on intersectionality (**Box 5.1**), Fatima begins to appreciate how the lingering trauma of these events has had a profound impact on perceptions and practices regarding reproductive health.

Fatima is surprised to find that they will not be providing direct care to pregnant women. Rather, intervention is delivered by Liberian nurses and social workers who are familiar with local customs, beliefs, and vernacular. Interventionists are fluent in Liberian English and represent the two largest ethnic groups in Liberia, Kpelle and Bassa. Fatima still has plenty to do by observing focus groups intended to continually improve cultural acceptability of the intervention curriculum and participating in conversations between intervention staff and community stakeholders about issues of confidentiality, privacy, and respect.

Fatima wakes up before sunrise each day because the intervention sessions are held early in the morning before participants leave for work in the fields. Each time the team moves on to a new village, they meet with the village chief to request permission to conduct the intervention (Johnson et al., 2008). Requesting permission is consistent with local custom, as is offering the chief a small token of appreciation for their cooperation and assistance. As the semester abroad ends, Fatima reflects on the assumptions they held before stepping foot in Liberia. On the flight back to the United States, Fatima sets a professional intention to be more self-aware of their biases and strive to take a culturally humble approach to the practice of public health.

BOX 5.1 INTERSECTIONALITY

Intersectionality is a theoretical framework that promotes understanding of how multiple social identities (e.g., race/ethnicity, gender, age, socioeconomic status, sexuality, geography, Indigenous status, religion) interact and overlap with individuals' experiences to influence inequitable health outcomes (Kapilashrami & Hankivsky, 2018). Intersectionality operates within systems of privilege and oppression (i.e., sexism, racism, classism).

In other words, intersectionality highlights how individuals' health status and access to health resources are affected by multiple and complex sources of oppression that cannot be unraveled or considered separately.

Global Mental Health

As highlighted in the preceding case study, health needs, perceptions, and outcomes are influenced by development and culture. The intervention Fatima traveled to Liberia to work on was developed in response to a specific set of developmental, cultural, and historical factors for a group with specific intersecting sets of identity. This case study also highlights the importance of focusing health behavior change efforts on not only physical health, but mental health as well. According to the Global Burden of Disease Study, widely considered to the be most comprehensive worldwide assessment of morbidity and mortality, mental health disorders account for more than 10% of the global burden of disease (Vos et al., 2020). This means 1 out of every 100 individuals in the world are affected by some mental, neurological, or substance use disorder. Considering that mental health conditions tend to affect familial and social networks, as well as ability to engage in employment and education, the real impact is likely much higher.

The significant physical, social, and economic burden of mental illness is further compounded by the lack of mental health workers worldwide; the WHO estimates fewer than 10 per 100,000 population (Hanna et al., 2018). Access is even further skewed in low- and middle-income countries. The already strained mental health system experienced another blow with the onset of the COVID-19 pandemic, which exacerbated many determinants of poor mental health (Santomauro et al., 2021).

COVID-19 Pandemic

The COVID-19 global pandemic is an example of a recent global health event where cultural influences were an important part of engagement in health behaviors. For example, in the United States, there were over 103 million documented cases of COVID-19 and over 1 million deaths attributed to the virus from March 2020 to March 2023 (coronavirus.jhu. edu/region/united-states, accessed 04.01.23). Early in the pandemic, most countries across the world implemented lockdown policies, resulting in business closures and/or operating limits, which resulted in employment layoffs, reductions in wages, and overall economic instability of the global economy (Gissandaner et al., 2023). Access to healthcare was also impacted as outpatient medical appointments were cancelled early in the pandemic and in some cases were eventually transitioned to telehealth appointments if those resources were available to medical providers and patients (Thomas et al., 2022). In addition, ED usage decreased for non-COVID-19-related health concerns, potentially due to fear of exposure to the virus (Wong et al., 2020). However, these behaviors may have led to increased healthcare risk for some conditions (e.g., cancer, stroke). Social isolation and delayed healthcare have led to increased symptoms of mental health concerns and more severe health complications (Vahratian et al., 2021).

The role of culture is relevant to mitigation strategies, screening, and treatment of COVID-19. Culturally accepted ways of greeting, such as shaking hands, kissing, and hugging, are thought to contribute to the spread of viruses, including COVID-19, which resulted in many countries encouraging changing customary cultural practices (e.g., elbow or fist bump replacing shaking hands) for primary prevention of virus transmission (Bruns et al., 2020). Access to various religious practices and rituals, including funeral and mourning rituals, were also modified, changed, or cancelled due to lockdown and isolation precautions (Bruns et al., 2020). The acceptance of other transmission mitigation strategies, such as mask use and vaccine administration, was also impacted by cultural beliefs and practices.

One cultural dimension important to consider is collectivism versus individualism, or the view of the self as interdependent compared with the view of the self as independent

(Lu et al., 2021). Research in all 50 U.S. states and in countries throughout the world revealed that mask usage during the COVID-19 pandemic was significantly higher in more collectivist cultures compared with individualistic cultures (Lu et al., 2021). Many collectivist countries throughout the world were able to initially contain the spread of COVID-19 during early parts of the pandemic, which exemplified members of collectivist cultures coming together to combat the virus (Lu et al., 2021). Cultural factors are important to consider in regard to preparing to respond and combat future worldwide pandemics.

The development of vaccines to specifically target COVID-19 began soon after the virus began spreading across the globe. Vaccines first became available for U.S. adults in December 2020, were expanded for children >12 years in May 2021, and further expanded to children >5 years in November 2021 (CDC, 2022b; FDA, 2022). Despite vaccine availability, a sizable proportion of the U.S. population remained unvaccinated at the end of the pandemic. The estimated initial vaccine acceptance rate in the United States was about 56% (Sallam, 2021), which was one of the lowest rates among highly developed nations. More recent data from April 2023 indicated that over 81% of the total U.S. population have received at least one dose of a COVID-19 vaccine (coronavirus.jhu.edu/region/united-states, accessed 04.04.23; CDC, 2022a; Diesel et al., 2021). Initially, parents' acceptance of COVID-19 vaccines for their children ranged from 72% to 89% in other countries, whereas only 46% of U.S. parents indicated being likely to vaccinate their children for COVID-19 (Sallam, 2021; Szilagyi, Shah et al., 2021). During the COVID-19 pandemic, the amount of information available from national, public health, healthcare, political, news, and other social media outlets led to widespread confusion about public health recommendations and led to misinformation and mistrust about effective medical treatments, such as medications to treat symptoms and vaccines to minimize transmission and reduce morbidity and mortality (French et al., 2020). The cultural context of politicization may have led to vaccine hesitancy in some countries and has been detailed specific to the U.S. context (Bolsen & Palm, 2022). In fact, political affiliation and trust are additional factors associated with the likelihood that U.S. adults would receive the COVID-19 vaccine. Specifically, those who identified as Republican were significantly more likely to say they were not getting the COVID-19 vaccine compared with those identifying as Democrat (Khubchandani et al., 2021). Political beliefs are thought to develop during adolescence and early adulthood when there are less political discussions with parents and increased consumption of political information (Niemi & Klingler, 2012). This period of development results in an increase in political efficacy, but also increases in distrust of the government (Niemi & Klinger, 2012). Lack of trust regarding the process used to develop vaccines and lack of trust in government approval of vaccines were found to be strongly associated with decreased likelihood of getting a COVID-19 vaccine, and trust accounted for most of the demographic differences found (e.g., age, race, education; Szilagyi, Thomas et al., 2021). Therefore, the sociopolitical environment during the COVID-19 pandemic, as well as the stage of political development, may have interacted to influence perceptions regarding risk of the virus, sources of information sought out, and safety and effectiveness of mitigation, prevention, and treatment strategies.

CONCLUSION

Health behavior change is a complex and highly individualistic process. As our world becomes more and more diverse, experiences of health, as well as developmental and cultural practices, will become more diverse as well. Despite individual and group differences, the pursuit of health equity is a commonality for all humans. Further appreciation of intersectionality of culture and development by healthcare practitioners, researcher, and policy makers is critical in achieving health equity.

> **SUMMARY KEY POINTS**
> - Developmental and cultural factors influence physical and mental health, as well as the effectiveness of health behavior change strategies.
> - Developmental milestones and developmental transitions are key times when multiple aspects of functioning and health may be impacted.
> - The intersection, or interaction, between development and cultural factors is important to consider.
> - Health behavior change strategies should be developed and implemented with development and cultural factors applicable to the specific population in mind.

> **DISCUSSION QUESTIONS**
> 1. In what ways do you feel developmental and cultural influences impacted you and/or your community's response to the COVID-19 pandemic? How can this inform responses to future pandemics?
> 2. What aspects of identity development do you believe are most relevant to your health and health-related behaviors?
> 3. Can you think of an example of how you might develop a culturally competent intervention for increasing physical activity?
> 4. How might a researcher employ cultural humility when working with an unfamiliar population?
> 5. Review the definitions of culture in Table 5.2. Which definition aligns with your personal definition of culture? How would you define culture for yourself and your community?

A robust set of instructor resources designed to supplement this text is located at http://connect.springerpub.com/content/book/978-0-8261-4265-8. Qualifying instructors may request access by emailing textbook@springerpub.com.

REFERENCES

Alesina, A., & Giuliano, P. (2015). Culture and institutions. *Journal of Economic Literature, 53*(4), 898–944.

Association, A. P. (2023). *Health advisory on social media use in adolescence*. https://www.apa.org/topics/social-media-internet/health-advisory-adolescent-social-media-use.pdf

Barkham, M., Broglia, E., Dufour, G., Fudge, M., Knowles, L., Percy, A., Turner, A., & Williams, C. (2019). Towards an evidence-base for student wellbeing and mental health: Definitions, developmental transitions and data sets. *Counseling Psychotherapy Research, 19*, 351–357.

Bejarano, C. M., Marker, A. M., & Cushing, C. C. (2019). Cognitive-behavioral therapy for pediatric obesity. In R. D. Friedberg & J. K. Paternostro (Eds.), *Handbook of cognitive behavioral therapy for pediatric medical conditions* (pp. 369–383). Springer Nature.

Beyens, I., Keijsers, L., & Coyne, S. M. (2022). Social media, parenting, and well-being. *Current Opinion in Psychology, 47*, 101350.

Biggs, B. K., Rodgers, K. V., Nayman, S. J., Hofschulte, D. R., Loncar, H., Kumar, S., Lynch, B. A., Rajjo, T. I., & Wilson, D. K. (2023). Translation of a family-based behavioral intervention for adolescent obesity using the RE-AIM framework and common steps from adaptation frameworks. *Translational Behavioral Medicine, 13*, 700–709. https://doi.org/10.1093/tbm/ibad022

Bolsen, T., & Palm, R. (2022). Politicization and COVID-19 vaccine resistance in the US. *Molecular Biology and Clinical Medicine in the Age of Politicization, 188*, 81–100. https://doi.org/10.1016/bs.pmbts.2021.10.002

Branje, S. (2022). Adolescent identity development in context. *Current Opinion in Psychology, 45*, 101286.

Braveman, P. (2006). Health disparities and health equity: concepts and measurement. *Annual Review of Public Health, 27*, 167–194.

Brottman, M. R., Char, D. M., Hattori, R. A., Heeb, R., & Taff, S. D. (2020). Toward cultural competency in health care: A scoping review of the diversity and inclusion education literature. *Academic Medicine, 95*(5), 803–813.

Bruns, D. P., Kraguljac, N. V., & Bruns, T. R. (2020). COVID-19: Facts, cultural considerations, and risk of stigmatization. *Journal of Transcultural Nursing, 31*(4), 326–332. https://doi.org/10.1177/1043659620917724

Callands, T. A., Hylick, K., Desrosiers, A., Gilliam, S. M., Taylor, E. N., Hunter, J. J., & Hansen, N. B. (2023). The feasibility and acceptability of Project POWER: A mindfulness-infused, cognitive-behavioral group intervention to address mental and sexual health needs of young pregnant women in Liberia. *BMC Pregnancy and Childbirth, 23*(1), 1–12.

CDC. (2022a). *COVID-19 vaccinations in the United States.*

CDC. (2022b). *Stay up to date with your COVID-19 vaccines.* https://www.cdc.gov/coronavirus/2019-ncov/vaccines/stay-up-to-date.html

CDC. (2022c). *What is health equity?* https://www.cdc.gov/healthequity/whatis/index.html

Charmaraman, L., Hernandez, J. M., & Hodes, R. (2022). Marginalized and understudied populations using digital media. In Jacqueline Nesi, Eva H. Telzer, & Mitchell J. Prinstein (Ed.), *Handbook of adolescent digital media use and mental health*, 188. Cambridge University Press.

Cookson, D., Jolley, D., Dempsey, R. C., & Povey, R. (2021). A social norms approach intervention to address misperceptions of anti-vaccine conspiracy beliefs amongst UK parents. *PLoS One, 16*(11), e0258985. https://doi.org/10.1371/journal.pone.0258985

Davis, A. M., Beaver, G., Gillette, M. D., Nelson, E.-L., Fleming, K., Romine, R. S., Sullivan, D. K., Lee, R., Gabriel, K. P., Dean, K., Murray, M., & Faith, M. (2019). iAmHealthy: Rationale, design and application of a family-based mHealth pediatric obesity intervention for rural children. *Contemporary Clinical Trials, 78*, 20–26. https://doi.org/10.1016/j.cct.2019.01.001

Diesel, J., Sterrett, N., Dasgupta, S., Kriss, J. L., Barry, V., Vanden Esschert, K., Whiteman, A., Cadwell, B. L., Weller, D., Qualters, J. R., Harris, L., Bhatt, A., Williams, C., Fox, L. M., Meaney Delman, D., Black, C. L., & Barbour, K. E. (2021). COVID-19 vaccination coverage among adults – United States, December 14, 2020-May 22, 2021. *Morbidity and Mortality Weekly Report, 70*(25), 922–927. https://doi.org/10.15585/mmwr.mm7025e1

Donenberg, G. R., Atujuna, M., Merrill, K. G., Emerson, E., Ndwayana, S., Blachman-Demner, D., & Bekker, L. G. (2021). An individually randomized controlled trial of a mother-daughter HIV/STI prevention program for adolescent girls and young women in South Africa: IMARA-SA study protocol. *BMC Public Health, 21*, 1708. https://doi.org/10.1186/s12889-021-11727-3

Education, C. D. O. (2019). *Responsive early education for young children and families experiencing homelessness.* CDE Press.

Erikson, E. H. (1968). *Identity youth and crisis.* WW Norton & Company.

FDA. (2022). *Pfizer-BioNTech COVID-19 vaccine.*

French, J., Deshpande, S., Evans, W., & Obregon, R. (2020). Key guidelines in developing a pre-emptive COVID-19 vaccination uptake promotion strategy. *International Journal of Environmental Research and Public Health, 17*(16). https://doi.org/10.3390/ijerph17165893

Garrett, L. (2007). The challenge of global health. *Foreign Affairs, 86*(1), 14–38.

Gissandaner, T. D., Lim, C. S., Sarver, D. E., Brown, D., McCulloh, R., Malloch, L., & Annett, R. D. (2023). Impact of COVID-19 on families with children: Examining sociodemographic differences. *Journal of Developmental & Behavioral Pediatrics, 44*(2), e88–e94. https://doi.org/10.1097/DBP.0000000000001147

Gómez, C. A., Kleinman, D. V., Pronk, N., Gordon, G. L. W., Ochiai, E., Blakey, C., Johnson, A., & Brewer, K. H. (2021). Practice full report: Addressing health equity and social determinants of health through healthy people 2030. *Journal of Public Health Management and Practice, 27*(6), S249.

Graham, A. L., Amato, M. S., Cha, S., Jacobs, M. A., Bottcher, M. M., & Papandonatos, G. D. (2021). Effectiveness of a vaping cessation text message program among young adult e-cigarette users: A randomized clinical trial. *JAMA Internal Medicine, 181*(7), 923–930. https://doi.org/10.1001/jamainternmed.2021.1793

Hanna, F., Barbui, C., Dua, T., Lora, A., van Regteren Altena, M., & Saxena, S. (2018). Global mental health: How are we doing? *World Psychiatry, 17*(3), 367.

Hines, M. (2020). Human gender development. *Neuroscience & Biobehavioral Reviews, 118*, 89–96. https://doi.org/10.1016/j.neubiorev.2020.07.018

Hoebel, E. A., & Frost, E. L. (1976). *Cultural and social anthropology.* McGraw-Hill.

Hofstede, G. (1997). *Cultures and organizations: Software of the mind.* McGraw Hill.

Hutchins, H. J., Wolff, B., Leeb, R., Ko, J. Y., Odom, E., Willey, J., Friedman, A., & Bitsko, R. H. (2020). COVID-19 mitigation behaviors by age group – United States, April-June 2020. *Morbidity and Mortality Weekly Report, 69*(43), 1584–1590. https://doi.org/10.15585/mmwr.mm6943e4

Ihmeideh, F., & Alkhawaldeh, M. (2017). Teachers' and parents' perceptions of the role of technology and digital media in developing child culture in the early years. *Children and Youth Services Review, 77*, 139–146.

Jamison, D. T., Summers, L. H., Alleyne, G., Arrow, K. J., Berkley, S., Binagwaho, A., Bustreo, F., Evans, D., Feachem, R. G., & Frenk, J. (2013). Global health 2035: A world converging within a generation. *The Lancet, 382*(9908), 1898–1955.

Johnson, K., Asher, J., Rosborough, S., Raja, A., Panjabi, R., Beadling, C., & Lawry, L. (2008). Association of combatant status and sexual violence with health and mental health outcomes in postconflict Liberia. *JAMA, 300*(6), 676–690.

Kapilashrami, A., & Hankivsky, O. (2018). Intersectionality and why it matters to global health. *The Lancet, 391*(10140), 2589–2591.

Keles, B., McCrae, N., & Grealish, A. (2020). A systematic review: The influence of social media on depression, anxiety and psychological distress in adolescents. *International Journal of Adolescence and Youth, 25*(1), 79–93.

Khubchandani, J., Sharma, S., Price, J. H., Wiblishauser, M. J., Sharma, M., & Webb, F. J. (2021). COVID-19 vaccination hesitancy in the United States: A rapid national assessment. *Journal of Community Health, 46*, 270–277. https://doi.org/10.1007/s10900-020-00958-x

Koplan, J. P., Bond, T. C., Merson, M. H., Reddy, K. S., Rodriguez, M. H., Sewankambo, N. K., & Wasserheit, J. N. (2009). Towards a common definition of global health. *The Lancet, 373*(9679), 1993–1995.

Lim, C. S., Schneider, E. M., & Janicke, D. M. (2018). Developmental influences on behavior change: Children, adolescents, emerging adults, and the elderly. In M. E. Hilliard, K. A. Riekert, J. K. Ockene, & L. Pbert (Eds.), *The handbook of health behavior change* (Vol. 5, pp. 75–101). Springer.

Lu, J. G., Jin, P., & English, A. S. (2021). Collectivism predicts mask use during COVID-19. *Proceedings of the National Academy of Sciences of the United States of America, 118*(23), e2021793118. https://doi.org/10.1073/pnas.2021793118

Mantena, S., Rogo, K., & Burke, T. F. (2020). Re-examining the race to send ventilators to low-resource settings. *Respiratory Care, 65*(9), 1378–1381.

Marcolino, M. S., Oliveira, J. A. Q., D'Agostino, M., Ribeiro, A. L., Alkmim, M. B. M., & Novillo-Ortiz, D. (2018). The impact of mHealth interventions: Systematic review of systematic reviews. *JMIR mHealth and uHealth, 6*(1), e8873.

Martinez, M. A., Osornio, A., Halim, M. L. D., & Zosuls, K. M. (2020). Gender: Awareness, identity, and stereotyping. In *Encyclopedia of infant and early childhood development* (2nd ed., Vol. 2). Elsevier.

Matsumoto, D. (2007). Culture, context, and behavior. *Journal of Personality, 75*(6), 1285–1320.

Moffitt, U., & Rogers, L. O. (2022). Studying ethnic-racial identity among White youth: White supremacy as a developmental context. *Journal of Research on Adolescence, 32*(3), 815–828.

Mousavi, M. S., Shahriari, M., Salehi, M., & Kohan, S. (2019). Gender identity development in the shadow of socialization: A grounded theory approach. *Archives of Women's Mental Health, 22*(2), 245–251. https://doi.org/10.1007/s00737-018-0888-0

Neblett, E. W., Jr., Rivas-Drake, D., & Umaña-Taylor, A. J. (2012). The promise of racial and ethnic protective factors in promoting ethnic minority youth development. *Child Development Perspectives, 6*(3), 295–303.

Nielsen, M. W., Stefanick, M. L., Peragine, D., Neilands, T. B., Ioannidis, J. P. A., Pilote, L., Prochaska, J. J., Cullen, M. R., Einstein, G., Klinge, I., LeBlanc, H., Paik, H. Y., & Schiebinger, L. (2021). Gender-related variables for health research. *Biology of Sex Differences, 12*(1), 23. https://doi.org/10.1186/s13293-021-00366-3

Niemi, R. G., & Klingler, J. D. (2012). The development of political attitudes and behaviour among young adults. *Australian Journal of Political Science, 47*, 31–54. https://doi.org/10.1080/10361146.2011.643167

Paudel, S., Jancey, J., Subedi, N., & Leavy, J. (2017). Correlates of mobile screen media use among children aged 0–8: A systematic review. *BMJ Open, 7*(10), e014585.

Prensky, M. (2001). Digital natives, digital immigrants part 2: Do they really think differently? *On the Horizon, 9*, 1–6. https://doi.org/10.1108/10748120110424843

Rosal, M. C., Wang, M. L., & Bodenlos, J. S. (2014). *Culture, behavior, and health.* In K. A. Riekert, J. K. Ockene, & L. Pbert (Eds.), *The handbook of health behavior change* (4th ed., pp. 109–136). Springer Publishing Company.

Sallam, M. (2021). COVID-19 vaccine hesitancy worldwide: A concise systematic review of vaccine acceptance rates. *Vaccines (Basel), 9*(2), 160. https://doi.org/10.3390/vaccines9020160

Santomauro, D. F., Herrera, A. M. M., Shadid, J., Zheng, P., Ashbaugh, C., Pigott, D. M., Abbafati, C., Adolph, C., Amlag, J. O., & Aravkin, A. Y. (2021). Global prevalence and burden of depressive and anxiety disorders in 204 countries and territories in 2020 due to the COVID-19 pandemic. *The Lancet, 398*(10312), 1700–1712.

Scullin, M. K., Jones, W. E., Phenis, R., Beevers, S., Rosen, S., Dinh, K., Kiselica, A., Keefe, F. J., & Benge, J. F. (2022). Using smartphone technology to improve prospective memory functioning: A randomized controlled trial. *Journal of the American Geriatrics Society*, 70(2), 459–469. https://doi.org/10.1111/jgs.17551

Shahin, W., Kennedy, G. A., & Stupans, I. (2019). The impact of personal and cultural beliefs on medication adherence of patients with chronic illnesses: A systematic review. *Patient Preference and Adherence*, 13, 1019–1035.

Shannon, H., Bush, K., Villeneuve, P. J., Hellemans, K. G., & Guimond, S. (2022). Problematic social media use in adolescents and young adults: Systematic review and meta-analysis. *JMIR Mental Health*, 9(4), e33450.

Sheldrick, R. C., Schlichting, L. E., Berger, B., Clyne, A., Ni, P., Perrin, E. C., & Vivier, P. M. (2019). Establishing new norms for developmental milestones. *Pediatrics*, 144(6), e20190374. https://doi.org/10.1542/peds.2019-0374

Shih, S., & Cohen, L. L. (2020). A systematic review of medication adherence interventions in pediatric sickle cell disease. *Journal of Pediatric Psychology*, 45(6), 593–606. https://doi.org/10.1093/jpepsy/jsaa031

Stark, L. J., Spear Filigno, S., Bolling, C., Ratcliff, M. B., Kichler, J. C., Robson, S. M., Simon, S. L., McCullough, M. B., Clifford, L. M., Odar Stough, C., Zion, C., & Ittenbach, R. F. (2018). Clinic and home-based behavioral intervention for obesity in preschoolers: A randomized trial. *The Journal of Pediatrics*, 192, 115–121 e111. https://doi.org/10.1016/j.jpeds.2017.09.063

Sue, D. W., & Sue, D. (1999). *Counseling the culturally different: Theory and practice*. John Wiley & Sons Inc.

Szilagyi, P. G., Shah, M. D., Delgado, J. R., Thomas, K., Vizueta, N., Cui, Y., Vangala, S., Shetgiri, R., & Kapteyn, A. (2021). Parents' intentions and perceptions about COVID-19 vaccination for their children: Results from a national survey. *Pediatrics*, 148(4), e2021052335. https://doi.org/10.1542/peds.2021-052335

Szilagyi, P. G., Thomas, K., Shah, M. D., Vizueta, N., Cui, Y., Vangala, S., Fox, C., & Kapteyn, A. (2021). The role of trust in the likelihood of receiving a COVID-19 vaccine: Results from a national survey. *Preventive Medicine*, 153, 106727. https://doi.org/10.1016/j.ypmed.2021.106727

The U.S. Surgeon General's Advisory. (2023). *Social media and youth mental health*. https://www.hhs.gov/sites/default/files/sg-youth-mental-health-social-media-advisory.pdf

Thomas, E. E., Taylor, M. L., Ward, E. C., Hwang, R., Cook, R., Ross, J. A., Webb, C., Harris, M., Hartley, C., Carswell, P., Burns, C. L., & Caffery, L. J. (2022). Beyond forced telehealth adoption: A framework to sustain telehealth among allied health services. *Journal of Telemedicine and Telecare*, 30(3), 559–569. https://doi.org/10.1177/1357633X221074499

Vahratian, A., Blumberg, S. J., Terlizzi, E. P., & Schiller, J. S. (2021). Symptoms of anxiety or depressive disorder and use of mental health care among adults during the COVID-19 pandemic – United States, August 2020-February 2021. *Morbidity and Mortality Weekly Report*, 70(13), 490–494. https://doi.org/10.15585/mmwr.mm7013e2

Vinck, P., & Pham, P. N. (2013). Association of exposure to intimate-partner physical violence and potentially traumatic war-related events with mental health in Liberia. *Social Science & Medicine*, 77, 41–49. https://doi.org/10.1016/j.socscimed.2012.10.026

Vos, T., Lim, S. S., Abbafati, C., Abbas, K. M., Abbasi, M., Abbasifard, M., Abbasi-Kangevari, M., Abbastabar, H., Abd-Allah, F., & Abdelalim, A. (2020). Global burden of 369 diseases and injuries in 204 countries and territories, 1990–2019: A systematic analysis for the Global Burden of Disease Study 2019. *The Lancet*, 396(10258), 1204–1222.

WHO. (2011). *mHealth: new horizons for health through mobile technologies*.

WHO. (2019). *Guidelines on physical activity, sedentary behaviour and sleep for children under 5 years of age*. World Health Organization.

Wong, L. E., Hawkins, J. E., Langness, S., Murrell, K. L., Iris, P., & Sammann, A. (2020). Where are all the patients? Addressing COVID-19 fear to encourage sick patients to seek emergency care. *NEJM Catalyst*, 1(3), 1–12.

CHAPTER 6

MEASURING HEALTH BEHAVIORS AT THE INDIVIDUAL AND COMMUNITY LEVELS

ALEXANDRA D. MONZON, JESSICA S. PIERCE, LINDSAY A. TALIAFERRO, AND RACHEL M. WASSERMAN

LEARNING OBJECTIVES

- Incorporate the social-ecological framework into health behavior assessment to identify potential measures of health behavior and factors that influence health behaviors at the individual, community, and population levels.
- Distinguish between objective and subjective as well as direct and indirect measures of health behavior and community-level factors and discuss the benefits and downsides of each.
- Describe psychometric and measurement design characteristics of health behavior instruments, including validity, reliability, sensitivity, and specificity.
- Discuss the implications of technological and medical advancement on the development of new methods to measure health behaviors.
- Recognize the strengths and weaknesses of various methods for measuring health behaviors and related factors, and discuss which might be more useful for specific situations.

INTRODUCTION

Accurate behavioral measurement is essential to many clinical and research activities related to health behavior change. First, public health efforts by agencies, such as the Centers for Disease Control and Prevention (CDC), rely on health surveillance for tracking changes in the health and behaviors of a specific population over time. Second, health behavior screening identifies or classifies individuals for targeted research or care delivery. Third, health behavior researchers often study associations among environmental characteristics, health behaviors, and clinical outcomes in individuals and communities. Fourth, behavior change interventions may include monitoring health behaviors and providing feedback. Fifth, clinicians and researchers use health behavior assessments to determine the impact of clinical interventions on key health behaviors and outcomes. Finally, population health assessments may identify structural factors that influence health and health behavior at the community level, identify specific community needs, and evaluate health outcomes related to changes in policy, physical environment, and community-based strategies.

This chapter focuses on both individual-level and community-level assessment strategies. For individual-level assessment strategies, examples will focus on several domains of health behaviors with cross-cutting applicability for common health concerns: eating behaviors, physical activity, sleep, and medical treatment engagement. Assessment of eating includes the frequency, amount, and nutritional characteristics of foods ingested. Physical activity assessment encompasses the frequency, duration, intensity, and types of energy-expending activities in which individuals engage. Behavioral sleep measurement encompasses nocturnal and daytime sleep habits along with sleep environment. Measurement of medical treatment engagement comprises assessing the frequency, quantity, timing, and duration of activities required for disease management, including taking prescribed medications and completing disease management therapies. Several non–patient-centered terms (e.g., adherence, compliance) have historically been used to describe how an individual manages a disease or chronic health condition. However, this chapter will use the term *engagement* when discussing medical treatment to acknowledge an individual's choice and autonomy with self-management decisions. For community-level strategies, examples will focus on factors that affect health behaviors, such as social determinants of health (SDOH), and population health outcomes. Assessing SDOH considers the environmental and structural conditions (i.e., economic stability, education access and quality, healthcare access and quality, neighborhood and built environment, and social and community content) that affect health behavior. Population health includes public health surveillance, which aims to quantify and track the distribution of risk and protective factors and health outcomes in a population to identify modifiable factors that influence the health of a population or community.

SOCIAL-ECOLOGICAL MODEL AND INTERSECTIONALITY: EXAMINING EFFECTS OF SYSTEMS OF OPPRESSION AND PRIVILEGE ON HEALTH OUTCOMES

Acknowledging contextual factors that influence health remains essential when assessing health behaviors at the individual and community levels. The social-ecological model reflects how individuals and communities are embedded within larger social systems and help explain the complex association between individual health behaviors and health outcomes (Sallis & Owen, 2015). This model indicates that many factors affect health and behavior change, not just a person's intent. Researchers have applied the social-ecological models to identify multilevel risks for adverse health outcomes, explore factors underpinning social inequities and health disparities, and assess an individual's risk and protection within a broader network, community, and public policy context (Baral et al., 2013). Further, at the structural level, systems of oppression and privilege interact with other multilevel factors that contribute to and maintain health inequalities.

Intersectionality is a theory that helps describe how intersections between multiple structural systems of oppression and privilege can create risk of health disparities at any level of the social-ecological model (see arrow in **Figure 6.1**), particularly for individuals with multiple minoritized identities. Health systems are driven by established sociopolitical structures, which are rooted in historical and contemporary systems of oppression and power (Young et al., 2020). Disparities in health outcomes across populations, especially those among populations with multiple minoritized identities (e.g., age, class, gender, sexual orientation), reflect systemic structural level factors such as differential barriers and facilitators associated with accessing and utilizing health services. Health inequities will continue to persist if health behaviors are assessed without acknowledging health equity within the context of social and structural systems. **Figure 6.1** illustrates these concepts using COVID-19-related mask wearing and social distancing behaviors as an example. While this chapter focuses on specific measurement tools and methodologies at the individual and community levels, researchers are encouraged to incorporate a broader sociopolitical context when assessing health behavior change.

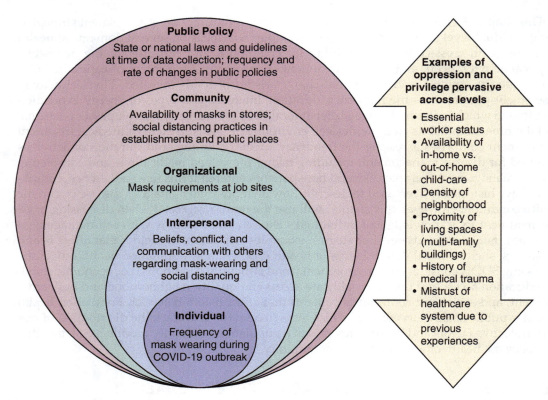

FIGURE 6.1 Application of the social-ecological model to measure factors related to mask wearing and social distancing behaviors during the COVID-19 outbreak.

CONSIDERATIONS FOR ASSESSMENT SELECTION

When selecting any health behavior assessment measure, researchers/clinicians need to consider the measures of psychometric properties and the rigor of the methods used to develop and test an instrument. Psychometric properties represent the ability of an instrument to make accurate and consistent measurements. Specifically, the validity of a measure represents the degree to which an instrument measures what it aims to measure. The reliability of a measure represents the production of consistent results when the instrument is completed in similar conditions. Sensitivity describes the ability of a measure to detect "true positives," and specificity describes the ability of a measure to detect "true negatives." In addition to psychometric properties, health behavior clinicians and researchers may consider various methods to enhance their measurement of health behaviors. For example, triangulating multiple sources of individual- and community-level data may provide a more comprehensive assessment of health behaviors than a single source (Raghunathan et al., 2021). Most assessment measures will involve some degree of missing data, and combining multiple sources of data could provide a more complete assessment of certain health outcomes. Further, using a person's ecological context, such as their surroundings and current environment, is helpful when interpreting individual data (Do et al., 2022). Ecological information can provide more nuanced information regarding the effects of environment over time on changes in health behaviors and/or health outcomes. Another important consideration involves balancing the collection of maximally informative, comprehensive data versus minimizing burden on participants and resources to conduct the assessment. Collecting longitudinal or repeated assessments using a multimethod, multi-informant assessment approach can increase the validity of conclusions drawn from data (Bufferd et al., 2014). However, overburdening participants with multiple assessments can lead to fatigue and may discourage participants from completing all measures or returning for follow-up. Some researchers suggest carefully evaluating the essential purpose of a study to help limit the assessment battery to the maximally informative and minimally burdensome combination of measures by prioritizing more intensive measures for constructs related to a study's primary aims (Sternfeld & Goldman-Rosas, 2012).

INDIVIDUAL-LEVEL HEALTH BEHAVIOR MEASUREMENT METHODOLOGIES

Subjective and objective assessment strategies can measure individual-level health behavior using individual self-reports, in vivo observations, biomarker assays, or electronically collected objective measures. *Objective* measures of health behaviors take two forms: direct observation (e.g., video recording) or indirect inference of a behavior based on concrete outcomes of the behavior (e.g., blood assays, body weight, pharmacy refill records). *Subjective* measures of health behaviors rely on individuals (e.g., oneself, clinician, parent, spouse) to report the occurrence of health behaviors. Subjective measures ask people to provide data on their or others' engagement in health behaviors and may be administered in various formats, for example, rating forms, interviews, and daily/weekly diaries. We describe and summarize the benefits and drawbacks of these various methods in the following sections and in **Table 6.1**.

Direct Objective Measures of Individual-Level Health Behavior

Direct measures of behavior monitor the occurrence of behaviors as they happen. In *behavioral observation* methods, a trained observer watches an individual, either live or via recording, and keeps count of each target behavior as it happens. Observation can occur in a naturalistic setting (e.g., at home or school) or in a staged scenario (e.g., eating a meal in a research lab), and observers track the frequency and duration of specific behaviors over a set period of time. Observers may keep track of behaviors with simple counts, rating scales, or coding systems. Behavioral observation may also include devices that electronically monitor a behavior. These technologies may include electronic pill bottles, medical devices, accelerometers, electronic scales, biosensors that attach to the body and record physiological measurements such as body position or oxygen level, or wearable cameras that record the occurrence of specific health behaviors. In the following sections, we provide examples of each measurement type for four health behaviors: diet, physical activity, sleep, and treatment (e.g., medication) engagement.

Regarding diet, researchers often use direct observation to assess eating through the remote food photography method (RFPM; Martin et al., 2012). Through this method, individuals can send researchers photos of foods they eat from their phones, along with detailed descriptions of their food content and intake, before and after meals. Researchers train study participants to standardize the distance and angle of photographs to facilitate serving size calculations. Traditionally, dietitians analyze photographs. However, more recently, phone applications can identify the type, volume, and nutritional content of foods, and wearable sensors can automate dietary intake data collection (Mortazavi & Gutierrez-Osuna, 2023).

For physical activity, researchers often employ pedometers, accelerometers, and actigraphy for participants to wear on their bodies during everyday activities to measure the acceleration of their physical movements. These devices can calculate and track the amount, types, intensity, and duration of activity (Hills et al., 2014). Devices, such as Fitbit (Fitbit Inc., San Francisco, CA), Jawbone UP Trackers (Jawbone Inc., San Francisco, CA), and Garmin VivoSmart (Garmin Ltd, Schaffhausen, Switzerland), can become part of more extensive health behavior monitoring programs that document fitness activities and link with data about other health behaviors (e.g., weight from electronic scales, sleep quality from actigraphy, user-inputted data about food intake). Such devices can capture multiple measures of health behaviors in a single system and verify self-reported data through electronic capture.

TABLE 6.1 Summary of Individual-Level Assessment Methods

METHOD	DESCRIPTION	BENEFITS	DRAWBACKS
Objective (direct)	Measurement of behavior as it occurs	• Measures behavior itself rather than by-product or report of behavior • Higher validity/accuracy than subjective data	• Long observation period needed to capture sufficient behavior sample • Potential for person to change their behavior if they know it is being recorded/observed
Behavioral observation (e.g., video-taped family meals)	Live or recorded activity watched and coded for frequency/length of target behaviors	• Greatest certainty of data's validity • Minimal risk for coder bias	• Time, resources to train coders so that they reliably code in the same way/agree upon how certain behaviors should be coded • Risk of human error in coding
Electronic monitoring (e.g., Fitbit or medicine bottle caps that track when open/close)	Occurrence of target behaviors captured and documented by technologies	• Low burden, integrates easily into regular activities • Ability to collect data remotely • Large amount of data collected • Reduced risk of human error	• Still may not be entirely accurate (e.g., Fitbit may not track steps if on a treadmill, and medication ingestion is not necessarily certain even if the cap is taken off) • Expense of devices and software • Risk of device malfunction, damage, or loss • Resources needed for data management
Objective (indirect)	Measurement of the by-products of a previous behavior	• Often more feasible to collect than observation data • Higher validity than subjective data	• Assumes that behavior has caused or contributed to the measured outcome • May be influenced by other factors aside from health behavior
Biochemical analysis (e.g., a blood or urine test to show how much of a substance is currently in the body)	Measurement of physiological markers associated with health behaviors, not a measure of health behaviors	• Often collected in routine clinical care • High reliability and validity (for recent/short-term behaviors)	• Expense, resources needed to collect and analyze samples (e.g., blood or urine) • Influence of individual differences (e.g., differences in metabolism can affect how long a substance stays in one's body) • Potential participant discomfort (e.g., blood draws)

METHOD	DESCRIPTION	BENEFITS	DRAWBACKS
Manual measurements (e.g., counting the number of pills left in the bottle)	Counts of physical products of health behaviors	• Minimal risk for rater bias • Straightforward data collection	• Risk of human error in counting • Time-intensive • Potential for person to change their behavior or manipulate the data (e.g., "pill dumping") because they know it is being monitored
Subjective (indirect)	Reports of health behaviors by individuals (self or others)	• Ease of data collection • Wide range of constructs can be assessed	• Do not measure behavior itself • Susceptible to reporter bias or fabricated/inaccurate data
Rating forms (self)	Own behavior in the past reported by the individual using a questionnaire or rating form	• Ease of data collection • Low resource needs • Can survey large samples • Can assess large periods of time	• Requires literacy, fluency in survey language • Difficult/impossible to request clarification, can lead to missing or inaccurate responses • Risk of rater bias or memory errors with longer recall period
24-hour recall interviews (self)	Specific health behaviors that occurred during the previous day reported by the individual	• Short recall period—reduced risk of bias or memory errors	• Time-intensive for participant and research team • May be biased by unique circumstances of previous day
Daily diaries/logs (self)	Specific health behaviors that occurred each day tracked by the individual	• Short recall period • Brief/easy to complete • Useful for behaviors that typically occur daily	• Rely on participant remembering to complete daily • Risk for participant completing entries that they missed, rather than doing it once a day
Ecological momentary assessment (self)	Individual prompted throughout the day to track or report on specific behaviors that are currently occurring or occurred in the immediate past	• Very short recall period • Assessment of behaviors in context of natural events/settings • Ease/convenience of data collection	• Risk for missing data due to nonresponses to prompts • May disrupt activities • Potential for person to change their behavior if they are being asked about it/reminded of it frequently

Regarding sleep behaviors, polysomnography, a lab-based assessment, is considered the "gold standard" of sleep measurement. Researchers often use polysomnography to diagnose sleep disorders by recording brain waves, oxygen levels in the blood, heart rate, breathing, and eye and leg movements (Rundo & Downey, 2019). Researchers often choose actigraphy to measure sleep duration and timing of sleep onset in individuals without sleep disorders, as this method is less intrusive, more ecologically valid, and provides continuous data collection over several days or weeks (Conley et al., 2019). However, because wake/sleep patterns are based on movement, actigraphy may overestimate sleep duration in people with longer sleep onset periods and periods of resting while awake (Van De Water et al., 2011). Due to this concern, recommendations suggest investigators collect subjective assessments of sleep behaviors in conjunction with actigraphy (Meltzer et al., 2012). Several other measures of sleep duration are available, but they need further validation, including bed motion sensors, eyelid movement sensors, sleep switch (i.e., a sensor for determining periods of sleep when the device is pinched and relaxed), and a noncontact biomotion sensor that uses Doppler radar to detect chest movement (Van De Water et al., 2011).

For medical treatment engagement, behavioral observation is known as "directly observed therapy" (DOT). Due to the inherent behavioral impact of being observed, researchers often consider DOT an intervention more than an assessment (Hart et al., 2010). Medication electronic monitoring devices capture and time-stamp the opening or actuation of medication packages. Examples include Medication Event Monitoring System (MEMS) caps for pill bottles (Aardex Group Ltd., Switzerland), Med-eMonitor "smart pillboxes" (InforMedix, Rockville, MD), Propeller Health devices for inhaled medications (Propellor Health, Madison, WI), and GlucoMe Insulin Pen Monitor cap for insulin pens (GlucoMe, Israel). Medical devices such as blood glucose meters, insulin pumps, and continuous positive airway pressure (CPAP) machines track health behaviors such as checking blood glucose, administering a pill or inhaler, and starting/stopping the CPAP machine. A large literature base supports the reliability and validity of electronic monitors for treatment engagement assessment and demonstrates a strong association with various health outcomes (Anghel et al., 2019; Aylward et al., 2015; Patton et al., 2017).

Indirect Objective Measures of Individual-Level Health Behavior

Indirect measures assess an outcome that results from a behavior after it has occurred. Objective indirect measures include analysis of biochemical markers produced from a behavior or manual counts of behavior by-products (e.g., leftover food, medications). Manual measurements include counts of the physical products of health behaviors, and biochemical analysis tracks physiological markers associated with health behaviors.

Regarding diet, biomarkers of vegetable and fruit consumption, including carotenoid concentrations, are assessed either with a blood sample or a noninvasive laser (Hosseini et al., 2018). However, such biomarkers are more appropriate for assessing intraindividual differences (e.g., individual changes over time due to intervention) rather than interindividual differences (e.g., comparing geographic populations). Other methods include using a weighed food inventory, in which a meal is weighed before and after eating. Benefits of indirect individual-level measures include low cost and precise measurements. However, the downsides of these measures include intrusiveness and burden for participants, as well as the potential for repeated measurements to impact eating behavior.

For physical activity, doubly labeled water represents the gold standard criterion against which other measures of physical activity are commonly validated (Dugas et al., 2011). This method involves measuring body fluid samples after drinking enriched water to determine the rates at which the body is expelling enriched oxygen and hydrogen isotopes over a 1- to 3-week observation period, which indicates energy expenditure (Westerterp, 2017).

Regarding sleep, measures of salivary melatonin, leptin, ghrelin, and other metabolic and inflammatory responses may represent valuable indirect measures of sleep duration, as hormone levels fluctuate within individuals throughout the sleep–wake cycle (Rynders et al., 2020).

However, these hormone biomarkers are not strongly related to subjective measures of alertness and sleepiness, and they are not recommended as a direct measure of sleep duration or sleepiness.

For medical treatment engagement, assessment methods often include biochemical analysis to quantify the concentration of a drug's metabolic by-products in the body by analyzing blood, saliva, or urine (Hommel et al., 2009). While biochemical analysis constitutes an objective value representing the amount of medication in one's body, it does not account for individual (e.g., metabolism) or drug-specific factors (e.g., half-life, the timing of administration) that can impact a drug's bioavailability (Gonzalez & Schneider, 2011). Pill counting is a common manual measurement approach in which researchers estimate the number of consumed medications during a given interval when counting pills at two timepoints (Conn & Ruppar, 2017). However, this method does not confirm patients used medications as prescribed. Pharmacy refill records represent another form of indirect measurement of remaining medication doses. For example, researchers can calculate the medication possession ratio by comparing the amount of medication prescribed with the days' supply of medication dispensed over a set period to determine the rate at which an individual uses the existing supply (Conn & Ruppar, 2017).

Subjective Measures of Individual-Level Health Behavior

Subjective measures rely on individuals (e.g., oneself, clinician, parent, spouse) to report the occurrence of health behaviors. On self-report rating forms, the length of the recall period can impact accuracy because, as memory lapses, intervening events, attitudes about a behavior, social desirability bias, and emotional state can all impact retrospective accounts (Jones & Johnston, 2011). Although shorter recall periods tend to yield data demonstrating higher validity, no optimal recall time range exists for all behaviors or measures (Stull et al., 2009). Researchers have developed strategies involving shorter recall periods to address this challenge, such as 24-hour recall interviews that assess health behaviors over the 24 hours before an interview. Using logs or diaries, participants can also track target behaviors daily. Detailed questions can accompany these log entries. However, because this method is repeated over several days, the more information collected at each entry, the greater the burden for participants and higher likelihood of missing data. With technological advances, participants may complete daily behavior tracking more conveniently online or with mobile devices. Using ecological momentary assessment (EMA), participants receive prompts (e.g., by alarm or text message) to report or track targeted behaviors throughout the day, occurring randomly, at set intervals, or following specific events such as meals (Doherty et al., 2020).

Regarding diet, self-report measures of eating behaviors use short-term recall periods (e.g., daily diaries, 24-hour recall interviews) or real-time reports. Food frequency questionnaires and diet history interviews are commonly used to assess an individual's average amounts and types of food eaten over a long period (i.e., several months/years) and can be adapted for specific study aims (England et al., 2015). For physical activity, self-report activity measures assess global trends in one's activity level, historical patterns (e.g., spanning more than 1 year to lifetime), or specific activities over a particular period (Sternfeld & Goldman-Rosas, 2012). While global measures (e.g., typical day or week) are useful for population-level surveillance, they may not detect an incremental change, and recall methods spanning a specific and relatively brief period (e.g., the previous week) are commonly used to assess short-term variations in behavior (Hallal et al., 2012). Compared with direct, objective measures of physical activity, self-report measures can over- or underestimate activity levels, raising questions about reliability and validity, and making it difficult to correct for measurement error (Prince et al., 2008).

Regarding sleep behaviors, two commonly used self-report measures are the Epworth Sleepiness Scale (ESS; Johns, 1991), which assesses daytime sleepiness, and the Pittsburgh Sleep Quality Index (Buysse et al., 1989), which assesses one's nocturnal sleep schedule, how long it takes to fall asleep, sleep duration and disturbances (e.g., feeling too hot/cold), use of sleep medications, and daytime dysfunction. Self-report questionnaires designed for youth also exist to address sleep quality, quantity, daytime sleepiness, sleep habits/hygiene, and cognitions about sleep specifically among children and adolescents (Erwin & Bashore, 2017). However, due to limited consciousness during sleep, self-reporting some behaviors (snoring, restlessness, duration and frequency of nighttime waking) may not prove valid.

For medical treatment engagement, self-report measures may glean global ratings of health behaviors (e.g., sedentary behavior) or assess specific disease management behaviors (e.g., insulin use). Several self-report measures of treatment engagement exist (Stirratt et al., 2015), and data from questionnaires and diaries often significantly correlate with other measures of treatment engagement and health status (Kichler et al., 2012). However, many measures have insufficient psychometric properties, including poor sensitivity and specificity (Koschack et al., 2010), and overreporting adherence is common (Nieuwkerk et al., 2010). A major challenge involves obtaining average estimates of treatment engagement when an individual engages differently with the various components of a regimen or when engagement varies over time (Garfield et al., 2011).

CASE STUDY 6.1: EXAMPLE OF OBJECTIVE HEALTH DATA AND SUBJECTIVE MEASURES IN PARENTS AND YOUTH WITH TYPE 1 DIABETES

Youth with type 1 diabetes mellitus (T1D) are at risk of experiencing nighttime hypoglycemia, and many parents report significant anxiety at night regarding glucose management. A recent study aimed to examine the relationship between parent/caregiver fear of nighttime hypoglycemia and nighttime glucose levels as measured by continuous glucose monitors (CGMs; Monzon et al., 2023). The study team collected objective health data from 116 children and adolescents with T1D via their CGM device that provided a continuous measure of glucose levels for a 14-day period. The study team calculated the percent of time that an individuals' nighttime glucose values were within the hypoglycemic range (i.e., <70 mg/dL), within the target range (i.e., 70–180 mg/dL), and within the hyperglycemic range (i.e., >180 mg/dL), and the mean and standard deviation for all nighttime glucose levels. Parents and caregivers completed the self-report Hypoglycemia Fear Survey for Parents (HFS-P; Clarke et al., 1998) with a recently created subscale that assessed specific worries related to nighttime hypoglycemia. The results of the study suggested that parents of youth with T1D may report higher fear of hypoglycemia if they observe greater fluctuations in their child's nighttime glucose levels, regardless of the percent of time their child's glucose levels are in the hypoglycemic range (Monzon et al., 2023). This case study includes the use of a subjective measure of fear of hypoglycemia and an objective measure of blood glucose levels. In addition, it highlights how subjective and objective measures may be uniquely beneficial for measuring different aspects of health behavior (e.g., managing blood glucose levels) and factors related to it.

COMMUNITY AND POPULATION-LEVEL HEALTH BEHAVIOR MEASUREMENT METHODOLOGIES

MacQueen and colleagues (2001, p. 1936) define *community* as "a group of people with diverse characteristics who are linked by social ties, share common perspectives, and engage in joint action in geographical locations or settings." Alternatively, Kindig and Stoddart (2003, p. 381) define *population health* as "the health outcomes of a group of individuals, including the distribution of such outcomes within the group" and they argue that "the field of population health includes health outcomes, patterns of health determinants, and policies and interventions that link these two." For the purposes of this chapter, we discuss measure of community-level factors such as social contextual data that may *influence* health behaviors and rate of health behavior change. For population-level measures, we discuss common measures of health behaviors that are aggregated at the community level (Table 6.2).

Objective Measures of Community Factors

Use of geographic information systems (GIS) technology has greatly increased over the last several decades to assess various public health outcomes. GIS technology combines complex algorithms, spatial analysis, geostatistics, and modeling of health, population, and environmental data to evaluate relationships between health-related variables and environmental risks (Fletcher-Lartey & Caprarelli, 2016). For example, GIS can visually display health service utilization in a given community, while considering factors related to locational constraints (e.g., public transportation) that could limit an individual from acquiring adequate healthcare (Musa et al., 2013). Further, researchers can assess social and cultural variables through GIS, similar to environmental covariates, to understand the distribution of SDOH, specific health disparities, and potential targets for intervention in a given area or community (Sharifi et al., 2016; Shi et al., 2022). Built environment and neighborhood characteristics also represent frequently assessed variables at the community level when assessing health behaviors. For example, researchers have utilized computer vision modeling techniques (i.e., object recognition, object detection, and scene labeling) and publicly available Google Street View images to assess various indicators of a neighborhood's or community's built environment (Nguyen et al., 2018), such as food desserts. To assess consumer and community food environments in stores and restaurants, researchers have also employed the Nutrition Environment Measurement Survey (NEMS; Glanz et al., 2023), which is a store audit tool that captures a wide range of food items sold in stores and uses a ranked score to assess the health value of a store. Data from the NEMS describe the availability, price, quality of food inside a store, and number and type of stores (i.e., grocery stores or convenience stores) in a particular area. For public safety assessments at the community level, researchers may utilize information from government agencies, for example, crime data, and employ mapping techniques to capture these data in a specific area (Khan et al., 2017).

In addition to measuring objective physical environment indicators of health behaviors, researchers have begun to measure stigmatizing social environments, or structural stigma, that assesses societal-level conditions, cultural norms, and institutional policies that constrain opportunities, resources, and well-being of stigmatized groups (Hatzenbuehler & Link, 2014). Examples of these measures may include quantifying state discriminatory and nondiscrimination laws and policies, the proportion of elected government officials that identify with a stigmatized or minoritized group, the density of individuals with a stigmatized or minoritized identity within a community, the quality of benefits and protections afforded to individuals with stigmatized or minoritized identities, the availability of city and state services for stigmatized or minoritized groups, and commitment of community leadership toward equitable and inclusive practices and services (Lattanner et al., 2021). In addition, measures of structural racism (e.g., State Racism Index) and sexual and gender identity discrimination (e.g., State Equality Index) assess racial/ethnic/gender/sexual identity structural discrimination at the neighborhood, community, and state levels. Measures of structural racism may include rates of fatal police shootings, residential segregation, incarceration, educational attainment, economic indicators and disparities, and employment status among different racial and ethnic groups (Mesic et al., 2018). Measuring these forms of discrimination and stigma at the community and population level is particularly important when considering factors that influence health behaviors. Growing evidence suggests that structural factors, such as racism, heterosexism, cisgenderism, classism, and sexism, and stigma significantly contribute to health inequities for minoritized groups that range from individual vulnerability to illness from chronic stress to premature mortality at a population level (Richman & Hatzenbuehler, 2014).

TABLE 6.2 Summary of Community-/Population-Level Assessment Methods

METHOD	DESCRIPTION	BENEFITS	DRAWBACKS
Objective (direct)	Measurement of behavior as it occurs	• Measures the behavior itself rather than by-product or report of behavior • Higher validity/accuracy than subjective data	• Long observation period needed to capture sufficient behavior sample • Potential for person to change their behavior if they know it is being recorded/observed
Population level (e.g., aggregated individual-level data from Fitbit)	Individual-level data grouped and analyzed based on defined "communities"	• Similar benefits as in Table 6.1—electronic monitoring • Allows for comparison across groups of individuals • Allows for tracking of behaviors and outcomes over time	• Similar drawbacks as in Table 6.1—electronic monitoring • Can help assess group differences, but not the reasons or factors as to why there might be group differences
Objective (indirect)	Measurement of the by-products of a previous behavior	• Often more feasible to collect than observation data • Higher validity than subjective data	• Assumes that the behavior has caused or contributed to the measured outcome • May be influenced by other factors aside from health behavior
Population level (e.g., EMR of labs, diagnoses, or vital reports)	Measurement of physiological markers associated with health behaviors, not a measure of health behaviors; aggregated across groups of individuals	• Often collected in routine clinical care • Data already collected into the medical record	• Data entered into the EMR not always accurate, as errors do occur • Not all health systems include the same measurements or record the same information • Data may not be up-to-date, as information is only entered into the electronic medical record at medical visits • Not all health systems use the same medical record

METHOD	DESCRIPTION	BENEFITS	DRAWBACKS
Community-level social contextual factors (e.g., geocoding, distance to nearest grocery store/market)	Using information about the environment to determine factors that may affect health behavior (e.g., access to nutritious food options)	• National databases, such as the national environment survey, publicly available • May help better understand why there are group- or population-level differences in health behaviors and health outcomes	• Less control over how data are collected • Publicly available data sets may not include or be able to provide data specific to the exact location (e.g., some use zip code, but there can be much variability in one zip code) • May not represent the most up-to-date information (e.g., may not reflect neighborhoods or environments that are quickly changing or experienced a natural disaster)
Subjective (indirect)	Reports of health behaviors by individuals (self or others)	• Ease of data collection • Wide range of constructs can be assessed	• Do not measure behavior itself • Susceptible to reporter bias or fabricated/inaccurate data
Community-level social contextual factors (e.g., community needs survey, interviews with community leaders, individual assessments of experiences with structural discrimination)	Own opinion and experiences with the environment or community reported by the individual	• Ease of data collection • Low resource needs • Can survey large samples • Can assess large periods of time	• Requires literacy, fluency in survey language • Difficult/impossible to request clarification, can lead to missing or inaccurate responses • Risk of rater bias or memory errors with longer recall period
Population level (e.g., large-scale, national surveys and phone interviews by the CDC, such as the BRFSS, YRBSS, and PLACES)	Aggregated information across individuals in a large geographic area that is often collected by government agencies or government-funded projects	• Publicly available data sets, e.g., via the CDC website • Can be used to assess group differences in frequency of health behaviors (e.g., YRBSS asks about frequency of alcohol use among high school-age youth)	• Less control over how data are collected • Less control over which individuals are invited to participate in the survey • May be some bias in who completes the survey and truthfulness in the reporting of the data, based on differences in trust in government agencies and how the data will be used/analyzed

BRFSS, Behavioral Risk Factor Surveillance System; CDC, Centers for Disease Control and Prevention; EMR, electronic medical record; PLACES, Population Level Analysis and Community Estimates; YRBSS, Youth Risk Behavior Surveillance System.

CASE STUDY 6.2: EXAMPLE OF OBJECTIVE MEASURES OF NEIGHBORHOOD AND BUILT ENVIRONMENT

To examine childhood obesity disparities, one study evaluated which racial/ethnic disparities in elevated child body mass index (BMI) are explained by neighborhood socioeconomic status (SES) and built environment (Sharifi et al., 2016). To construct measures of neighborhood SES and built environment, researchers used GIS software to link area-based socioeconomic measures, food environment, and the physical activity environment of participants to individuals' residential addresses. SES was characterized by linked area-based measures from the American Community Survey on median household income and percent of adults without a high school diploma. The study used spatial data sets to characterize the food environment by calculating the distance to the nearest fast-food and non–fast-food restaurants, supermarket (≥50 employees), and small food store (<50 employees) from each address. In addition, they calculated recreational open space density (a count of open spaces for recreation such as parks), intersection density (the number of intersections per square kilometer where three or more road segments come together), residential density (the number of housing units per square kilometer of the census tract), and land use mix (the level of variety of businesses in an area among five land use types: food, retail, services, cultural/educational, and physical activity). The results of the study suggest that neighborhood SES may be an important mediator of racial/ethnic disparities among children with obesity, while features of the built environment, related to food and physical activity, contribute to the observed obesity disparities, but to a lesser degree than neighborhood SES (Sharifi et al., 2016). One strength of this study was the examination of health outcome data (BMI, via electronic medical record) along with several community-level factors that may *influence* behaviors relevant to obesity, such as nutrition and physical activity. Still, while this study included objective measures, none of these measured health behavior directly.

Objective Measures of Population-Level Outcomes

Researchers can aggregate individual-level direct objective measures to analyze health outcomes on a population level. For example, use of physical activity monitors in population-based research has increased significantly in the past two decades. These studies seek to characterize physical activity in a population at a specific timepoint to provide group mean data and prevalence estimates. Matthews et al. (2012) provide guidelines for using activity monitors in population-based research, including consideration of the type of device; placement on the body; measurement scale (e.g., number of days to include); plan for distributing, tracking, and receiving monitors; and increasing monitor use. When individual-level data are aggregated across a group of people, based on geographic location, for example, this information may be helpful in characterizing the health behaviors of the community, thus could be compared with other communities.

Subjective Measures of Community-Level Factors

Researchers and community leaders can conduct a community needs or health assessment to identify areas of health improvement using individual-level subjective techniques discussed earlier. These assessments may involve interviews with community leaders, key informants, and community members, or administering self-report measures that assess a wide range of health behaviors or use of community programs (e.g., physical activity, nutrition, tobacco use, chronic disease management, after-school programs, preventive health or wellness activities). Regarding self-report assessments of perceived structural racism, heterosexism/homophobia, cisgenderism, sexism, classism, and so on, and stigma, researchers have administered measures assessing individuals' perceptions of structural discrimination, perceived discrimination, and stigma within their communities, as well as attitudes of individuals within a geographic community toward members of minoritized and stigmatized groups, which they then aggregate at the community level (Hatzenbuehler, 2017).

Subjective Measures of Population-Level Factors

Many population-based assessments utilize individual self-report measures administered on a large scale to capture the health behaviors of a given community. The CDC often employs self-report measures of health behaviors aggregated at the population level to provide national, state, and local data on chronic diseases, risk factors, and outcomes. For example, the Behavioral Risk Factor Surveillance System (BRFSS; Mokdad, 2009) represents one of the largest health survey systems, continuously conducted in all 50 states. This telephone survey collects data from U.S. adult residents regarding their health-related risk behaviors, chronic health conditions, and use of preventive services. Similarly, the Youth Risk Behavior Surveillance System (YRBSS) national survey assesses a broad range of health behaviors (e.g., behaviors that contribute to unintentional injury and violence, tobacco use, alcohol and other drug use, sexual behaviors that contribute to unintended pregnancy and sexually transmitted infection [STI]/HIV infection, dietary behaviors, physical inactivity) among high school students from both public and private schools in the United States (Underwood et al., 2020). Another example is the Population Level Analysis and Community Estimates (PLACES) project through the CDC, which provides health data for small areas across the United States by linking geocoded health self-report surveys and high spatial resolution population demographic and socioeconomic data (Greenlund, 2022). These surveys and findings are used to inform and assess public health programs and funding priorities.

CONSIDERATIONS AND FUTURE DIRECTIONS IN MEASURING HEALTH BEHAVIOR

No measure of health behavior is perfect, and individual investigators and practitioners must determine the most appropriate measures of health behavior, given their primary hypotheses, need for accuracy, burden on participants, and available resources. Technological advances allow for creative and novel methods of measuring health behavior, and researchers/clinicians/public health practitioners should thoughtfully choose a measure (novel or well-established) based on the measure's appropriateness for a particular purpose. The increasingly widespread use of electronic health records (EHRs) brings great potential to systematically collect and evaluate health and health behavior data in research and clinical practice (Estabrooks et al., 2012). Healthcare systems can integrate questionnaires into the EHR (e.g., via patient access portals, at kiosks or tablets during medical visits) to collect data efficiently, systematically, and consistently (Glasgow & Emmons, 2011). However, several risks and challenges accompany this technological advance. Most EHRs are not designed to incorporate information about health behavior; thus, integrating behavioral health tools creates an additional burden on the research/practitioner team (Cifuentes et al., 2015). The use of different measures used at different institutions or by different providers can limit opportunities to compare data across large groups of people. Finally, researchers/clinicians/public health practitioners must consider privacy and confidentiality concerns, as all providers with access to a person's EHR may see sensitive information collected in behavioral research (e.g., high-risk behaviors).

In addition to technological advances, future studies in health behavior research can consider using valid parallel measures to capture common elements of intersectional stigma and discrimination to better understand the multiple, complex factors affecting health disparities and health inequities across populations. Many systems, particularly healthcare, are rooted in policies that uphold discriminatory, stigmatizing, and colonial practices, which disproportionally impact adverse health outcomes for minoritized and marginalized groups (Doubeni et al., 2021; Laurencin & McClinton, 2020). For example, the U.S. Preventive Services Task Force has identified differences in the quality and frequency of preventive health screenings across

114 | • THEORIES, FRAMEWORKS, AND MEASURES RELEVANT TO HEALTH BEHAVIORS

racial groups, and underrepresentation of racial and ethnic minority groups in health research (Doubeni et al., 2021). Health disparities are perpetuated across populations and health conditions when practices rooted in stigma and discrimination are embedded in U.S. institutions as macro-level structural determinants of health (Johnson-Agbakwu et al., 2022). Further, most health behavior data collected at the state and national level do not disaggregate data for racial and ethnic (or sexual and gender identity) subgroups, and parallel data assessing historical, cultural, and sociopolitical stigma and discrimination often do not exist (Sabado-Liwag et al., 2022). To fully understand and appreciate relationships between systems of oppression on various health outcomes for minoritized populations, researchers can consider incorporating valid measures that assess multiple forms of stigma and discrimination to comprehensively understand health disparities and the overall impact of structural factors on health behavior.

SUMMARY KEY POINTS

- Social-ecological models help describe how policy, community, organizational, and interpersonal systems, including structural systems of oppression and privilege, impact health behaviors and disparities in health outcomes.

- Assessments across all levels (individual, community, and population) can be subjective or objective and can be measured in a number of ways, including paper-and-pencil rating forms/surveys/interviews, in vivo observations, biomarker assays, electronic wearable devices, electronic medical record, geocoding, and so forth.

- Psychometrics, such as validity, reliability, sensitivity, and specificity, help determine the strengths and limitations of a particular measure.

- As technology evolves, we may find new ways of combining and triangulating measures of health behaviors, community factors, and health outcomes across levels of the social-ecological model (e.g., using wearable devices to assess individual behaviors *and* location in which those behaviors take place).

- No measure of health behavior is perfect, and individual investigators must determine the most appropriate measures of health behavior given the primary hypothesis, need for accuracy, burden on the participants, and available resources.

DISCUSSION QUESTIONS

1. Consider a health concern that is relevant to your community. If you were asked to participate in a measurement of your own health behavior regarding this health concern, how would you feel about being asked to have your behavior observed objectively versus subjectively? Indirectly versus directly? Would some forms of measurement feel more invasive than others? What would make invasive forms of measurement feel "worth it" in order for you to participate?

2. Review Case Study 6.2, "Example of Objective Measures of Neighborhood and Built Environment." Imagine you live in a neighborhood with a high percentage of adults without a high school diploma; no nearby supermarkets or parks; and a high rate of obesity, type 2 diabetes, and heart disease. A new fast-food chain restaurant expresses interest in opening a location in your neighborhood. The restaurant advertises itself as offering "fresh" and "healthy" options. How would you feel about this restaurant opening near you? How would the opening of such a location affect your life and health, along with the health of your neighbors? What information would you need to form an opinion?

(continued)

DISCUSSION QUESTIONS (*continued*)

3. Consider a hypothetical pandemic much like COVID-19 where populations are advised by the government to socially distance and stay home aside from participating in essential activities. During this pandemic, a group of health researchers launch a study where they ask participants to wear a device that tracks their location at all times. Participants are also asked to log how many people they come into contact with per day. How would you predict a population's willingness to participate in such a study during this hypothetical time? What would be some potential concerns that would deter participants? Would you participate if asked?

4. Do you have any ethical concerns in measuring health-related risk behaviors? Are some populations, such as children, more prone to ethical concerns than others?

5. Review Figure 6.1. How well do you think public policy addressed the needs of the most privileged and most oppressed members of your community? What were the gaps in need that were not addressed? What resources would have helped those who needed assistance the most during the height of the COVID-19 pandemic?

A robust set of instructor resources designed to supplement this text is located at http://connect.springerpub.com/content/book/978-0-8261-4265-8. Qualifying instructors may request access by emailing textbook@springerpub.com.

REFERENCES

Anghel, L. A., Farcas, A. M., & Oprean, R. N. (2019). An overview of the common methods used to measure treatment adherence. *Medicine and Pharmacy Reports, 92*(2), 117–122. https://doi.org/10.15386/mpr-1201

Aylward, B. S., Rausch, J. R., & Modi, A. C. (2015). An examination of 1-year adherence and persistence rates to antiepileptic medication in children with newly diagnosed epilepsy. *Journal of Pediatric Psychology, 40*(1), 66–74. https://doi.org/10.1093/jpepsy/jsu010

Baral, S., Logie, C. H., Grosso, A., Wirtz, A. L., & Beyrer, C. (2013). Modified social ecological model: A tool to guide the assessment of the risks and risk contexts of HIV epidemics. *BMC Public Health, 13*(1), 482. https://doi.org/10.1186/1471-2458-13-482

Bufferd, S. J., Dougherty, L. R., Olino, T. M., Dyson, M. W., Laptook, R. S., Carlson, G. A., & Klein, D. N. (2014). Predictors of the onset of depression in young children: A multi-method, multi-informant longitudinal study from ages 3 to 6. *Journal of Child Psychology and Psychiatry, 55*(11), 1279–1287. https://doi.org/10.1111/jcpp.12252

Buysse, D. J., Reynolds, C. F., Monk, T. H., Berman, S. R., & Kupfer, D. J. (1989). The Pittsburgh Sleep Quality Index: A new instrument for psychiatric practice and research. *Psychiatry Research, 28*(2), 193–213. https://doi.org/10.1016/0165-1781(89)90047-4

Cifuentes, M., Davis, M., Fernald, D., Gunn, R., Dickinson, P., & Cohen, D. J. (2015). Electronic health record challenges, workarounds, and solutions observed in practices integrating behavioral health and primary care. *The Journal of the American Board of Family Medicine, 28*(Suppl. 1), S63–S72. https://doi.org/10.3122/jabfm.2015.S1.150133

Clarke, W. L., Gonder-Frederick, L. A., Snyder, A. L., & Cox, D. J. (1998). Maternal fear of hypoglycemia in their children with insulin dependent diabetes mellitus. *Journal of Pediatric Endocrinology and Metabolism, 11*(Suppl. 1), 189–194. https://doi.org/10.1515/jpem.1998.11.s1.189

Conley, S., Knies, A., Batten, J., Ash, G., Miner, B., Hwang, Y., Jeon, S., & Redeker, N. S. (2019). Agreement between actigraphic and polysomnographic measures of sleep in adults with and without chronic conditions: A systematic review and meta-analysis. *Sleep Medicine Reviews, 46*, 151–160. https://doi.org/10.1016/j.smrv.2019.05.001

Conn, V. S., & Ruppar, T. M. (2017). Medication adherence outcomes of 771 intervention trials: Systematic review and meta-analysis. *Preventive Medicine, 99,* 269–276. https://doi.org/10.1016/j.ypmed.2017.03.008

Do, B., Zink, J., Mason, T. B., Belcher, B. R., & Dunton, G. F. (2022). Physical activity and sedentary time among mothers of school-aged children: Differences in accelerometer-derived pattern metrics by demographic, employment, and household factors. *Women's Health Issues, 32*(5), 490–498. https://doi.org/10.1016/j.whi.2022.03.005

Doherty, K., Balaskas, A., & Doherty, G. (2020). The design of ecological momentary assessment technologies. *Interacting with Computers, 32*(1), 257–278. https://doi.org/10.1093/iwcomp/iwaa019

Doubeni, C. A., Simon, M., & Krist, A. H. (2021). Addressing systemic racism through clinical preventive service recommendations from the US Preventive Services Task Force. *JAMA, 325*(7), 627–628. https://doi.org/10.1001/jama.2020.26188

Dugas, L. R., Harders, R., Merrill, S., Ebersole, K., Shoham, D. A., Rush, E. C., Assah, F. K., Forrester, T., Durazo-Arvizu, R. A., & Luke, A. (2011). Energy expenditure in adults living in developing compared with industrialized countries: A meta-analysis of doubly labeled water studies. *The American Journal of Clinical Nutrition, 93*(2), 427–441. https://doi.org/10.3945/ajcn.110.007278

England, C. Y., Andrews, R. C., Jago, R., & Thompson, J. L. (2015). A systematic review of brief dietary questionnaires suitable for clinical use in the prevention and management of obesity, cardiovascular disease and type 2 diabetes. *European Journal of Clinical Nutrition, 69*(9), 977–1003. Article 9. https://doi.org/10.1038/ejcn.2015.6

Erwin, A. M., & Bashore, L. (2017). Subjective sleep measures in children: Self-report. *Frontiers in Pediatrics.* https://doi.org/10.3389/fped.2017.00022

Estabrooks, P. A., Boyle, M., Emmons, K. M., Glasgow, R. E., Hesse, B. W., Kaplan, R. M., Krist, A. H., Moser, R. P., & Taylor, M. V. (2012). Harmonized patient-reported data elements in the electronic health record: Supporting meaningful use by primary care action on health behaviors and key psychosocial factors. *Journal of the American Medical Informatics Association, 19*(4), 575–582. https://doi.org/10.1136/amiajnl-2011-000576

Fletcher-Lartey, S. M., & Caprarelli, G. (2016). Application of GIS technology in public health: Successes and challenges. *Parasitology, 143*(4), 401–415. https://doi.org/10.1017/S0031182015001869

Garfield, S., Clifford, S., Eliasson, L., Barber, N., & Willson, A. (2011). Suitability of measures of self-reported medication adherence for routine clinical use: A systematic review. *BMC Medical Research Methodology, 11*(1), 149. https://doi.org/10.1186/1471-2288-11-149

Glanz, K., Fultz, A. K., Sallis, J. F., Clawson, M., McLaughlin, K. C., Green, S., & Saelens, B. E. (2023). Use of the nutrition environment measures survey: A systematic review. *American Journal of Preventive Medicine, 65*(1), 131–142. https://doi.org/10.1016/j.amepre.2023.02.008

Glasgow, R., & Emmons, K. M. (2011). The public health need for patient-reported measures and health behaviors in electronic health records: A policy statement of the Society of Behavioral Medicine. *Translational Behavioral Medicine, 1*(1), 108–109. https://doi.org/10.1007/s13142-011-0017-3

Gonzalez, J. S., & Schneider, H. E. (2011). Methodological issues in the assessment of diabetes treatment adherence. *Current Diabetes Reports, 11*(6), 472–479. https://doi.org/10.1007/s11892-011-0229-4

Greenlund, K. J. (2022). PLACES: Local data for better health. *Preventing Chronic Disease, 19,* 210459. https://doi.org/10.5888/pcd19.210459

Hallal, P. C., Andersen, L. B., Bull, F. C., Guthold, R., Haskell, W., & Ekelund, U. (2012). Global physical activity levels: Surveillance progress, pitfalls, and prospects. *The Lancet, 380*(9838), 247–257. https://doi.org/10.1016/S0140-6736(12)60646-1

Hart, J. E., Jeon, C. Y., Ivers, L. C., Behforouz, H. L., Caldas, A., Drobac, P. C., & Shin, S. S. (2010). Effect of directly observed therapy for highly active antiretroviral therapy on virologic, immunologic, and adherence outcomes: A meta-analysis and systematic review. *Journal of Acquired Immune Deficiency Syndromes (1999), 54*(2), 167–179. https://doi.org/10.1097/QAI.0b013e3181d9a330

Hatzenbuehler, M. L. (2017). Advancing research on structural stigma and sexual orientation disparities in mental health among youth. *Journal of Clinical Child and Adolescent Psychology, 46*(3), 463–475. https://doi.org/10.1080/15374416.2016.1247360

Hatzenbuehler, M. L., & Link, B. G. (2014). Introduction to the special issue on structural stigma and health. *Social Science & Medicine, 103,* 1–6. https://doi.org/10.1016/j.socscimed.2013.12.017

Hills, A. P., Mokhtar, N., & Byrne, N. M. (2014). Assessment of physical activity and energy expenditure: An overview of objective measures. *Frontiers in Nutrition, 1.* https://www.frontiersin.org/articles/10.3389/fnut.2014.00005

Hommel, K. A., Davis, C. M., & Baldassano, R. N. (2009). Objective versus subjective assessment of oral medication adherence in pediatric inflammatory bowel disease. *Inflammatory Bowel Diseases, 15*(4), 589–593. https://doi.org/10.1002/ibd.20798

Hosseini, B., Berthon, B. S., Saedisomeolia, A., Starkey, M. R., Collison, A., Wark, P. A. B., & Wood, L. G. (2018). Effects of fruit and vegetable consumption on inflammatory biomarkers and immune cell populations: A systematic literature review and meta-analysis. *The American Journal of Clinical Nutrition, 108*(1), 136–155. https://doi.org/10.1093/ajcn/nqy082

Johns, M. W. (1991). A new method for measuring daytime sleepiness: The Epworth Sleepiness Scale. *Sleep, 14*(6), 540–545. https://doi.org/10.1093/sleep/14.6.540

Johnson-Agbakwu, C. E., Ali, N. S., Oxford, C. M., Wingo, S., Manin, E., & Coonrod, D. V. (2022). Racism, COVID-19, and health inequity in the USA: A call to action. *Journal of Racial and Ethnic Health Disparities, 9*(1), 52–58. https://doi.org/10.1007/s40615-020-00928-y

Jones, M., & Johnston, D. (2011). Understanding phenomena in the real world: The case for real time data collection in health services research. *Journal of Health Services Research & Policy, 16*(3), 172–176. https://doi.org/10.1258/jhsrp.2010.010016

Khan, M. A., Saeed, N., Ahmad, A. W., & Lee, C. (2017). Location awareness in 5G networks using RSS measurements for public safety applications. *IEEE Access, 5*, 21753–21762. https://doi.org/10.1109/ACCESS.2017.2750238

Kichler, J. C., Kaugars, A. S., Maglio, K., & Alemzadeh, R. (2012). Exploratory analysis of the relationships among different methods of assessing adherence and glycemic control in youth with type 1 diabetes mellitus. *Health Psychology, 31*, 35–42. https://doi.org/10.1037/a0024704

Kindig, D., & Stoddart, G. (2003). What is population health?. American Journal of Public Health, 93(3), 380–383. https://doi.org/10.2105/ajph.93.3.380

Koschack, J., Marx, G., Schnakenberg, J., Kochen, M. M., & Himmel, W. (2010). Comparison of two self-rating instruments for medication adherence assessment in hypertension revealed insufficient psychometric properties. *Journal of Clinical Epidemiology, 63*(3), 299–306. https://doi.org/10.1016/j.jclinepi.2009.06.011

Lattanner, M. R., Ford, J., Bo, N., Tu, W., Pachankis, J. E., Dodge, B., & Hatzenbuehler, M. L. (2021). A contextual approach to the psychological study of identity concealment: Examining direct, interactive, and indirect effects of structural stigma on concealment motivation across proximal and distal geographic levels. *Psychological Science, 32*(10), 1684–1696. https://doi.org/10.1177/09567976211018624

Laurencin, C. T., & McClinton, A. (2020). The COVID-19 pandemic: A call to action to identify and address racial and ethnic disparities. *Journal of Racial and Ethnic Health Disparities, 7*(3), 398–402. https://doi.org/10.1007/s40615-020-00756-0

MacQueen, K.M., McLellan, E., Metzger, D.S., Kegeles, S., Strauss, R.P., Scotti, R., Blanchard, L., & Trotter, R.T. (2001) What is community? An evidence-based definition for participatory public health. American Journal of Public Health, 91(12):1929-38. https://doi.org/10.2105/ajph.91.12.1929.

Martin, C. K., Correa, J. B., Han, H., Allen, H. R., Rood, J. C., Champagne, C. M., Gunturk, B. K., & Bray, G. A. (2012). Validity of the Remote Food Photography Method (RFPM) for estimating energy and nutrient intake in near real-time. *Obesity, 20*(4), 891–899. https://doi.org/10.1038/oby.2011.344

Matthews, C. E., Hagströmer, M., Pober, D. M., & Bowles, H. R. (2012). Best practices for using physical activity monitors in population-based research. *Medicine and Science in Sports and Exercise, 44*(1 Suppl. 1), S68–S76. https://doi.org/10.1249/MSS.0b013e3182399e5b

Meltzer, L. J., Montgomery-Downs, H. E., Insana, S. P., & Walsh, C. M. (2012). Use of actigraphy for assessment in pediatric sleep research. *Sleep Medicine Reviews, 16*(5), 463–475. https://doi.org/10.1016/j.smrv.2011.10.002

Mesic, A., Franklin, L., Cansever, A., Potter, F., Sharma, A., Knopov, A., & Siegel, M. (2018). The relationship between structural racism and black-white disparities in fatal police shootings at the state level. *Journal of the National Medical Association, 110*(2), 106–116. https://doi.org/10.1016/j.jnma.2017.12.002

Mokdad, A. H. (2009). The behavioral risk factors surveillance system: Past, present, and future. *Annual Review of Public Health, 30*(1), 43–54. https://doi.org/10.1146/annurev.publhealth.031308.100226

Monzon, A. D., McDonough, R., Cushing, C. C., Clements, M., & Patton, S. R. (2023). Examining the relationship between nighttime glucose values in youth with type 1 diabetes and parent fear of nighttime hypoglycemia. *Pediatric Diabetes, 2023*, e9953662. https://doi.org/10.1155/2023/9953662

Mortazavi, B. J., & Gutierrez-Osuna, R. (2023). A review of digital innovations for diet monitoring and precision nutrition. *Journal of Diabetes Science and Technology, 17*(1), 217–223. https://doi.org/10.1177/19322968211041356

Musa, G. J., Chiang, P.-H., Sylk, T., Bavley, R., Keating, W., Lakew, B., Tsou, H.-C., & Hoven, C. W. (2013). Use of GIS mapping as a public health tool—From cholera to cancer. *Health Services Insights, 6*, 111–116. https://doi.org/10.4137/HSI.S10471

Nguyen, Q. C., Sajjadi, M., McCullough, M., Pham, M., Nguyen, T. T., Yu, W., Meng, H.-W., Wen, M., Li, F., Smith, K. R., Brunisholz, K., & Tasdizen, T. (2018). Neighbourhood looking glass: 360o automated characterisation of the built environment for neighbourhood effects research. *Journal of Epidemiology and Community Health, 72*(3), 260–266. https://doi.org/10.1136/jech-2017-209456

Nieuwkerk, P. T., de Boer-van der Kolk, I. M., Prins, J. M., Locadia, M., & Sprangers, M. A. (2010). Self-reported adherence is more predictive of virological treatment response among patients with a lower tendency towards socially desirable responding. *Antiviral Therapy, 15*(6), 913–916. https://doi.org/10.3851/IMP1644

Patton, S. R., Driscoll, K. A., & Clements, M. A. (2017). Adherence to insulin pump behaviors in young children with type 1 diabetes mellitus: Opportunities for intervention. *Journal of Diabetes Science and Technology, 11*(1), 87–91. https://doi.org/10.1177/1932296816658901

Prince, S. A., Adamo, K. B., Hamel, M. E., Hardt, J., Gorber, S. C., & Tremblay, M. (2008). A comparison of direct versus self-report measures for assessing physical activity in adults: A systematic review. *International Journal of Behavioral Nutrition and Physical Activity, 5*(1), 56. https://doi.org/10.1186/1479-5868-5-56

Raghunathan, T., Ghosh, K., Rosen, A., Imbriano, P., Stewart, S., Bondarenko, I., Messer, K., Berglund, P., Shaffer, J., & Cutler, D. (2021). Combining information from multiple data sources to assess population health. *Journal of Survey Statistics and Methodology, 9*(3), 598–625. https://doi.org/10.1093/jssam/smz047

Richman, L. S., & Hatzenbuehler, M. L. (2014). A multilevel analysis of stigma and health: Implications for research and policy. *Policy Insights from the Behavioral and Brain Sciences, 1*(1), 213–221. https://doi.org/10.1177/2372732214548862

Rundo, J. V., & Downey, R. (2019). Polysomnography. In K. H. Levin & P. Chauvel (Eds.), *Handbook of clinical neurology* (Vol. 160, pp. 381–392). Elsevier. https://doi.org/10.1016/B978-0-444-64032-1.00025-4

Rynders, C. A., Morton, S. J., Bessesen, D. H., Wright, K. P., Jr., & Broussard, J. L. (2020). Circadian rhythm of substrate oxidation and hormonal regulators of energy balance. *Obesity, 28*(S1), S104–S113. https://doi.org/10.1002/oby.22816

Sabado-Liwag, M. D., Manalo-Pedro, E., Taggueg, R., Bacong, A. M., Adia, A., Demanarig, D., Sumibcay, J. R., Valderama-Wallace, C., Oronce, C. I. A., Bonus, R., & Ponce, N. A. (2022). Addressing the interlocking impact of colonialism and racism on Filipinx/a/o American health inequities. *Health Affairs, 41*(2), 289–295. https://doi.org/10.1377/hlthaff.2021.01418

Sallis, J. F., & Owen, N. (2015). Ecological models of health behavior. In V. Viswanath, B. K. Rimer, & K. Glanz (Eds.), *Health behavior: Theory, research, and practice* (5th ed., pp. 43–64). Jossey-Bass.

Sharifi, M., Sequist, T. D., Rifas-Shiman, S. L., Melly, S. J., Duncan, D. T., Horan, C. M., Smith, R. L., Marshall, R., & Taveras, E. M. (2016). The role of neighborhood characteristics and the built environment in understanding racial/ethnic disparities in childhood obesity. *Preventive Medicine, 91*, 103–109. https://doi.org/10.1016/j.ypmed.2016.07.009

Shi, Q., Herbert, C., Ward, D. V., Simin, K., McCormick, B. A., Iii, R. T. E., & Zai, A. H. (2022). COVID-19 variant surveillance and social determinants in Central Massachusetts: Development study. *JMIR Formative Research, 6*(6), e37858. https://doi.org/10.2196/37858

Sternfeld, B., & Goldman-Rosas, L. (2012). A systematic approach to selecting an appropriate measure of self-reported physical activity or sedentary behavior. *Journal of Physical Activity and Health, 9*(s1), S19–S28. https://doi.org/10.1123/jpah.9.s1.s19

Stirratt, M. J., Dunbar-Jacob, J., Crane, H. M., Simoni, J. M., Czajkowski, S., Hilliard, M. E., Aikens, J. E., Hunter, C. M., Velligan, D. I., Huntley, K., Ogedegbe, G., Rand, C. S., Schron, E., & Nilsen, W. J. (2015). Self-report measures of medication adherence behavior: Recommendations on optimal use. *Translational Behavioral Medicine, 5*(4), 470–482. https://doi.org/10.1007/s13142-015-0315-2

Stull, D. E., Leidy, N. K., Parasuraman, B., & Chassany, O. (2009). Optimal recall periods for patient-reported outcomes: Challenges and potential solutions. *Current Medical Research and Opinion, 25*(4), 929–942. https://doi.org/10.1185/03007990902774765

Underwood, J. M., Brener, N., Thornton, J., Harris, W. A., Bryan, L. N., Shanklin, S. L., Deputy, N., Roberts, A. M., Queen, B., Chyen, D., Whittle, L., Lim, C., Yamakawa, Y., Leon-Nguyen, M., Kilmer, G., Smith-Grant, J., Demissie, Z., Jones, S. E., Clayton, H., & Dittus, P. (2020). Overview and methods for the youth risk behavior surveillance system—United States, 2019. *MMWR Supplements, 69*(1), 1–10. https://doi.org/10.15585/mmwr.su6901a1

Van De Water, A. T. M., Holmes, A., & Hurley, D. A. (2011). Objective measurements of sleep for non-laboratory settings as alternatives to polysomnography—A systematic review. *Journal of Sleep Research, 20*(1pt2), 183–200. https://doi.org/10.1111/j.1365-2869.2009.00814.x

Westerterp, K. R. (2017). Doubly labelled water assessment of energy expenditure: Principle, practice, and promise. *European Journal of Applied Physiology, 117*(7), 1277–1285. https://doi.org/10.1007/s00421-017-3641-x

Young, R., Ayiasi, R. M., Shung-King, M., & Morgan, R. (2020). Health systems of oppression: Applying intersectionality in health systems to expose hidden inequities. *Health Policy and Planning, 35*(9), 1228–1230. https://doi.org/10.1093/heapol/czaa111

PART II: PRIORITIZED BEHAVIORS FOR PRIMARY PREVENTION OF DISEASE

CHAPTER 7

DIETARY BEHAVIOR CHANGE

TRACY E. CRANE AND SAMANTHA WERTS-PELTER

LEARNING OBJECTIVES

- Identify barriers to dietary behavior change present at the individual, social, and environmental levels.
- Understand why the distribution of educational materials alone is unlikely to promote change in eating behaviors.
- Recognize the relevance of behavioral theories and constructs in the promotion of eating behaviors.
- Understand behavioral approaches used in patient-centered counseling to promote changes in eating behaviors.
- Observe how electronic and/or mobile technology has contributed to eating behavior change at the individual, group, or community level.

INTRODUCTION

The recurring National Health and Nutrition Examination Survey (NHANES) data (National Center for Health Statistics, 2023), based on self-reported dietary intake, suggest that Americans are on average consuming diets incongruent with the Dietary Guidelines for Americans (Dietary Guidelines for Americans 2020–2025, 2020). Importantly, the quality of dietary intake, measured as overall diet pattern score, is well below what is considered healthy in relation to chronic disease risk reduction. Intake of dietary fat, saturated fat, sodium, and sugar-sweetened beverages exceeds recommendations, and intake of fiber, fruits and vegetables, and omega-3 fatty acids is well below the estimated levels for optimal health (U.S. Department of Agriculture, 2022). Alarmingly, these patterns have persisted for several decades and are a major contributor to the current epidemic of overweight/obesity and obesity-related chronic diseases such as diabetes, cardiovascular disease, as well as several cancers (Centers for Disease Control and Prevention, 2023). This disconnect between what we choose to eat and the well-substantiated risk for disease when less healthy food selections are made has led to an increased interest in eating behavior. Food choices are complex and represent a variety of motivational and contributing factors, such as taste/satisfaction, culture, psychosocial distress, and health, thus making absolute and sustained behavior change challenging. The food environment and regulatory processes also have a large influence on individual dietary behaviors.

Humans must eat to survive and be healthy; thus, avoidance is not a sustainable approach to positive eating behavior change. Eating behaviors require multiple choices repeated on a daily, if not hourly, basis. Each stimulus to eat, from hunger to visual cues, smells, or taste, often acts to promote greater intake of food. The increasing abundance and availability of foods (e.g., 24-hour food delivery) have also promoted greater intake over time. However, beyond abundance and repeated exposures, research suggests that the decision to select healthier, less energy-dense foods is both biological and behavioral.

This chapter serves to inform approaches to dietary behavior change by briefly reviewing the biology of eating; the relevant behavioral theories, constructs, and strategies that have been effectively applied for changing eating behaviors; as well as the modification of environment to promote healthy eating behaviors. The content is largely concentrated on individual behavior change as this has historically been the focus of most interventions. However, there is increasing awareness that policy- and population-level change, frequently implemented within a community, workplace, or clinic, will also be necessary to achieve the magnitude of sustained change in eating behavior necessary to make whole person wellness a reality at the population level. Finally, this chapter explores the role of electronic and mobile technology (mHealth) in promoting healthy eating behaviors.

THE BIOLOGY OF EATING

The drive to consume energy is largely driven by paracrine, endocrine, metabolic, and hormonal signaling pathways (Nogueiras, 2021). These complex pathways secrete signals that communicate hunger and satiety to regulate energy balance in our bodies. **Figure 7.1** illustrates several of these key regulatory factors within the brain and gastrointestinal tract that regulate energy balance and appetite control (Blundell et al., 2020). While the human body

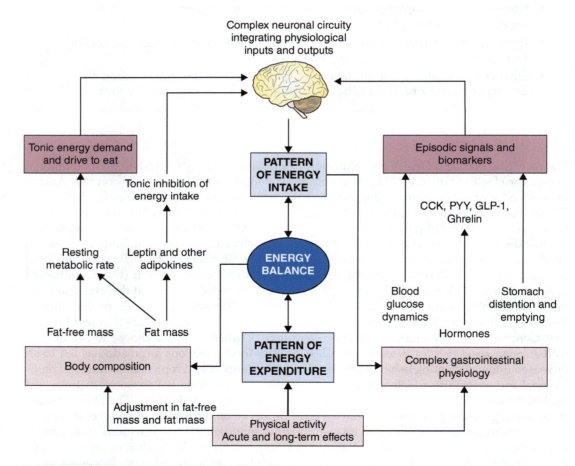

FIGURE 7.1 Biology of eating behavior.
CCK, cholecystokinin; GLP-1, glucagon-like peptide-1; PYY, pancreatic polypeptide.
Source: Adapted from Blundell, J. E., Gibbons, C., Beaulieu, K., Casanova, N., Duarte, C., Finlayson, G., Stubbs, R. J., & Hopkins, M. (2020). The drive to eat in homo sapiens: Energy expenditure drives energy intake. *Physiology & Behavior, 219*, 112846. https://doi.org/10.1016/j.physbeh.2020.112846.

has sophisticated regulatory feedback systems to optimize energy control, behavioral factors have a profound impact on these systems, particularly within the human brain and gastrointestinal tract. Furthermore, research on self-regulation of appetite suggests this is a complex pathophysiology, and the heterogeneity of the biological influences on eating behavior at the individual level demonstrates that behavioral therapy to promote changes in eating behavior will also have highly variable responses and is consistently demonstrated in both practice and clinical trial research (Dohle et al., 2018).

THE BEHAVIOR OF EATING

Beyond biology, there is a significant, not fully understood role for behavior in food choices. Behavioral influences on intake include conditioned responses such as food preferences, aversions, and satiations, as well as cognitive behavioral factors such as social influences, cultural norms, and esthetics. In addition, ecological influences such as relative energy densities and nutrient drivers must also be considered when examining the role of behavior on dietary choices. To illustrate in a more applied way, behavioral influences include a variety of factors, such as stimulus response (chocolate as a "comfort food"), knowledge ("Consume calcium-rich dairy for bone health"), social influences ("Mom said eat your vegetables"), behavioral norms (daily lattes), role modeling ("Grandpa always avoided salt"), aversions/ attitudes ("olives make me ill"), and even reinforcement ("Coffee/beer taste wonderful").

Approaches to help individuals modify their eating behaviors generally support attainment of the Dietary Guidelines for Americans, or some adaptation thereof, and require behavioral treatment or other interventions. New approaches, such as nutritional coaching, are person-centered and are likely to be more sustainable than traditional methods of diet restriction alone (Dayan et al., 2019). Effective behavioral treatment must be goal-directed, process-oriented, and advocate for small rather than large change. Frequently, the approach will integrate multiple components, from self-monitoring to stimulus control and cognitive restructuring.

Individual Dietary Behavior Change

Individual behaviors surrounding food choices may reflect personal health behavior, health-related behavior change, or health (dietary) protective behavior. Personal health behavior reflects food choices that result in a direct effect on the individual's health. These behaviors may or may not be driven by a desire to improve one's health. Food choices are more commonly the result of taste, habits, availability, beliefs, and attitudes that may indirectly alter health status despite the original or primary motivational factor driving the eating behavior. Health-related behavior change differs from personal health behavior as it captures behaviors of others that indirectly improve the target individual's health status. This would include the behaviors of friends, family members, or perhaps even administrators and policy makers that affect the eating behavior of others. For example, the dietary behaviors of children and adolescents are largely dependent on those of their primary caregivers. Depending on life stage, a multigenerational or community-based dietary intervention may be more successful at eliciting dietary behavior change than an individually focused strategy. Health-protective eating behaviors are behaviors that are undertaken with the primary, if not the sole, intent of improving a specific health indicator (e.g., serum cholesterol, blood pressure), whether it is risk reduction for disease or control/treatment of disease.

Historically, changing dietary behaviors at the individual level has relied on trained professionals (registered dietitian, nutritionists, medical doctors, registered nurses, etc.) who provide education on specific facts and/or knowledge for the individual using an advice-giving mode to elicit the desired change. While this approach may result in short-term modest improvements in food choices in a small percentage of individuals, there is a significant body of literature demonstrating that these approaches to behavior change fail in terms of magnitude of change needed as well as the duration of change realized. Those trained in behavioral medicine understand that these approaches often fail to engage the patient in the decision-making process or to ensure that the patient has made a conscientious effort to determine the value of specific dietary behavior changes in the context of their own risk–benefit evaluation. Reliance on trained professionals to provide nutrition education is not generally feasible for medically underserved and underresourced communities with limited access to healthcare professionals. It also does little to address the systemic barriers to healthy eating, such as food accessibility, cost, and marketing. Yet, beyond nutritional counseling, these approaches are broadly applied in many behavioral healthcare practices. A more productive patient-centered approach that engages the patient in developing plans and motivation for change has been demonstrated to be effective (Martins & McNeil, 2009; Ockene et al., 1999) and should be considered for long-term, sustainable change.

Common Barriers to Healthy Eating

Beyond imparting knowledge and engaging the patient, efforts have also been undertaken to identify barriers to making healthy food choices (Table 7.1). These barriers may be present at the individual, social, or environmental level, or a combination thereof. Recent research

TABLE 7.1 Barriers to Change in Eating Behaviors to Achieve Recommended Diet Intake Patterns for Optimal Health

Individual	Lack of knowledge
	Financial/food insecurity
	Lack of or limited motivation
	Low perceived risk; insufficient benefit
	Hunger
	Taste
	Lack of awareness; mindfulness
	Habituation of food intake
	Stress/coping
Social	Cultural norms
	Holiday or religious practices
	Family composition/social isolation
	Meals consumed at home or away from home
	Shared meal environment
	Food-related memories
	Lack of social support for healthy behaviors
	Social media as venue to promote food intake; share recipes
Environmental	Food accessibility; lack of supermarkets
	Food policy and regulation
	External stimuli
	Food marketing
	Frequency of food exposures
	Quality of food exposures

evaluating social influence on intake suggests that people will adapt their food choices based on the choices of others or to present a more favorable impression of themselves (Higgs & Ruddock, 2020). There is also inequitable access to fresh, healthy food across different socio-economic, racial, ethnic, and geographic lines that influences individual eating behaviors. For example, low-income and marginalized neighborhoods are more likely to be targeted by sugar subsidies and other discriminatory food regulation policies that result in a greater availability of sugary beverages and snacks instead of nutrient-dense foods (O'Hara & Toussaint, 2021). It is important to consider how societal and environmental inequities may be influencing individual dietary habits and how addressing upstream determinants can positively support nutrition.

Habituation as a Determinant of Dietary Behavior

Epstein and colleagues suggest that habituation of intake is an important determinant of food selection and thus may be an important determinant of resistance to change (Epstein et al., 2009). Food intake, in this context, is the result of repeated exposure to orosensory cues that drive the decision to eat. These same cues may drive decisions related to stoppage of eating and thus contribute to an individual's propensity toward obesity. To dishabituate a behavior is challenging in that it requires both an awareness of the habit and cues stimulating a specific eating decision and the capacity to alter or override these habit-associated cues to make a different decision around the food behavior. To dishabituate, stimuli need to be removed or altered. For example, stimuli include, but are not limited to, who the meal is shared with, time of day, sensory influences (McCrickerd & Forde, 2016), and related factors that may promote what has been labeled as "mindless eating" (Ogden et al., 2013). One example of a common habituated dietary pattern is eating popcorn during a movie. People often eat larger quantities of popcorn and other candies and snacks when they are distracted by other sensory cues. To promote dishabituation of this eating behavior, one intervention may include replacing less nutrient-dense foods, like buttered popcorn, with healthier alternatives, such as plain popcorn or carrot sticks.

PROMOTION OF HEALTHY EATING

Role of Diet Education

There are several approaches to behavior change. Commonly, healthcare providers employ one-way delivery of information, or education, to help patients change eating behavior. For example, clinicians may provide dietary handouts explaining how to reduce dietary fat, salt/sodium, or even portion sizes. Lack of information is a barrier to effective change in dietary behaviors. Evidence exists to suggest that filling knowledge gaps can enhance diet change toward healthier food choices, as has been demonstrated with teacher-delivered nutrition education programs for elementary-age students (Cotton et al., 2020) and education interventions to improve nutrition knowledge in athletes (Tam et al., 2019). However, these materials are frequently printed in mass without formative work to determine patient understanding, interpretation, and/or ability to employ the information to change their dietary behavior. In some cases, the materials are not adapted to different cultural norms or expectations, or may reflect a relatively verbatim translation without modification for cultural context. Seldom is health literacy evaluated during the development of educational materials, resulting in handouts that frequently include medical terminology, mathematical computations, and reading levels that are beyond the literacy level of the target population. Further, this unidirectional approach is unlikely to result in long-term effectiveness given the complexity of eating behavior and the multiplicity of factors that contribute to the individual's risk-to-benefit assessment that can lead to significant changes in food choices. Dissemination of information without application of behavioral theory is likely to ignore important psychological, social (inter- and intrapersonal), environmental, cultural, and even economic constraints (Walters et al., 2020).

Importantly, even if the information provided through education fills a gap in the patient's knowledge, there is limited evidence that education alone impacts behavior change in relation to achieving complex healthy eating goals.

Behavior Theories and Constructs

Promoting healthy eating is complex, and it is clear that a number of behavioral theories inform on best practice to support healthy food choices. However, these theories must be integrated into a larger context of eating behavior to have relevance in the context of the scientific study of eating behavior. In 2015, the University College of London published an informative conference proceeding focused on establishing a framework for the application of behavioral theories to effectively intervene on dietary selections and eating practices (Atkins & Michie, 2015). **Figure 7.2** illustrates the framework, integrating the multiple and varied sources of behavior, intervention functions, and policy.

A number of behavior change theories have been applied to dietary behavior. Commonly applied theories and constructs are described in **Table 7.2** (see the chapters in Part I, "Theories, Frameworks, and Measures Relevant to Health Behaviors," for a more in-depth discussion). Dietary behavior is not only complex in terms of the individual decision to eat or not eat a given food item. This decision-making process is repeated multiple times throughout a day and continuously in an individual's lifetime. Theories developed to help individuals change eating behavior must consider multiple factors at the individual, social unit, and population level that influence and inform each decision to consume or not consume food (**Figure 7.3**).

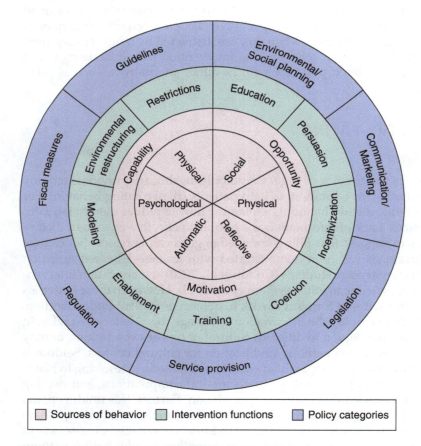

FIGURE 7.2 The behavior change wheel.
Source: From Michie S., Atkins L. & West, R. (2014). *The Behaviour Change Wheel: A Guide to Designing Interventions.* London: Silverback Publishing.

7 • DIETARY BEHAVIOR CHANGE **125**

TABLE 7.2 Behavior Theories Applied to Dietary Change

THEORY	BASIS	STRATEGIES	APPLICATIONS TO DIETARY CHANGE
Health belief model	An individual must feel personally threatened or susceptible to a disease and believe that the benefits of acting outweigh the risks/costs.	Cues that promote eating behavior change under this model: • Individual experiences a family member or close friend diagnosed with a disease • Media campaign or report suggesting disease risk • Notification by a healthcare provider that risk is elevated	A cluster, randomized controlled trial in Kenya found that a culturally sensitive diabetes education intervention utilizing the health belief model to increase diabetes knowledge and awareness significantly increased the perceived susceptibility to diabetes, increased the perceived benefit of eating a healthy diet, and significantly improved dietary intake (Githinji et al., 2022).
Social cognitive theory	Eating behavior is thought to be a function of modeling or observed learning, which is then reinforced to promote self-efficacy.	Individuals learn how to make a specific dietary behavior change through observation and experiential learning, such as: • Cooking demonstration • Grocery store food purchasing trips • Role-playing	The PAWS program was an after-school dietary intervention for adolescents utilizing peer-led and adult-led education to improve self-efficacy related to healthy eating and found significant increases in whole grain intake (Muzaffar et al., 2019).
Self-determination theory	Reinforcement and environmental contingencies are highly effective in influencing behavior but must remain in effect for behavior to be sustained.	Counseling or health coaching that applies this theory will likely incorporate: • Autonomy-supportive behaviors that address the patient's current perspectives and emotions • Problem-solving • Identification of patient aspirations in relation to goal setting • Integration of competence support	The Fit U intervention conducted with Latinx college students utilized self-monitoring of dietary behavior augmented by culturally tailored motivational feedback and goal setting to improve dietary intake. Participants in the intervention significantly improved their perceived dietary competence and significantly improved their consumption of fruit and vegetables (Blow et al., 2022).

(continued)

TABLE 7.2 Behavior Theories Applied to Dietary Change (*continued*)			
THEORY	**BASIS**	**STRATEGIES**	**APPLICATIONS TO DIETARY CHANGE**
Transtheoretical model	Behavior change involves a sequence of "events" or stages that build toward sustained behavior change.	Can be applied to: • Screen patients for eligibility in interventions or dietary change programs • Identify which stage of change the individual is currently in, such as the contemplation or preparation stage • Incorporate stage-specific tactics to encourage participant behavior change	A 7-month, randomized controlled trial conducted in Brazil tested a transtheoretical model-based nutritional intervention on fruit and vegetable intake. The intervention included workshops, motivational messaging, and educational materials designed for each stage of change. They found that the intervention materials successfully promoted progression through the stages of change and increased fruit and vegetable intake (Mendonça et al., 2022).

PAWS, Peer-education About Weight Steadiness.

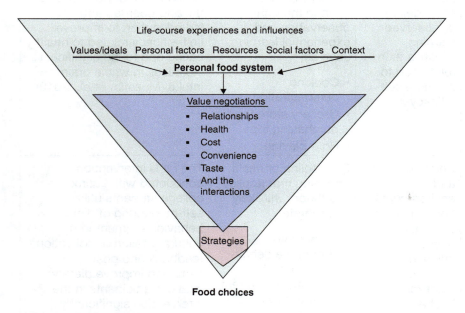

FIGURE 7.3 The food choice model.
Sources: Furst, T., Connors, M., Bisogni, C. A., Sobal, J., & Falk, L. W. (1996). Food choice: a conceptual model of the process. Appetite, 26(3), 247-265. Adapted from Foster, G. D., Makris, A. P., & Bailer, B. A. (2005). Behavioral treatment of obesity. *The American Journal of Clinical Nutrition, 82*(1 Suppl.), 230S–235S. https://doi.org/10.1093/ajcn/82.1.230S.

Of note, the application of theories to promote eating behavior change is reportedly inconsistent, and interventions that do apply theory may not change eating behavior any more so than interventions that do not (Dalgetty et al., 2019).

Although many different terms and phrases are used, there are several concepts that are consistent across theories. First, awareness is critical for change to take place. The individual must first understand the need for change. Next, support is critical in not only initial change but especially for long-term, sustained changes. Support is needed not only in the form of other individuals offering assistance and encouragement, but in one's environment as well. These supports can in turn support the confidence that an individual has in their ability to change. With these in place, the likelihood of change is significantly increased. Many of the behavioral approaches outlined next are intended to directly impact awareness, support, and confidence.

BEHAVIORAL APPROACHES: TOWARD HEALTHIER DIETARY CHOICES

Goal Setting

Goal setting is an important component of dietary behavior change. Goals not only provide the necessary clarity regarding structure, specificity, and expected outcomes, they also support self-efficacy over time. Goal setting should include both short- and long-term goals. Short-terms goals, if achieved, should promote the eventual achievement of long-term goals as well. Short-term goals should follow the SMART goal model (**S**pecific, **M**easurable, **A**ttainable, **R**ealistic, **T**imely) to be effective in promoting the desired behavior change and be developed in collaboration with the person to individualize the goal to address barriers identified that may hinder their success in achieving the goal. For example, a short-term goal to eat vegetables every day is unlikely to be successful if the individual has reported that there are no available vegetable options to eat at their place of work where they spend 8 hours each day. Instead, the short-term goal should be developed to address this barrier to dietary behavior change and could be revised to: "I will eat two servings of vegetables during each workday. I will prepare the vegetables at home and take them with me to work. These will include raw carrot or celery sticks that I keep at my desk, a salad I prepare, or a leftover vegetable dish from dinner that I will reheat in the break area microwave at lunch time." This level of specificity promotes behavior change in a way that is attainable and realistic within the individual's "influences" on dietary decision-making, has a set timeline, and success can be measured. Although goal setting is infrequently studied as a "stand-alone" behavioral component, it has been demonstrated that personalized goal setting has the greatest potential impact on behavior change. Goal setting is most effective when accompanied with self-monitoring (White et al., 2020).

Self-Monitoring

Self-monitoring in the context of diet is the act of recording a specific dietary behavior on an ongoing basis. The value of self-monitoring lies in repeated awareness or cues for healthy decisions. However, the recorded self-monitoring information must align with the short- and long-term goals that have been set. For example, recording all foods consumed may be relevant when energy intake goals have been set for weight loss, but may overburden patients and have less relevance when the target behavior is reduced sodium intake for blood pressure control. In this situation, having individuals record only sodium content from labels of foods consumed and/or use of saltshaker/packets may have more relevance and be more feasible and sustainable for self-monitoring behavior. Components of eating behavior that are frequently self-monitored for diet change include not only tracking of overall diet and specific nutrients (sodium, fiber, fat, fruit, and vegetables), but also meal spacing, location, timing, rate of eating, and stimulus control.

Self-monitoring can be challenging to initiate. Matching the approach to the individual can facilitate success in this area. For example, a younger person may have resisted writing down all foods consumed in a diary format but may wish to use a smartphone app to record intake and find the immediate evaluation of outcome (sum of sodium intake throughout the day), motivating them to continue self-monitoring. The frequency of self-monitoring is also important. The general practice is to recommend that dietary monitoring be completed daily at least in the initial change period (6–12 weeks). After this point, self-monitoring frequency may be reduced without marked recidivism in behavior, but should not be eliminated as a behavior change strategy all together. Self-monitoring should also be increased in frequency and adjusted in context as new barriers to change are identified and new approaches to achieving long-term health goals are set. With recent advances in mHealth technology, the use of electronic applications for self-monitoring has become more common. Recent systematic reviews suggest that the use of mHealth self-monitoring tools is correlated with greater adherence to lifestyle tracking than traditional paper tracking and greater adherence to lifestyle interventions (Cavero-Redondo et al., 2020; Patel et al., 2021). Another systematic review suggested any self-monitoring, regardless of method applied, can support regulation of food intake (Semper et al., 2016). A caveat to the use of digital self-monitoring is that there is limited evidence in underserved and underrepresented populations and there is a potential to promote health inequities if proper adaptation and resource availability are not considered (Paldan et al., 2018).

Social Support

Support is an important factor for behavior change and increased duration of change over time. It may be in the form of groups, as has been commonly employed in several long-term dietary trials requiring substantial dietary change, including the Women's Health Initiative Dietary Modification Trial (Anderson et al., 2003), the PREDIMED-Plus trial (Fernandez-Lazaro et al., 2022), and the Look AHEAD trial (Look AHEAD Research Group, 2003). Attendance at group sessions has also been associated with greater adherence to dietary goals (Tinker et al., 2007). There is also evidence that group counseling may be more effective than individual phone-based counseling for weight control (Befort et al., 2010).

Beyond group support, perceived support from clinic or study staff throughout trial participation has been shown to promote greater change in eating behaviors. These changes were found to be strongly related to enhanced self-efficacy. Frequency and quality of contact as well as extended duration of contact each may have independent effects on dietary behavior change, and both appear to be integral to the achievement and maintenance of dietary behavioral goals (Ross Middleton et al., 2012).

Additionally, Perri and colleagues have evaluated social support for healthy behaviors and identified an important role for friends and family. This work suggests that family and friend support is associated with greater success in weight loss (Kiernan et al., 2012).

Problem-Solving and Decision-Making

Behavioral approaches to dietary change generally address the issue of problem-solving early in the counseling process. The important issue here is for the patient, rather than the clinician, to identify problems. This is important if there is to be ownership of the short-term goals required to address the problems as identified. Problem-solving requires the use of both cognitive behavioral techniques that not only address the person's perceived barriers to behavior change, but also their prior or planned approaches to overcome these barriers to promote the achievement of dietary goals. The discussion may begin with an open listing of barriers, followed by a review of usual daily activities around food that may help identify additional barriers. Developing a diagram of the behavior chain surrounding food choices can help the individual identify barriers that are not as readily apparent without reviewing a typical day's activity and how these may inform eating choices. Case study 7.1 provides an example as to how a behavior chain might be developed in conversation with the patient.

Once barriers have been identified, the discussion can then focus on identifying approaches previously employed that were successful in promoting healthy eating, and specific new strategies that the patient identifies as adoptable for use in meeting dietary behavioral goals. The role of the counselor is to facilitate the identification of barriers as well as change strategies. Problem-solving is not a stand-alone technique, but rather is generally applied within a larger behavioral plan to promote dietary change.

CASE STUDY 7.1: BARRIERS TO HEALTHY EATING

Sarah is an elementary school teacher and a single mother of three. She spends much of her time planning healthy meals for her children but is having a hard time prioritizing her own food intake. On a typical day, she wakes up at 5:30 a.m. and has 30 minutes to get ready for her day before waking up her kids and getting them ready for school. Most of her morning is spent preparing breakfast for her kids and packing their lunches. She skips breakfast and tells herself she will eat something when she gets to work. At work, her morning is filled with teaching, and by the time she has a chance to stop and eat something she is usually starving and quickly grabs a bag of pretzels from the vending machine.

Today, Sarah has lunch monitor duty at school and does not have a chance to eat the salad she packed for lunch until her class goes to gym class later in the day. By this point, she is stressed from her busy workday and still hungry since she has not had enough to eat. She stops by the teachers' lounge and grabs a chocolate bar from the candy jar. Her oldest child was named student of the month today, so on the way home from school she stops at the grocery store and lets the kids pick out a carton of ice cream for dessert. Since Sarah is feeling guilty about eating the chocolate bar at school, she decides to choose a low-calorie option for herself. While the kids do their homework, Sarah jumps on the treadmill for 20 minutes and then makes dinner for her and her family. By 7 p.m., Sarah is starving and decides to take out the ice cream she purchased. She ends up eating half of the carton because she is so hungry and feels defeated about her food choices for the day.

Sarah's experience is like what many people experience when making food choices. People are faced with several decisions about their dietary intake each day and several face unforeseen barriers to making healthy choices. **Figure 7.4** helps to identify where her barriers are for healthy eating and helps to more readily create goals that can address these challenges.

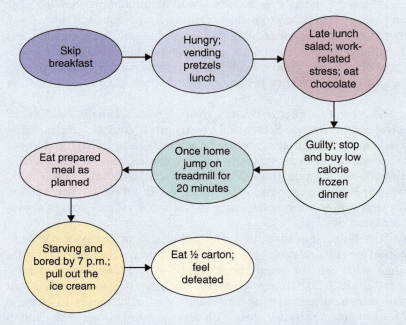

FIGURE 7.4 Sarah's food behavior decision-making: Identifying barriers to change.
Source: Adapted from Foster, G. D., Makris, A. P., & Bailer, B. A. (2005). Behavioral treatment of obesity. *The American Journal of Clinical Nutrition, 82*(1, Suppl.), 230S–235S. https://doi.org/10.1093/ajcn/82.1.230S.

Intuitive Eating

Eating behavior related to the treatment of obesity is complex. Historically, approaches have centered on energy restriction. These programs, such as intermittent fasting and time-restricted eating, have demonstrated effectiveness, but longer term weight maintenance has been challenging to achieve (Fanti et al., 2021; Nordmo et al., 2020). Intuitive eating has emerged as an alternative approach to intake restriction (Cadena-Schlam & López-Guimerà, 2015). Intuitive eating relies on internal cues and biological regulation of food intake to control overall consumption. Compared with more traditional energy restriction approaches, these approaches have been found to result in higher retention, greater reduction in anxiety and depression, and increased self-esteem, as well as potential superiority in terms of longer term weight control (Babbott et al., 2023; Linardon et al., 2021). However, intuitive eating and mindful eating programs lack evidence derived from scientifically rigorous studies, and additional evidence is needed to determine the impact of these approaches on dietary behaviors and health outcomes (Grider et al., 2021).

Motivational Interviewing

Motivational interviewing (MI) has demonstrated efficacy, perhaps superior to other strategies, in changing behaviors associated with improved health (Bischof et al., 2021). MI is one of the most widely applied strategy to dietary behavior change (Barnes & Ivezaj, 2015). For example, research on the utilization of MI for lifestyle behavior change with adult cancer survivors has shown effectiveness in various settings and with different cancer types and care trajectories (Seven et al., 2022).

MI is a collaborative, person-centered form of guiding individuals to elicit and strengthen motivation for change (Miller & Moyers, 2007). MI helps individuals identify and resolve ambivalence with behaviors targeted for change and centers on motivational processes that facilitate the desired change. MI by nature is a conversation between the patient and the healthcare provider that honors autonomy and is evocative (www.motivationalinterviewing.org). An effective MI interaction has been described to include eight tasks: openness of discussion, proficiency in patient-centered counseling, identifying change and sustain talk, eliciting and strengthening change talk, reflectively hearing sustain and resistance talk, recognizing readiness toward the development of a change plan, consolidating commitment, and transitioning and blending MI techniques with other effective behavioral approaches and strategies (Miller & Moyers, 2007).

MI centers on *resolving ambivalence for effective behavior change while building motivation and encouraging autonomy*. Considering these are behavioral versus physiological outcomes, the results of MI may vary based on the desired intervention target. For example, MI has demonstrated success with dietary behavior change for fruits and vegetables; however, it has documented less success with body weight outcomes (Makin et al., 2021; Michalopoulou et al., 2022). As long-term, sustainable behavior change can be difficult without patient investment, it is important to prioritize and center intervention targets (behavior vs. physiological outcome) based on patient needs and desires.

Importantly, a 2023 systematic review identified that cultural adaptation of MI techniques, specifically adaptation for cultural context, content, and concepts, is more successful at eliciting behavior change with diverse populations compared with control and non-adapted methods (Self et al., 2023). A 2020 narrative systematic review also identified that acknowledgment of culture and incorporation of considerations for variances in cultural norms when utilizing MI lead to greater effectiveness with diverse populations (Bahafzallah et al., 2020). Culturally adapted health coaching has great implications for health equity and may improve the retention, adherence, and engagement of individuals to dietary change programming.

Technology and Mobile Health Strategies

The wealth of new innovations, apps, and devices for dietary assessment, self-monitoring, and behavior change has presented many opportunities as well as new challenges in dietary behavior change. The use of mobile or electronic technology is now considered a relatively routine component of many of the dietary interventions tested to promote eating behavior change (Schoeppe et al., 2016). In 2016, West and Michie published the first guide to digital behavior interventions in healthcare (West & Michie, 2016). This guide seeks to set a best-practice approach and provide the evaluator framework to ensure rigorous study of the efficacy and effectiveness of mobile approaches to behavior change, including assessment of acceptability, practicality, effectiveness, affordability, safety, and equity. A 2019 systematic review found that app-based mHealth interventions for improving dietary behaviors and nutrition-related outcomes are effective and feasible (Villinger et al., 2019).

In the past 5 years, the evidence supporting the achievement of behavior change with technological approaches has increased substantially. New research also highlights the sustainability of behavior change after interventions utilizing mHealth technologies. For example, a 4-year follow-up of the GISMAL (Grupo de Investigación en Salud Móvil en America Latina) study in Peru, which assessed the effects of a 1-year mHealth intervention on blood pressure and body weight in low-resource settings, found that reductions in participant body weight and body mass index (BMI) were sustained up to 5 years postrandomization (Bernabe-Ortiz et al., 2020). The theoretical model that has the most relevance here is likely the diffusion of innovations theory, although several studies using these methods also report use of the social cognitive theory, the transtheoretical model (TTM), and the precaution adoption process (Norman et al., 2007). It should be noted that a 2023 systematic review including 30 studies on digital behavior change interventions to increase vegetable intake found a risk of bias that was quite high at greater than 80%. Few interventions included a behavioral theory and/or involved stakeholders/end users in the intervention design (Livingstone et al., 2023). Beyond theory, mHealth interventions may also have greater success at promoting dietary and physical activity behavior change with attention to user engagement, credibility, interactivity, and persuasion science (Dounavi & Tsoumani, 2019). While mHealth has the potential to increase access to evidence-based remote intervention, there are important considerations for how equitably these types of interventions are disseminated, such as digital literacy, broadband access, technical support, and digital device ownership (Lyles et al., 2021). Lack of consideration for these elements when implementing mHealth-based dietary intervention may perpetuate the barriers that underresourced and marginalized communities face.

Earlier dietary studies focused primarily on the use of telephone-based counseling and CD-ROM delivery of information. More recently, efforts are ongoing to expand to smartphone applications and game-based multimodality interventions to promote dietary behavior change (Eicher-Miller et al., 2021; Srivastava et al., 2022); however, there is a paucity of research providing comparative effectiveness between the methodological approaches employed. In general, evidence does support the ability to promote behavior change using electronic and mobile technology-based approaches, and modest evidence exists for diet-specific approaches (Schoeppe et al., 2016; Villinger et al., 2019).

In terms of smartphone apps, an effort to standardize the evaluation, and thus indirectly the potential effectiveness, has resulted in the development of the Mobile App Rating Scale. Using this scale, Bardus and colleagues suggested that weight management apps were generally of moderate quality and would be expected to promote self-monitoring of eating behavior and ultimately support weight control (Bardus et al., 2016). Others express concern regarding the quality and lack of regulatory oversight to ensure consumers have the tools needed to support weight loss-associated eating (and physical activity) behavior change (McKay et al., 2019). A 2019 systematic review of web- and smartphone-based dietary interventions found that accessible mHealth technologies did promote eating behavior change toward weight management, but that additional research should examine user engagement techniques (Young et al., 2019).

The use of mHealth/eHealth in behavior science is challenged by a rapidly changing technological environment in relation to available apps, devices, and delivery systems, such that by the time a study is complete and reported in the literature, newer, more novel, and perhaps more easily implemented devices and apps may be available. Further, across cultural, gender, education, and age groups, adoption of individual devices and apps can vary widely not only in relation to technology commonly used but also to the frequency of use and time to full adoption. These factors challenge the external validity of the research being done to evaluate e-technology for behavior change, including dietary change.

PROMOTING DIETARY BEHAVIOR CHANGE IN SELECT SETTINGS

Communities/Schools

Owing to the fact that our communities influence our food choices and indirectly food intake, several community and/or school-based interventions have been tested to determine the potential to influence foods consumed in the context of the "real world." These interventions have included menu labeling (Rincón-Gallardo Patiño et al., 2020; Shangguan et al., 2019), portion control, restriction of sale (Gonçalves et al., 2021), and promotion of store-based interventions for health promotion (Mah et al., 2019). Such approaches have shown none to modest effects on intake, generally in relation to slight reductions in total energy intake, increased fruit/vegetable intake, or lower fat, sugar, or salt intake. More recent school-based mHealth interventions incorporating mobile technology, wearables, and/or internet components were found to be effective at increasing fruit and vegetable intake in the short term and only with small effect sizes (Champion et al., 2019). None of the community/school-based approaches have demonstrated effectiveness in relation to longer term, disease-specific outcomes.

Workplace

Among adults, the workplace encompasses a significant portion of an individual's eating experience. Eating behaviors in the workplace are increasingly being evaluated in terms of opportunities to promote healthy choices. Ranging from modifying cafeteria meals to restricting vending machine choices, the workplace holds potential to alter food choices. Food-based interventions in the workplace are one aspect of the "choice architecture" approach to enhancing the health of employees. A 2019 systematic review of systematic reviews suggested that well-designed interventions that incorporate employee feedback in the planning and implementation stages, obtain management support, tailor the intervention to the specific workplace environment, and intervene at multiple levels of the socioecological model (i.e., individual, community, and institution; Schliemann & Woodside, 2019) were more successful. Additional research demonstrates that mHealth tools such as wearables and mobile applications may be an effective approach to dietary intervention in workplace environments if personalization and user-centered approaches are designed with daily work routines in mind (Pan et al., 2022).

Clinics

In addition to individual- and group-specific counseling efforts designed to support healthy eating choices, the clinical environment can serve as an additional reinforcement for patients. First and foremost, healthcare providers must receive adequate training on the importance of diet in health as well as effective methods to promote improvements in eating behaviors. Yet deficiencies in current training programs continue to be identified (Crowley et al., 2019). Providers must also develop competence in addressing eating behaviors with their patients and avoid disparagement of those who report less nutrient-dense diets or who are obese, a common and generally socially acceptable prejudice in the current healthcare system (Butsch et al., 2020; Mastrocola et al., 2020). Empathy in encounters is central to meaningful interactions toward change in eating behaviors. Healthcare providers should ask patients their own perceptions about their weight or dietary behaviors and build from the response, affirm and normalize the difficulty in making and sustaining changes in eating behavior, and listen carefully using a patient-centered approach, such as MI.

Beyond developing an empathetic initial encounter, the physical office can be modified to deliver an attitude of empathy, education, and self-empowerment. First, evaluate the clinic in relation to physical attributes (e.g., room to wait comfortably, chairs without arms, scales that can weigh individuals with severe obesity, examination gowns that fit all sizes, and use of large blood pressure cuffs). Second, provide access to relevant educational resources (healthy food choice/behavior pamphlets, websites, diet assessment/monitoring applications) using mHealth, posters on the clinic walls promoting healthy food, and even an office policy to restrict unhealthy food and beverages in the clinic setting. Third, provide clinic staff the opportunity, support, and recognition for advancing their skills in behavioral counseling to support patients who select to undertake change in eating behaviors. Consider encouraging clinic staff to adopt dietary behavior change personally to gain empathy and experience with the process. Fourth, understand and communicate the importance of realistic expectations.

Finally, routine integration of healthy lifestyle promotion into health services is needed if we are to succeed in improving the health of the population. Strategies should engage the healthcare providers, managers, researchers, and patient representatives using a socioecological model wherein the healthcare system is actively partnered, individual behavior change is supported, and educational limitations are overcome to achieve optimal dietary health.

CONCLUSION/GAPS IN CURRENT KNOWLEDGE

Changing dietary behaviors is challenging. Numerous factors contribute to every food choice, including what, how much, when, and why we choose to eat. Complicating the matter more is that eating is a required behavior. Thus, the decision must be repeated several times a day throughout a person's life; abstinence, employed for behavior modification of tobacco, drugs, or alcohol use, is not generally plausible except perhaps in relation to individual food omissions in the diet.

Current evidence suggests that clear and specific goals that are identified and defined by the individual, as well as self-monitoring of the behavioral goals established, are a necessary component of any successful change in eating behavior. These goals should be complemented with clear antecedents to provide the "how to" for successful eating behavior change in the context of the individual's life circumstances. Additionally, relapse prevention and recovery is an essential phase in any long-term plan for sustained eating behavior change.

Promoting healthy food choices and related eating behaviors for patients is critical to reducing obesity, obesity-related chronic diseases, and a variety of other clinical diagnoses. Despite the challenges, when patients can change eating behaviors to healthier choices, there is a clear benefit that translates to numerous disease-specific outcomes.

SUMMARY KEY POINTS

- Changing dietary behavior is complex and requires long-term, dynamic, and multi-level approaches and strategies that consider the intra- and interpersonal determinants of dietary intake, as well as the food environment, policy, and socioeconomic influences on diet.
- No single behavioral theory works best; theories should be adapted to the individual intervention and/or patient or setting/environment.
- Patient-centered counseling, including MI, is one of the most tested and effective strategies for dietary behavior change to date, but many providers lack sufficient training to effectively apply such strategies in practice.
- To promote change in dietary behavior, clinicians should help individuals set clear and specific goals, promote self-monitoring, recognize the role of social support and use it to enhance change in eating behavior, review the mechanisms for behavior and behavior change (antecedents), and focus on preventing relapse.
- Mobile and electronic technologies may facilitate changes in eating behavior that support health.
- Efforts to identify and determine "best practice" regarding behavioral theories, constructs, and strategies to help improve dietary behaviors need to be continued.

DISCUSSION QUESTIONS

1. Consider the factors that determine your own eating behavior. What would you find difficult to change?
2. After reading this chapter, what do you think the best approach is for introducing dietary change with an individual who is ambivalent to increasing their fruit and vegetable intake?
3. What are some strategies that could be considered to encourage healthy eating for individuals who do not have as much control over their food environment, such as children or older adults living in community homes?
4. How might the approach to influencing dietary change differ based on culture, socioeconomic status, age, or geographic location?
5. In your experience, do you agree that patient-centered counseling is the most effective method for influencing dietary behavior change? Why or why not?

A robust set of instructor resources designed to supplement this text is located at http://connect.springerpub.com/content/book/978-0-8261-4265-8. Qualifying instructors may request access by emailing textbook@springerpub.com.

REFERENCES

Anderson, G. L., Manson, J., Wallace, R., Lund, B., Hall, D., Davis, S., Shumaker, S., Wang, C.-Y., Stein, E., & Prentice, R. L. (2003). Implementation of the women's health initiative study design. *Annals of Epidemiology*, 13(9 Suppl.), S5–S17. https://doi.org/10.1016/s1047-2797(03)00043-7

Atkins, L., & Michie, S. (2015). Designing interventions to change eating behaviours. *Proceedings of the Nutrition Society*, 74(2), 164–170. https://doi.org/10.1017/S0029665115000075

Babbott, K. M., Cavadino, A., Brenton-Peters, J., Consedine, N. S., & Roberts, M. (2023). Outcomes of intuitive eating interventions: A systematic review and meta-analysis. *Eating Disorders, 31*(1), 33–63. https://doi.org/10.1080/10640266.2022.2030124

Bahafzallah, L., Hayden, K. A., Raffin Bouchal, S., Singh, P., & King-Shier, K. M. (2020). Motivational interviewing in ethnic populations. *Journal of Immigrant and Minority Health, 22*(4), 816–851. https://doi.org/10.1007/s10903-019-00940-3

Bardus, M., van Beurden, S. B., Smith, J. R., & Abraham, C. (2016). A review and content analysis of engagement, functionality, aesthetics, information quality, and change techniques in the most popular commercial apps for weight management. *International Journal of Behavioral Nutrition and Physical Activity, 13*(1), 35. https://doi.org/10.1186/s12966-016-0359-9

Barnes, R. D., & Ivezaj, V. (2015). A systematic review of motivational interviewing for weight loss among adults in primary care. *Obesity Reviews, 16*(4), 304–318. https://doi.org/10.1111/obr.12264

Befort, C. A., Donnelly, J. E., Sullivan, D. K., Ellerbeck, E. F., & Perri, M. G. (2010). Group versus individual phone-based obesity treatment for rural women. *Eating Behaviors, 11*(1), 11–17. https://doi.org/10.1016/j.eatbeh.2009.08.002

Bernabe-Ortiz, A., Pauschardt, J., Diez-Canseco, F., & Miranda, J. J. (2020). Sustainability of mHealth effects on cardiometabolic risk factors: Five-year results of a randomized clinical trial. *Journal of Medical Internet Research, 22*(4), e14595. https://doi.org/10.2196/14595

Bischof, G., Bischof, A., & Rumpf, H.-J. (2021). Motivational interviewing: An evidence-based approach for use in medical practice. *Deutsches Ärzteblatt International, 118*(7), 109–115. https://doi.org/10.3238/arztebl.m2021.0014

Blow, J., Sagaribay, R., & Cooper, T. V. (2022). A pilot study examining the impact of a brief health education intervention on food choices and exercise in a Latinx college student sample. *Appetite, 173*, 105979. https://doi.org/10.1016/j.appet.2022.105979

Blundell, J. E., Gibbons, C., Beaulieu, K., Casanova, N., Duarte, C., Finlayson, G., Stubbs, R. J., & Hopkins, M. (2020). The drive to eat in homo sapiens: Energy expenditure drives energy intake. *Physiology & Behavior, 219*, 112846. https://doi.org/10.1016/j.physbeh.2020.112846

Butsch, W. S., Kushner, R. F., Alford, S., & Smolarz, B. G. (2020). Low priority of obesity education leads to lack of medical students' preparedness to effectively treat patients with obesity: Results from the U.S. medical school obesity education curriculum benchmark study. *BMC Medical Education, 20*(1), 23. https://doi.org/10.1186/s12909-020-1925-z

Cadena-Schlam, L., & López-Guimerà, G. (2015). Intuitive eating: An emerging approach to eating behavior. *Nutrición Hospitalaria, 31*(3), 995–1002. https://doi.org/10.3305/nh.2015.31.3.7980

Cavero-Redondo, I., Martinez-Vizcaino, V., Fernandez-Rodriguez, R., Saz-Lara, A., Pascual-Morena, C., & Álvarez-Bueno, C. (2020). Effect of behavioral weight management interventions using lifestyle mHealth self-monitoring on weight loss: A systematic review and meta-analysis. *Nutrients, 12*(7), 1977. https://doi.org/10.3390/nu12071977

Centers for Disease Control and Prevention. (2023, March 2). *National Center for Chronic Disease Prevention and Health Promotion.* https://www.cdc.gov/chronicdisease/index.htm

Champion, K. E., Parmenter, B., McGowan, C., Spring, B., Wafford, Q. E., Gardner, L. A., Thornton, L., McBride, N., Barrett, E. L., Teesson, M., Newton, N. C., Chapman, C., Slade, T., Sunderland, M., Bauer, J., Allsop, S., Hides, L., Stapinksi, L., Birrell, L., & Mewton, L. (2019). Effectiveness of school-based eHealth interventions to prevent multiple lifestyle risk behaviours among adolescents: A systematic review and meta-analysis. *The Lancet Digital Health, 1*(5), e206–e221. https://doi.org/10.1016/S2589-7500(19)30088-3

Cotton, W., Dudley, D., Peralta, L., & Werkhoven, T. (2020). The effect of teacher-delivered nutrition education programs on elementary-aged students: An updated systematic review and meta-analysis. *Preventive Medicine Reports, 20*, 101178. https://doi.org/10.1016/j.pmedr.2020.101178

Crowley, J., Ball, L., & Hiddink, G. J. (2019). Nutrition in medical education: A systematic review. *The Lancet Planetary Health, 3*(9), e379–e389. https://doi.org/10.1016/S2542-5196(19)30171-8

Dalgetty, R., Miller, C. B., & Dombrowski, S. U. (2019). Examining the theory-effectiveness hypothesis: A systematic review of systematic reviews. *British Journal of Health Psychology, 24*(2), 334–356. https://doi.org/10.1111/bjhp.12356

Dayan, P. H., Sforzo, G., Boisseau, N., Pereira-Lancha, L. O., & Lancha, A. H. (2019). A new clinical perspective: Treating obesity with nutritional coaching versus energy-restricted diets. *Nutrition, 60*, 147–151. https://doi.org/10.1016/j.nut.2018.09.027

Dietary Guidelines for Americans 2020–2025. (2020). *Dietary guidelines for Americans.* https://www.dietaryguidelines.gov/resources/2020-2025-dietary-guidelines-online-materials

Dohle, S., Diel, K., & Hofmann, W. (2018). Executive functions and the self-regulation of eating behavior: A review. *Appetite, 124*, 4–9. https://doi.org/10.1016/j.appet.2017.05.041

Dounavi, K., & Tsoumani, O. (2019). Mobile health applications in weight management: A systematic literature review. *American Journal of Preventive Medicine, 56*(6), 894–903. https://doi.org/10.1016/j.amepre.2018.12.005

Eicher-Miller, H. A., Prapkree, L., & Palacios, C. (2021). Expanding the capabilities of nutrition research and health promotion through mobile-based applications. *Advances in Nutrition, 12*(3), 1032–1041. https://doi.org/10.1093/advances/nmab022

Epstein, L. H., Temple, J. L., Roemmich, J. N., & Bouton, M. E. (2009). Habituation as a determinant of human food intake. *Psychological Review, 116*(2), 384–407. https://doi.org/10.1037/a0015074

Fanti, M., Mishra, A., Longo, V. D., & Brandhorst, S. (2021). Time-restricted eating, intermittent fasting, and fasting-mimicking diets in weight loss. *Current Obesity Reports, 10*(2), 70–80. https://doi.org/10.1007/s13679-021-00424-2

Fernandez-Lazaro, C. I., Toledo, E., Buil-Cosiales, P., Salas-Salvadó, J., Corella, D., Fitó, M., Martínez, J. A., Alonso-Gómez, Á. M., Wärnberg, J., Vioque, J., Romaguera, D., López-Miranda, J., Estruch, R., Tinahones, F. J., Lapetra, J., Serra-Majem, L., Bueno-Cavanillas, A., Tur, J. A., Martín Sánchez, V., . . . for the PREDIMED-Plus investigators. (2022). Factors associated with successful dietary changes in an energy-reduced Mediterranean diet intervention: A longitudinal analysis in the PREDIMED-Plus trial. *European Journal of Nutrition, 61*(3), 1457–1475. https://doi.org/10.1007/s00394-021-02697-8

Githinji, P., Dawson, J. A., Appiah, D., & Rethorst, C. D. (2022). A culturally sensitive and theory-based intervention on prevention and management of diabetes: A cluster randomized control trial. *Nutrients, 14*(23), 5126. https://doi.org/10.3390/nu14235126

Gonçalves, V. S. S., Figueiredo, A. C. M. G., Silva, S. A., Silva, S. U., Ronca, D. B., Dutra, E. S., & Carvalho, K. M. B. (2021). The food environment in schools and their immediate vicinities as-soci-ated with excess weight in adolescence: A systematic review and meta-analysis. *Health & Place, 71*, 102664. https://doi.org/10.1016/j.healthplace.2021.102664

Grider, H. S., Douglas, S. M., & Raynor, H. A. (2021). The influence of mindful eating and/or intuitive eating approaches on dietary intake: A systematic review. *Journal of the Academy of Nutrition and Dietetics, 121*(4), 709–727.e1. https://doi.org/10.1016/j.jand.2020.10.019

Higgs, S., & Ruddock, H. (2020). Social influences on eating. In H. L. Meiselman (Ed.), *Handbook of eating and drinking: Interdisciplinary perspectives* (pp. 277–291). Springer Publishing Company. https://doi.org/10.1007/978-3-030-14504-0_27

Kiernan, M., Moore, S. D., Schoffman, D. E., Lee, K., King, A. C., Taylor, C. B., Kiernan, N. E., & Perri, M. G. (2012). Social support for healthy behaviors: Scale psychometrics and prediction of weight loss among women in a behavioral program. *Obesity, 20*(4), 756–764. https://doi.org/10.1038/oby.2011.293

Linardon, J., Tylka, T. L., & Fuller-Tyszkiewicz, M. (2021). Intuitive eating and its psychological cor-relates: A meta-analysis. *International Journal of Eating Disorders, 54*(7), 1073–1098. https://doi.org/10.1002/eat.23509

Livingstone, K. M., Rawstorn, J. C., Partridge, S. R., Godrich, S. L., McNaughton, S. A., Hendrie, G. A., Blekkenhorst, L. C., Maddison, R., Zhang, Y., Barnett, S., Mathers, J. C., Packard, M., & Alston, L. (2023). Digital behaviour change interventions to increase vegetable intake in adults: A systematic review. *International Journal of Behaviour Nutrition and Physical Activity, 20*(1), 36. https://doi.org/10.1186/s12966-023-01439-9

Look AHEAD Research Group. (2003). Look AHEAD (Action for Health in Diabetes): Design and methods for a clinical trial of weight loss for the prevention of cardiovascular disease in type 2 diabetes. *Controlled Clinical Trials, 24*(5), 610–628. https://doi.org/10.1016/s0197-2456(03)00064-3

Lyles, C. R., Wachter, R. M., & Sarkar, U. (2021). Focusing on digital health equity. *JAMA, 326*(18), 1795–1796. https://doi.org/10.1001/jama.2021.18459

Makin, H., Chisholm, A., Fallon, V., & Goodwin, L. (2021). Use of motivational interviewing in behavioural interventions among adults with obesity: A systematic review and meta-analysis. *Clinical Obesity, 11*(4), e12457. https://doi.org/10.1111/cob.12457

Mah, C. L., Luongo, G., Hasdell, R., Taylor, N. G. A., & Lo, B. K. (2019). A systematic review of the effect of retail food environment interventions on diet and health with a focus on the enabling role of public policies. *Current Nutrition Reports, 8*(4), 411–428. https://doi.org/10.1007/s13668-019-00295-z

Martins, R. K., & McNeil, D. W. (2009). Review of motivational interviewing in promoting health behaviors. *Clinical Psychology Review, 29*(4), 283–293. https://doi.org/10.1016/j.cpr.2009.02.001

Mastrocola, M. R., Roque, S. S., Benning, L. V., & Stanford, F. C. (2020). Obesity education in medical schools, residencies, and fellowships throughout the world: A systematic review. *International Journal of Obesity, 44*(2), 269–279. https://doi.org/10.1038/s41366-019-0453-6

McCrickerd, K., & Forde, C. (2016). Sensory influences on food intake control: Moving beyond palatability. *Obesity Reviews, 17*(1), 18–29. https://doi.org/10.1111/obr.12340

McKay, F. H., Wright, A., Shill, J., Stephens, H., & Uccellini, M. (2019). Using health and well-being apps for behavior change: A systematic search and rating of apps. *JMIR MHealth and UHealth, 7*(7), e11926. https://doi.org/10.2196/11926

Mendonça, R. de D., Mingoti, S. A., Gazzinelli Bethony, M. F., Martinez-Gonzalez, M. A., Bes-Rastrollo, M., & Lopes, A. C. S. (2022). Intervention for promoting intake of fruits and vegetables in

Brazilians: A randomised controlled trial. *Public Health Nutrition, 25*(3), 781–793. https://doi.org/10.1017/S1368980021004341

Michalopoulou, M., Ferrey, A. E., Harmer, G., Goddard, L., Kebbe, M., Theodoulou, A., Jebb, S. A., & Aveyard, P. (2022). Effectiveness of motivational interviewing in managing overweight and obesity: A systematic review and meta-analysis. *Annals of Internal Medicine, 175*(6), 838–850. https://doi.org/10.7326/M21-3128

Miller, W. R., & Moyers, T. B. (2007). Eight stages in learning Motivational Interviewing. *Journal of Teaching in the Addictions*, (5), 3–17.

Muzaffar, H., Nikolaus, C. J., Ogolsky, B. G., Lane, A., Liguori, C., & Nickols-Richardson, S. M. (2019). Promoting cooking, nutrition, and physical activity in afterschool settings. *American Journal of Health Behavior, 43*(6), 1050–1063. https://doi.org/10.5993/AJHB.43.6.4

National Center for Health Statistics. (2023, January 5). *Diet/nutrition*. https://www.cdc.gov/nchs/fastats/diet.htm

Nogueiras, R. (2021). MECHANISMS IN ENDOCRINOLOGY: The gut–brain axis: Regulating energy balance independent of food intake. *European Journal of Endocrinology, 185*(3), R75–R91. https://doi.org/10.1530/EJE-21-0277

Nordmo, M., Danielsen, Y. S., & Nordmo, M. (2020). The challenge of keeping it off, a descriptive systematic review of high-quality, follow-up studies of obesity treatments. *Obesity Reviews, 21*(1), e12949. https://doi.org/10.1111/obr.12949

Norman, G. J., Zabinski, M. F., Adams, M. A., Rosenberg, D. E., Yaroch, A. L., & Atienza, A. A. (2007). A review of eHealth interventions for physical activity and dietary behavior change. *American Journal of Preventive Medicine, 33*(4), 336–345. https://doi.org/10.1016/j.amepre.2007.05.007

Ockene, I. S., Hebert, J. R., Ockene, J. K., Saperia, G. M., Stanek, E., Nicolosi, R., Merriam, P. A., & Hurley, T. G. (1999). Effect of physician-delivered nutrition counseling training and an office-support program on saturated fat intake, weight, and serum lipid measurements in a hyperlipidemic population: Worcester Area Trial for Counseling in Hyperlipidemia (WATCH). *Archives of Internal Medicine, 159*(7), 725–731. https://doi.org/10.1001/archinte.159.7.725

Ogden, J., Coop, N., Cousins, C., Crump, R., Field, L., Hughes, S., & Woodger, N. (2013). Distraction, the desire to eat and food intake. Towards an expanded model of mindless eating. *Appetite, 62*, 119–126. https://doi.org/10.1016/j.appet.2012.11.023

O'Hara, S., & Toussaint, E. C. (2021). Food access in crisis: Food security and COVID-19. *Ecological Economics, 180*, 106859. https://doi.org/10.1016/j.ecolecon.2020.106859

Paldan, K., Sauer, H., & Wagner, N.-F. (2018). Promoting inequality? Self-monitoring applications and the problem of social justice. *AI & SOCIETY, 38*, 2597–2607. https://doi.org/10.1007/s00146-018-0835-7

Pan, S., Ren, X., Vos, S., & Brombacher, A. (2022). Digital tools to promote healthy eating for working-age individuals: A scoping review. *The Ninth International Symposium of Chinese CHI*, 1–8. https://doi.org/10.1145/3490355.3490356

Patel, M. L., Wakayama, L. N., & Bennett, G. G. (2021). Self-monitoring via digital health in weight loss interventions: A systematic review among adults with overweight or obesity. *Obesity, 29*(3), 478–499. https://doi.org/10.1002/oby.23088

Rincón-Gallardo Patiño, S., Zhou, M., Da Silva Gomes, F., Lemaire, R., Hedrick, V., Serrano, E., & Kraak, V. I. (2020). Effects of menu labeling policies on transnational restaurant chains to promote a healthy diet: A scoping review to inform policy and research. *Nutrients, 12*(6), 1544. https://doi.org/10.3390/nu12061544

Ross Middleton, K., Patidar, S., & Perri, M. (2012). The impact of extended care on the long-term maintenance of weight loss: A systematic review and meta-analysis. *Obesity Reviews, 13*(6), 509–517. https://doi.org/10.1111/j.1467-789X.2011.00972.x

Schliemann, D., & Woodside, J. V. (2019). The effectiveness of dietary workplace interventions: A systematic review of systematic reviews. *Public Health Nutrition, 22*(5), 942–955. https://doi.org/10.1017/S1368980018003750

Schoeppe, S., Alley, S., Van Lippevelde, W., Bray, N. A., Williams, S. L., Duncan, M. J., & Vandelanotte, C. (2016). Efficacy of interventions that use apps to improve diet, physical activity and sedentary behaviour: A systematic review. *International Journal of Behavioral Nutrition and Physical Activity, 13*(1), 127. https://doi.org/10.1186/s12966-016-0454-y

Self, K. J., Borsari, B., Ladd, B. O., Nicolas, G., Gibson, C. J., Jackson, K., & Manuel, J. K. (2023). Cultural adaptations of motivational interviewing: A systematic review. *Psychological Services, 20*, 7–18. https://doi.org/10.1037/ser0000619

Semper, H., Povey, R., & Clark-Carter, D. (2016). A systematic review of the effectiveness of smartphone applications that encourage dietary self-regulatory strategies for weight loss in overweight and obese adults. *Obesity Reviews, 17*(9), 895–906. https://doi.org/10.1111/obr.12428

Seven, M., Reid, A., Abban, S., Madziar, C., & Faro, J. M. (2022). Motivational interviewing interventions aiming to improve health behaviors among cancer survivors: A systematic scoping review. *Journal of Cancer Survivorship, 17*, 795–804. https://doi.org/10.1007/s11764-022-01253-5

Shangguan, S., Afshin, A., Shulkin, M., Ma, W., Marsden, D., Smith, J., Saheb-Kashaf, M., Shi, P., Micha, R., Imamura, F., & Mozaffarian, D. (2019). A meta-analysis of food labeling effects on consumer diet behaviors and industry practices. *American Journal of Preventive Medicine, 56*(2), 300–314. https://doi.org/10.1016/j.amepre.2018.09.024

Srivastava, R., Kushwaha, S., Khanna, P., Gupta, M., Bharti, B., & Jain, R. (2022). Comprehensive overview of smartphone applications delivering child nutrition information. *Nutrition, 103–104*, 111773. https://doi.org/10.1016/j.nut.2022.111773

Tam, R., Beck, K. L., Manore, M. M., Gifford, J., Flood, V. M., & O'Connor, H. (2019). Effectiveness of education interventions designed to improve nutrition knowledge in athletes: A systematic review. *Sports Medicine, 49*(11), 1769–1786. https://doi.org/10.1007/s40279-019-01157-y

Tinker, L. F., Rosal, M. C., Young, A. F., Perri, M. G., Patterson, R. E., Van Horn, L., Assaf, A. R., Bowen, D. J., Ockene, J., & Hays, J. (2007). Predictors of dietary change and maintenance in the Women's Health Initiative Dietary Modification Trial. *Journal of the American Dietetic Association, 107*(7), 1155–1166. https://doi.org/10.1016/j.jada.2007.04.010

United States Department of Agriculture. (2022). *What we eat in America.* https://www.ars.usda.gov /northeast-area/beltsville-md-bhnrc/beltsville-human-nutrition-research-center/food-surveys -research-group/docs/wweianhanes-overview/

Villinger, K., Wahl, D. R., Boeing, H., Schupp, H. T., & Renner, B. (2019). The effectiveness of app-based mobile interventions on nutrition behaviours and nutrition-related health outcomes: A systematic review and meta-analysis. *Obesity Reviews, 20*(10), 1465–1484. https://doi.org/10.1111/obr.12903

Walters, R., Leslie, S. J., Polson, R., Cusack, T., & Gorely, T. (2020). Establishing the efficacy of interventions to improve health literacy and health behaviours: A systematic review. *BMC Public Health, 20*(1), 1040. https://doi.org/10.1186/s12889-020-08991-0

West, R., & Michie, S. (2016). *A guide to development and evaluation of digital behaviour interventions in healthcare.* Silverback Publishing.

White, N. D., Bautista, V., Lenz, T., & Cosimano, A. (2020). Using the SMART-EST goals in lifestyle medicine prescription. *American Journal of Lifestyle Medicine, 14*(3), 271–273. https://doi.org/10 .1177/1559827620905775

Young, C., Campolonghi, S., Ponsonby, S., Dawson, S. L., O'Neil, A., Kay-Lambkin, F., McNaughton, S. A., Berk, M., & Jacka, F. N. (2019). Supporting engagement, adherence, and behavior change in online dietary interventions. *Journal of Nutrition Education and Behavior, 51*(6), 719–739. https://doi .org/10.1016/j.jneb.2019.03.006

CHAPTER 8

PHYSICAL ACTIVITY

JYLANA L. SHEATS, SANDRA J. WINTER, AND ABBY C. KING

LEARNING OBJECTIVES

- Describe the epidemiology, significance, and measurement of physical activity behavior.
- Identify frameworks and perspectives that can be used to broaden the targets and contexts of physical activity interventions.
- Explain individual, social, and built environment factors that contribute to physical activity behavior.
- Explain and critically assess disparities and inequities influencing physical activity behavior.
- Discuss how information and communication technologies (ICT) can be used to promote physical activity.
- Discuss challenges and opportunities in the field of physical activity research.

INTRODUCTION

Physical activity is defined as "any bodily movement produced by skeletal muscles that result in energy expenditure" (Caspersen et al., 1985, p. 126), whereas *exercise* is typically defined as a subset of physical activity that involves "planned, structured, and repetitive bodily movements done to improve or maintain one or more components of physical fitness" (Caspersen et al., 1985, p. 126). This chapter provides an overview of the significance, implications for health and well-being, challenges and inequities, intervention strategies, and future directions regarding physical activity behavior.

EPIDEMIOLOGY AND SIGNIFICANCE

History and Development of Physical Activity Research

Historically, physical activity research has been grounded in exercise science, a subfield of kinesiology, particularly as it relates to the examination of vigorous-intensity physical activity, moderate-intensity physical activity, and low-intensity physical activity (Keadle et al., 2021).

Supported in part by NIH Grant R01AG071490 from the National Institute on Aging (PI: King A.C.), NIH Grant 1R44AG071211-01A1 from the National Institute on Aging (PI: Fauci M.), and Grant P30DK092924 from Diabetes Research for Equity through the Advanced Multilevel Science Center for Diabetes Translational Research.

Today, physical activity research has expanded and shifted more toward the multidisciplinary field of public health (John et al., 2020), which has foundations in epidemiology, social and behavioral sciences (e.g., psychology), environmental health science, and other disciplines (Keadle et al., 2021). There has also been a stream of research on the negative effects of prolonged periods of physical inactivity, operationalized as sedentary behavior, which includes "any waking behavior characterized by a low level of energy expenditure while sitting, reclining, or lying" (U.S. Department of Health and Human Services [DHHS], 2018, p. 21), such as television viewing, playing video games, using a computer, sitting at school or work, and sitting while commuting. It is important to note that sedentary behaviors are relatively complex and should not simply be thought of as an absence of physical activity.

The broad concept of "active living" recognizes that physical activity can be classified into four different domains: (a) leisure time, (b) occupational, (c) domestic or household, and (d) transportation (Whitfield et al., 2020). Research into the various domains and modes of physical activity has been facilitated by improvements in self-reported, observational, and device-based physical activity assessment, as well as a growing body of literature on the effects of the built environment on physical activity levels. The primary types of self-report physical activity measures are diaries/logs, structured interviews, and surveys/questionnaires (Marasso et al., 2021). While not an exhaustive list, examples of national population-level surveys to surveil physical activity include the Behavioral Risk Factor Surveillance System (BRFSS), the National Health Interview Survey (NHIS), the National Health and Nutrition Examination Survey (NHANES), the Youth Risk Behavior Surveillance System (YRBSS), the National Survey of Children's Health (NSCH), and the National Household Travel Survey (NHTS). Data on the type of physical activity (e.g., aerobic vs. muscle-strengthening), dose (frequency, duration, intensity), and domain (i.e., leisure time, occupational, domestic, and transportation) are collected via self-report from samples of the U.S. population across the life course (Centers for Disease Control and Prevention [CDC], 2021; Wons et al., 2023). For global self-report measurement of physical activity, the International Physical Activity Questionnaire (IPAQ) is often utilized and recognized as the most widely used long- and short-form physical activity questionnaire (Kim et al., 2013). However, it should be kept in mind that the IPAQ was developed originally as an epidemiological measure at the population level, rather than a measure aimed specifically at capturing individual-level physical activity changes in response to interventions. Quantitative and qualitative data collected through these large epidemiological surveys help (a) ensure that there are standardized metrics for the subjective measurement of physical activity behavior across population studies; and (b) provide a mechanism to assess physical activity trends and the extent to which national guidelines, which are more extensively covered later in this chapter, are being achieved. In contrast, device-based measures often do not involve self-reported data. Instead, data are captured through devices that record physical activity in real time and in the context in which the behavior occurs (e.g., pedometers to measure daily step counts, accelerometers in wearable devices/activity trackers/mobile phones to measure the volume and intensity of movement/activity). Examples of other device-based tools to measure physical activity include heart rate monitors and multisensory devices (e.g., acceleration, heat, heart, sweat) that can be combined with location capabilities, such as global positioning systems (GPS), as well as indirect calorimetry and the doubly labeled water method (Cosoli et al., 2020; Wons et al., 2023). Regarding device-based tools, there is an increasing amount of attention focused on user characteristics, such as the amount of melanin concentration in the skin (i.e., skin tone), high-density hair follicles, and device placement (wrist, hip, stomach, ankle), all of which may impact device accuracy in measuring physical activity (Cosoli et al., 2020). Other common advantages and disadvantages to using self-report and device-based measures are shown in Table 8.1.

TABLE 8.1 Advantages and Disadvantages of Self-Report and Device-Based Physical Activity Measures

MEASURE TYPE	COMMON ADVANTAGES	COMMON DISADVANTAGES
Self-report measures	• Convenient, cost-effective, unobtrusive, low participant burden, and scalable • Obtain data on the frequency, duration, intensity, type of physical activity, and context	• Potential for overestimation of physical activity dosage due to recall bias, response bias, and social desirability bias • Inability to accurately estimate physical activity, duration, and intensity • Low correlations with objective measures of physical activity
Device-based measures	• Modern accelerometers cited as being smaller, less expensive, and user-friendly • More accurate measures of energy expenditure • Can be used to validate self-report measures	• Potentially expensive and intrusive and can be difficult to scale • Often requires complex data and statistical methods for analysis • Lack of sustained user engagement • Greater potential for technology issues

Sources: From Gorzelitz, J., Peppard, P. E., Malecki, K., Gennuso, K., Nieto, F. J., & Cadmus-Bertram, L. (2018). Predictors of discordance in self-report versus device-measured physical activity measurement. *Annals of Epidemiology, 28*(7), 427–431. https://doi.org/10.1016/j.annepidem.2018.03.016; Keusch, F., Wenz, A., & Conrad, F. (2022). Do you have your smartphone with you? Behavioral barriers for measuring everyday activities with smartphone sensors. *Computers in Human Behavior, 127*, 107054. https://doi.org/10.1016/j.chb.2021.107054; Wons, O., Lampe, E., Boyajian, L., Patarinski, A. G., & Juarascio, A. (2023). A research approach to self-report and objective measurements of physical activity in eating disorders. In V. B. Patel, & V. R. Preedy (Eds.), *Eating Disorders,* 413–432. https://doi.org/10.1007/978-3-031-16691-4_58.

PHYSICAL AND MENTAL HEALTH-RELATED OUTCOMES

The panel of experts on the national Physical Activity Guidelines Advisory Committee has advised that physical activity is "one of the most important actions that people of all ages can take to improve their health." Studies show that physical activity reduces the risk of all-cause and specific-cause mortality and demonstrates positive benefits in adults (Jakicic et al., 2019). Table 8.2 describes some of the major diseases and health conditions significantly positively impacted by regular participation in physical activity behaviors highlighted in the Physical Activity Guidelines for Americans (DHHS, 2018).

TABLE 8.2 Types of Diseases and Health Conditions That Benefit From Physical Activity

DISEASE OR CONDITION TYPE	DESCRIPTION OF HEALTH BENEFITS ASSOCIATED WITH REGULAR PHYSICAL ACTIVITY
Cardiorespiratory health	Prevention or management of cardiovascular disease (e.g., diseases of the heart, lungs, and blood vessels)
Cardiometabolic health	Prevention or management of heart disease, stroke, and type 2 diabetes; related risk factors (e.g., hypertension, high cholesterol, overweight and obesity); and related weight management behaviors
Bone and musculoskeletal health	Improved bone, joint, and muscle health (e.g., bone density, structure, and strength; osteoarthritis; muscle mass)

(continued)

TABLE 8.2 Types of Diseases and Health Conditions That Benefit From Physical Activity (*continued*)

DISEASE OR CONDITION TYPE	DESCRIPTION OF HEALTH BENEFITS ASSOCIATED WITH REGULAR PHYSICAL ACTIVITY
Functional ability and fall prevention	Greater capacity to perform activities of daily living (i.e., fundamental everyday tasks, or behaviors, such as hygiene, getting dressed, and eating) and lower risk of hip fracture among older adults
Brain health	Improved cognitive function, executive function, sleep, and sense of quality of life, as well as lower risk of dementia and Alzheimer disease, depression, and trait, or long-term, anxiety
Cancer	Lower risk of developing specific types of cancer (e.g., bladder, breast, colon, endometrium, esophagus, kidney, lung, stomach)

Important biomarkers of chronic disease risk have also been linked with physical activity levels, including body weight, body composition, blood pressure, blood cholesterol, insulin sensitivity, autonomic nervous system regulation, and bone and muscle strength, among adults and youth, respectively (DHHS, 2018). A dose–response relationship between physical activity and health status exists, where individuals at the most inactive portion of the curve have the greatest health risks (Jakicic et al., 2019). While typically increasing as a function of age, health risks that are a result of being physically inactive are evident across demographic characteristics such as race/ethnicity, sex/gender, education, income, and body weight (DHHS, 2018).

THE PREVALENCE OF PHYSICAL ACTIVITY AMONG AMERICANS AND SUMMARY OF THE PHYSICAL ACTIVITY GUIDELINES FOR AMERICANS

Physical activity health behavior change research and practice continue to be informed by an examination of how much physical activity (i.e., dose–response), of what type (aerobic, ambulatory, strength-training, and balance activities), and at what intensity (low, moderate, moderate-vigorous, vigorous, maximal effort) are required to achieve which kind of health benefit (e.g., improvements to metabolic or cardiorespiratory systems, or strength, functioning, and balance improvements; Wake, 2022). Current evidence suggests that the health-enhancing benefits of physical activity, including all-cause mortality, can be realized in bouts of activity of *any duration*, whereas previous research recommended a minimum of 10-minute episodes (or bouts) to obtain health benefits (Jakicic et al., 2019).

Over the last two decades, there has been a growing recognition of the negative health effects linked with prolonged sedentary behaviors (e.g., sitting, television viewing, and prolonged screen time), independent of physical activity levels. Sedentary behavior is associated with increased risk of obesity-related diseases such as type 2 diabetes, cardiovascular disease, and all-cause mortality (DHHS, 2018; Park et al., 2020). There is also evidence of a significant dose–response relationship between sedentary behavior and all-cause mortality and cardiovascular disease mortality (DHHS, 2018). High U.S. population levels of sitting watching television or videos (i.e., at least 2 hours per day) are associated with being male, non-Hispanic Black, having obesity, and/or being physically inactive. However, when comparing trends across U.S. population subgroups, the data are comparable (Yang et al., 2019). While there is no determination of a recommended daily sedentary duration, time, and frequency (DHHS, 2018), it has been suggested at an individual level to reduce prolonged periods of sitting and replace sedentary behavior with low-impact physical activity (Park et al., 2020). It is also advisable to develop multilevel interventions that include self-monitoring (Compernolle et al., 2019), with future research needed to further investigate a dose–response association between sedentary behavior and key health outcome and explore differences and similarities across demographic variables (Saunders et al., 2020).

The national Physical Activity Guidelines (DHHS, 2018) provide recommendations for Americans across the life course. These guidelines, summarized in **Figure 8.1**, describe the recommended mode, frequency, duration, and intensity needed to achieve health benefits.

The Physical Activity Guidelines (DHHS, 2018) posit that physical activity can be safe for all and increase gradually over time. To safely engage in physical activity behaviors and reduce the risk of injury or other adverse events, the guidelines note that one's chosen physical activity should consider fitness level, health status, and health goals. For those with chronic health conditions or symptoms, consultation with a healthcare professional or physical activity specialist is recommended (DHHS, 2018).

Despite the documented health benefits of physical activity, most Americans do not meet national guidelines, with differences being reported across demographic variables. Decreases in physical activity and increases in sedentary behavior have been shown across the life course, including in patients with a range of health issues (Dempsey et al., 2020). One-quarter of adults aged 18 years and older are physically inactive (25.3%), reporting no participation "in any physical activities outside of work over the last month" (CDC, 2022), and only 23% of children in the United States meet the guidelines (Friel et al., 2020).

The increasing prevalence of Americans failing to meet the guidelines combined with the risks of being too inactive to protect their health has contributed to physical inactivity being recognized in the United States and worldwide as a key behavioral risk factors for the development of chronic disease, alongside tobacco use and poor diet (Everest et al., 2022). The

PRESCHOOL-AGED CHILDREN (3–5 YEARS)	CHILDREN AND ADOLESCENTS (6–17 years)	ADULTS* (18–64 years)	OLDER ADULTS* (65 years and older)
Engage in a **variety of types of physical activity** throughout the day.	At least **60 minutes** (1 hour) or more of **moderate-to-vigorous physical activity or vigorous-intensity aerobic physical activity** on most days of the week. Children and adolescents activities should include **muscle-strengthening** physical activity on at least 3 days a week as well as **bone-strengthening activities**.	At least **150 to 300 minutes** (2.5 hours to 5 hours) **per week** of **moderate-intensity** physical activity **OR** **75 minutes to 150 minutes** (1 hour 15 minutes to 2 hours 30 minutes) per week of **vigorous-intensity** aerobic physical activity On **2 or more days** a week, moderate or greater intensity **muscle-strengthening activities** that involve all major muscle groups	At least **150 to 300 minutes** (2.5 hours to 5 hours) **per week** of **moderate-intensity** physical activity **OR** **75 minutes to 150 minutes** (1 hour 15 minutes to 2 hours 30 minutes) per week of **vigorous-intensity** aerobic physical activity On **2 or more days** a week, moderate or greater intensity **muscle-strengthening activities** that involve all major muscle groups If able, engage in **multicomponent physical activity** (e.g., **balance training** and **aerobic and muscle-strengthening activities**). *Physical activity should be done based on fitness level and/or with consideration of one's ability and health conditions

FIGURE 8.1 Physical Activity Guidelines for Americans by age group.
Source: From U.S. Department of Health and Human Services. (2018). *Physical activity guidelines for Americans.* https://health.gov/sites/default/files/2019-09/Physical_Activity_Guidelines_2nd_edition.pdf

144 II • PRIORITIZED BEHAVIORS FOR PRIMARY PREVENTION OF DISEASE

2018 Physical Activity Guidelines for Americans provide detailed recommendations for individuals across the life course (Figure 8.1). Understanding that population subgroups may have different needs, the 2018 Physical Activity Guidelines also provide guidance for women during pregnancy and the postpartum period, adults with chronic health conditions, and adults with disabilities (DHHS, 2018). The next section will examine the various multilevel factors that influence physical activity levels.

FACTORS CONTRIBUTING TO REGULAR PHYSICAL ACTIVITY

"Simply moving more" for any duration has positive benefits for health and well-being (DHHS, 2018). The benefits of physical activity extend to individuals of all ages regardless of race and ethnicity group or socioeconomic status (SES; DHHS, 2018). Yet physical activity behavior is both complex and multidimensional. As noted earlier, an abundance of scientific evidence shows that regularly engaging in physical activity leads to substantial improvements in physical health, brain health, cognitive function, and overall quality of life; lower healthcare costs (DHHS, 2018); and extended life expectancy (Lee et al., 2022). Several factors, however, can influence whether physical activity behavior—either formal (exercise) or informal—occurs. Socioecological perspectives posit that behaviors, including physical activities, are influenced by the intersection of individual, social, community, and societal factors (King et al., 2019; Rhodes et al., 2019). This framing supports a better understanding of the multidimensional and multilevel influencing factors associated with adherence to or participation in physical activity behavior, as well as their intersection.

The next section provides an overview of individual, social, and built environment factors associated with regular physical activity. An understanding of potential influencing factors may provide insight on areas for future research and assist program planners, interventionists, and policy makers in the development of individual- to population-based strategies to promote and improve physical activity behaviors across the life course.

Individual-Level Factors

Among U.S. adults, nonmodifiable factors associated with physical activity include, but are not limited to, race and ethnicity, gender, age, SES, physical function and health status, and psychosocial factors (Bennie et al., 2019; DHHS, 2018). For example, in a systematic review, it was found that being non-White is associated with having low levels of physical activity (Lounassalo et al., 2019). Regarding gender, men typically have been found to be more physically active than women, but there is evidence of within-group race and ethnicity-based differences related to gender. When stratified by race and ethnicity, Latinx men are cited as being the least physically active subgroup of adults (23.5%) relative to their White (30.5%), Asian (30.2%), and Black (29.7%) counterparts who do not meet the Physical Activity Guidelines. White women, meanwhile, are more likely to meet the national guidelines for physical activity relative to Latinx (18.0%), Black (16.5%), and Asian (16.7%) women (Bennie et al., 2019; Elgaddal et al., 2022). Research on race- or ethnicity-based differences in physical activity among children, however, is mixed and may be the result of self-reported versus device-based measurement (Lee & Gao, 2021). Older adults (aged 65 years and older) comprise the fastest growing age group in the United States (Population Reference Bureau, 2023) and are more likely to report being physically inactive (31.9%) relative to middle-aged adults (26.2%; CDC, 2019; Cunningham et al., 2020). In a comprehensive review, Franco and colleagues (2015) identified six themes related to barriers to physical activity among older adults, including the following: (a) social influences, (b) physical limitations, (c) competing priorities, (d) access difficulties, (e) lack of clarity related to personal benefits of physical activity, and (f) negative motivational and belief sets. Other major factors that present unique challenges for older adults' participation in physical activities include current health status and changes in health (Stojanovic et al., 2023), chronic pain, and reduced physical or cognitive function. Notably, increasing age throughout the life course is often linked with declines in physical activity levels. For example, consistent findings in the literature demonstrate that as children mature to adolescence they often become less physically active, with girls declining at a younger age than boys (Farooq et al., 2020). In addition to physiological, behavioral, and psychosocial factors, physical activity researchers have identified genetic and evolutionary factors that may contribute to the propensity for being physically active or inactive as well (Bauman et al., 2012). For example, prior engagement in physical activity during adolescence is correlated with later engagement in physical activity in adulthood (Bauman et al., 2012). Across all race and ethnicities, genders, and age groups, data show that in the United States physical activity is low among people living with disabilities. Today, 61 million adults (CDC, 2023) and 3 million children (U.S. Census Bureau, 2021) in the United States live with a disability. National surveillance data indicate that 46.8% of adults living with disabilities do not meet the national guidelines for physical activity (CDC, 2023). Adults with disabilities are more likely to have obesity and chronic conditions (i.e., heart disease, stroke, diabetes, cancer, asthma, arthritis) than adults without disabilities, making regular physical activity participation even more critical (CDC, 2023) given the physical health, psychological, and social benefits (DHHS, 2018). Children living with disabilities also do not engage in adequate levels of physical activity based on combined 2016 and 2017 data from the NSCH data set (Case et al., 2020).

Psychosocial variables, such as attitude, exercise-related self-efficacy (i.e., confidence in one's capability to engage in exercise), and self-determination, are linked with higher levels of physical activity among adults (Erturan et al., 2020; Wang et al., 2022). Furthermore, individuals' expectations for, and their realization of, positive outcomes related to being physically active, having positive intentions to perform physical activity, and perceiving that enjoyment comes from physical activity are associated with increased levels of physical activity (Bauman et al., 2012; DHHS, 2018). Among children and adolescents, psychosocial and behavioral factors such as one's intention to be active, perceived barriers, perceived competence, parent attitudes about, and social support for physical activity, dietary factors, and sedentary behaviors are associated with physical activity levels (DHHS, 2018; Xu et al., 2020).

In an assessment of the relationship between key SES indicators (i.e., education, income, employment status) and physical activity time allocation across domains (leisure, housework, and paid work), there is evidence that individuals with less education tend to be less active overall, although they often report more time in household activities relative to those with higher education levels. In contrast, with higher income individuals, there is a greater ability to outsource housework and childcare and spend more time in leisure-time physical activity due to increased time, skills, access to physical activity-supportive settings, and knowledge (Cusatis & Garbarski, 2019).

CASE STUDY 8.1: PEOPLE LIVING WITH DISABILITIES

National data show that 46.8% of adults living with disabilities in the United States have not met the national guidelines for physical activity (CDC, 2023). Children living with disabilities similarly are less likely to engage in physical activity relative to children without disabilities (Carbone et al., 2021). Researchers have argued for cross-sector collaboration and increased availability of and accessibility to community-based physical activity opportunities for people living with disabilities (Herbison et al., 2023). Herbison and colleagues (2023) applied the World Café method, a participatory approach that facilitates the exploration and discussion of topics among diverse groups (Table 8.3; Löhr et al., 2020). They convened a meeting with direct and indirect stakeholders (N = 45) with the goal of solution-finding to address issues related to accessing community-based physical activity opportunities to facilitate social participation and diminish social isolation among people living with physical disabilities. Participants included people living with

(continued)

CASE STUDY 8.1: PEOPLE LIVING WITH DISABILITIES (*continued*)

TABLE 8.3 Themes to Enhance Social Participation and Reduce Social Isolation Among People Living With Disabilities Extracted From the World Café

SOLUTION THEMES	PRACTICAL EXAMPLES
Representation and visibility	Prioritize hiring people living with disabilities.
Finances	Lower direct costs for program participants.
Connection and social support	Foster social networks that provide informational support.
Education and programming	Increase awareness of existing disability services and resources.
Government programs and policies	Enforce accessibility standards for indoor and outdoor spaces.

Source: Content extracted from Herbison, J. D., Osborne, M., Andersen, J., Lepage, P., Pagé, V., Levasseur, C., Beckers, M., Gainforth, H. L., Lamontagne, M.-E, & Sweet, S. N. (2023). Strategies to improve access to physical activity opportunities for people with physical disabilities. *Translational Behavioral Medicine, 13*(7), 486–500. https://doi.org/10.1093/tbm/ibac119.

disabilities, current patients in a rehabilitation hospital, a kinesiologist, practitioners, graduate students, and representatives from organizations and government agencies serving people with disabilities. Participants shared lived experiences within the context of their respective role and capacities and engaged in a process that supported the coproduction of knowledge. Together they created 17 practical strategies situated across five themes described in Table 8.3. Herbison and colleagues (2023) posited that the strategies can be used to inform the design and implementation of solutions (e.g., programs, intervention, policies), funding proposals, and obtain buy-in from decision-making entities to improve access to physical activity opportunities.

SOCIAL DETERMINANTS OF HEALTH

Context matters—and to fully address all the determinants of physical activity behavior across the life course, consideration of the social determinants of health (SDOH) is critical. SDOH are the "conditions in the environments in which people are born, live, learn, work, play, worship, and age that affect a wide range of health, functioning, and quality-of-life outcomes and risks" (Gómez et al., 2022, p. S249, S251). The next section explores the social factors that play a role in promoting and/or hindering physical activity levels.

Social Factors

In addition to individual-level factors, social factors such as social support and social networks can influence physical activity behavior (Heredia et al., 2020; King et al., 2019). Relationships are inherently a critical element of social support, as social support encompasses a network of friends, family, tangible and intangible resources, and actions available in times of need (National Cancer Institute, 2023). There are two primary dimensions of social support: (a) structural and (b) functional support. *Structural support* refers to the strength and quality of one's social network, whereas *functional support* refers to the provision of support by one's social network (e.g., emotional, informational, material/tangible, appraisal; Li &Wang, 2021). Receiving positive social support from family, friends, coworkers, and other people in an individual's environment is consistently associated with increased levels of physical activity (Bauman et al., 2012; Xu et al., 2020). For example, engaging in physical activity with neighbors and there being a sense of community social cohesion are associated with improvements in physical activity among Black adults in Southern United States (Islam et al., 2022). When examining social support and physical activity among a subsample of Black women (N = 187) who had been active for 6 months or greater, Affuso and colleagues (2022) demonstrated the value of identifying and understanding the nuances of social support. While study outcomes among the sample varied, they also found that motivating factors among this population included the health of family members (vs. being motivated by family members), and being held accountable by friends motivated physical activity behavior and maintenance. The power of social support was observed among a sample of Indigenous people as well. Ironside and colleagues (2021) found that engagement in physical activity behavior was associated with greater community, family, and perceived social support, as well as individual-level factors (i.e., experiences with discrimination, attending residential school, and being in foster care).

There is also evidence for a relationship between social support via companionship and leisure-time physical activity. For example, among a sample of Latinx individuals, having an exercise partner and the ability to name two or more supporters increased the likelihood of leisure-time physical activity (Soto et al., 2018). The COVID-19 pandemic presented unique challenges in building and sustaining relationships, and social isolation (lack of companionship and perceived isolation) was abundant (Hwang et al., 2020). The related social distancing mandates and city- to statewide lockdowns had major implications for worldwide health and well-being given the closure of public and private spaces for physical activity, such as schools and universities, gyms, and recreation centers, as well as local parks and other green spaces, which often limited access to physical activity opportunities (Amini et al., 2021). Unfortunately, companionship is not always available. In one study, dogs were found to be important sources of social support when contact with other humans was limited or not possible during the COVID-19 pandemic lockdowns (Bowen et al., 2021). The potential social support for physical activity through human–animal companionship is an increasing area of interest. Human–animal interactions have benefits that cut across physical, mental, and social "spheres of human functioning" (Hoy-Gerlach et al., 2020). Studies have shown that this type of bond and companionship promotes increased physical activity, provides social support (Westgarth et al., 2019), is a source of social interaction, and has positive effects on mental health, well-being, and quality of life (e.g., feelings of isolation, depression; Marquez et al., 2020).

Social networks have been evaluated as a distinct area relating to social contexts and are centered on the structural elements of social relationships. Such networks have been shown to be important in facilitating physical activity behavior, particularly among Black Americans and older adults, respectively (Flórez et al., 2018). In a systematic review, Prochnow and Patterson (2022) found that physical activity was influenced by the homophilic nature, size, and composition of and exposure to social networks. For women, physical activity behaviors have been found to reflect the behavior of their best friend (Montgomery et al., 2021). In exploring the influence of gender differences within the context of adolescent peer relationships, one study found that male physical activity behaviors were associated with the physical activity behaviors occurring in their friend group. Among Latinx adults, there was a positive association between having a larger social network and meeting the Physical Activity Guidelines for leisure-time physical activity (Marquez et al., 2014). Similarly, Mötteli and Dohle (2020) examined the personal networks of nonexercisers and exercisers. Having more exercisers in one's network was associated with higher levels of physical activity. Given the above types of findings, Zimmer and colleagues (2022) recommended that when working with older adults in physical activity programs, it is important to (a) facilitate relationships that will provide social support, (b) promote cultural awareness and acceptance to foster engagement as well as the development of meaningful relationships, and (c) encourage supportive relationships where the emotional and tangible needs of older adults can be achieved.

Built Environment Factors

Growing recognition exists concerning the associations between physical activity and individual-, social-, and built environment-level factors (Bauman et al., 2012; Bonaccorsi et al., 2020). Built environments are human-made surroundings that influence behaviors and other domains, and include land use (e.g., open space, green space, connectivity), transportation systems (both motorized and active), buildings (home, schools, worksites, retail shops, food stores), and infrastructure (e.g., transportation systems, water supply, energy networks). Demonstrated to be a key driver of physical activity, common built environment categories and attributes are described in **Table 8.4** (Fonseca et al., 2022).

Both perceived (e.g., self-report instruments such as the Neighborhood Environment Walkability Scale [NEWS]; Adams et al., 2009) and device-based and related measures capturing built environment design and infrastructure elements of neighborhoods and communities (e.g., geographic information system [GIS], housing density, street connectivity, location of shopping and other destinations) have been linked with variations in physical activity (Althoff et al., 2017; Peters et al., 2020) and sedentary behavior. In the secondary analysis of a systematic review, researchers examined neighborhood environments and physical activity among children using GIS (Smith et al., 2022). Findings illuminated the value of a comprehensive urban design and provided evidence of associations between having a range of destinations in proximal distance to the neighborhood, shorter distances to schools, and traffic safety with children's active travel. Neighborhood attributes that positively impact adults' physical activity are having access to facilities, destinations, and programs; land-use mix and street connectivity; street lighting; safety (from crime, traffic); availability of open spaces; pedestrian-friendly infrastructure; and aesthetically pleasing scenery (Bonaccorsi et al., 2020; Mooney et al., 2020). Examples of features with negative associations are poor access to shopping centers, barriers to walking/cycling, being unsafe (crime), stray dogs, traffic, vandalism, littering, street lighting, lack of aesthetically pleasing scenery, and noise (Bonaccorsi et al., 2020).

TABLE 8.4 Common Built Environment Categories and Attributes

BUILT ENVIRONMENT CATEGORY	ATTRIBUTE
Land-use density	Residential, population, amenity (number, distance), job
Land-use diversity	Land-use mix, retail floor area
Accessibility	Access to amenities and places of interest, transport, car parking, central business district, and other attractions
Street network connectivity	Density (intersection, street), blocks, link to node, continuity, integration, network microanalysis, cul-de-sacs, directness, impedance
Pedestrian facility and comfort	Sidewalk characteristics, slopes, environment
Safety and security	Traffic safety (volume, speed, number of lanes, accidents, calming devices), crime security
Streetscape design	Aesthetics, enclosure, complexity, human scale, imageability, transparency

Source: Data from Fonseca, F., Ribeiro, P. J., Conticelli, E., Jabbari, M., Papageorgiou, G., Tondelli, S., & Ramos, R. A. (2022). Built environment attributes and their influence on walkability. *International Journal of Sustainable Transportation, 16*(7), 660–679. https://doi.org/10.1080/15568318.2021.1914793.

Neighborhood factors associated with physical activity behavior among older adults include having access to neighborhood amenities, access to parks, traffic, and overall safety (Lee & Fan, 2023). Althoff and colleagues (2017) used real-world, smartphone-based accelerometry data from more than two million people worldwide and found that built environments are particularly influential for women's walking/physical activity behavior. General safety, verbal harassment, and physical harm and violence (assault, gun violence, gang-related activities) are neighborhood-level factors shown to influence activity among Black Americans, Hispanic/Latinx, and individuals in low-income communities (Bantham et al., 2021; Payán et al., 2019). Access becomes an issue when communities such as these are underserved and underresourced with unequal opportunities (e.g., access to gyms, parks, and recreation facilities) for physical activity relative to higher income, predominantly White neighborhoods (Bantham et al., 2021; Payán et al., 2019). The impact of built environments on physical activity may be particularly pronounced for rural communities and population subgroups, such as older adults, women, and historically marginalized (e.g., economically, socially) populations (Lee & Fan, 2023; Payán et al., 2019; Tuckett et al., 2020). Those residing in rural communities have high rates of physical inactivity and are less likely to meet recommendations compared with their urban and suburban counterparts. More research is needed to fully understand neighborhood-level determinants of physical activity in rural communities, but lack of opportunities and recreation spaces (indoor, outdoor) for physical activity, geographic isolation, perceived safety, and a host of other factors exacerbate these rates (Meyer et al., 2016).

In summary, there are many factors at the individual, social, and environmental levels that affect physical activity levels. Exploring physical activity at these levels with consideration of race and ethnicity, gender, age, and class, ability, and/or other critical factors is essential to help ensure that equity is at the forefront as solutions are identified and implemented.

CASE STUDY 8.2: CITIZEN SCIENCE AS A TOOL TO ASSESS WALKABILITY

Citizen science is a participatory approach to research where members of the public are directly involved in at least one phase of the scientific process with the goal of collaboration and increasing knowledge and understanding around an important problem(s) (Mintz & Couch, 2022). The *Our Voice* initiative (med.stanford.edu/ourvoice .html) is an equity-based citizen science methodology. Through *Our Voice,* local "citizen scientists" (i.e., community residents) utilize the Discovery Tool mobile application to document features of their communities that impact their ability to lead healthy lives by capturing geocoded photos and narratives (text, audio) and rating neighborhood features. Citizen scientists then review their own findings, prioritize areas for change, and learn how to mobilize local decision-makers to promote improvements that will support community health (King, Campero et al., 2020; Tuckett et al., 2018).

GirlTrek (www.girltrek.org) is the largest public health nonprofit for Black women and girls in the United States, founded by T. Morgan Dixon and Vanessa Garrison in 2010. With over 1,371,776 members today, GirlTrek encourages women to use walking behavior as a practical first step to engage in self-care, reclaim their neighborhoods, and promote and ignite healthy lifestyles, families, and communities (GirlTrek, 2023; Our Voice, n.d.). In 2017, they engaged with the HARTS Lab to use the *Our Voice* approach. As part of the effort, groups of Black women in eight U.S. cities were trained to use the Discovery Tool to assess walkability and collect data to advance changes in neighborhood-built environments (Our Voice, n.d.). Read the *GirlTrek Multi-City Walkability Assessment* project overview and outcomes at med.stanford.edu/ourvoice/our-projects/united-states /girltrek---our-voice-collaboration.html.

PHYSICAL ACTIVITY INTERVENTIONS

Acknowledgment of the influence of context and differences across and within subgroups of the population is important in the development and implementation of successful physical activity interventions. The next section provides an overview of evidence-based behavioral, social, informational, environmental, and policy-based approaches to address physical inactivity.

Behavioral and Social Approaches

Theories and models of behavior change help not only to "explain, predict, and understand health behavior" (Hayden, 2022), but also to guide intervention and program design, components, and messaging. Behavioral interventions, based on the social cognitive theory and its derivatives (Beauchamp et al., 2019; Rhodes et al., 2019), apply theory in teaching individuals skills (e.g., goal setting, problem-solving) and positive beliefs that aid in the adoption and maintenance of physical activity behaviors, and aim to enhance immediate social and environmental circumstances that support and facilitate their practice. Common components of individual-level, theoretically based behavioral interventions include goal setting and self-regulation, provision of accurate information about the benefits of physical activity, and awareness enhancement (i.e., increasing awareness of opportunities to be active). Receiving reliable personalized feedback about progress, building social support for regular physical activity, and engaging in active problem-solving related to barriers to physical activity are additional self-regulatory strategies shown to improve physical activity participation (Beauchamp et al., 2019; King et al., 2019; McEwan et al., 2022).

Behavioral and social interventions typically utilize a combination of cognitive and behavioral strategies that can be delivered through a range of communication channels (Hicks et al., 2022). These channels include in-person programs (Carraça et al., 2021), phone-based programs (Swoboda et al., 2017), print and other mass media (Marcus et al., 2007), and digital/health information and communication technologies (ICT; Carraça et al., 2021). Health ICT may be classified into categories of web-based programs, such as social media (Hicks et al., 2022; Vereen et al., 2023), cell phone- and smartphone-based programs (Laranjo et al., 2021; Sheats et al., 2018), embodied conversational agents (Milne-Ives et al., 2020), handheld computers/tablets (Afaneh et al., 2022; Wood et al., 2015), gamification and wearables (Mazeas et al., 2022), and interactive voice response "telehealth" systems (King, King et al., 2020; Milne-Ives et al., 2020). These provide a range of possible intervention delivery modalities.

Social interventions are designed to provide individuals with strategies for receiving and giving support and encouragement to and from family, friends, coworkers, and others. Family-based social support interventions have shown increased participation around physical activity. Similarly, social support interventions in community settings that have focused on strengthening existing or new relationships and social networks for behavior change outside of the family (e.g., at worksites or in other community settings) have generally been found to be effective (Kahn et al., 2002). *Social network interventions* are defined as "purposeful efforts to use social networks or social network data to generate social influence, accelerate behavior change, improve performance, and/or achieve desirable outcomes among individuals, communities, organizations, or populations" (Valente, 2012, p. 49). As noted in a review by Hunter and colleagues (2019), individuals are inherently embedded within social networks, and that utilizing these networks may be especially important for health behavior. However, this line of research is still emerging, with social network analysis and data being underused and social network interventions remaining scant (Hunter et al., 2019). Expanding the context within which we examine and design interventions addressing social factors has the potential to help us better understand and address the dynamic social factors that influence physical activity behavior.

Informational and Technology-Based Approaches

Informational interventions use educational strategies to target constructs related to behavior change. Specifically, knowledge, attitudes, beliefs, and related mind-sets about the benefits of regular physical activity are key factors to target to initiate behavior change. Examples of interventional messages include notifying people of the locations of current relevant opportunities for physical activity within their community and strategies for accessing these opportunities (e.g., pertinent public transit information). Other strategies include providing people with normative information regarding how and where others around them are engaging in physical activity, and instructions to help enable them to increase their regular physical activity levels. While education alone is insufficient to elicit changes in physical activity, educational approaches can provide a foundation for further intervention and influence upstream factors related to motivation (e.g., attitudes and beliefs).

Other types of useful information include educating people on the benefits of being physically active. Such benefits include, but are not limited to, both immediate (acute) benefits of a physical activity episode (e.g., increased energy, positive mood, cognitive function, fun, social connection) as well as longer term benefits (e.g., improved health and daily function, wellness, and quality of life; decreased risk of a range of diseases; DHHS, 2018). Evidence on large-scale, community-wide education campaigns delivered through more traditional channels, such as print, television, and radio, has led to increases in knowledge about exercise and physical activity, as well as intentions to be more physically active (Guide to Community Preventive Services, 2012). Two crucial strategies are translating content/materials into the language(s) of the population of interest, using inclusive language and ensuring that intervention contents are between a sixth- and seventh-grade reading level.

The use of ICT (e.g., mobile and smartphones, communication-based connectivity, and networked devices) spans the age, income, and education continua and is vastly growing (Hicks et al., 2022). Smartphones, miniature devices, sensor technology, low-power wireless connectivity, and cloud services have forged the way for a growing digital health market where these technologies are being used to promote health as a behavior change intervention medium (e.g., to distribute health information or change behavior through tailored messages; Hicks et al., 2022). Yet longer term engagement with, and the ongoing use of, health-promoting technologies is challenging, particularly when technologies focus on engagement with the device more so than engagement in the health behavior of interest (Cole-Lewis et al., 2019; Mazeas et al., 2022). Studies have shown that the effects of technology-based and gamified interventions may improve physical activity regardless of age or health status (Mazeas et al., 2022). Specific technology-enabled areas of promise include the use of the following:

- Ecological momentary assessments and just-in-time adaptive interventions (JITAIs) to facilitate the provision of real-time, contextually relevant data both from and to users (Hardeman et al., 2019)

- Social media and social networks to support physical activity initiation and maintenance, particularly among populations experiencing health disparities (Vereen et al., 2023)

- Integration of game-like elements to promote engagement and potentially increase the dose of health-enhancing exercise (Mazeas, 2022)

- Augmented and virtual reality platforms as an effective strategy for increasing physical activity behavior across the age continuum (Ng et al., 2019)

- Easy-to-use mobile apps capturing multidimensional information that reflects the actual physical activity-relevant "lived experiences" of community members across different age groups, geographies, and circumstances (King, Campero et al., 2020)

Interventionist and program planners should harness the power of these technologies, and the health behavior change theory, to promote regular physical activity. For example, in a review of technologies for the prevention and treatment of cardiovascular disease in adults (Winter et al., 2016), 108 of the 240 relevant intervention articles targeted physical activity. Of these, 57 (62%) used behavior change theory, with the most common theories being the social cognitive theory (28%), the stages of change theory (14%), and the theory of planned behavior (9%). The most common behavior change techniques applied based on the CALO-RE taxonomy developed by Michie et al. (2013) were prompting self-monitoring of behavior (58%), providing feedback on performance (49%), and behavioral goal setting (48%). Promising digital intervention components to promote physical activity among children and adolescents include self-monitoring of physical activity and sedentary behavior; use of smartphone apps or web-based devices that monitor and track behaviors, goals, and achievements; and exergames (i.e., games that combine exercise and play; Mazeas et al., 2022).

Moving forward, whether print, digital, or otherwise, information and technology-based health promotion efforts should focus on being user-centered to ensure the greatest reach and impact (Sheats et al., 2018). Further, more scientifically rigorous research is needed to determine the most effective components and modes of delivery of health-promoting technology interventions. To increase the rigor of studies evaluating technologies to promote physical activity, it has been recommended to use effective comparison groups, adequate power analyses, a combination of device-based and self-report measurement of physical activity, larger effect sizes, and longer term follow-up to assess the maintenance of behavior changes (King et al., 2019; Mazeas et al., 2022). Conducting more agile, solution-oriented science that keeps pace with the rapid advancements in technology development is important as well.

Environmental and Policy-Based Approaches

Environmental and policy-based interventions aim to alter some aspect of the physical or policy environment. This is done often as a means for reducing systemic barriers to physical activity. Incorporating environmental strategies into health promotion efforts may result in more effective community health interventions that support and sustain positive health behaviors across a wider segment of the community. Examples of specific environmental/policy approaches that may improve levels of physical activity are incorporating sidewalk and bike lanes into community design and urban planning, providing funds for hiking and walking trails as part of highway projects, designing safe routes for walking or bicycling to school (Rodriguez et al., 2019), developing "complete street" policies (e.g., increasing street aesthetics and safety for pedestrians and cyclists though foliage, crosswalks, speed bumps, traffic lights, roundabouts), and providing incentives for the establishment of mixed-use developments involving both residential and commercial destinations. Additional research is needed to better understand and measure the scale and impacts of the built environment, and the extent to which local contexts, the intersection of the natural environment, built environment, and physical activity, and cultural influences moderate physical activity behavior (Bonaccorsi et al., 2020).

Environmental interventions have the potential to complement informational, social, and behavioral interventions (Rodriguez Espinosa et al., 2023). Given their scale and scope, their population reach could be greater in addition to their potential for benefiting all individuals in a community. Interventions to promote physical activity in specific community settings, such as schools and worksites, also have the potential for broad impact. However, the need for better controlled, scientifically rigorous studies remains. Research has shown that for several population segments, effective physical activity interventions will likely need to contain multiple program components, including school, family, and/or community member involvement (Rodriguez Espinosa et al., 2023). Successful school-based physical activity interventions have also incorporated environmental and policy strategies to extend the reach of and involve others potentially influential in a child's physical activity behavior (Cassar et al., 2019). A well-designed curriculum combined with engagement and collaboration with teachers has been shown to be efficacious for increasing physical activity (e.g., moderate to vigorous physical activity; Lerum et al., 2019). Because the efficacy of school-based interventions has been reported to be, at times, inconsistent, further systematic research in this area is indicated.

Like school settings for children, worksites present a potentially convenient setting for health promotion programming for working-age adults. In a systematic review, enablers within worksites that supported health behaviors (including physical activity) included implementing motivational strategies (installing bike racks) and counseling, providing financial rewards and incentives (group-based more so than individual rewards), and designing multicomponent interventions (e.g., supportive environments and policy actions). Some described barriers are time (work schedules), workplace culture, job-related fatigue, working multiple shifts, and workloads (Worley et al., 2022). Example strategies to promote physical activity in worksites include incorporating structured physical activity breaks during the workday, promoting the use of stairs rather than elevators, locating parking lots farther away from the worksite to encourage more walking, and providing tailored motivational programs based on behavior change theory. Evidence also supports the use of environmental cues and point-of-decision prompts in successfully promoting physical activity in such settings (King et al., 2019).

In summary, a comprehensive approach that appropriately targets behavioral, informational, social, environmental, and policy-based interventions is indicated to improve and better understand the complex factors that affect physical activity behavior.

FUTURE DIRECTIONS IN PHYSICAL ACTIVITY PROMOTION

Several emerging directions in the physical activity promotion arena are summarized in the following sections. These approaches have the potential to broaden both the overall impact and population "reach" of interventions in the field.

Stealth Interventions

"Stealth" health promotion interventions typically refer to interventions that are carried out for a particular nonhealthy purpose, but have as a side effect the promotion of healthy behaviors (Manika et al., 2021). For example, Skouteris and colleagues (2013) utilized tools from the field of social marketing to increase children's motivation to engage in healthy behaviors (i.e., healthy eating and physical activity behaviors) by way of an environmental sustainability social movement. It was through their innovative approach that they simultaneously supported the uptake of healthy behaviors at the individual level and increased children's awareness in a way that has the potential to lead to sustainable practices that may impact environmental health. Another example is the implementation of a culturally informed obesity prevention study for Mexican American girls where the primary intervention was folkloric dance, with no specific mention of "physical activity" or "exercise" (Azevedo et al., 2013). This type of intervention design may provide motivation for physical activity and improve knowledge, skills, attitudes, and physical activity behaviors overall.

Multiple Behavior Change Interventions

Heart disease, cancer, and stroke remain the leading chronic diseases among U.S. adults and the leading causes of death. Currently, over half of adults (51.8%) have at least one chronic condition, with over one-quarter (27.2%) being diagnosed with multiple chronic conditions (Boersma et al., 2021; DHHS, 2018). There is a substantial body of literature on both single and multiple behavior change interventions (King et al., 2019). Multiple health behavior change interventions can target several health behaviors either simultaneously (i.e., at the same time) or sequentially (i.e., by starting with one health behavior and subsequently adding others; King et al., 2013). Compared with single behavior change interventions, multiple health behavior interventions have the potential to be as, or more, effective in changing health behaviors. They can also provide a better use of resources and maximize health promotion contact opportunities, have greater real-world applicability, and be more relevant for behaviors that co-occur (Duan et al., 2021). Successfully changing one health behavior may lead to increased confidence and self-efficacy that other health behaviors can be successfully changed, particularly if the change process for the different health behaviors is similar (Duan et al., 2021). It is also possible that multiple health behavior change interventions may not be as effective as single health behavior change interventions because such approaches can be overwhelming and confusing, and different behaviors may require different behavior change strategies. Single health behavior change interventions facilitate a greater focus on specific content, can be more comprehensive for a particular health behavior, and may be less cognitively demanding than combined health behavior change interventions (King et al., 2019). Additional research is required to better understand the potential of multiple behavior change interventions to improve health behaviors and outcomes, particularly for different populations.

BROADENING THE TARGETS AND CONTEXTS OF PHYSICAL ACTIVITY INTERVENTIONS

The adoption and maintenance of health-promoting physical activity are complex and warrant examination from a broad perspective. Possible approaches include using a social-ecological perspective (Rhodes et al., 2019), incorporating an interdisciplinary and multisector approach, examining physical activity across the life course, and considering a variety of physical activity modes (frequency, intensity, duration, and type) and domains (leisure, occupational, household, and transport-related activities).

Applying a Social-Ecological Framework

Health behavior change can be usefully studied by applying a social-ecological framework that considers not only an individual's behavior, but also the contexts in which an individual lives (Rhodes et al., 2019). For example, an individual may set personal goals to be more physically active, but these goals may be thwarted by a lack of social support and encouragement from family and friends, an absence of wellness programs available at school or in the workplace, a lack of appropriate recreational facilities in the neighborhood, and/or an absence of state and local policies that make travel by foot or bicycle safe and easy. Broadening the targets of physical activity research and interventions to incorporate a more holistic, social-ecological perspective requires a multisector approach that includes professionals not only from public health and healthcare, but also from parks and recreation, law enforcement, education, transportation, urban planning, education, policy, and business (DHHS, 2018). Support for the different levels that comprise such a social-ecological approach can be found in the literature (Rhodes et al., 2019). In addition, a growing literature supports the systematic inclusion of the actual "lived experiences" of residents themselves as part of this mix (King, Campero et al., 2020).

Utilizing a Life-Course Perspective

The life-course approach is an alternative or complementary framework in which to consider physical activity. The 2018 Physical Activity Guidelines for Americans provide information for children and adolescents aged 6 to 17, adults aged 18 to 64, older adults aged 65 and older, and special populations such as pregnant women and people with disabilities and chronic medical conditions (DHHS, 2018). Rarely, however, are interventions developed that target or include more than one age group or population. Doing so could potentially harness social and contextual forces shared across age groups and life stages, with broadened intervention impacts a possible consequence.

CHALLENGES AND OPPORTUNITIES IN THE FIELD OF PHYSICAL ACTIVITY RESEARCH

There are multiple factors that affect the adoption and maintenance of regular physical activity over the life course, including biological and sociocultural determinants, some of which are invariant (e.g., age and gender) and some are modifiable (e.g., behavioral patterns and several social and environmental contexts; Bauman et al., 2012; DHHS, 2018). Like other health behaviors and conditions, while short-term adoption of increased physical activity can often be achieved by many individuals, longer term maintenance of a more active lifestyle typically proves far more challenging (Fleig et al., 2013). Further research is needed regarding how best to maintain physical activity behavior over the longer term. To do this typically requires extending study periods, which necessitates a greater investment of resources (both financial and human). Currently, funding agencies do not typically support studies of a sufficient length to evaluate maintenance strategies and relapse prevention over time.

The body of knowledge regarding health behavior change research that targets physical activity is ever increasing. One of the challenges facing researchers in this field is to determine appropriate ways of summarizing and integrating the literature. Meta-analyses are increasingly being used to combine and compare the results of different studies, but if not conducted properly meta-analyses can result in spurious results (Sox & Goodman, 2012). Common areas of bias include inadequate or inconsistent protocols for the identification and selection of studies, integrating studies in which methods are far from homogeneous, insufficient availability of data on study methods and results, and using incorrect statistical tests to analyze the integrated data (Dwan et al., 2013).

Despite the growing body of knowledge regarding evidence-based interventions to promote physical activity previously discussed, less is known about how to effectively disseminate proven interventions in community and healthcare settings (King et al., 2019). Successful dissemination of an effective intervention typically requires a comprehensive approach that targets external validity as well as internal validity. In their Advisory Committee Highlights from the Physical Activity Guidelines report, King and colleagues (2019) emphasize the need for targeted dissemination efforts for underserved population subgroups. This approach not only helps ensure that all subgroups benefit from evidence-based practices, but it can also serve as a mechanism to understand which intervention strategies and combination of strategies work for whom and why. Leveraging the promise of community-engaged citizen science has been effective at contextualizing the multilevel social and structural determinants of health among marginalized and underserved populations (King, Campero et al., 2020) and could help facilitate engagement, build trust, and ultimately inform physical activity intervention and program design.

Increasing globalization made possible by improved transportation and communication, urbanization, and unhealthy lifestyles (poor diet, sedentary behaviors) are contributing to increases in the prevalence and incidence of chronic diseases worldwide. Innovative population-based strategies such as health education campaigns utilizing technology, social media, and "edutainment" (Nam & Choi, 2023), as well as fiscal and regulatory measures in combination with health behavior change, are urgently needed to improve health in the United States and on a global scale. Practitioners and researchers in developed countries have substantial knowledge regarding physical activity behavior change accumulated over the past half century that can be shared with their counterparts in developing countries.

CONCLUSION

In summary, although engaging in even reasonably modest amounts of physical activity on a regular basis has been shown to have important health benefits across the life span, promoting physical activity adoption and sustained maintenance remains challenging. An individual's ability to engage regularly in physical activity and reduce sedentary time is affected not only by personal characteristics but also by the social, built, and policy environments in which the individual lives, works, studies, and plays. A comprehensive approach to promoting regular physical activity is therefore required that intervenes across the range of social-ecological levels and across the life course. Adequately translating, disseminating, and scaling up successful physical activity health behavior change research and best practices continue to challenge researchers and practitioners alike. To address these issues, a social ecological, multidisciplinary approach that incorporates broader perspectives, with input from healthcare providers, researchers, local government, nonprofit organizations, and community members themselves, is strongly recommended. Finally, harnessing the power of technology to accelerate and sustain positive physical activity behavior change is an area that holds much promise for the future, regardless of age or local circumstances. Through this wide array of approaches and perspectives, creating and sustaining a physically active population may be more fully realized.

SUMMARY KEY POINTS

- Engaging in regular physical activity is beneficial across the life course to achieve optimal health, and has implications for disease prevention, all-cause mortality, and overall quality of life. It is recommended that adults achieve 150 to 300 minutes of physical activity per week, with even short bouts improving health and well-being.
- There are advantages and disadvantages of self-report and device-based measures of physical activity behavior.
- From a social ecological lens, factors at the individual, interpersonal, community, and societal/environmental level have the potential to impact physical activity behavior.
- Advances in technology, from wearables to the advent of augmented reality, present opportunities that enhance physical activity behavior monitoring and interventions. However, equitable access to technology must be considered for maximal reach and impact.
- Providing the opportunity to codesign interventions (digital or nondigital) using design thinking and human-centered design, for example, may support broader integration and sustainability.
- To facilitate behavior change, cocreation, public engagement, and meaningful collaborations between researchers, practitioners, policy makers, and community members are essential to effectively address disparities in physical activity behavior and related health outcomes.

DISCUSSION QUESTIONS

1. Review the solution themes and their respective examples in Table 8.3. Provide practical examples of how each theme might be implemented within the context of your community.

2. People living with disabilities make up one subgroup of the population that has issues accessing community-based physical activity opportunities. List two other subgroups of the population that may experience access issues and explain why. Assess the extent to which individual-level factors have the potential to impact their levels of physical and/or inactivity.

3. Imagine that you were going to implement the World Café methodology in your community. As part of this, evaluate who the relevant stakeholders might be (e.g., nonprofit [including academia], for-profit/private, government). List the names of at least five individuals, groups, and cross-sector stakeholders that you would consider inviting to hear their lived experiences and with whom you would codesign solutions. Make it a goal to include stakeholders who represent multiple levels of the social-ecological model. Critique and explain the relative value, or importance, that each stakeholder would bring to the discussion?

4. With the *Our Voice* methodology in mind, take a brief walk in your community. Identify neighborhood features that promote and hinder physical activity.

5. What solutions could you imagine to better promote physical activity in your community? How would your selected solutions impact different population subgroups in your community and what might any unintended consequences be? How might you address those unintended consequences, if any?

A robust set of instructor resources designed to supplement this text is located at http://connect.springerpub.com/content/book/978-0-8261-4265-8. Qualifying instructors may request access by emailing textbook@springerpub.com.

REFERENCES

Adams, M. A., Ryan, S., Kerr, J., Sallis, J. F., Patrick, K., Frank, L. D., & Norman, G. J. (2009). Validation of the Neighborhood Environment Walkability Scale (NEWS) items using geographic information systems. *Journal of Physical Activity and Health, 6*(s1), S113–S123. https://doi.org/10.1123/jpah.6.s1.s113

Afaneh, H., Fernes, P. K., Lewis, E. C., King, A. C., Banchoff, A., & Sheats, J. L. (2022). Our voice NOLA: Leveraging a community engaged citizen science method to contextualize the new orleans food environment. *International Journal of Environmental Research and Public Health, 19*(22), 14790. https://doi.org/10.3390/ijerph192214790

Affuso, O., Kinsey, A. W., Whitt-Glover, M. C., Segar, M., & Bowen, P. (2022). Social environments and physical activity among active black women. *American Journal of Health Promotion, 36*(8), 1275–1283. https://doi.org/10.1177/08901171221102139. Epub 2022 May 17.

Althoff, T., Sosič, R., Hicks, J. L., King, A. C., Delp, S. L., & Leskovec, J. (2017). Large-scale physical activity data reveal worldwide activity inequality. *Nature, 547*(7663), 336–339. https://doi.org/10.1038/nature23018

Amini, H., Habibi, S., Islamoglu, A. H., Isanejad, E., Uz, C., & Daniyari, H. (2021). COVID-19 pandemic-induced physical inactivity: The necessity of updating the Global Action Plan on Physical Activity 2018–2030. *Environmental Health and Preventive Medicine, 26*(1), 1–3. https://doi.org/10.1186/s12199-021-00955-z

Azevedo, K. J., Mendoza, S., Fernández, M., Haydel, K. F., Fujimoto, M., Tirumalai, E. C., & Robinson, T. N. (2013). Turn off the TV and dance! Participation in culturally tailored health interventions: Implications for obesity prevention among Mexican American girls. *Ethnicity & Disease, 23*(4), 452.

Bantham, A., Ross, S. E. T., Sebastião, E., & Hall, G. (2021). Overcoming barriers to physical activity in underserved populations. *Progress in Cardiovascular Diseases, 64*, 64–71. https://doi.org/10.1016/j.pcad.2020.11.002

Bauman, A. E., Reis, R. S., Sallis, J. F., Wells, J. C., Loos, R. J., & Martin, B. W. (2012). Correlates of physical activity: Why are some people physically active and others not? *The Lancet, 380*(9838), 258–271. https://doi.org/10.1016/S0140-6736(12)60735-1

Beauchamp, M. R., Crawford, K. L., & Jackson, B. (2019). Social cognitive theory and physical activity: Mechanisms of behavior change, critique, and legacy. *Psychology of Sport and Exercise, 42*, 110–117. https://doi.org/10.1016/j.psychsport.2018.11.009

Bennie, J. A., De Cocker, K., Teychenne, M. J., Brown, W. J., & Biddle, S. J. (2019). The epidemiology of aerobic physical activity and muscle-strengthening activity guideline adherence among 383,928 US adults. *International Journal of Behavioral Nutrition and Physical Activity, 16*, 1–11. https://doi.org/10.1186/s12966-019-0797-2

Boersma, P., Cohen, R. A., Zelaya, C. E., & Moy, E. (2021). Multiple chronic conditions among veterans and nonveterans: United States, 2015–2018. *National Health Statistics Reports*, (153), 1–13.

Bonaccorsi, G., Manzi, F., Del Riccio, M., Setola, N., Naldi, E., Milani, C., Giorgetti, D., Dellisanti, C., & Lorini, C. (2020). Impact of the built environment and the neighborhood in promoting the physical activity and the healthy aging in older people: An umbrella review. *International Journal of Environmental Research and Public Health, 17*(17), 6127. https://doi.org/10.3390/ijerph17176127

Bowen, J., Bulbena, A., & Fatjó, J. (2021). The value of companion dogs as a source of social support for their owners: Findings from a pre-pandemic representative sample and a convenience sample obtained during the COVID-19 lockdown in Spain. *Frontiers in Psychiatry, 12*, 622060. https://doi.org/10.3389/fpsyt.2021.622060

Carbone, P. S., Smith, P. J., Lewis, C., & LeBlanc, C. (2021). Promoting the participation of children and adolescents with disabilities in sports, recreation, and physical activity. *Pediatrics. 148*(6), e2021054664. https://doi.org/10.1542/peds.2021-054664.

Carraça, E., Encantado, J., Battista, F., Beaulieu, K., Blundell, J., Busetto, L., van Baak, M., Dicker, D., Ermolao, A., Farpour-Lambert, N., Pramono, A., Woodward, E., Bellicha, A., & Oppert, J. M. (2021). Effective behavior change techniques to promote physical activity in adults with overweight or obesity: A systematic review and meta-analysis. *Obesity Reviews, 22*, e13258. https://doi.org/10.1111/obr.13258

Case, L., Ross, S., & Yun, J. (2020). Physical activity guideline compliance among a national sample of children with various developmental disabilities. *Disability and Health Journal, 13*(2), 100881. https://doi.org/10.1016/j.dhjo.2019.100881

Cassar, S., Salmon, J., Timperio, A., Naylor, P. J., Van Nassau, F., Contardo Ayala, A. M., & Koorts, H. (2019). Adoption, implementation and sustainability of school-based physical activity and sedentary behaviour interventions in real-world settings: A systematic review. *International Journal of Behavioral Nutrition and Physical Activity, 16*(1), 1–13. https://doi.org/10.1186/s12966-019-0876-4

Caspersen, C. J., Powell, K. E., & Christenson, G. M. (1985). Physical activity, exercise, and physical fitness: Definitions and distinctions for health-related research. Public Health Reports, 100(2), 126.

Centers for Disease Control and Prevention. (2019). *Behavioral risk factor surveillance system survey data*. U.S. Department of Health and Human Services, Centers for Disease Control and Prevention.

Centers for Disease Control and Prevention. (2021). *Surveillance systems*. https://www.cdc.gov/physicalactivity/data/surveillance.htm

Centers for Disease Control and Prevention. (2022). *CDC releases updated maps of American's high levels of physical inactivity*. https://www.cdc.gov/media/releases/2022/p0120-inactivity-map.html

Centers for Disease Control and Prevention. (2023). *National center on birth defects and developmental disabilities, division of human development and disability*. Disability and Health Data System (DHDS) Data [online]. https://dhds.cdc.gov

Cole-Lewis, H., Ezeanochie, N., & Turgiss, J. (2019). Understanding health behavior technology engagement: Pathway to measuring digital behavior change interventions. *JMIR Formative Research, 3*(4), e14052. https://doi.org/10.2196/14052

Compernolle, S., DeSmet, A., Poppe, L., Crombez, G., De Bourdeaudhuij, I., Cardon, G., van der Ploeg, H. P., & Van Dyck, D. (2019). Effectiveness of interventions using self-monitoring to reduce sedentary behavior in adults: A systematic review and meta-analysis. *International Journal of Behavioral Nutrition and Physical Activity, 16*(1), 1–16. https://doi.org/10.1186/s12966-019-0824-3

Cosoli, G., Spinsante, S., & Scalise, L. (2020). Wrist-worn and chest-strap wearable devices: Systematic review on accuracy and metrological characteristics. *Measurement, 159*, 107789.

Cunningham, C., O' Sullivan, R., Caserotti, P., & Tully, M. A. (2020). Consequences of physical inactivity in older adults: A systematic review of reviews and meta-analyses. *Scandinavian Journal of Medicine & Science in Sports, 30*(5), 816–827. https://doi.org/10.1111/sms.13616

Cusatis, R., & Garbarski, D. (2019). Different domains of physical activity: The role of leisure, housework/care work, and paid work in socioeconomic differences in reported physical activity. *SSM-Population Health, 7*, 100387. https://doi.org/10.1016/j.ssmph.2019.100387

Dempsey, P. C., Matthews, C. E., Dashti, S. G., Doherty, A. R., Bergouignan, A., Van Roekel, E. H., Dunstan, D. W., Wareham, N. J., Yates, T. E., Wijndaele, K., & Lynch, B. M. (2020). Sedentary behavior and chronic disease: Mechanisms and future directions. *Journal of Physical Activity and Health, 17*(1), 52–61. https://doi.org/10.1123/jpah.2019-0377

Duan, Y., Shang, B., Liang, W., Du, G., Yang, M., & Rhodes, R. E. (2021). Effects of eHealth-based multiple health behavior change interventions on physical activity, healthy diet, and weight in people with noncommunicable diseases: Systematic review and meta-analysis. *Journal of Medical Internet Research, 23*(2), e23786. https://doi.org/10.2196/23786

Dwan, K., Gamble, C., Williamson, P. R., & Kirkham, J. J. (2013). Systematic review of the empirical evidence of study publication bias and outcome reporting bias–An updated review. *PLoS One, 8*(7), e66844. https://doi.org/10.1371/journal.pone.0066844

Elgaddal, N., Kramarow, E. A., & Reuben, C. (2022). Physical activity among adults aged 18 and over: United States, 2020. *NCHS Data Brief, 443*, 1–8.

Erturan, G., McBride, R., & Agbuga, B. (2020). Self-regulation and self-efficacy as mediators of achievement goals and leisure time physical activity: A proposed model. *Pedagogy of Physical Culture and Sports, 24*(1), 12–20.

Everest, G., Marshall, L., Fraser, C., & Briggs, A. (2022). *Addressing the leading risk factors for ill health* [Online]. The Health Foundation. https://www.health.org.uk/publications/reports/addressing-the-leading-risk-factors-for-ill-health

Farooq, A., Martin, A., Janssen, X., Wilson, M. G., Gibson, A. M., Hughes, A., & Reilly, J. J. (2020). Longitudinal changes in moderate-to-vigorous-intensity physical activity in children and adolescents: A systematic review and meta-analysis. *Obesity Reviews, 21*(1), e12953. https://doi.org/10.1111/obr.12953

Fleig, L., Pomp, S., Schwarzer, R., & Lippke, S. (2013). Promoting exercise maintenance: How interventions with booster sessions improve long-term rehabilitation outcomes. *Rehabilitation Psychology, 58*(4), 323. https://psycnet.apa.org/doi/10.1037/a0033885

Flórez, K. R., Richardson, A. S., Ghosh-Dastidar, M. B., Troxel, W., DeSantis, A., Colabianchi, N., & Dubowitz, T. (2018). The power of social networks and social support in promotion of physical activity and body mass index among African American adults. *SSM - Population Health, 4*, 327–333. https://doi.org/10.1016/j.ssmph.2018.03.004

Fonseca, F., Ribeiro, P. J., Conticelli, E., Jabbari, M., Papageorgiou, G., Tondelli, S., & Ramos, R. A. (2022). Built environment attributes and their influence on walkability. *International Journal of Sustainable Transportation, 16*(7), 660–679. https://doi.org/10.1080/15568318.2021.1914793

Franco, M. R., Tong, A., Howard, K., Sherrington, C., Ferreira, P. H., Pinto, R. Z., & Ferreira, M. L. (2015). Older people's perspectives on participation in physical activity: A systematic review and thematic synthesis of qualitative literature. *British Journal of Sports Medicine, 49*(19), 1268–1276.

Friel, C. P., Duran, A. T., Shechter, A., & Diaz, K. M. (2020). US children meeting physical activity, screen time, and sleep guidelines. *American Journal of Preventive Medicine, 59*(4), 513–521. https://doi.org/10.1016/j.amepre.2020.05.007

GirlTrek. (2023). *GirlTrek.* https://www.girltrek.org

Gómez, C. A., Kleinman, D. V., Pronk, N., Gordon, G. L. W., Ochiai, E., Blakey, C., Johnson, A., & Brewer, K. H. (2021). Practice full report: Addressing health equity and social determinants of health through healthy people 2030. *Journal of Public Health Management and Practice, 27*(6), S249. https://doi.org/10.1097/PHH.0000000000001297

Gorzelitz, J., Peppard, P. E., Malecki, K., Gennuso, K., Nieto, F. J., & Cadmus-Bertram, L. (2018). Predictors of discordance in self-report versus device-measured physical activity measurement. *Annals of Epidemiology, 28*(7), 427–431. https://doi.org/10.1016/j.annepidem.2018.03.016

Hardeman, W., Houghton, J., Lane, K., Jones, A., & Naughton, F. (2019). A systematic review of just-in-time adaptive interventions (JITAIs) to promote physical activity. *International Journal of Behavioral Nutrition and Physical Activity, 16*(1), 1–21. https://doi.org/10.1186/s12966-019-0792-7

Hayden, J. (2022). *Introduction to health behavior theory.* Jones & Bartlett Learning.

Herbison, J. D., Osborne, M., Andersen, J., Lepage, P., Pagé, V., Levasseur, C., Beckers, M., Gainforth, H. L., Lamontagne, M.-E, & Sweet, S. N. (2023). Strategies to improve access to physical activity opportunities for people with physical disabilities. *Translational Behavioral Medicine, 13*(7), 486–500. https://doi.org/10.1093/tbm/ibac119

Heredia, N., Nguyen, N., & McNeill, L. H. (2020). The importance of the social environment in achieving high levels of physical activity and fruit and vegetable intake in African American church members. *American Journal of Health Promotion, 34*(8), 886–893. https://doi.org/10.1177/0890117120925361

Hicks, J. L., Boswell, M. A., Althoff, T., Crum, A. J., Ku, J. P., Landay, J. A., Moya, P. M. L., Murnane, E. L., Snyder, M. P., King, A. C., & Delp, S. L. (2022). Leveraging mobile technology for public health promotion: A multidisciplinary perspective. *Annual Review of Public Health, 44*, 131–150. https://doi.org/10.1146/annurev-publhealth-060220-041643

Hoy-Gerlach, J., Rauktis, M., & Newhill, C. (2020). (Non-human) animal companionship: A crucial support for people during the COVID-19 pandemic. *Society Register, 4*(2), 109–120. https://doi.org/10.14746/sr.2020.4.2.08

Hwang, T. J., Rabheru, K., Peisah, C., Reichman, W., & Ikeda, M. (2020). Loneliness and social isolation during the COVID-19 pandemic. *International Psychogeriatrics, 32*(10), 1217–1220. https://doi.org/10.1017/S1041610220000988

Ironside, A., Ferguson, L. J., Katapally, T. R., Hedayat, L. M., Johnson, S. R., & Foulds, H. J. A. (2021). Social determinants associated with physical activity among Indigenous adults at the University of Saskatchewan. *Applied Physiology, Nutrition, and Metabolism, 46*(10), 1159–1169. https://doi.org/10.1139/apnm-2020-0781

Islam, S. J., Kim, J. H., Baltrus, P., Topel, M. L., Liu, C., Ko, Y. A., Mujahid, M. S., Vaccarino, V., Sims, M., Mubasher, M., Khan, A., Ejaz, K., Searles, C., Dunbar, S., Pemu, P., Taylor, H. A., Quyyumi, A. A., & Lewis, T. T. (2022). Neighborhood characteristics and ideal cardiovascular health among Black adults: Results from the Morehouse-Emory Cardiovascular (MECA) Center for Health Equity. *Annals of Epidemiology, 65*, 120-e1. https://doi.org/10.1016/j.annepidem.2020.11.009

Jakicic, J. M., Kraus, W. E., Powell, K. E., Campbell, W. W., Janz, K. F., Troiano, R. P., Sprow, K., Torres, A., & Piercy, K. L. (2019). Association between bout duration of physical activity and health: Systematic review. *Medicine and Science in Sports and Exercise, 51*(6), 1213. https://doi.org/10.1249/MSS.0000000000001933

John, J. M., Haug, V., & Thiel, A. (2020). Physical activity behavior from a transdisciplinary biopsychosocial perspective: A Scoping Review. *Sports Med Open, 6*(1), 49. https://doi.org/10.1186/s40798-020-00279-2

Kahn, E. B., Ramsey, L. T., Brownson, R. C., Heath, G. W., Howze, E. H., Powell, K. E., Stone, E. J., Rajab, M. W., & Corso, P. (2002). The effectiveness of interventions to increase physical activity. A systematic review. *American Journal of Preventive Medicine, 22*(4 Suppl), 73–107. https://doi.org/10.1016/s0749-3797(02)00434-8

Keadle, S. K., Bustamante, E. E., & Buman, M. P. (2021). Physical activity and public health: Four decades of progress. *Kinesiology Review, 10*(3), 319–330. https://doi.org/10.1123/kr.2021-0028

Keusch, F., Wenz, A., & Conrad, F. (2022). Do you have your smartphone with you? Behavioral barriers for measuring everyday activities with smartphone sensors. *Computers in Human Behavior, 127*, 107054. https://doi.org/10.1016/j.chb.2021.107054

Kim, Y., Park, I., & Kang, M. (2013). Convergent validity of the international physical activity questionnaire (IPAQ): Meta-analysis. *Public Health Nutrition, 16*(3), 440–452. https://doi.org/10.1017/S1368980012002996

King, A. C., Campero, I., Sheats, J. L., Sweet, C. M. C., Espinosa, P. R., Garcia, D., Hauser, M., Done, M., Patel, M. L., Parikh, N. M., Corral, C., & Ahn, D. K. (2020). Testing the effectiveness of physical activity advice delivered via text messaging vs. human phone advisors in a Latino population: The

On The Move randomized controlled trial design and methods. *Contemporary Clinical Trials, 95,* 106084. https://doi.org/10.1016/j.cct.2020.106084

King, A. C., Castro, C. M., Buman, M. P., Hekler, E. B., Urizar, G. G., Jr., & Ahn, D. K. (2013). Behavioral impacts of sequentially versus simultaneously delivered dietary plus physical activity interventions: The CALM trial. *Annals of Behavioral Medicine, 46*(2), 157–168. https://doi.org/10.1007/s12160-013 -9501-y

King, A. C., King, D. K., Banchoff, A., Solomonov, S., Ben Natan, O., Hua, J., Gardiner, P., Goldman Rosas, L., Espinosa, P. R., Winter, S. J., Sheats, J., Salvo, D., Aguilar-Farias, N., Stathi, A., Akira Hino, A., Porter, M. M., & Our Voice Global Citizen Science Research Network. (2020). Employing participatory citizen science methods to promote age-friendly environments worldwide. *International Journal of Environmental Research and Public Health, 17*(5), 1541. https://doi.org/10.3390 /ijerph17051541

King, A. C., Whitt-Glover, M. C., Marquez, D. X., Buman, M. P., Napolitano, M. A., Jakicic, J., Fulton, J. E., Tennant, B. L., & 2018 Physical Activity Guidelines Advisory Committee. (2019). Physical activity promotion: Highlights from the 2018 physical activity guidelines advisory committee systematic review. *Medicine & Science in Sports & Exercise, 51*(6), 1340–1353. https://doi.org/10.1249 /MSS.0000000000001945

Laranjo, L., Ding, D., Heleno, B., Kocaballi, B., Quiroz, J. C., Tong, H. L., Chahwan, B., Luisa Neves, A., Gabarron, E., Phuong Dao, K., Rodrigues, D., Costa Neves, G., Antunes, M. L., Coiera, E., & Bates, D. W. (2021). Do smartphone applications and activity trackers increase physical activity in adults? Systematic review, meta-analysis and metaregression. *British Journal of Sports Medicine, 55*(8), 422–432. http://doi.org/10.1136/bjsports-2020-102892

Lee, D. H., Rezende, L. F. M., Joh, H. K., Keum, N., Ferrari, G, Rey-Lopez, J. P., Rimm, E.B., Tabung, F. K., & Giovannucci, E. L. (2022). Long-Term Leisure-Time physical activity intensity and allcause and cause-specific mortality: A prospective cohort of US adults. *Circulation, 146*(7), 523-534. https://doi.org/10.1161/CIRCULATIONAHA.121.058162

Lee, J. E., & Gao, Z. (2021). Racial difference in children's physical activity and psychosocial beliefs in physical education. *JTRM in Kinesiology.* http://www.sports-media.org/index.php/jtrm-in -kinesiology/49-racial-difference-in-children-s-physical-activity-and-psychosocial-beliefs-in -physical-education

Lee, Y. H., & Fan, S. Y. (2023). Psychosocial and environmental factors related to physical activity in middle-aged and older adults. *Scientific Reports, 13*(1), 7788.

Lerum, Ø., Bartholomew, J., McKay, H., Resaland, G. K., Tjomsland, H. E., Anderssen, S. A., Leirhaug, P. E.; & Moe, V. F. (2019). Active smarter teachers: Primary school teachers' perceptions and maintenance of a school-based physical activity intervention. *Translational Journal of the American College of Sports Medicine, 4*(17), 141–147. https://doi.org/10.1249/TJX .0000000000000104

Li, H., & Wang, C. (2021). The relationships among structural social support, functional social support, and loneliness in older adults: Analysis of regional differences based on a multigroup structural equation model. *Frontiers in Psychology, 12,* 732173. https://doi.org/10.3389/fpsyg .2021.732173

Löhr, K., Weinhardt, M., & Sieber, S. (2020). The "World Café" as a participatory method for collecting qualitative data. *International Journal of Qualitative Methods, 19.* https://doi.org/10.1177 /1609406920916976

Lounassalo, I., Salin, K., Kankaanpää, A., Hirvensalo, M., Palomäki, S., Tolvanen, A., Yang, X., & Tammelin, T. H. (2019). Distinct trajectories of physical activity and related factors during the life course in the general population: A systematic review. *BMC Public Health, 19,* 1–12. https://doi .org/10.1186/s12889-019-6513-y

Manika, D., Blokland, Y., Smith, L., Mansfield, L., & Klonizakis, M. (2021). Using stealth marketing techniques to increase physical activity and decrease sedentary time in the workplace: A feasibility study investigating the spill-overs of employee pro-environmental behaviour. *International Journal of Business Science and Applied Management, 16*(1), 28–49.

Marasso, D., Lupo, C., Collura, S., Rainoldi, A., & Brustio, P. R. (2021). Subjective versus objective measure of physical activity: A systematic review and meta-analysis of the convergent validity of the Physical Activity Questionnaire for Children (PAQ-C). *International Journal of Environmental Research and Public Health, 18*(7), 3413. https://doi.org/10.3390/ijerph18073413

Marcus, B. H., Napolitano, M. A., King, A. C., Lewis, B. A., Whiteley, J. A., Albrecht, A. E., Parisi, A. F., Bock, B. C., Pinto, B. M., Sciamanna, C. A., Jakicic, J. M., & Papandonatos, G. D. (2007). Examination of print and telephone channels for physical activity promotion: Rationale, design, and baseline data from Project STRIDE. *Contemporary Clinical Trails, 28*(1), 90–104. https://doi.org/10.1016/j .cct.2006.04.003

Marquez, B., Elder, J. P., Arredondo, E. M., Madanat, H., Ji, M., & Ayala, G. X. (2014). Social network characteristics associated with health promoting behaviors among Latinos. *Health Psychology, 33*(6), 544. https://psycnet.apa.org/doi/10.1037/hea0000092

Marquez, D. X., Aguiñaga, S., Vásquez, P. M., Conroy, D. E., Erickson, K. I., Hillman, C., Stillman, C. M., Ballard, R. M., Sheppard, B. B., Petruzzello, S. J., King, A. C., & Powell, K. E. (2020). A systematic review of physical activity and quality of life and well-being. *Translational Behavioral Medicine, 10*(5), 1098–1109. https://doi.org/10.1093/tbm/ibz198

Mazeas, A., Duclos, M., Pereira, B., & Chalabaev, A. (2022). Evaluating the effectiveness of gamification on physical activity: Systematic review and meta-analysis of randomized controlled trials. *Journal of Medical Internet Research, 24*(1), e26779. https://doi.org/10.2196/26779

McEwan, D., Rhodes, R. E., & Beauchamp, M. R. (2022). What happens when the party is over?: Sustaining physical activity behaviors after intervention cessation. *Behavioral Medicine, 48*(1), 1–9. https://doi.org/10.1080/08964289.2020.1750335

Meyer, M. R. U., Moore, J. B., Abildso, C., Edwards, M. B., Gamble, A., & Baskin, M. L. (2016). Rural active living: A call to action. *Journal of Public Health Management and Practice: JPHMP, 22*(5), E11. https://doi.org/10.1097/PHH.0000000000000333

Michie, S., Richardson, M., Johnston, M., Abraham, C., Francis, J., Hardeman, W., Eccles, M. P., Cane, J., & Wood, C. E. (2013). The behavior change technique taxonomy (v1) of 93 hierarchically clustered techniques: Building an international consensus for the reporting of behavior change interventions. *Annals of Behavioral Medicine, 46*(1), 81–95. https://doi.org/10.1007/s12160-013-9486-6

Milne-Ives, M., de Cock, C., Lim, E., Shehadeh, M. H., de Pennington, N., Mole, G., Normando, E., & Meinert, E. (2020). The effectiveness of artificial intelligence conversational agents in health care: Systematic review. *Journal of Medical Internet Research, 22*(10), e20346. https://doi.org/10.2196/20346

Mintz, E., & Couch, J. (2022). Biomedical citizen science at the National Institutes of Health. *Citizen Science: Theory and Practice, 7*(1), 37. http://doi.org/10.5334/cstp.543

Montgomery, S. C., Donnelly, M., Badham, J., Kee, F., Dunne, L., & Hunter, R. F. (2021). A multimethod exploration into the social networks of young teenagers and their physical activity behavior. *BMC Public Health, 21*, 1–18. https://doi.org/10.1186/s12889-020-10081-0

Mooney, S. J., Hurvitz, P. M., Moudon, A. V., Zhou, C., Dalmat, R., & Saelens, B. E. (2020). Residential neighborhood features associated with objectively measured walking near home: Revisiting walkability using the Automatic Context Measurement Tool (ACMT). *Health & Place, 63*, 102332. https://doi.org/10.1016/j.healthplace.2020.102332

Mötteli, S., & Dohle, S. (2020). Egocentric social network correlates of physical activity. *Journal of Sport and Health Science, 9*(4), 339–344. https://doi.org/10.1016/j.jshs.2017.01.002

Nam, S. & Choi, H. (2023). Edutainment content production platform based on activity control using skeleton tracking. https://sensors.myu-group.co.jp/article.php?ss=4267

National Cancer Institute. (2023). *Social support.* https://www.cancer.gov/publications/dictionaries/cancer-terms/def/social-support

Ng, Y. L., Ma, F., Ho, F. K., Ip, P., & Fu, K. W. (2019). Effectiveness of virtual and augmented reality-enhanced exercise on physical activity, psychological outcomes, and physical performance: A systematic review and meta-analysis of randomized controlled trials. *Computers in Human Behavior, 99*, 278–291. https://doi.org/10.1016/j.chb.2019.05.026

Our Voice. (n.d.). *GirlTrek multi-city walkability assessments (2017).* Our Voice: Citizen Science for Health Equity. Retrieved May 8, 2023, from https://med.stanford.edu/ourvoice/our-projects/united-states/girltrek---our-voice-collaboration.html

Park, J. H., Moon, J. H., Kim, H. J., Kong, M. H., & Oh, Y. H. (2020). Sedentary lifestyle: Overview of updated evidence of potential health risks. *Korean Journal of Family Medicine, 41*(6), 365. https://doi.org/10.4082%2Fkjfm.20.0165

Payán, D. D., Sloane, D. C., Illum, J., & Lewis, L. B. (2019). Intrapersonal and environmental barriers to physical activity among Blacks and Latinos. *Journal of Nutrition Education and Behavior, 51*(4), 478–485. https://doi.org/10.1016/j.jneb.2018.10.001

Peters, M., Muellmann, S., Christianson, L., Stalling, I., Bammann, K., Drell, C., & Forberger, S. (2020). Measuring the association of objective and perceived neighborhood environment with physical activity in older adults: Challenges and implications from a systematic review. *International Journal of Health Geographics, 19*(1), 1–20. https://doi.org/10.1186/s12942-020-00243-z

Population Reference Bureau. (2023). *U.S. Growing bigger, older, and more diverse.* https://www.prb.org/resources/u-s-growing-bigger-older-and-more-diverse/

Prochnow, T., & Patterson, M. S. (2022). Assessing social network influences on adult physical activity using social network analysis: A systematic review. *American Journal of Health Promotion, 36*(3), 537-558. https://doi.org/10.1177/08901171211060701

Rhodes, R. E., McEwan, D., & Rebar, A. L. (2019). Theories of physical activity behaviour change: A history and synthesis of approaches. *Psychology of Sport and Exercise, 42*, 100–109. https://doi.org/10.1016/j.psychsport.2018.11.010

Rodriguez, N. M., Arce, A., Kawaguchi, A., Hua, J., Broderick, B., Winter, S. J., & King, A. C. (2019). Enhancing safe routes to school programs through community-engaged citizen science: Two pilot investigations in lower density areas of Santa Clara County, California, USA. *BMC Public Health, 19*, 1–11. https://doi.org/10.1186/s12889-019-6563-1

Rodriguez Espinosa, P., King, A. C., Blanco-Velazquez, I., Banchoff, A. W., Campero, M. I., Chen, W. T., & Rosas, L. G. (2023). Engaging diverse midlife and older adults in a multilevel participatory physical activity intervention: Evaluating impacts using Ripple Effects Mapping. *Translational Behavioral Medicine, 13*(9), 666–674. https://doi.org/10.1093/tbm/ibad018

Saunders, T. J., McIsaac, T., Douillette, K., Gaulton, N., Hunter, S., Rhodes, R. E., Prince, S. A., Carson, V., Chaput, J.-P., Chastin, S., Giangregorio, L., Janssen, I., Katzmarzyk, P. T., Kho, M. E., Poitras, V. J., Powell, K. E., Ross, R., Ross-White, A., Tremblay, M. S., & Healy, G. N. (2020). Sedentary behaviour and health in adults: An overview of systematic reviews. *Applied Physiology, Nutrition, and Metabolism, 45*(10), S197–S217. https://doi.org/10.1139/apnm-2020-0272

Sheats, J. L., Petrin, C., Darensbourg, R. M., & Wheeler, C. S. (2018). A Theoretically-Grounded investigation of perceptions about healthy eating and mHealth support among African American men and women in New Orleans, Louisiana. *Family & Community Health, 41*(2), S15. https://doi.org/10.1097/FCH.0000000000000177

Skouteris, H., Cox, R., Huang, T., Rutherford, L., Edwards, S., & Cutter-Mackenzie, A. (2013). Promoting obesity prevention together with environmental sustainability. *Health Promotion International, 29*(3), 454–462. https://doi.org/10.1093/heapro/dat007

Smith, M., Mavoa, S., Ikeda, E., Hasanzadeh, K., Zhao, J., Rinne, T. E., Donnellan, N., Kyttä, M., & Cui, J. (2022). Associations between children's physical activity and neighborhood environments using GIS: A secondary analysis from a systematic scoping review. *International Journal of Environmental Research and Public Health, 19*(3), 1033. https://doi.org/10.3390/ijerph19031033

Soto, S. H., Arredondo, E. M., Haughton, J., & Shakya, H. (2018). Leisure-time physical activity and characteristics of social network support for exercise among Latinas. *American Journal of Health Promotion, 32*(2), 432–439. https://doi.org/10.1177/0890117117699927

Sox, H. C., & Goodman, S. N. (2012). The methods of comparative effectiveness research. *Annual Review of Public Health, 33*, 425–445. https://doi.org/10.1146/annurev-publhealth-031811-124610

Stojanovic, M., Babulal, G. M., & Head, D. (2023). Determinants of physical activity engagement in older adults. *Journal of Behavioral Medicine, 46*(5), 1–13. https://doi.org/10.1007/s10865-023-00404-y

Swoboda, C. M., Miller, C. K., & Wills, C. E. (2017). Frequency of diet and physical activity goal attainment and barriers encountered among adults with type 2 diabetes during a telephone coaching intervention. *Clinical Diabetes, 35*(5), 286–293. https://doi.org/10.2337/cd17-0023

Tuckett, A. G., Freeman, A., Hetherington, S., Gardiner, P. A., King, A. C., & Burnie Brae Citizen Scientists. (2018). Older adults using our voice citizen science to create change in their neighborhood environment. *International Journal of Environmental Research and Public Health, 15*(12), 2685. https://doi.org/10.3390/ijerph15122685

U.S. Census Bureau. (2021). Childhood disability in the United States: 2019. https://www.census.gov/library/publications/2021/acs/acsbr-006.html

U.S. Department of Health and Human Services. (2018). *Physical activity guidelines for Americans*. https://health.gov/sites/default/files/2019-09/Physical_Activity_Guidelines_2nd_edition.pdf

Valente, T. W. (2012). Network interventions. science, 337(6090), 49-53.

Vereen, R. N., Kurtzman, R., & Noar, S. M. (2023). Are social media interventions for health behavior change efficacious among populations with health disparities?: A meta-analytic review. *Health Communication, 38*(1), 133–140. https://doi.org/10.1080/10410236.2021.1937830

Wake, A. D. (2022). Protective effects of physical activity against health risks associated with type 1 diabetes: "Health benefits outweigh the risks". *World Journal of Diabetes, 13*(3), 161. https://doi.org/10.4239/wjd.v13.i3.161

Wang, Y., Li, P., Zhang, B., & Han, Y. (2022). Does cognitive attitude matter when affective attitude is negative in physical activity behavior change? *Research Quarterly for Exercise and Sport, 94*(4), 1053–1061. https://doi.org/10.1080/02701367.2022.2111021

Westgarth, C., Christley, R. M., Jewell, C., German, A. J., Boddy, L. M., & Christian, H. E. (2019). Dog owners are more likely to meet physical activity guidelines than people without a dog: An investigation of the association between dog ownership and physical activity levels in a UK community. *Scientific Reports, 9*(1), 1–10. https://doi.org/10.1038/s41598-019-41254-6

Whitfield, G. P., Ussery, E. N., & Carlson, S. A. (2020). Peer reviewed: Combining data from assessments of leisure, occupational, household, and transportation physical activity among US adults, NHANES 2011–2016. *Preventing Chronic Disease, 17*, 200137. https://doi.org/10.5888/pcd17.200137

Winter, S. J., Sheats, J. L., & King, A. C. (2016). The use of behavior change techniques and theory in technologies for cardiovascular disease prevention and treatment in adults: A comprehensive review. *Progress in Cardiovascular Diseases, 58*(6), 605–612. https://doi.org/10.1016/j.pcad.2016.02.005

Wood, F. G., Alley, E., Baer, S., & Johnson, R. (2015). Interactive multimedia tailored to improve diabetes self-management. *Nursing Clinics of North America, 50*(3), 565–576. https://doi.org/10.1016/j.cnur.2015.05.009

Wons, O., Lampe, E., Boyajian, L., Patarinski, A. G., & Juarascio, A. (2023). A research approach to self-report and objective measurements of physical activity in eating disorders. In V. B. Patel & V. R. Preedy (Eds.), *Eating Disorders*, 413–432. https://doi.org/10.1007/978-3-031-16691-4_58

Worley, V., Fraser, P., Allender, S., & Bolton, K. A. (2022). Describing workplace interventions aimed to improve health of staff in hospital settings–a systematic review. *BMC Health Services Research*, 22(1), 459. https://doi.org/10.1186/s12913-021-07418-9

Xu, L., Rogers, C. R., Halliday, T. M., Wu, Q., & Wilmouth, L. (2020). Correlates of physical activity, psychosocial factors, and home environment exposure among US adolescents: Insights for cancer risk reduction from the FLASHE study. *International Journal of Environmental Research and Public Health*, 17(16), 5753. https://doi.org/10.3390/ijerph17165753

Yang, L., Cao, C., Kantor, E. D., Nguyen, L. H., Zheng, X., Park, Y., Giovannucci, E. L., Matthews, C. E., Colditz, G. A., & Cao, Y. (2019). Trends in sedentary behavior among the US population, 2001–2016. *JAMA*, 321(16), 1587–1597. https://doi.org/10.1001/jama.2019.3636

Zimmer, C., McDonough, M. H., Hewson, J., Toohey, A. M., Din, C., Crocker, P. R., & Bennett, E. V. (2022). Social support among older adults in group physical activity programs. *Journal of Applied Sport Psychology*, 35(4), 658–679. https://doi.org/10.1080/10413200.2022.2055223

CHAPTER 9

TOBACCO, ALCOHOL, AND OTHER DRUGS

OLUWOLE JEGEDE, JOYCE RIVERA, MARK JENKINS, AND AYANA JORDAN

LEARNING OBJECTIVES

- Understand the prevalence of tobacco, alcohol, and drug use and cessation.
- Identify the biological, psychological, and social factors that influence tobacco, alcohol, and drug use and dependence.
- Describe intervention approaches that can be used to help people change tobacco, alcohol, and drug use behavior.
- Describe different interventions for individuals who drink alcohol or take drugs excessively.
- Understand the theoretical and practice bases of the interventions.
- Evaluate the evidence for the effectiveness of the interventions.

INTRODUCTION

In this chapter we have included collected expertise from a variety of addiction experts, including physicians, clinicians, citizen scientists, academicians, researchers, and people in recovery. The information contained therein provides a nuanced perspective of how various people in the field understand substance use and the tensions that may arise in considering problematic use versus functional use. There is also a higher level overview of tobacco, alcohol, and other substances, providing real-world applicability of all. Finally, there is a necessary discretion of special populations that must be considered with striving for health equity in treating people with substance use disorders (SUD).

GENERAL PRINCIPLES

Substance Use Disorder: Diagnostic Criteria (Box 9.1)

SUBSTANCE USE: CHAOTIC OR FUNCTIONAL?

What is a drug? Why do people use drugs? Responses to this question are as varied as the number of people pooled and all responses would be valid. People who use drugs (PWUD) take them because drugs work; drugs work for whatever it is PWUD need them to work for until drugs no longer work. The above framing is important and must be understood as the point in which practitioners begin to engage people who experience and suffer from SUDs and where most opinions, observations, and stigma are based or have been handed down to PWUD and people with SUDs from clinicians and practitioners.

BOX 9.1 DIAGNOSTIC CRITERIA FOR SUBSTANCE USE DISORDER

The following are the 11 criteria to diagnose a person with substance use disorder (SUD) according to the *Diagnostic and Statistical Manual of Mental Disorders*, Fifth Edition, Text Revised (*DSM-5-TR*; APA, 2022):

1. The substance is frequently taken in larger quantities or for a longer time than intended.
2. There is a continuing desire or unsuccessful attempts to cut down or control substance use.
3. A large amount of time is spent in activities necessary to acquire the substance, use the substance, or recover from its effects.
4. There is a craving, or a strong desire, to use the substance.
5. There is recurrent substance use that leads to failure to meet significant obligations at the workplace, in school, or at home.
6. There is continued substance use in spite of continued or recurring social or interpersonal difficulties as a result of, or made worse by, the effects of the substance.
7. Previously valued social, work, or recreational activities are abandoned or decreased due to substance use.
8. There is recurring substance use in settings or situations in which it is physically dangerous.
9. Substance use is continued in spite of the individual's awareness of having a continuing or recurring physical or psychological difficulty most likely caused by or made worse by the substance.
10. There is a need for significantly increased quantities of the substance to reach intoxication or other intended effects, or notably decreased effects with continued use of the same amount of the substance (i.e., tolerance).
11. There are two components of withdrawal symptoms, either of which meet the overall criterion for withdrawal symptoms:
    a. There is a required number of withdrawal symptoms that occur when substance use is cut back or stopped following a long period of use or a period of heavy use.
    b. The substance or a related substance is used to alleviate, get over, or avoid withdrawal symptoms.

    To diagnose someone with any SUD, at least two criteria must be met. If two to three criteria are met, this indicates mild disease, four to five is moderate, and six or greater is considered severe SUD. These criteria have been simplified and categorized into three main areas—craving, control, and consequences (**Figure 9.1**)—by addiction medicine doctors Jeanette Tetrault, MD, and Kenneth Morford, MD.

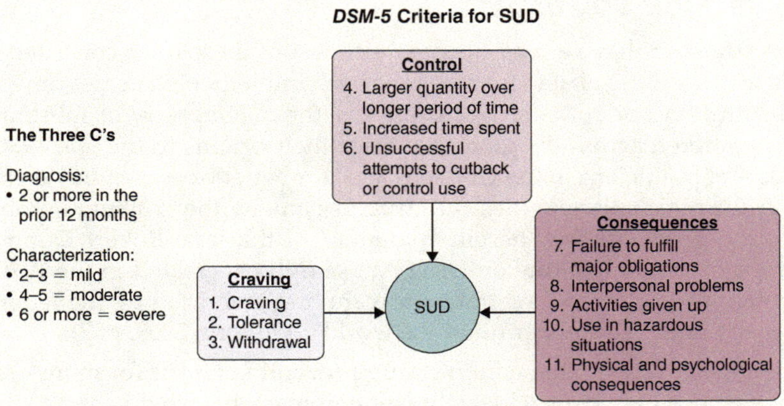

FIGURE 9.1 The 3Cs of substance use disorder.
DSM-5, *Diagnostic and Statistical Manual of Mental Disorders*, Fifth Edition; SUD, substance use disorder.
Source: Image courtesy of Jeanette Tetrault, MD, and Kenneth Morford, MD.

To understand chaotic versus functional substance use, we must first deconstruct what that means. We are a drug-using society, although we do not readily admit it. Take coffee for instance. Coffee is used (to various levels) by many American adults, but rarely thought of as a drug and certainly not something to be consumed in a chaotic fashion. Interestingly, however, caffeine-related disorders are listed in the latest iteration of the *Diagnostic and Statistical Manual of Mental Disorders* (5th ed.; *DSM-5*; APA, 2022). Yet, if you speak to many people who consume coffee and ask how much and how often they drink a day, they will likely not readily accept a diagnosis of a caffeine-related disorder or be surprised that there can be negative effects related to ongoing use (Ágoston et al., 2018). Can people who only function with caffeine be described as chaotic use?

To understand substance use, we must describe the nuanced difference between chaotic and functional use. First, substance use must be separated from SUD, and second we must acknowledge that substance use occurs on a spectrum. For example, an individual who reports periods of heavier than their usual use of a substance might be considered to have chaotic use by some, or manageable use by others, if there are no negative consequences associated with that use. Chaotic substance use needs to be considered on an individual level along with assessment of the impact on that individual's psychosocial function. One person's marker of heavy usage may be quite typical and light for another.

Risk Reduction Versus Harm Reduction

It is important to understand the difference between risk reduction and actual harm reduction. For example, giving out naloxone and fentanyl test strips while still advocating for an abstinence-based recovery implies risk reduction, which may be a component of harm reduction, but we need to go a bit further to encompass the full spirit at the core of harm reduction. For example, a true respite center could be something similar to the managed alcohol programs (MAP) model in Canada that was established for people with alcohol use disorder (AUD) and experiencing chronic homelessness (Landefeld et al., 2023). MAP is an alcohol harm reduction program that helps manage alcohol consumption by providing eligible individuals with regular doses of alcohol as part of a structured program, in addition to housing, jobs, and other social services (Smith-Bernardin et al., 2022). This model, built on the understanding that the abstinence model was not working and that they needed to work with people with AUD, and in the true harm reduction spirit, in other words, MAP exemplifies the core spirit of harm reduction by meeting people where they were. The model of respite centers have become necessary, whether an individual with SUD wants to stay for an evening or until they find stable housing.

Substance Use Prevention Strategies

Substance use prevention strategies have a long history, but most of these have consisted of prohibitions against the use of various substances that have been implemented across time by governments, religious institutions, or both. In the current era, the rich tapestry of substance use prevention programs scattered across the globe can trace their origins to the late 1960s, when health professionals and politicians in the United States, for better or worse, made connections between rising crime rates in inner cities and drug use among the growing number of incarcerated men, as an outcome of the "heroin epidemic" of that era. Robert Dupont, MD, the first Director of the National Institute on Drug Abuse (NIDA) created in the 1970s, recounted the moment when drug prevention strategies were first embraced by the federal government as necessary, and later "adopted around the world" (DuPont, 2009, p. 7):

> Prior to the Executive Order of 1971, the nation's drug prevention efforts for more than half a century had been almost exclusively law enforcement, what became known as "supply reduction." . . . the federal government [was now] committed to an entirely new, "balanced" drug abuse prevention strategy. That meant that treatment, prevention, and research gained equal footing with law enforcement in U.S. drug abuse prevention policy.

Of course, the idea that with the stroke of a pen, drug use prevention was on "equal footing" with law enforcement in the suppression of illegal drug use and distribution was, and is, astonishing, but this period marked the official involvement of the U.S. federal government (and subsequently, state and local governments) into the field of drug use prevention.

The U.S. government's initial embrace of substance use prevention programs was narrowly focused; the Narcotic Treatment Administration (NTA) was established in the early 1970s by policy makers and professionals to address the connections they had made between crime and heroin use, but they "struggled to develop effective interventions without sufficient guidance or knowledge of how drug-using behaviors began or how these behaviors progressed" (Sloboda et al., 2009, p. 179). As Dupont (2009) noted, their exclusive focus on heroin was quickly seen as too short-sighted and the agency expanded its horizons, opening the door to what became a vast landscape of drug prevention strategies and programs aimed at all manner of substances.

In the wake of this expanded focus, researchers and professionals who established fledgling drug prevention programs in the 1970s and 1980s tended to focus on identifying "risk" and "protective" factors that predisposed particular populations to substance use and abuse, especially adolescents, but their "failure to demonstrate the effectiveness of prevention programming resulted in a moratorium" on research and new programs in the United States (Sloboda et al., 2009), at least until the crack epidemic of the late 1980s when the urgency of the circumstances placed new demands on the government's responsiveness to the problem.

Social Determinants of Substance Use

Substance use prevention programs have often relied on individual-level approaches to understand problems related to substance use and to fashion solutions. This is especially true in the United States, where individualist orientation predisposes policy makers and practitioners to construct programs that focus on individuals, and which tend to blame their personal shortcomings and deficiencies for failures to achieve success. This individualist orientation was especially true of the first generation of prevention programs that relied on a "risk and protective factors" approach to programming, and beginning in the 1980s it was an approach that was fed by new ideas about biological and psychosocial root causes. It was also an approach that led to a focus on subgroups of people that exhibited "signs or symptoms" of using controlled or illegal substances as the appropriate targets of these programs (Evans et al., 1978; Haggerty & Mrazek, 1994; Sloboda et al., 2009).

Variations of victim-blaming presented as "evidence-based" substance use prevention programming continue to dominate the landscape, both nationally and internationally, yet beginning in the late 1970s, researchers began to recognize the power of social determinants in substance use (Evans et al., 1978). While still representing a sliver of government's overall spending on substance use prevention, a generation of "community-based prevention" programs grew from research that focused on social determinants of substance use (especially the influence of media on peers), and which showed that "substance use and other risky life-style behaviors" could be prevented (Sloboda et al., 2009).

The usefulness of social determinants in helping to make sense of attitudes, orientations, and behaviors surrounding substance use and to fashion effective prevention programs is evidenced by the increasing number of books and papers devoted to the topic, and yet even researchers who explicitly write about social determinants of substance use are affected by the individualist-oriented environment in which they operate. For example, a recent study of more than 900 papers devoted to examining the role of social determinants in substance use prevention programs found that there were an extraordinarily large number of social determinants that operated at different levels and affected lives in different ways, but Ronzani and colleagues (2023, p. 9) also found that "[t]here is a predominance of studies focused in microsocial factors and on individuals, in detriment of more complex analysis that approach the drug use as a social and collective issue, showing not only the strength of individualist and essentialist perspective in that field, but also pointing to the nefarious effects of the responsibilities in relation to people that come from that epistemological tradition" (Dimenstein et al., 2017). This perspective even turns the individual into a target for the treatment, going against the literature of this field of knowledge, which points to a better effectiveness of actions based in the community and local environment.

The "more complex analysis that approaches drug use as a social and collective issue" that Ronzani et al. call for—an analysis that draws our attention to the intersection of culture, history, and how a community delivers care—is in short supply, but badly needed. Part of the problem is that the intersection of multiple dynamic factors cannot be analyzed or effectively modeled using the types of quantitative analyses that are part and parcel of corporate healthcare, and institutional bureaucracies are slow to respond to new or novel methods that threaten to displace proven methods and techniques of program evaluation that consistently point the finger of blame at "patients" and not their circumstances.

HARM REDUCTION

Harm Reduction: Overview of Historical Origins

Across the world and throughout the ages, all but the early Inuit have found flora and fauna to alter their consciousness (Weil & Rosen, 2004). Recreational substance use is a pervasive and enduring human pastime that, for the most part, has been safely managed; not all drug use is misuse. Mind-altering and medical plants and drugs often have beneficial and promising outcomes; less often, they lead to detrimental ones. Harm reduction may take a variety of forms in different cultures and subcultures, but they share similar features that distinguish them from other forms of drug regulation. Responsive to the European antiauthoritarian youth movement in the 1960s, the antipsychiatry movements, and the failure of the traditional, medical-psychiatric approach to alcohol, the Dutch pioneered a "society-oriented drug care" approach in the 1970s as part of a continuum of drug care (a similar approach was also tried during this period in Liverpool, England). This approach introduced concepts like "self-help," "social reinsertion," "the client is expert," "normalize illegal drug use," and "do not medicalize, criminalize, stigmatize," among others. By the 1980s, the relationship between injection drug use and HIV added further urgency for governments to embrace, finance, and expand harm reduction approaches. By the 1990s, more countries in Europe and around the globe began harm reduction programs.

By the time the first cases were reported in the United States in 1981, injection-related HIV had already been spreading among intravenous (IV) drug users for nearly a decade (Des Jarlais et al., 1989). The incidence was highest in those states at the forefront of the "war on drugs" and criminalized possession of needles and/or syringes as well as other injection supplies (New York State, e.g., was infamous for its "draconian" Rockefeller drug laws). Predictably the 11 U.S. states with prohibitionist laws imposing artificial scarcity of injection equipment had the highest incidence of injection-related HIV/AIDS cases (Lurie & Drucker, 1997). In 1988 alone, the number of new HIV infections approached a million people in the United States; drug prohibition policies were not a solution, they were part of the problem (Moss & Bacchetti, 1989). From punitive prohibition emerged activist-driven syringe exchanges who coined the harm reduction approach of "working with drug users where they're at" as an effective means of saving lives (Brooner et al., 1998; Vlahov & Junge, 1998). Indeed, by 2021, with an estimated 1.2 million people in the United States living with HIV, only 7% of the new infections were drug injectors (CDC, 2023a).

Harm Reduction: Lessons Learned

Over the 30+ years that harm reduction has been practiced, some lessons have been learned and some core characteristics have emerged (MacCoun, 1998). Harm reduction practice involves the mediation of drug use through the provision of self-management strategies that are immediately effective in reducing personal and communal harm (Majoor & Rivera, 2003). Today, we view it simply as leading with empathy, practicing mercy, and providing safety. Services that are anonymous and free are essential components of the engagement and retention process. Successful harm reduction strategies and interventions fall into the following five generic categories (Majoor & Rivera, 2003).

- *Palliative care:* Low-threshold services that take care of participants' basic and acute needs, including food, showers, hot/cold drinks, syringes, condoms, clothes, shoes/boots, and sleeping bags. A roof to sleep under brings a sense of safety and self-worth that lays cornerstones for changing high-risk behaviors.

- *Stress reduction:* Bodily relaxation is a precondition that enables behavior changes. A holistic health approach to health and well-being may include strategies such as the creation of a "sanctuary" space, and the use of acupuncture, massage, yoga, and relaxation techniques that reduce stress.

- *Education and information:* To make participants their own change agents, harm reduction agencies focus on building information resources that make a difference in everyday decision-making. Up-to-date knowledge that is presented in various modalities and in linguistically and culturally appropriate ways helps participants more effectively navigate difficulties and addresses concerns.

- *Healing and empowerment:* Healing from past wounds and gathering power for upcoming changes characterize the later stages of the harm reduction working alliance. Support groups, social skills training, and individual mental health services are available for crisis intervention, assessment of psychiatric disorders, and to help participants gain more self-awareness through regular counseling.

- *Social integration:* Interventions that are aimed at reintegrating participants back into society are initiated via effective case management, but the most essential component is the support of "natural" groups, like the family. This means that the harm reduction agency must be a "family" center to be effective in its mission to support participants in their journey back into society.

Current Progress in Harm Reduction

Substantially reduced rates of HIV and viral hepatitis C infection among drug users are among the most prominent outcomes achieved by harm reduction programs around the world (Broz et al., 2021). Harm reduction programs in the United States have spearheaded the use of naloxone (Narcan) to counteract opioid-related overdoses and have saved countless lives and lowered emergency and hospital costs nationwide (Strang et al., 2019), while globally overdose prevention centers have demonstrated the effectiveness of supervised injection to reducing unintended overdose (Dow-Fleisner et al., 2022; Lambdin et al., 2022; Nolan et al., 2022; Roux et al., 2023). In addition, people who participate in harm reduction programs are more likely to reduce use and injection of drugs (Hagan et al., 2000) and are five times more likely to initiate SUD treatment than nonparticipants (Kidorf et al., 2009).

The Future of Harm Reduction: Integration and Specialization (Box 9.2)

Harm reduction proponents have helped the United States turn a corner on decades of drug-related harms that are associated with prohibitive, punitive drug policies. Not only did increasing access to sterile syringes prevent HIV and hepatitis C virus and other bloodborne diseases, but these strategies also broke the negative framing of drug use, and it is no small victory that we view drug users as whole persons not behaviors and that we differentiate between drug use and misuse. A new rigor in policy directs service provision in ethical directions of care, services, and research.

BOX 9.2 INNOVATIONS IN HARM REDUCTION SERVICES

- *Drug user health hubs:* create an integrated network of services including office-based buprenorphine, medical cannabis, HCV and STI treatment, wound care, and seamless referrals to other providers (Javed et al., 2020)

- *Women-of-substance health hubs:* center women as the primary hub in their family system, with the focus on providing safety and building agency by recognizing the unique burdens experienced by women who use drugs; resources including privileged spaces, reproductive care, mental health, childcare and related resources, and advocacy

- Real-time drug testing availability to PWUD (Burr et al., 2014)

- *Overdose prevention centers:* have staff trained to reverse opioid-related overdoses and have a significant role to play in reversing the upward trend of overdoses in the United States

- *Expanding access to harm reduction services:* pharmacy sales of naloxone without a prescription, home and mail delivery, syringe vending machines, and integrating syringe access to drug injectors within hospital systems (Broz et al., 2021)

HCV, hepatitis C virus; PWUD, people who use drugs; STI, sexually transmitted infection.

CASE STUDY 9.1: RASHAD'S STORY

Rashad is a 24-year-old Black man who is very well-known to the emergency service of the local hospital, having made several visits to the ED over the last few months. Rashad is diagnosed with schizophrenia and cocaine use disorders and has made frequent visits to the ED. Typically, he presents with complaints of depression, resulting in overnight stays until he is discharged.

Today's visit feels markedly different from his previous ones. During this visit, he shares that he is experiencing command auditory hallucinations; "the voices are telling me to kill myself," he says. The resident doctor on call conducts a thorough evaluation of Rashad's condition. The doctor considers Rashad's history of cocaine use, with evidence from a positive urine test, and suggests that the emergence of auditory hallucinations, accompanied by suicidal ideation, could easily be explained by the patient's drug use and likely not a result an exacerbation of a primary psychotic illness. The doctor is leaning toward discharging the patient.

TOBACCO, ALCOHOL, AND OTHER SUBSTANCE USE DISORDERS

Tobacco Use and Tobacco Use Disorder: Diagnostic Principles

Tobacco use is a major public health concern, with devastating consequences, and addressing use is critical to prevent morbidity and mortality worldwide (Giulietti et al., 2020). As with all harmful substance use, it is important to accurately diagnose the problem (tobacco use vs. tobacco use disorder [TUD]) so that an appropriate treatment plan can be put in place, in collaboration with the patient. It is important to note that everyone that uses tobacco does not meet the criteria for TUD; however, it is important to assess and diagnose an addiction when present. Unfortunately, clinicians do not always identify or follow criteria to establish a TUD diagnosis, which leads to ill-constructed treatment planning, ineffective treatment, and frustration for both the patient and the clinician alike. To this end, following the *DSM-5* criteria for SUD is key to diagnosing someone with TUD (see Box 9.1).

Epidemiology of Tobacco Use

Tobacco use is the leading cause of preventable disease worldwide (Samet, 2013) and the principal cause of disability and death in the United States (Cornelius et al., 2022). Even though the way tobacco is used has changed over the years and cigarette smoking has declined over several decades, an array of combustible and noncombustible tobacco products have been produced and popularized (Cornelius et al., 2022). Examples of combustible tobacco products in addition to cigarettes include cigars and cigarillos, whereas smokeless noncombustible options include nicotine vaping and heated tobacco products.

In the 2020 National Health Interview Survey, an estimated 47 million adults in the United States were using commercial tobacco products, with the most popular being cigarettes (12.5%), electronic cigarettes (e-cigarettes; 3.7%), cigars (3.5%), smokeless tobacco (2.3%), and pipes (1.1%; Cornelius et al., 2022). Approximately, three million middle and high school students use tobacco products, and one in four of people who do not smoke are exposed to secondhand smoke (inhalation via another person's use; CDC, 2023b). Finally, tobacco use is a leading cause of mortality and morbidity and is known to lead to negative health consequences such as heart disease, stroke, lung diseases, type 2 diabetes, and rheumatoid arthritis. Further, 80% to 90% of lung cancer deaths are linked to tobacco use, and nearly 8 in 10 cases of chronic obstructive pulmonary disease (COPD) are caused by smoking tobacco (CDC, 2023b). Another often-overlooked consequence of smoking is the damage to the health of the teeth and gums, leading to periodontal disease and gum loss (NIDCR, 2023).

Neurobiology of Tobacco Addiction

Nicotine is the psychoactive agent in tobacco that increases the likelihood of someone developing a habit (Markou, 2008). Dependence on nicotine is thought to be the primary driver of TUD, making it difficult to stop use long term. Much of the literature on the neurobiology of TUD is focused on understanding how nicotine acts in the brain to identify targets for decreasing cravings and long-term TUD treatment. Research in animal models have identified glutamate, γ-aminobutyric acid (GABA), cholinergic, and dopamine neurotransmitter interactions in the ventral tegmental area (VTA), the amygdala, and the prefrontal cortex (PFC) as the primary areas where nicotine has its effects (Markou, 2008). Many of the treatments for TUD are geared at decreasing glutamate or increasing GABA transmission to decrease the rewarding effects of nicotine (Markou, 2008).

Clinical Evaluation to Facilitate Tobacco Use Disorder Treatment

There are many different approaches to helping someone with TUD treatment; however, there are evidence-based therapies that can be used. One, such as MI or motivational interviewing (Miller & Rollnick, 2002), is an approach used to assess motivation, and in

172 II • PRIORITIZED BEHAVIORS FOR PRIMARY PREVENTION OF DISEASE

partnership with the person to enable behavior change that is durable. MI will be covered in greater detail in the next section. Another approach is use of the Screening, Brief Intervention, and Referral to Treatment (SBIRT; SAMHSA, 2017), or screening, brief intervention, and referral to treatment. SBIRT allows the provider to quickly assess the severity of tobacco or other substance use, focus on increasing insight and awareness regarding tobacco use and motivation toward behavior change, and referral to treatment when those identified need more extensive treatment with access to specialty care. MI can be integrated into SBIRT to increase the likelihood of lasting change. Regardless of the approach taken, some overarching practice guidelines established by the National Institutes of Health for the treatment of TUD include the following (Clinical Practice Guideline Treating Tobacco Use and Dependence 2008 Update Panel, Liaisons, and Staff, 2008):

- Assessing for tobacco use and establishing a TUD based on the *DSM-5* criteria
- Advising the person to stop using tobacco
- Assessing the willingness of the person to stop using tobacco
- Assisting those who are willing to help stop tobacco use
- Arranging for follow-up to prevent relapse
This framework is commonly referred to as the "5 As" to help stop the use of tobacco.

Motivational Interviewing for Tobacco Use Disorder Treatment

MI is an evidence-based technique that can be used for a variety of behavioral health conditions to help reduce and stop unwanted behavior to elicit lasting change (Miller & Rollnick, 2002). Even though MI was originally developed to treat addiction, it is an effective tool for many patient populations. MI uses a guiding style of communication to empower people to change in a respectful and curious manner. MI is practiced with an underlying spirit, often referred to as the "MI spirit," a collaborative style or way of being with people. The core elements of MI include partnership, evocation, acceptance, and compassion (Levounis et al., 2017). Partnership underscores the collaborative nature between an MI practitioner and the person; evocation underscores that people already possess within themselves what is needed for change; acceptance refers to the MI practitioner taking on a nonjudgmental stance and accepting the person's decision once they have all the information to change or not change; compassion speaks to the MI practitioner always seeking to promote and center the well-being and priorities of the person above all else (MINT, 2019). In addition to the "MI spirit," there are core skills known as the OARS: **O**pen-ended questions, **A**ffirmation, **R**eflections, and **S**ummarizing (Levounis et al., 2017). Box 9.3 is a short example of questions that are often used in an MI-based clinical interview.

BOX 9.3 EXAMPLE QUESTIONS USED IN A MOTIVATIONAL INTERVIEWING-BASED CLINICAL INTERVIEW

- Can you tell me about the pros and cons of making the choice to stop using tobacco?
- On a scale of 1–10, how confident are you in your ability to make this change? What factors contribute to that level of confidence?
- How would your life look different if you successfully made this change?
- What self-care strategies can you incorporate into your plan to manage stress or challenges that may arise during the change process?

Medications for Tobacco Use Disorder

There are seven Food and Drug Administration (FDA)-approved medications for TUD that can largely be organized into three broader categories. These broader categories include nicotine replacement therapy (NRT) and medications, bupropion, and varenicline. NRT comes in five forms, namely a transdermal patch, gum, lozenge, oral inhaler, and nasal spray. The more common forms of NRT and medication options for the treatment of TUD are included in Table 9.1, along with doses, side effects, and relative contraindications.

TABLE 9.1 FDA-Approved Medications for Tobacco Use Disorder				
NRT PATCH	**NRT GUM**	**NRT LOZENGE**	**BUPROPION**	**VARENICLINE**
Mechanism of action				
Full agonist at nicotinic receptors	Full agonist at nicotinic receptors	Full agonist at nicotinic receptors	Reuptake inhibitor at NE and dopaminergic receptors, antagonist at nicotine receptors	Partial agonist at nicotinic receptors
Doses				
21 mg, 14 mg, 7 mg >10 cigarettes daily: 21 mg patch 4–6 weeks, then 14 mg 2 weeks, then 7 mg 2 weeks <10 cigarettes daily: 14 mg for 6 weeks, then 7 mg for 2 weeks One patch daily upper body, rotating placements	2 mg and 4 mg 1 piece every 1–2 hours for the first 6 weeks, then 1 piece 2–4 hours for 3 weeks, then 1 piece every 4–8 hours for 3 weeks "Park and chew" method Max of 24 pieces per day	2 mg and 4 mg 1 lozenge every 1–2 hours for the first 6 weeks, then 1 lozenge every 2–4 hours for 3 weeks, then 1 lozenge every 4–8 hours for 3 weeks	150 mg daily for 3 days, then increase to 150 mg BID Begin 1–2 weeks before quit date	0.5 mg days 1–3, 0.5 mg BID day 4–7, then 1 mg BID Begin 1 week before quit date
Side effects				
• Local skin reaction • Insomnia (can take off at bedtime>	• Hiccups • Dyspepsia • Mouth soreness	• Nausea • Hiccups • Heartburn • Headache	• Insomnia • Dry mouth • Nervousness • Nausea • Seizures (risk is 0.1%)	• Nausea • Sleep disturbance • Headache
Relative contraindications				
• Severe eczema • Psoriasis	• Should not eat or drink 15 minutes prior to or during use	• Should not eat or drink 15 minutes prior to or during use	• Seizure disorder • Eating disorder • Alcohol withdrawal	• Severe renal impairment

FDA, Food and Drug Administration; NE, norepinephrine; nrt, nicotine replacement therapy.
Source: Modified with permission from Dr. Jeanette Tetrault and Dr. Kenneth Morford.

CASE STUDY 9.2: TASHA'S STORY

Tasha started vaping tobacco in the 11th grade after she got introduced to the JUUL flavored cartridges, with mint being her favorite flavor. In 2022, the FDA banned all JUUL e-cigarette devices, so she began smoking menthol cigarettes that she could easily buy illegally from the street. By the time she was 19 years old, Tasha was smoking menthol cigarettes daily. Last year, Tasha started cosmetology school, now smoking 1.5 packs of menthol cigarettes daily, and at the time found out she was pregnant.

She attempted to stop smoking cigarettes on her own, but after relentless headaches, difficulty sleeping, decreased concentration, and restlessness, she started smoking again. Tasha then began to feel enormous guilt and melancholy as she understood smoking was bad for her baby but was unable to stop. Tasha has since given birth to her baby, who was born underweight and had to spend time in the neonatal intensive care unit but continues to smoke—although Tasha smokes less (1 pack of cigarettes daily instead of 1.5).

Today, we meet Tasha at her baby's 3-month follow up appointment and the doctor is trying to engage her in a conversation to help her stop smoking cigarettes given the risks to herself and her newborn child.

Alcohol Use and Alcohol Use Disorder

DIAGNOSTIC PRINCIPLES

Alcohol use is highly prevalent in the United States and around the world. Like any other substance use, it is helpful and clinically meaningful to consider alcohol use on a spectrum, from no use to varying degrees of use, to heavy use and the development of AUD at the top of the diagnostic pyramid. The U.S. Preventive Services Task Force (USPSTF) recommends screening of alcohol use in adults and pregnant women in primary care settings and brief behavioral counseling to people who engage in risky drinking behaviors (U.S. Preventive Services Task Force et al., 2018). Screening for alcohol use includes the use of the Alcohol Use Disorders Identification Test–Consumption (AUDIT-C) and the National Institute on Alcohol Abuse and Alcoholism (NIAAA)-recommended Single Alcohol Screening Question (SASQ). Both instruments have good specificity and sensitivity in detecting unhealthy alcohol use in diverse populations. The AUDIT-C has three questions about frequency of alcohol use, typical amount of alcohol use, and occasions of heavy use.

The SASQ asks "how many times in the past year have you had five [for men] or four [for women and all adults older than 65 years] or more drinks in a day?" Another commonly used screening tool is the Cut down, Annoyed, Guilty, Eye-opener (CAGE) tool, which detects only alcohol dependence rather than the full spectrum of unhealthy alcohol use. A positive screen on any of these instruments should prompt further evaluation of the patient for an AUD. The diagnosis of AUD is based on the criteria set by the latest iteration of the *Diagnostic and Statistical Manual of Mental Disorders*, Fifth Edition, Text Revised (*DSM-5-TR*). The *DSM-5* has a set of 11 criteria that divide AUD into mild, moderate, or severe disorders based on the number of met criteria (2–3, 4–5, and 6 or more symptoms, respectively). Emerging literature has shown racial and ethnic disparities in the diagnosis of AUD. A recent study shows that Black and Hispanic military veterans were more likely to be diagnosed with AUD than their White counterparts, even at the same level of alcohol consumption, with Black men having 23% to 109% greater odds of an AUD diagnosis (Vickers-Smith et al., 2023).

EPIDEMIOLOGY OF ALCOHOL USE

According to the National Survey on Drug Use and Health (NSDUH), in 2021, 10.6% of individuals aged 12 and older in the United States (29.5 million people) had AUD in the past year. Within this age group, 12.1% were male and 9.1% were female. Among this age group, 47.5%

(133.1 million people) drank alcohol in the past month, with the highest users (51.9%) among those aged 26 or older. Racial differences were also observed in the NSDUH national data, showing that past-year AUD was lowest among Asian people (6.0%) compared with other racial or ethnic groups aged 12 or older (10.1% among Black people and 15.6% among Native American or Alaska Native people; NSDUH, 2021).

Alcohol use can lead to serious acute and long-term medical and psychological consequences. It is also a major cause of disability and severe economic strain worldwide. An estimated 5.1% of the global burden of disease and injury, equivalent to 132.6 million disability-adjusted life years (DALYs), was due to alcohol use, according to the World Health Organization (WHO, 2019).

PHARMACOLOGY OF ALCOHOL

The potential toxicity of alcohol has been shown to be related to the process of its metabolism and its metabolites. Alcohol is metabolized mainly in the liver through oxidation into acetaldehyde and acetate via an active constitutive aldehyde dehydrogenase pathway and inducible microsomal ethanol oxidizing system (MEOS) elimination pathway. ADH and MEOS convert alcohol into acetaldehyde, which is further metabolized by aldehyde dehydrogenases (ALDHs) into acetate (Wallner & Olsen, 2008). About 40% of Asian people (Japanese, Chinese, and Koreans) have an inactive ALDH2*2 mutation that results in much more acetaldehyde after drinking than normal (Duranceaux et al., 2006; Schuckit, 2009). Alcohol exerts its myriad effects through its activation of the brain reward systems via numerous neurotransmitter systems.

TREATMENT FOR ALCOHOL USE DISORDER

Motivational Interviewing for Alcohol Use Disorder Treatment. Miller and Rollnick (2002) defined *MI* as "a client-centered, directive method for enhancing intrinsic motivation to change by exploring and resolving ambivalence" (Miller & Rollnick, 2002, p. 25). SBIRT is a very well-researched approach to implementing universal screening based on the MI principles. After screening for alcohol use, clinicians are encouraged to place individuals in categories based on their pattern of use as such categorization enables allocation of intervention. Categories include no risk (no alcohol use), low risk (those with a moderate drinking pattern), at risk (those above the moderate drinking level, i.e., binge drinking and heavy drinking pattern), high risk (those with both binge and heavy drinking patterns), and finally those who fall in the AUD category. SBIRT is particularly useful among individuals who fall in the at-risk and high-risk categories for alcohol use.

MEDICATIONS FOR ALCOHOL USE DISORDER

The FDA-approved medications for AUD include disulfiram, acamprosate, and naltrexone (oral and long-acting injectable), but other medications often used on an off-label basis include topiramate and gabapentin.

Disulfiram inhibits the enzyme aldehyde dehydrogenase, which catalyzes the oxidation of acetaldehyde to acetic acid. The ingestion of alcohol while on disulfiram elevates the blood acetaldehyde concentration (as the enzyme aldehyde dehydrogenase is inhibited), resulting in disulfiram–ethanol reaction (DER), including warmth and flushing of the skin, tachycardia, palpitations, hypotension, nausea, vomiting, shortness of breath, sweating, dizziness, blurred vision, and confusion. Disulfiram must be used with caution in patients with severe cardiovascular disease, who are pregnant, and who have psychosis. Acamprosate increases GABA neurotransmission. Acamprosate is excreted unmetabolized and therefore it is required to check renal function (baseline creatinine) before medication initiation. Naltrexone exerts its effects via mu-opioid receptor blockade, thus reducing the reinforcing effects of alcohol. Common adverse effects include gastrointestinal (GI) symptoms including nausea, vomiting, decreased appetite, and abdominal pain, as well as injection site symptoms including nodule swelling, tenderness, and pain.

Cannabis Use and Cannabis Use Disorder

DIAGNOSTIC PRINCIPLES

The increase in the prevalence of cannabis use has been reported across all age groups. It is estimated that 10% to 30% of people with a past-year cannabis use will meet the criteria for cannabis use disorder (CUD; Budney et al., 2019; Leung et al., 2020). It is therefore important for clinicians to recognize cannabis use as a precursor to CUD, with CUD as a primary diagnosis or as a co-occurring disorder to other psychiatric or medical conditions. CUD is diagnosed clinically by a thorough evaluation of the patient's presenting symptoms based on the *DSM-5-TR* criteria. The clinical evaluation of cannabis use and CUD involves clarifying the pattern of use and establishing a diagnosis based on set criteria. It bears emphasis, however, that cannabis use or a positive cannabis urine toxicology does not equate to criteria for CUD.

EPIDEMIOLOGY OF CANNABIS USE DISORDER

Cannabis is one of the most used psychoactive substances in the United States and around the world. According to the NSDUH, in the United States, 18.7% of people aged 12 or older (52.5 million people) have used cannabis in the past year, including 10.5% of adolescents. However, only 5.8% (or 16.3 million people) met the *DSM-5* criteria for CUD in the past year, with 4.6% (10.2 million) people being adolescents aged 12 to 17 years old. The risk of CUD increases with early age of initiation and frequency of use during adolescence (Leung et al., 2020).

Recent evidence shows that the diagnosis of CUD has steadily increased in the United States, with Black/African American individuals having consistently higher prevalence than other racial/ethnic groups (Hasin et al., 2022). Consistent with the general population, between 2005 and 2019, the percentages of veterans diagnosed with CUD in the <35, 35–64, and ≥65 years age groups increased from 1.70%, 1.59%, and 0.03% to 4.84%, 2.86%, and 0.74%, respectively (Hasin et al., 2022). Possible explanations for this increase include changing laws and regulations; decreasing perception of risk; increasing cannabis potency; and use of cannabis to self-treat pain, mood, and anxiety (Botsford et al., 2020; Hasin et al., 2020, 2022).

CANNABIS LEGALIZATION: IMPACT OF REGULATION ON RELATED USE

There has been an increased wave of nonmedical and recreational cannabis legalization across the country. Recreational cannabis use has been legalized in 23 states, and about half of the adult U.S population currently reside in a state where individuals at least 21 years old can legally obtain cannabis products.

Observable changes in the wake of this regulatory product changes include increased potency, range of product formulations and routes to deliver the product faster. While the impact on the perception of risk, other substance use, psychiatric disorders, and associated morbidity is emerging in the literature, it stands to reason that the impact of increased cannabis legislation and regulation warrants concern about an increase in potential for the development of CUD especially among adolescents and young adults. Taken together, the increased legislation of cannabis in the country is likely to make individuals have a reduced perception of risk and may use highly potent products, more frequently, via faster longer acting routes of use and at younger ages. Thus, the transition from cannabis use to CUD especially in people with risk factors such as adolescents, psychotic disorders, and family history of psychotic disorders should be leveraged to inform regulatory policy:

- Increased delta-9-tetrahydrocannabinol (THC) potency and dose
- Route of use (smoking and vaping vs. edibles)
- Increased access and availability of high-potency cannabis
- Aggressive cannabis marketing through advertising on TV, radio, billboards, or social media, or by sponsorship at cultural and sports events

The changing terrain of cannabis legislation, however, raises new questions about racial/ethnic disparities in the application of the legislation given the historical precedent of drug-related mass incarceration and racial-based disparate applications of the legal system.

PHARMACOLOGY OF CANNABIS: THE ENDOCANNABINOID SYSTEM

There are over 700 varieties of the cannabis plant, with hundreds of unique cannabinoids, noncannabinoid terpenes, and flavonoids. THC is the primary psychoactive component, but there are other cannabinoids, including cannabidiol (CBD), delta-8-THC, cannabinol, cannabigerol, cannabichromene, and delta-9-tetrahydrocannabivarin (Haney, 2022). The endocannabinoid system (ECS) is an ubiquitous lipid signaling neuromodulatory network that plays major roles in many different functional processes in the brain, including the regulation of emotions, motivation, and cognition. The ECS is composed of endogenously produced cannabinoids (endocannabinoids), cannabinoid receptors (CB1 and CB2), and the enzymes responsible for the synthesis and degradation of endocannabinoids. Anandamide (AEA) and 2-arachidonoylglycerol (2-AG), the main endocannabinoids, are small molecules derived from arachidonic acid. Other less studied N-acylethanolamines include N-stearoylethanolamide (SEA), N-palmitoylethanolamide (PEA), and N-oleoylethanolamide (OEA). Cannabinoid receptors are G protein-coupled receptors and are differentially distributed throughout the brain and periphery. The cannabinoid receptor type 1 (CB1r) is most abundant in the central nervous system (CNS), expressed in the basal ganglia, cerebellum, PFC, nucleus accumbens, hippocampus, and stress response-related areas including the central amygdala and the paraventricular nucleus of the hypothalamus (Navarrete et al., 2020). The cannabinoid receptor type 2 (CB2r) is predominantly distributed within tissues of the immune system. Unlike the CB1r, CB2rs are less commonly expressed in healthy CNS but highly upregulated in glial cells under neuropathological conditions, such as in senile plaques in Alzheimer disease, activated microglial cells, macrophages in multiple sclerosis, and spinal cord in amyotrophic lateral sclerosis (Xin et al., 2020). In addition, CB2r has been proposed to be highly inducible in conditions such as anxiety and addictive disorders (Xin et al., 2020).

TREATMENTS FOR CANNABIS USE DISORDER

There are no FDA-approved medications for the treatment of CUD. However, buspirone has shown some efficacy for cannabis dependence (reduction in positive urine drug screens and to have shorter time to first negative urinary drug screen compared with placebo) in a small randomized controlled trial (RCT), although no significant differences between treatment groups were observed (McRae-Clark et al., 2009).

Controlled human laboratory studies and small open-label clinical trials suggest that dronabinol may also be useful. Preclinical studies have suggested the potential of fatty acid amide hydrolase (FAAH) inhibitors such as URB597, endocannabinoid-metabolizing enzymes, and nicotinic alpha7 receptor antagonists such as methyllycaconitine (MLA; (Weinstein & Gorelick, 2011). Other medications that have shown potential in the treatment of CUD include gabapentin (Mason et al., 2012), N-acetyl cysteine (NAC; Gray et al., 2012), naltrexone (Haney et al., 2015), varenicline (McRae-Clark et al., 2021), nabilone (Haney et al., 2013), and CBD (Freeman et al., 2020).

Withdrawal symptoms of cannabis can be a source of significant distress and return to cannabis use. These symptoms include irritability, anxiety, insomnia, decreased appetite, depressed mood, and somatic symptoms like abdominal pain, tremors, fever, and headaches. Cannabis withdrawal has been managed with dronabinol (Haney et al., 2003), nabiximols, mirtazapine, zolpidem, benzodiazepines, and guanfacine. Overall, behavioral treatments are the mainstay treatments for CUD, including cognitive behavioral therapy (CBT), motivational enhancement therapy (MET), and contingency management (CM).

Opioids and Synthetic Opioids

The unprecedented rise in drug overdose deaths over the last few years has been linked to the surge in the availability in highly potent synthetic opioids (HPSO) such as fentanyl and fentanyl analogs in drug supplies. The landscape of drug supplies has evolved quite significantly with the admixture of HPSO in almost any other substances, including cocaine and heroin. Emerging literature has also shown worsening racial disparities in opioid-related overdose mortality, with increasing rates in the Black/African American communities due in part to the rise in fentanyls (Friedman & Hansen, 2022).

DIAGNOSTIC PRINCIPLES

Opioid use disorder (OUD), like other SUDs, is a chronic relapsing disorder initially driven by activation of the brain reward systems, but later leading to activation of antireward neurocircuits that drive adverse emotional states and relapse (Strang et al., 2020). The proportion of individuals who develop OUD after infrequent use is unclear and variable. Various risk factors for developing OUD have been described in literature, including opioid availability, rate of opioid pain prescriptions, social stressors (including systemic racism), peer pressures, co-occurring psychiatric disorders, social determinants of health (poverty, poor neighborhoods), and chronic noncancer pain (Strang et al., 2020). OUD addiction develops in a hypothesized three-stage model: binge/intoxication, withdrawal/negative affect, and preoccupation/anticipation. The neurocircuitry involved in these domains include the basal ganglia mediating binge/intoxication stage, the extended amygdala mediating the withdrawal/negative affect stage, and the PFC mediating the preoccupation/anticipation stage (Koob & Moal, 1997). Chronic opioid use results in a dysfunctional state that ultimately leads to opioid addiction.

EPIDEMIOLOGY OF OPIOID USE

In the United States, according to the NSDUH, among people aged 12 or older in 2021, 3.3% (9.2 million people) *misused* opioids in the past year and 2% (5.6 million people) had an OUD in the past year. The most common reason for misusing prescription pain medications was to relieve physical pain (64.3%). Other reasons included "to feel good or get high" (10.7%) and "to relax or relieve tension" (7.3%).

Opioid-related mortality has been on the rise from 21,089 in 2010 to 47,600 in 2017. However, 68,630 and 80,411 deaths were reported in 2020 and 2021; the highest rate of increase was in minoritized communities. Trends of opioid overdose death rates in Black/African Americans continue to rise, across age groups (Larochelle et al., 2021). Recent literature has also indicated that males are significantly more susceptible than females to overdose caused by opioids and stimulant drugs (Butelman et al., 2023).

PHARMACOLOGY OF OPIOIDS

Opioids act at three opioid receptors: delta, kappa, and mu. Opioid agonists bind to G protein-coupled receptors to cause cellular hyperpolarization. Most clinically relevant opioid analgesics bind to μ(*mu*)-opioid peptide (MOP) receptors in the central and peripheral nervous system in an agonist manner to elicit analgesia.

MEDICATIONS FOR OPIOID USE DISORDER

FDA-approved medications for OUD include buprenorphine, methadone, and naltrexone. The patient's medical history, clinical presentation, and preference must be considered in the medication choice.

Buprenorphine: Buprenorphine is a partial mu agonist with a maximal dose-effect ceiling that is below significant respiratory depression. Buprenorphine provides relief from opioid withdrawal symptoms through agonist effect.

Initiation dose must be well-timed to when the patient is already in moderate opioid withdrawal (Clinical Opioid Withdrawal Scale [COWS] is an 11-item clinician-administered tool that helps determine the stage and severity of opioid withdrawal; Wesson & Ling, 2003). There is a risk of precipitated withdrawals in patients who have recently used full agonist opioids (e.g., heroin, oxycodone, etc.). Higher doses of buprenorphine may be required in individuals using high-potency synthetic opioids such as fentanyl.

Methadone: Methadone is a long-acting full agonist at the mu-opioid receptor. Methadone treatment is associated with high rates of treatment retention, reduced mortality, and HIV seroconversion. Methadone is tightly regulated in the United States and only dispensed out of federal opioid treatment programs (OTPs). Overdose is a risk on methadone especially in the first week of treatment and in individuals who are also using other drugs, such as alcohol or benzodiazepines.

Cocaine Use and Cocaine Use Disorder

In 2021, 1.7% (4.8 million) of people older than 12 years old used cocaine in the past year, mostly among people aged 18 to 25. In the same year, about 0.4% of the population used crack cocaine in the past year. Interestingly, however, cocaine use in the past year among people aged 12 or older did not differ among racial or ethnic groups, but Black people (0.9%) were more likely to use crack in the past year compared with Hispanic or Asian people (both 0.1%).

DIAGNOSTIC PRINCIPLES

Cocaine use disorder diagnosis is a clinical diagnosis following the diagnostic criteria set by the *DSM-5-TR*. Like other SUD, the diagnosis of cocaine use disorder goes beyond cocaine use but encompasses loss of control and impact on the daily lives. The routes of use include intranasal (sniffing or snorting), smoking (as the free base known as crack cocaine), and IV.

PHARMACOLOGY OF COCAINE

Cocaine blocks the reuptake of serotonin, noradrenaline, and dopamine, thus exerting a strong psychoactive effect. The euphoria experienced by users is from the blockade of the presynaptic dopamine transporter (DAT) in the synaptic cleft, which causes an increase in extracellular dopamine.

TREATMENTS FOR COCAINE USE DISORDER

There are no FDA-approved medications for treating cocaine use disorder. In a recent large systematic review, only CM was significantly associated with an increased likelihood of having a negative test result for the presence of cocaine (OR: 2.13; 95% CI: 1.62–2.80; Bentzley et al., 2021). However, pharmacological strategies targeting a variety of neurobiological targets such as dopamine, GABA, and norepinephrine are being utilized clinically and in research.

Emerging Drugs: Xylazine

The emergence of xylazine in illicit drug supplies across the United States has been a major public health concern. Xylazine's novelty was recognized as a preferred adulterant among people who inject drugs (PWID) in Puerto Rico as an addition to fentanyl (Reyes et al., 2012). Curiously, the pattern of xylazine prevalence and spread has suggested an ethnographic association with fentanyl as xylazine overdose-related deaths have occurred almost exclusively in connection to fentanyl (Friedman et al., 2022; Shover et al., 2020).

Xylazine (street name "Tranq"), a methyl benzene (1,3-dimethylbenzene) that is substituted by a 5,6-dihydro-4H-1,3-thiazin-2-ylnitrilo group at position 2, is a clonidine analog that acts as an agonist at alpha-2 adrenoceptors. Xylazine has no FDA-approved indications in humans; it is a nonopioid large animal tranquilizer (anestesia de caballo), emetic, and sedative with analgesic and muscle relaxant properties. Earlier studies in Puerto Rico found that 90.6% of syringes containing xylazine also contained speedball and the results were replicated in

II • PRIORITIZED BEHAVIORS FOR PRIMARY PREVENTION OF DISEASE

Pennsylvania as fentanyl was found in 98.4% of xylazine-involved deaths. The use of xylazine in fentanyl drug supplies has been related to the possibility that xylazine tends to prolong the euphoric effects of fentanyl.

The main route of xylazine administration is injection (84.5%), inhalation (14%), and more than 40% in a mixture with speedball (Reyes et al., 2012). Of a drug-using sample in Puerto Rico health-related problems, 21.1% reported at least one overdose episode and 35.2% reported skin lesions (Reyes et al., 2012). Although human xylazine use was first reported in Puerto Rico among PWID in the 2010s, current data show that related mortality has moved to and continues to increase across the northeastern United States. In Pennsylvania, xylazine-related mortality increased from 2% to 26% between 2015 and 2020. In 2020, 19.3% of all drug overdose deaths in Maryland were related to xylazine, and 10.2% in Connecticut. A study of 10 jurisdictions showed that the prevalence rose from 0.36% in 2015 to 6.7% in 2020 (Friedman et al., 2022).

The full spectrum of xylazine toxicity remains unknown, but due to its partial alpha-2 adrenergic agonist properties it is known to produce marked hypotension and bradycardia (secondary to vagal stimulation) and its synergistic effects with opioids. Naloxone may not fully reverse overdose symptoms from xylazine, given that xylazine is not an opioid. A high prevalence of skin lesions among xylazine users resulting in cellulites, abscesses, and even limb losses has been reported several times. These extensive soft tissue lesions are hypothesized to be a result of direct soft tissue injury, compartment syndrome, necrosis from tissue hypoxemia, and reduced sensitivity to skin injury.

TREATMENT

Cases of suspected xylazine-related overdose may not be responsive to naloxone; in fact, suspected overdose unresponsive to naloxone should prompt suspicion for xylazine toxicity. In these cases, focus should be on optimizing respiration and blood pressure. Other care includes endotracheal intubation, IV fluid resuscitation, EKG, glucose monitoring, and electrolytes replacement. Most cases of xylazine toxicity involve an opioid (usually fentanyl); hence, naloxone should still be used in emergent situations.

SPECIAL POPULATIONS

There are vulnerable populations that must be included when discussing substance use and SUDs. These populations include but are not limited to (a) children and adolescents, (b) pregnant persons, and (c) racial and ethnic minoritized populations. Special considerations for each of the above will be discussed in brief in the following section.

Children and Adolescent Substance Use

The information contained herein is based on a 2022 systematic review about substance use in children and adolescents (Nebhinani et al., 2022). The most used substances worldwide in this population are alcohol, cannabis, and tobacco. Cannabis has increased drastically in the last 10 years, as many adolescents do not see cannabis as harmful. This may be related to the legalization of cannabis, along with increased visibility and accessibility to edibles and gummies containing THC, the active ingredient in cannabis. In the United States specifically, the Monitoring the Future Study indicates alcohol is the most used substance in adolescents, with over 50% of 18-year-old people reporting lifetime alcohol use. Cannabis (45%) and cigarettes (31%) were the next two used substances in this age range. Vaping/e-cigarettes were found to be a popular mode of tobacco use for adolescents, with the FDA banning products such as JUUL to prevent further use. Understanding the environmental and biological factors underlying substance use and subsequent addiction among children and emerging adolescents is essential given lifetime morbidity and mortality risk associated with SUDs.

Preventing substance use in a developing brain (up to age 25) is key, as we know there are neurobiological underpinnings of substance use. Substance misuse can disrupt three areas of the brain: the basal ganglia, the extended amygdala, and the PFC. This disruption leads to irresponsible decision-making, like continuing to use substances despite negative consequences. In addition to brain chemistry, other factors can lead to the development of an SUD. These factors include psychological and social influences, mental illness, and genetic predisposition. The strongest predictor of use in this population is parental use and early adverse childhood experiences or ACEs. Therefore, investing in programs that adequately support prevention, intensive and comprehensive screening efforts for substance use, and treatment to mitigate the harmful effects of ACEs is vital for these populations.

Pregnancy

Using substances during pregnancy is a major public health concern. Forray reviews key considerations in her 2016 seminal article (Forray, 2016), which outlines major points for providers to understand. The most frequently used substance in pregnancy is tobacco, followed by alcohol and cannabis. A mixture of substances, both licit and illicit, are also seen in this population. The reproductive years (18–44) present the highest risk for developing SUD, especially during years 18 through 29 (Forray, 2016). A study published in 2020 found that among those who used cannabis and alcohol during pregnancy, 74% also used tobacco as well, demonstrating the concern for polysubstance use (Ko et al., 2020). **Figure 9.2** outlines the percentages of polysubstance use in this population. Opioid use in pregnancy has increased exponentially, leading to higher rates of neonatal abstinence syndrome, but also unintended death of the mother and the fetus (Ko et al., 2020).

Screening for polysubstance use in this demographic is of utmost importance, given the risk of morbidity and mortality for both the mother and the developing fetus. As there are limited options for interventions during the prenatal period, ensuring the use of substances is decreased substantially or prevented altogether is paramount. Treatment during pregnancy is largely composed of behavioral and psychosocial interventions, with CM being shown to be the most successful of these options. CM is a behavioral therapy where people are rewarded (cash incentives, vouchers, items of value) for evidence of positive behavior change, hence "reinforcing" lasting change (Petry, 2011). Other common modalities include MI and CBT, a therapy that helps people understand how situations lead to undesirable thoughts and how to avoid these environmental triggers. For people using opioids specially, medications for OUD,

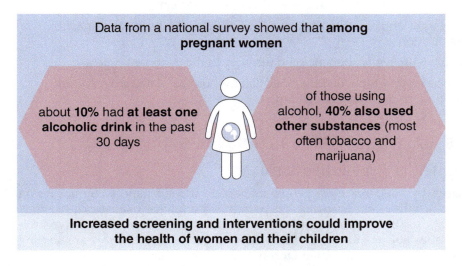

FIGURE 9.2 Alcohol use among pregnant women.
Source: From the National Survey on Drug Use and Health (NSDUH), United States, 2015–2018.

including methadone and buprenorphine, are the gold standard of care, shown to decrease mortality for both the mother and the fetus (Stover & Davis, 2015). Taken together, screening pregnant women, understanding which substances are being used, and tailoring treatments to effectively eliminate use are necessary to ensure favorable outcomes.

Racial and Ethnic Minoritized Populations

Considering the needs of people with poor health outcomes related to SUD is essential given the lasting impacts of racism (Jones, 2000), steeped in disadvantage. Racism, not race, causes disparate outcomes for racial and ethnic minoritized with SUD. Overwhelming evidence shows that structural and institutional factors are the biggest drivers of inequities among racial and minoritized populations (Jegede, Mathis, Youins, Guy, Gross, and Jordan, in press). For example, the addiction literature demonstrates that even though people racialized as Black now outpace White people in the rate of overdose deaths due to opioid use (Furr-Holden et al., 2021), Black people are less likely to be recommended for lifesaving medication for OUD (Lagisetty et al., 2019). Furthermore, despite equivocal or decreased substance use among racial and ethnic minoritized individuals, they are more likely to be criminalized for their use, as opposed to referral for treatment (James & Jordan, 2018).

Given these disparate outcomes, it is important for providers to have an understanding on how to interface with this population and the healthcare system for improved outcomes. We conclude this section by offering practices that can prevent health disparities in SUD for racial and ethnic minoritized people. These include understanding the impact of racism by screening for vulnerabilities in the social determinants of health using the social vulnerability tool (Bourgois et al., 2017), practicing structural competency (Metzl & Hansen, 2014), and collaborating with community to determine solutions. Considering diverse cultural views and community perspectives, especially those who have been historically excluded, is essential to developing community-supported solutions. Harm reduction is another strategy to achieve equity. Harm reduction seeks to optimize safety for people using substances, while reducing the harmful effects of minoritization, othering, and stigma. The following is a list of practices to consider when working with this population:

- Assess for structural vulnerability given disadvantage.
- Inquire how being racial and ethnically minoritized may have impacted their experience.
- Partner with community organizations well-versed on racism.
- Partner with legal organizations that can help address the negative impact of SUD criminalization.
- Involve people with lived experience and recovery in the treatment process.
- Ask about social supports beyond the clinic that may be useful for recovery (faith leaders, spiritual practices, extended family).

PREVENTION STRATEGIES FOR SUBSTANCE USE DISORDERS

General Principles of Preventive Care

It is abundantly clear, by now, that most people manage to use substances without losing control and without negative consequences. Yet persons with low-risk substance use may progress to problematic use and/or to dependent use (the triad use pattern). Preventive strategies to avoid substance abuse and reduce its health and social consequences are shifting from a focus on reducing supply and demand through law enforcement, to a recognition that the best results are achieved through integrated policies. We have gained insights into a wide range of risk factors for initiating, continuing, and engaging in harmful and dependent use.

9 • TOBACCO, ALCOHOL, AND OTHER DRUGS 183

Risk factors point to where to intervene, and at the forefront of prevention protective factors show us how to intervene.

These efforts include psychosocial approaches and recently the recognition that mental disorders and neurobiological hypotheses may not exclusively mediate problematic substance abuse, such as environmental factors related to early exposure to violence, growing up in environments lacking affection and caring, intense exposure to stress, and lack of social networks, especially if they cooccur in socially disorganized environment with easy availability of substances.

Harm Reduction as Path to Safety Optimization

Harm reduction has demonstrable effectiveness in reducing major health and social consequences. The field of drug treatment is amid a paradigm shift, with harm reduction strategies challenging treatment notions and strategies now understood to be dehumanizing, stigmatizing, and ineffective without constant external vigilance. The on-the-ground realities of persons dependent on drugs to which they have no legal access are a daunting maze of risks to life and freedom. Harm reduction may take a variety of forms in diverse cultures and subcultures. The diversity of meanings and activities is enormous, and while much remains to be written about the actual practices of reduction across the United States and the globe some core characteristics have emerged.

From the reality of the drug user, you can collaboratively work with them on the various aspects of life, intrinsically building their motivation to take their next steps, with self, family, children, and tangible safety, (e.g., housing, work, creativity). By making drug dependency better manageable you also make it safer. You co-create opportunities for the drug user to take optimal care of their health by reducing risks and practicing preventive care.

Harm reduction is rooted, therefore, in principles that align with both science and practice. Respecting the dignity of your patient is a *humanistic* value. Accepting the pervasiveness of mind-altering drugs with curiosity and without judgment is *pragmatic* realism. Drugs have beneficial effects, and they carry risks. Seek your patient's experience with both the benefits and risks of their drug use. Work together to reduce the identified negative effects of drugs. Those harms can be addressed through a continuum of interventions that may include attempts at incremental abstinence, including the use of medically assisted treatment like methadone or buprenorphine. Every patient requires an intervention that is immediately effective to reduce harm.

Harm reduction is an act of accepting life as it is, in social and economic ways for the dependent drug user, not as some other groups or institutions want it to be or become—humanizing the dehumanized by building their personal capacities, social resources, and mediating the patient's challenges with punitive bureaucracies. Street-level bureaucrats who in their professional roles can and do exercise authority over persons who use drugs may enact such authority with pragmatic grace and acceptance. Accepting the pervasiveness of mind-altering products also means that humans seek mind-altering opportunities in safety. Acknowledge the disproportionate social and economic reality of poor and minority drug users in our country.

Public Policies That Will Promote Health Equity in Substance Use Disorder Outcomes

The U.S. drug policy regime is still at a crossroads. Are we integrating harm reduction for fundamental change? Or are we appropriating harm reduction to soften punitive prohibition? These policy changes could begin to help us resolve the conundrum.

- Prevention research can profit from research on how drug users learn to protect themselves against the risks of substance use.
- Promoting healthy lifestyles, which include managed drug use strategies, is more effective than emphasizing what is forbidden and dangerous.

- Align the Controlled Substances Act with the diverse legal realities across the country, for example, status/number of states: legal (23), legal for medical use only (17), only low THC medically legal (5), and no program for legal THC (6).
- Align the Controlled Substances Act with the research efforts suggesting the effectiveness of 3,4-methylenedioxymethamphetamine (MDMA) in the treatment of posttraumatic stress disorder and psychotherapeutic efforts.
- Authorize pilot studies of overdose prevention centers within metropolitan statistical areas looking to understand, manage, and reduce the incidence of unintended opioid-related drug poisoning.

Any one of these policy changes could be used to help persuade policy entrepreneurs, funding sources, and the public that harm reduction programs are of value because they offer such advantages as best autonomy for the participant, healthier communities, and a humane and cost-effective solution for society.

SUBSTANCE USE: OTHER CONSIDERATIONS

GOMER: GET OUT OF MY EMERGENCY ROOM

Trainees and young clinicians starting their careers in addiction medicine ready to make a difference in the world learn quickly that there is an untold hierarchy of patient care and particularly how to deal with PWUD and the supposedly "drug-seeking" population. How PWUD are treated in the ED cannot be ignored, as many practitioners are instructed to get them out of the ED quickly. "GOMER"—"Get Out of My Emergency Room"—is a phenomenon described in Samuel Shem's novel *The House of God*, published in 1978, which tells the story of an intern's first year in training (Shem, 1978). GOMER refers to the experience of individuals who are labeled as "frequent flyers." Once labeled, this population will both be subjected to longer than usual wait times for basic services and then most often discharged (Redko et al., 2006). Quite often, people with SUDs (e.g., OUD) leave the ED because they begin to experience withdrawal symptoms, have experienced this behavior previously, or have heard of this and anticipate a repeat performance. They are fearful and want to be treated with compassion and not judged or treated differently because of their use. In the age of fentanyl, not being heard or treated on time and long wait times could lead to a possible fatal overdose. Sadly, these experiences are passed on to other members of their social circles. This dynamic has created a sad reality, where people from marginalized populations do not enter treatment through the front door.

In addition, minimal curriculum time is allocated in professional programs on SUD training and learning how to effectively address this population (Jegede et al., 2023), where GOMER thinking is not addressed and unfortunately perpetuated. A large part of deconstructing stigma deals with our understanding and how we are taught to look at specific substances, scenarios, and the systemic and racial bias associated with drug use. Thirty years ago, with lingering perceptions to date, cannabis was looked at as a gateway drug, whereas now it is largely accepted in society as "medicine" and acceptable recreation as only one-fourth of people (26.5%) perceived great risk from smoking marijuana once or twice a week according to the NSDUH (2021). In states such as Oregon where cannabis has been legal for personal use for several years, there was a correlation with lower overdose rates by 25% versus states that did not have recreational cannabis (Bachhuber et al., 2014). This trend may be due to people using cannabis for pain management instead of opioids.

Deconstructing Social Stigma: A Need for Social Breaks

Increasing evidence shows racial stigma associated with various substances. Whenever we talk about crack cocaine, for example, we think of racial and ethnic minoritized communities instead of substance use by all classes, races, and ethnicities. Beyond the racialization of substance use, medical equipment such as a syringe is stigmatized, given use by people with SUDs. The mental picture of someone using a syringe for anything other than a prescribed necessity immediately has a negative connotation. As such, simply acknowledging that America is indeed a society with PWUD and therefore those with SUDs are not inherently desperate or "dirty" may facilitate a shift in perspectives on drug use and begin to remove stigma.

There are no shortcuts to destigmatization. We must understand the needs for social breaks among PWUD (including injection drug users). Social breaks, such as chatting with peers, allow one to share experiences and feel part of a group, which can serve as a resource for safer use, recovery, and respite. As discussed earlier, the present healthcare systems often present barriers for people to get into treatment. Traditional addiction treatment models have barriers for many and do not work for some, especially from racial and ethnic minoritized backgrounds (Jordan et al., 2021). There is then an increasing need to elevate and implement harm reduction respite treatment sites that will allow people to have access to shelter, showers, food, counseling, and medication for addiction treatment (MAT).

We must create environments that foster safety and allow for open honest conversations where people can talk about their substance use, specifically what their substance use looks like daily (e.g., functional vs. chaotic use) and when and if they are ready to change or move toward recovery. Understanding why people use substances and supporting a choice to minimize harm and optimize the safety of substance use, known as harm reduction, also have merit to minimize unintended death (Marlatt, 1996). Harm reduction is a central topic of discussion given the trajectory of SUD fatalities associated.

"More Meds, Less Beds"

Furthermore, there is an increasing push in healthcare toward "More Meds, Less Beds" (Redko et al., 2006), which is an extension of racially biased treatment methods and lack the understanding of marginalized populations. While immediate access to MAT options like buprenorphine has a place in the SUD treatment arsenal, they may not always work well for transient populations or ambulatory participants who are unable to keep their medication safe or who lack external supports to access MAT on a regular basis. The urban center requires the increased presence and utilization of harm reduction programs. These programs have more access to individuals requiring basic, nonemergent healthcare treatment in the community since they often engage those who may not be receiving care elsewhere. In the struggle against opioid overdose mortality, easy accessibility to methadone as a medication for OUD, like buprenorphine, must be given a much-needed policy consideration. One example that has been tried in the community is the use of mobile methadone programs whereby individuals not otherwise enrolled in OTP can receive methadone as a humane approach to reduce the risk of an accidental fatal overdose (El-Sabawi et al., 2021).

Patients should be able to access a healthcare system where they have autonomy and input into their care and what they want to address, rather than being told what they need to address. EDs and medical systems should treat people who have substance use-related issues with the same level of care and concern as they would with someone who has a diabetic emergency or a heart attack. Finally, we need more street-based prescribers that do not necessarily park in one place but go out to the encampments and truly meet people where they are at.

Future Directions for Research

Research allows for adaptation of best practice, but researchers must do more than just ask questions and gather data. There must be a bidirectional approach where research participants can readily access resources that are helpful to PWUD. One way to employ an equity framework in community research is to plan for participant reimbursement to the equivalent of a livable wage, during the time the research is occurring, while also linking participants to a wide array of services that address the social determinants of health (True et al., 2017). Reimagining the role of researchers and practitioners in the community is essential when addressing people with SUDs. We must center relationships with communities and teach researchers and practitioners how to engage the whole person, rather than focus on substance use alone. There remains provider stigma attached to PWUD, indicating a need for researchers and practitioners to obtain more training on how to effectively partner with these populations for improved health outcomes.

SUMMARY KEY POINTS

- Substance use prevention has limited chances while housing insecurity, food insecurity, and economic inequities continue to outpace opportunities for building agency, families, and community.
- Increased access to prevention resources leads to reductions in disease and mortality.
- Integrating office-based buprenorphine into syringe services programs increases treatment retention.
- Peer workers, with appropriate support for managing their use, facilitate greater drug user referral and engagement in treatment.

DISCUSSION QUESTIONS

1. What are some of your assumptions about PWUD? Do you consider SUD as an individual's moral failure, or do you consider SUD as a chronic illness like diabetes or hypertension?
2. Where did you form these assumptions? Personal experience, home, school or work, and so forth?
3. What are your thoughts about harm reduction? How can harm reduction approaches both help reduce stigma and prevent drug overdose deaths in the community?
4. Imagine that on a very busy day with many patients to treat, you encounter a "frequent flyer" with SUD. How can this patient be treated compassionately and with dignity while other patients are also served?
5. Consider the effects of social isolation on individuals dealing with SUDs. How can these individuals be helped at every stage of treatment?

A robust set of instructor resources designed to supplement this text is located at http://connect.springerpub.com/content/book/978-0-8261-4265-8. Qualifying instructors may request access by emailing textbook@springerpub.com.

REFERENCES

Ágoston, C., Urbán, R., Richman, M. J., & Demetrovics, Z. (2018). Caffeine use disorder: An item-response theory analysis of proposed DSM-5 criteria. *Addictive Behaviors, 81*, 109–116. https://doi.org/10.1016/j.addbeh.2018.02.012

APA. (2022). *Diagnostic and statistical manual of mental disorders 5th edition—Text revised*. APA Publishing.

Bachhuber, M. A., Saloner, B., Cunningham, C. O., & Barry, C. L. (2014). Medical cannabis laws and opioid analgesic overdose mortality in the United States, 1999–2010. *JAMA Internal Medicine, 174*(10), 1668–1673. https://doi.org/10.1001/jamainternmed.2014.4005

Bentzley, B. S., Han, S. S., Neuner, S., Humphreys, K., Kampman, K. M., & Halpern, C. H. (2021). Comparison of treatments for cocaine use disorder among adults: A systematic review and meta-analysis. *JAMA Network Open, 4*(5), e218049. https://doi.org/10.1001/jamanetworkopen.2021.8049

Botsford, S. L., Yang, S., & George, T. P. (2020). Cannabis and cannabinoids in mood and anxiety disorders: Impact on illness onset and course, and assessment of therapeutic potential. *Am J Addict, 29*(1), 9–26. https://doi.org/10.1111/ajad.12963

Bourgois, P., Holmes, S. M., Sue, K., & Quesada, J. (2017). Structural vulnerability: Operationalizing the concept to address health disparities in clinical care. *Academic Medicine, 92*(3), 299–307. https://doi.org/10.1097/acm.0000000000001294

Brooner, R., Kidorf, M., King, V., Beilenson, P., Svikis, D., & Vlahov, D. (1998). Drug abuse treatment success among needle exchange participants. *Public Health Reports, 113*(Suppl. 1), 129.

Broz, D., Carnes, N., Chapin-Bardales, J., Des Jarlais, D. C., Handanagic, S., Jones, C. M., McClung, R. P., & Asher, A. K. (2021). Syringe services programs' role in ending the HIV epidemic in the US: Why we cannot do it without them. *American Journal of Preventive Medicine, 61*(5 Suppl. 1), S118–S129. https://doi.org/10.1016/j.amepre.2021.05.044

Budney, A. J., Sofis, M. J., & Borodovsky, J. T. (2019). An update on cannabis use disorder with comment on the impact of policy related to therapeutic and recreational cannabis use. *European Archives of Psychiatry and Clinical Neuroscience, 269*, 73–86. https://doi.org/10.1007/s00406-018-0976-1

Burr, C. K., Storm, D. S., Hoyt, M. J., Dutton, L., Berezny, L., Allread, V., & Paul, S. (2014). Integrating health and prevention services in syringe access programs: A strategy to address unmet needs in a high-risk population. *Public Health Reports, 129*(Suppl. 1), 26–32. https://doi.org/10.1177/00333549141291S105

Butelman, E. R., Huang, Y., Epstein, D. H., Shaham, Y., Goldstein, R. Z., Volkow, N. D., & Alia-Klein, N. (2023). Overdose mortality rates for opioids and stimulant drugs are substantially higher in men than in women: State-level analysis. *Neuropsychopharmacology, 48*, 1639–1647. https://doi.org/10.1038/s41386-023-01601-8

CDC. (2023a). *HIV surveillance report* (Diagnoses of HIV infection in the United States and dependent areas, 2021. https://www.cdc.gov/hiv/library/reports/hiv-surveillance/vol-34/index.html

CDC. (2023b, May 4, 2023). *Smoking and tobacco use.* https://www.cdc.gov/tobacco/data_statistics/index.htm

Clinical Practice Guideline Treating Tobacco Use and Dependence 2008 Update Panel, Liaisons, and Staff. (2008). A clinical practice guideline for treating tobacco use and dependence: 2008 update: A US public health service report. *American Journal of Preventive Medicine, 35*(2), 158–176. https://doi.org/10.1016/j.amepre.2008.04.009

Cornelius, M. E., Loretan, C. G., Wang, T. W., Jamal, A., & Homa, D. M. (2022). Tobacco product use among adults—United States, 2020. *Morbidity and Mortality Weekly Report, 71*(11), 397–405. https://doi.org/10.15585/mmwr.mm7111a1

Des Jarlais, D. C., Friedman, S. R., Novick, D. M., Sotheran, J. L., Thomas, P., Yancovitz, S. R., Mildvan, D., Weber, J., Kreek, M. J., & Maslansky, R. (1989). HIV-1 infection among intravenous drug users in Manhattan, New York City, from 1977 through 1987. *JAMA, 261*(7), 1008–1012. https://doi.org/10.1001/jama.261.7.1008

Dimenstein, M., Siqueira, K., Macedo, J. P., Leite, J., & Dantas, C. (2017). Determinação social da saúde mental: Contribuições à psicologia no cuidado territorial. *Arquivos Brasileiros de Psicologia, 69*(2), 72–87. http://pepsic.bvsalud.org/pdf/arbp/v69n2/06.pdf

Dow-Fleisner, S. J., Lomness, A., & Woolgar, L. (2022). Impact of safe consumption facilities on individual and community outcomes: A scoping review of the past decade of research. *Emerging Trends in Drugs, Addictions, and Health, 2*, 100046. https://doi.org/10.1016/j.etdah.2022.100046

DuPont, R. L. (2009). Reflections on the early history of National Institute on Drug Abuse (NIDA): Implications for today. *Journal of Drug Issues, 39*(1), 5–14. https://doi.org/10.1177/002204260903900101

Duranceaux, N. C., Schuckit, M. A., Eng, M. Y., Robinson, S. K., Carr, L. G., & Wall, T. L. (2006). Associations of variations in alcohol dehydrogenase genes with the level of response to alcohol in non-Asians. *Alcoholism: Clinical and Experimental Research, 30*(9), 1470–1478.

El-Sabawi, T., Baney, M., Canzater, S. L., & Weizman, S. R. (2021). The new mobile methadone rules and what they mean for treatment access. *Health Affairs Forefront.* https://www.healthaffairs.org/content/forefront/new-mobile-methadone-rules-and-they-mean-treatment-access

Evans, R. I., Rozelle, R. M., Mittelmark, M. B., Hansen, W. B., Bane, A. L., & Havis, J. (1978). Deterring the onset of smoking in children: Knowledge of immediate physiological effects and coping with peer pressure, media pressure, and parent modeling 1. *Journal of Applied Social Psychology, 8*(2), 126–135. https://doi.org/10.1111/j.1559-1816.1978.tb00771.x

Forray, A. (2016). Substance use during pregnancy. *F1000Research, 5.* https://doi.org/10.12688/f1000research.7645.1

Freeman, T. P., Hindocha, C., Baio, G., Shaban, N. D. C., Thomas, E. M., Astbury, D., Freeman, A. M., Lees, R., Craft, S., Morrison, P. D., Bloomfield, M. A. P., O'Ryan, D., Kinghorn, J., Morgan, C. J. A., Mofeez, A., & Curran, H. V. (2020). Cannabidiol for the treatment of cannabis use disorder: A phase

2a, double-blind, placebo-controlled, randomised, adaptive Bayesian trial. *Lancet Psychiatry, 7*(10), 865–874. https://doi.org/10.1016/s2215-0366(20)30290-x

Friedman, J., Montero, F., Bourgois, P., Wahbi, R., Dye, D., Goodman-Meza, D., & Shover, C. (2022). Xylazine spreads across the US: A growing component of the increasingly synthetic and polysubstance overdose crisis. *Drug and Alcohol Dependence, 233,* 109380. https://doi.org/10.1016/j.drugalcdep.2022.109380

Friedman, J. R., & Hansen, H. (2022). Evaluation of increases in drug overdose mortality rates in the US by race and ethnicity before and during the COVID-19 pandemic. *JAMA Psychiatry, 79*(4), 379–381. https://doi.org/10.1001/jamapsychiatry.2022.0004

Furr-Holden, D., Milam, A. J., Wang, L., & Sadler, R. (2021). African Americans now outpace whites in opioid-involved overdose deaths: A comparison of temporal trends from 1999 to 2018. *Addiction (Abingdon, England), 116*(3), 677–683. https://doi.org/10.1111/add.15233

Giulietti, F., Filipponi, A., Rosettani, G., Giordano, P., Iacoacci, C., Spannella, F., & Sarzani, R. (2020). Pharmacological approach to smoking cessation: An updated review for daily clinical practice. *High Blood Pressure & Cardiovascular Prevention, 27*(5), 349–362. https://doi.org/10.1007/s40292-020-00396-9

Gray, K. M., Carpenter, M. J., Baker, N. L., DeSantis, S. M., Kryway, E., Hartwell, K. J., McRae-Clark, A. L., & Brady, K. T. (2012). A double-blind randomized controlled trial of N-acetylcysteine in cannabis-dependent adolescents. *The American Jorunal of Psychiatry, 169*(8), 805–812. https://doi.org/10.1176/appi.ajp.2012.12010055

Hagan, H., McGough, J. P., Thiede, H., Hopkins, S., Duchin, J., & Alexander, E. R. (2000). Reduced injection frequency and increased entry and retention in drug treatment associated with needle-exchange participation in Seattle drug injectors. *Journal of Substance Abuse Treatment, 19*(3), 247–252. https://doi.org/10.1016/s0740-5472(00)00104-5

Haggerty, R. J., & Mrazek, P. J. (1994). Can we prevent mental illness? *Bulletin of the New York Academy of Medicine, 71*(2), 300–306.

Haney, M. (2022). Cannabis use and the endocannabinoid system: A clinical perspective. *American Journal of Psychiatry, 179*(1), 21–25. https://doi.org/10.1176/appi.ajp.2021.21111138

Haney, M., Cooper, Z. D., Bedi, G., Vosburg, S. K., Comer, S. D., & Foltin, R. W. (2013). Nabilone decreases marijuana withdrawal and a laboratory measure of marijuana relapse. *Neuropsychopharmacology, 38*(8), 1557–1565. https://doi.org/10.1038/npp.2013.54

Haney, M., Hart, C. L., Ward, A. S., & Foltin, R. W. (2003). Nefazodone decreases anxiety during marijuana withdrawal in humans. *Psychopharmacology, 165,* 157–165. https://doi.org/10.1007/s00213-002-1210-3

Haney, M., Ramesh, D., Glass, A., Pavlicova, M., Bedi, G., & Cooper, Z. D. (2015). Naltrexone maintenance decreases cannabis self-administration and subjective effects in daily cannabis smokers. *Neuropsychopharmacology, 40*(11), 2489–2498. https://doi.org/10.1038/npp.2015.108

Hasin, D. S., Saxon, A. J., Malte, C., Olfson, M., Keyes, K. M., Gradus, J. L., Cerdá, M., Maynard, C. C., Keyhani, S., & Martins, S. S. (2022). Trends in cannabis use disorder diagnoses in the US Veterans Health Administration, 2005–2019. *American Journal of Psychiatry, 179*(10), 748–757. https://doi.org/10.1176/appi.ajp.22010034

Hasin, D. S., Shmulewitz, D., Cerdá, M., Keyes, K. M., Olfson, M., Sarvet, A. L., & Wall, M. M. (2020). US adults with pain, a group increasingly vulnerable to nonmedical cannabis use and cannabis use disorder: 2001–2002 and 2012–2013. *American Journal of Psychiatry, 177*(7), 611–618. https://doi.org/10.1176/appi.ajp.2019.19030284

James, K., & Jordan, A. (2018). The opioid crisis in black communities. *The Journal of Law, Medicine & Ethics, 46*(2), 404–421. https://doi.org/10.1177/1073110518782949

Javed, Z., Burk, K., Facente, S., Pegram, L., Ali, A., & Asher, A. (2020). Syringe services programs: A technical package of effective strategies and approaches for planning, design, and implementation. https://stacks.cdc.gov/view/cdc/105304

Jegede, O., Na, P. J., Petrakis, I., & Muvvala, S. B. (2023). The current status of medical education on opioids. In Kelly E. Dunn (Ed.), *The Oxford Handbook of Opioids and Opioid Use Disorder*, Oxford Library of Psychology (online edn, Oxford Academic, 20 Apr. 2023), https://doi.org/10.1093/oxfordhb/9780197618431.013.5

Jones, C. P. (2000). Levels of racism: A theoretic framework and a gardener's tale. *American Journal of Public Health, 90*(8), 1212–1215. https://doi.org/10.2105/ajph.90.8.1212

Jordan, A., Babuscio, T., Nich, C., & Carroll, K. M. (2021). A feasibility study providing substance use treatment in the Black church. *J Subst Abuse Treat, 124,* 108218. https://doi.org/10.1016/j.jsat.2020.108218

Kidorf, M., King, V. L., Neufeld, K., Peirce, J., Kolodner, K., & Brooner, R. K. (2009). Improving substance abuse treatment enrollment in community syringe exchangers. *Addiction (Abingdon, England), 104*(5), 786–795. https://doi.org/10.1111/j.1360-0443.2009.02560.x

Ko, J. Y., Coy, K. C., Haight, S. C., Haegerich, T. M., Williams, L., Cox, S., Njai, R., & Grant, A. M. (2020). Characteristics of marijuana use during pregnancy—Eight states, pregnancy risk assessment monitoring system, 2017. *Morbidity and Mortality Weekly Report, 69*(32), 1058–1063. https://doi.org/10.15585/mmwr.mm6932a2

Koob, G. F., & Moal, M. L. (1997). Drug abuse: Hedonic homeostatic dysregulation. *Science, 278*(5335), 52–58. https://doi.org/10.1126/science.278.5335.52

Lagisetty, P. A., Ross, R., Bohnert, A., Clay, M., & Maust, D. T. (2019). Buprenorphine treatment divide by race/ethnicity and payment. *JAMA Psychiatry, 76*(9), 979–981. https://doi.org/10.1001/jamapsychiatry.2019.0876

Lambdin, B. H., Davidson, P. J., Browne, E. N., Suen, L. W., Wenger, L. D., & Kral, A. H. (2022). Reduced emergency department visits and hospitalisation with use of an unsanctioned safe consumption site for injection drug use in the United States. *Journal of General Internal Medicine, 37*(15), 3853–3860. https://doi.org/10.1007/s11606-021-07312-4

Landefeld, C. C., Pauly, B., Stockwell, T., Nance, M., & Smith-Bernardin, S. (2023). Managed alcohol programs: An innovative and evidence-based solution for adults with severe alcohol use disorder who are experiencing homelessness. *NEJM Catalyst Innovations in Care Delivery, 4*(2). https://catalyst.nejm.org/doi/full/10.1056/CAT.22.0301

Larochelle, M. R., Slavova, S., Root, E. D., Feaster, D. J., Ward, P. J., Selk, S. C., Knott, C., Villani, J., & Samet, J. H. (2021). Disparities in opioid overdose death trends by race/ethnicity, 2018–2019, from the HEALing Communities study. *American Journal of Public Health, 111*(10), 1851–1854. https://doi.org/10.2105/ajph.2021.306431

Leung, J., Chan, G. C., Hides, L., & Hall, W. D. (2020). What is the prevalence and risk of cannabis use disorders among people who use cannabis? A systematic review and meta-analysis. *Addictive Behaviors, 109*, 106479. https://doi.org/10.1016/j.addbeh.2020.106479

Levounis, P., Arnaout, B., & Marienfeld, C. (2017). *Motivational interviewing for clinical practice*. APA Publishing.

Lurie, P., & Drucker, E. (1997). An opportunity lost: HIV infections associated with lack of a national needle-exchange programme in the USA. *The Lancet, 349*(9052), 604–608. https://doi.org/10.1016/S0140-6736(96)05439-6

MacCoun, R. J. (1998). Toward a psychology of harm reduction. *American Psychologist, 53*(11), 1199–208. https://doi.org/10.1037//0003-066x.53.11.1199

Majoor, B., & Rivera, J. (2003). SACHR: An example of an integrated, harm reduction drug treatment program. *Journal of Substance Abuse Treatment, 25*(4), 257–262. https://doi.org/10.1016/s0740-5472(03)00086-2

Markou, A. (2008). Neurobiology of nicotine dependence. *Philosophical Transactions of the Royal Society B: Biological Sciences, 363*(1507), 3159–3168. https://doi.org/10.1098/rstb.2008.0095

Marlatt, G. A. (1996). Harm reduction: Come as you are. *Addictive Behaviors, 21*(6), 779–788. https://doi.org/10.1016/0306-4603(96)00042-1

Mason, B. J., Crean, R., Goodell, V., Light, J. M., Quello, S., Shadan, F., Buffkins, K., Kyle, M., Adusumalli, M., Begovic, A., & Rao, S. (2012). A proof-of-concept randomized controlled study of gabapentin: Effects on cannabis use, withdrawal and executive function deficits in cannabis-dependent adults. *Neuropsychopharmacology, 37*(7), 1689–1698. https://doi.org/10.1038/npp.2012.14

McRae-Clark, A. L., Carter, R. E., Killeen, T. K., Carpenter, M. J., Wahlquist, A. E., Simpson, S. A., & Brady, K. T. (2009). A placebo-controlled trial of buspirone for the treatment of marijuana dependence. *Drug Alcohol Depend, 105*(1–2), 132–138. https://doi.org/10.1016/j.drugalcdep.2009.06.022

McRae-Clark, A. L., Gray, K. M., Baker, N. L., Sherman, B. J., Squeglia, L., Sahlem, G. L., Wagner, A., & Tomko, R. (2021). Varenicline as a treatment for cannabis use disorder: A placebo-controlled pilot trial. *Drug Alcohol Depend, 229*(Pt B), 109111. https://doi.org/10.1016/j.drugalcdep.2021.109111

Metzl, J. M., & Hansen, H. (2014). Structural competency: Theorizing a new medical engagement with stigma and inequality. *Social Science & Medicine, 103*, 126–133. https://doi.org/10.1016/j.socscimed.2013.06.032

Miller, W. R., & Rollnick, S. (2002). *Motivational interviewing: Preparing people for change* (2nd ed.). Guilford Press.

MINT. (2019). *Understanding motivational interviewing*. https://motivationalinterviewing.org/understanding-motivational-interviewing

Moss, A. R., & Bacchetti, P. (1989). Natural history of HIV infection. *Aids, 3*(2), 55–61. https://doi.org/10.1097/00002030-198902000-00001

Navarrete, F., García-Gutiérrez, M. S., Jurado-Barba, R., Rubio, G., Gasparyan, A., Austrich-Olivares, A., & Manzanares, J. (2020). Endocannabinoid system components as potential biomarkers in psychiatry. *Frontiers in Psychiatry, 11*, 315. https://doi.org/10.3389/fpsyt.2020.00315

Nebhinani, N., Singh, P., & Mamta. (2022). Substance use disorders in children and adolescents. *Journal of Indian Association for Child and Adolescent Mental Health, 18*(2), 128–136. https://doi.org/10.1177/09731342221096503

NIDCR. (2023). *Periodontal (Gum) disease*. https://www.nidcr.nih.gov/health-info/gum-disease#:~:text=Periodontal%20(gum)%20disease%20is%20an,%2C%20red%2C%20and%20bleeding%20gums

Nolan, S., Kelian, S., Kerr, T., Young, S., Malmgren, I., Ghafari, C., Harrison, S., Wood, E., Lysyshyn, M., & Holliday, E. (2022). Harm reduction in the hospital: An overdose prevention site (OPS) at a Canadian hospital. *Drug and Alcohol Dependence, 239*, 109608. https://doi.org/10.1016/j.drugalcdep .2022.109608

NSDUH. (2021). *Key substance use and mental health indicators in the United States: Results from the 2021 National Survey on Drug Use and Health* (HHS Publication No. PEP22-07-01-005, NSDUH Series H-57). https://www.samhsa.gov/data/report/2021-nsduh-annual-national-report

Petry, N. M. (2011). Contingency management: What it is and why psychiatrists should want to use it. *The psychiatrist, 35*(5), 161–163. https://doi.org/ 10.1192/pb.bp.110.031831

Redko, C., Rapp, R. C., & Carlson, R. G. (2006). Waiting time as a barrier to treatment entry: Perceptions of substance users. *J Drug Issues, 36*(4), 831–852. https://doi.org/10.1177 /002204260603600404

Reyes, J. C., Negrón, J. L., Colón, H. M., Padilla, A. M., Millán, M. Y., Matos, T. D., & Robles, R. R. (2012). The emerging of xylazine as a new drug of abuse and its health consequences among drug users in Puerto Rico. *Journal of Urban Health, 89*(3), 519–526. https://doi.org/10.1007/s11524-011 -9662-6

Ronzani, T. M., Pereira, T. S., Castro, J. B., & Dimenstein, M. (2023). Social determinants and drug dependence: Systematic review of literature. *Psicologia: Teoria e Pesquisa, 39*, e39407. https://doi .org/10.1590/0102.3772e39407.en

Roux, P., Jauffret-Roustide, M., Donadille, C., Briand Madrid, L., Denis, C., Célérier, I., Chauvin, C., Hamelin, N., Maradan, G., & Carrieri, M. (2023). Impact of drug consumption rooms on non-fatal overdoses, abscesses and emergency department visits in people who inject drugs in France: Results from the COSINUS cohort. *International Journal of Epidemiology, 52*(2), 562–576. https://doi .org/10.1093/ije/dyac120

Samet, J. M. (2013). Tobacco smoking: The leading cause of preventable disease worldwide. *Thoracic Surgery Clinics, 23*(2), 103–112. https://doi.org/10.1016/j.thorsurg.2013.01.009

SAMHSA. (2017). *About screening, brief intervention, and referral to treatment (SBIRT)*. https://www .samhsa.gov/sbirt/about

Schuckit, M. A. (2009). Alcohol-use disorders. *The Lancet, 373*(9662), 492–501. https://doi.org/10.1016 /S0140-6736(09)60009-X

Shem, S. (1978). *The house of God: A novel*. Putnam Publishing Group.

Shover, C. L., Falasinnu, T. O., Dwyer, C. L., Santos, N. B., Cunningham, N. J., Freedman, R. B., Vest, N. A., & Humphreys, K. (2020). Steep increases in fentanyl-related mortality west of the Mississippi River: Recent evidence from county and state surveillance. *Drug and Alcohol Dependence, 216*, 108314. https://doi.org/10.1016/j.drugalcdep.2020.108314

Sloboda, Z., Cottler, L. B., Hawkins, J. D., & Pentz, M. A. (2009). Reflections on 40 years of drug abuse prevention research. *Journal of Drug Issues, 39*(1), 179–195. https://doi.org/10.1177 /002204260903900114

Smith-Bernardin, S. M., Suen, L. W., Barr-Walker, J., Cuervo, I. A., & Handley, M. A. (2022). Scoping review of managed alcohol programs. *Harm Reduction Journal, 19*(1), 82. https://doi.org/10.1186 /s12954-022-00646-0

Stover, M. W., & Davis, J. M. (2015). Opioids in pregnancy and neonatal abstinence syndrome. *Seminars in Perinatology, 39*(7), 561–565. https://doi.org/10.1053/j.semperi.2015.08.013

Strang, J., McDonald, R., Campbell, G., Degenhardt, L., Nielsen, S., Ritter, A., & Dale, O. (2019). Take-home naloxone for the emergency interim management of opioid overdose: The public health application of an emergency medicine. *Drugs, 79*, 1395–1418. https://doi.org/10.1007/s40265-019 -01154-5

Strang, J., Volkow, N. D., Degenhardt, L., Hickman, M., Johnson, K., Koob, G. F., Marshall, B. D. L., Tyndall, M., & Walsh, S. L. (2020). Opioid use disorder. *Nature Reviews Disease Primers, 6*(1), 3. https://doi.org/10.1038/s41572-019-0137-5

True, G., Alexander, L. B., & Fisher, C. B. (2017). Supporting the role of community members employed as research staff: Perspectives of community researchers working in addiction research. *Social Science & Medicine, 187*, 67–75. https://doi.org/10.1016/j.socscimed.2017.06.023

US Preventive Services Task Force; Curry, S. J., Krist, A. H., Owens, D. K., Barry, M. J., Caughey, A. B., Davidson, K. W., Doubeni, C. A., Epling, J. W., Jr., Kemper, A. R., Kubik, M., Landefeld, C. S., Mangione, C. M., Silverstein, M., Simon, M. A., Tseng, C.-W., & Wong, J. B. (2018). Unhealthy alcohol use in adolescents and adults: Screening and behavioral counseling interventions. *US Preventive Serivces Task Force recommendation Statement, 320*(18), 1899–1909. https://doi.org /10.1001/jama.2018.16789.

Vickers-Smith, R., Justice, A. C., Becker, W. C., Rentsch, C. T., Curtis, B., Fernander, A., Hartwell, E. E., Ighodaro, E. T., Kember, R. L., Tate, J., & Kranzler, H. R. (2023). Racial and ethnic bias in the diagnosis of alcohol use disorder in veterans. *The American Journal of Psychiatry, 180*(6), 426–436. https://doi.org/10.1176/appi.ajp.21111097

Vlahov, D., & Junge, B. (1998). The role of needle exchange programs in HIV prevention. *Public Health Reports, 113*(Suppl. 1), 75.

Wallner, M., & Olsen, R. W. (2008). Physiology and pharmacology of alcohol: The imidazobenzodiazepine alcohol antagonist site on subtypes of GABAA receptors as an opportunity for drug development? *British Journal of Pharmacology, 154*(2), 288–298. https://doi.org/10.1038/bjp.2008.32

Weil, A., & Rosen, W. (2004). *From chocolate to morphine: Everything you need to know about mind-altering drugs.* HMH.

Weinstein, A. M., & Gorelick, D. A. (2011). Pharmacological treatment of cannabis dependence. *Current Pharmaceutical Design, 17*(14), 1351–1358. https://doi.org/10.2174/138161211796150846

Wesson, D. R., & Ling, W. (2003). The clinical opiate withdrawal scale (COWS). *Journal of Psychoactive Drugs, 35*(2), 253–259. https://doi.org/10.1080/02791072.2003.10400007

World Health Organization. (2019). *Global status report on alcohol and health 2018.* World Health Organization.

Xin, Q., Xu, F., Taylor, D. H., Zhao, J. F., & Wu, J. (2020). The impact of cannabinoid type 2 receptors (CB2Rs) in neuroprotection against neurological disorders. *Acta Pharmacologica Sinica, 41*(12), 1507–1518. https://doi.org/10.1038/s41401-020-00530-2

CHAPTER 10

VACCINES

ABRAM L. WAGNER

LEARNING OBJECTIVES

- Discuss the role that governments, healthcare providers, and communities play in maintaining high vaccination coverage.
- Apply behavioral nudges to conversations between vaccination providers and patients.
- Use motivational interviewing in the context of vaccination.
- Explain the limits of health behavior models in explaining vaccination uptake.
- Define vaccine hesitancy.

WHAT ARE VACCINES?

Vaccines encompass a range of biological products that have been purposefully designed to induce active immunity in the recipient, or vaccinee. Vaccines derive from pathogens, but the pathogens have been processed—through attenuation, inactivation, or isolation of immunologically important subcomponents—so as to substantially reduce the likelihood of severe disease in the vaccinee (Wodi & Morelli, 2021).

Modern-day vaccination is a global enterprise. Epidemiologists research how viral, bacterial, or parasitic diseases cross borders and transmit among people. Basic scientists worldwide study these pathogens and identify antigen targets. Pharmaceutical companies use cross-national supply chains to source materials and manufacture vaccines. Clinical researchers assess the efficacy of vaccines in experimental clinical trials and their effectiveness in local settings through observation studies. The World Health Organization (WHO), along with country-specific National Immunization Technical Advisory Groups (NITAG), develops recommendations for use of these vaccines (Steffen et al., 2021).

The history of vaccination echoes these global patterns and highlights contributions from diverse populations. By the 1600s, people in South Asia and China had iterated upon the precursor to modern-day vaccination, smallpox variolation, which was a procedure of transferring pus or scabs from someone recovering from smallpox to another who had not previously been infected. Effective, and relatively safe compared with natural infection, variolation subsequently spread throughout Asia and Africa. Lady Mary Wortley Montagu brought the ideas of variolation from the Ottoman Empire to England in 1721, when she had her daughter undergo the procedure. Also in the early 1700s, Onesimus, an enslaved person in Massachusetts, introduced the idea of variolation, which had already spread into Africa, to Cotton Mather, an intellectual who tried to popularize the procedure throughout the American colonies (Plotkin & Plotkin, 2024).

The germ theory and other advances in immunology, virology, bacteriology, biotechnology, and engineering have pushed the crudeness of variation into a broad array of safe and effective vaccines. By the 1700s, several people, historically most notably Dr. Edward Jenner, had innovated upon the smallpox *variolation* to create a safer smallpox *vaccine* (which was derived instead from cowpox, thus vaccine's Latinate name deriving from vacca, or cow). Scientific greats such as Louis Pasteur, Thomas Francis, Pearl Kendrick, Grace Eldering, Jonas Salk, Albert Sabin, Maurice Hilleman, Michiaki Takahashi, and countless others dedicated their lives to studying vaccines and pushing the field to have the scientific advances that are available today (Plotkin & Plotkin, 2024).

The development and distribution of vaccines have led to a substantial decline in infectious disease morbidity and mortality. In the United States, from the immediate period prior to vaccination introduction to the early 2000s, there has been greater than 90% decline in cases and 99% decline in deaths due to diphtheria, tetanus, pertussis, polio, and measles, mumps, and rubella (MMR; Roush et al., 2007).

Cases and outbreaks of vaccine-preventable diseases have persisted in recent years at least in part due to purposefully unvaccinated individuals (Halsey & Salmon, 2015). For example, in 2017, an unvaccinated 6-year old child in Oregon had to be mechanically ventilated for 44 days after being infected with tetanus (Guzman-Cottrill et al., 2019). In an outbreak of measles at Disneyland in California in 2015, 49 were unvaccinated, of whom 12 were too young to be vaccinated and 28 were intentionally unvaccinated (Zipprich et al., 2015). In a 2017 outbreak of measles in Minnesota, most cases were children of Somali immigrants (Hall et al., 2017), and a large majority (71%) of Somali American parents had believed there was a connection between measles vaccination and autism (Christianson et al., 2020).

Although only smallpox has been eradicated globally, regional efforts to eliminate measles, rubella, and polio have succeeded, raising the prospect of their worldwide eradication (Dixon et al., 2021; Rachlin et al., 2022). Yet, in 2020, over 17 million children worldwide had not received the first dose of diphtheria, tetanus, and pertussis (DTP) vaccine, a commonly used marker of immunization service utilization, given its long history of use (Muhoza et al., 2021). Understanding who these children are and why they are not vaccinated is incredibly important to mitigate future outbreaks of vaccine-preventable disease. Moreover, from observed data (Dimitrova et al., 2023; Leslie et al., 2018) and mathematical models (Masters et al., 2020), we know that high vaccination coverage in a large geographic area could mask pockets of low vaccination coverage, where transmission of infections could still occur.

HOW DO GOVERNMENTS MAKE DECISIONS ABOUT VACCINES?

A goal of many governments is to increase vaccination coverage in the population. As one of the great public health achievements (Centers for Disease Control and Prevention [CDC], 1999b, 2011), vaccinations can further government goals to reduce mortality and morbidity among vulnerable populations, notably but not limited to children, and increase life spans. Government recommendations about vaccines are usually formalized through a NITAG, which in the United States is named the Advisory Committee on Immunization Practices (ACIP). NITAGs include various stakeholders and healthcare workers, but also nonspecialist members of the general population, who review the epidemiology of a vaccine-preventable disease, results from clinical trials, and cost-effectiveness analyses to provide independent input into the details of a vaccine recommendations.

A large consideration of NITAGs is whether to push toward local *elimination* or *control* of a particular vaccine-preventable disease. Elimination indicates disruption of transmission within a country, although imported cases and limited epidemiological chains of transmission from imported cases can still occur. Control is a more modest goal, whereby incidence is reduced but endemic transmission remains. Worldwide *eradication* of a disease, as has been done for smallpox, can only occur after it has been eliminated from every country. Beyond

194 II • PRIORITIZED BEHAVIORS FOR PRIMARY PREVENTION OF DISEASE

the greater financial resources needed to eliminate a disease, the decision to have a goal of control, but not elimination, could also be due to certain vaccines' limitations in effectiveness or preventing infection.

NITAGs also make decisions about who should be vaccinated. Their recommendations delineate medical contraindications to vaccination and the indicated age range, but also whether vaccination should be limited by other factors like prior immunity, risk profile, and chronic disease, notably immunodeficiencies.

NITAGs in different countries may come to different recommendations about the same vaccine as a result of varying local epidemiology of disease, results from within-country clinical trials, cost-effectiveness estimates, or other competing priorities. WHO also releases vaccine position papers (WHO, 2017). Vaccines that WHO recommends be included in every routine immunization program are a part of the Expanded Program on Immunization (EPI).

Different countries may have various sensitivities to safety signals during postmarketing surveillance of adverse events. For example, due to concerns about adverse events, Japan temporarily limited the use of the DTP vaccine in 1975, the MMR vaccine in 1993, and the human papillomavirus (HPV) vaccine in 2013 (Andreae et al., 2004; Haruyama et al., 2022). Subsequently, the uptake of these vaccines plummeted, and when alternative vaccines were provided (like single antigen vaccines) vaccinations were substantially delayed, leading to increases in infection, thousands more cases of clinical disease, and dozens of reported deaths from vaccine-preventable diseases (Andreae et al., 2004). In this way, government decisions about vaccines can have clear and wide-ranging impacts on population health.

Governments can decide to mandate vaccination. Vaccine mandates differ from recommendations in a number of ways. Recommendations are processed through an apolitical, scientific advisory body (the NITAG), whereas mandates are legislated. In the United States, different states have different laws about vaccine mandates, and these laws can vary in what vaccines are included, what exceptions, or waivers, are available, and how difficult it is to acquire a waiver. The political basis for vaccine mandates in the United States derives from the ruling of *Jacobson v. Massachusetts* in 1905, where the Supreme Court indicated that individual objections to a smallpox vaccination did not overrule political efforts to protect the public against an epidemic (Parmet et al., 2005). This original court case referred to a fine given to individuals unvaccinated, but vaccine mandates in the modern era often refer to requirements for children to be vaccinated prior to attending a day care or school.

All states allow for individuals with medical contraindications to not be vaccinated; many states also allow for "philosophical" or "religious" waivers as well (Salmon & Siegel, 2001). Given the ambiguity in their distinction, these two waivers can be grouped together as "nonmedical" exemptions. States vary in how difficult it is to obtain a nonmedical waiver. This range in difficulty could come from the availability of a preexisting form, whether the form needs to be notarized, whether the parent needs to have educational counseling at a health department, and whether it needs to be annually recertified (Bednarczyk et al., 2019). Removing nonmedical exemptions to vaccination is probably more effective at increasing vaccine coverage than keeping nonmedical exemptions but making them more difficult to obtain (Bednarczyk et al., 2019; Garnier et al., 2020; Mashinini et al., 2020).

Although vaccine mandates existed prior to the current routine childhood immunization series, the COVID-19 pandemic once again brought adult vaccine mandates to the forefront of public discourse. Although these mandates could prove useful in increasing vaccination coverage, some have argued that the mandates could be counterproductive because of the potential for harms (Jamrozik, 2022). For pandemic vaccines or other newly developed vaccines, there are also concerns that limited population data may be driving far-reaching policy decisions (Jamrozik, 2022).

Populations could react negatively to vaccine mandates, reducing long-term trust in public health and exacerbating existing inequities in health (Bardosh et al., 2022). Implementing policies with increased vaccination enforcement led to reduced overall vaccine acceptance in one study of COVID-19 vaccination in the United States, and this reduction was even greater for those who identified as vaccine-hesitant at the survey baseline (Eshun-Wilson et al., 2021). The impact of vaccine mandates likely differs by the degree of coercion of the mandate (Lytras et al., 2016). In a survey of individuals not yet vaccinated against SARS-CoV-2, many reported that a range of political efforts to promote vaccination would actually decrease their likelihood of getting vaccinated, and their responses differed by political affiliation and other indicators of socioeconomic status (Sargent et al., 2022). In one survey from the Kaiser Family Foundation, 25% of adult workers in the United States mentioned being subjected to a COVID-19 vaccine mandate and 5% mentioned leaving a job because of a vaccine mandate (Kaiser Family Foundation, 2021). These studies from the recent COVID-19 vaccine rollout highlight potential pitfalls in the use of vaccine mandates.

HOW CAN VACCINATION PROVIDERS INCREASE VACCINE UPTAKE?

After vaccines have been licensed and authorized for use in a country, vaccination decisions shift to individuals and their vaccination providers. There is a long documented history of physician–patient communication about vaccines; training manuals from early 19th-century France detail how medical doctors can convince patients to receive a smallpox vaccine (Szarke, 2022). Moreover, across a large body of research, a strong recommendation from vaccination providers has remained one of the most important predictors of whether an individual is vaccinated or not. In a meta-analysis of 62 studies of HPV vaccination, a physician recommendation had the strongest impact on parents getting their child vaccinated (Newman et al., 2018). Although often "vaccination provider" refers to a physician, studies show that nurses (Bowling, 2018) and pharmacists (Murray et al., 2021) can also provide impactful recommendations to individuals. Given changing immunization schedules, structural barriers to vaccination, and the need for advanced skills in risk communication surrounding vaccines, other possibilities would be to create a specialty position of vaccination counselor (Ulrich et al., 2022) or to rely on community organizations to promote vaccines (Shen et al., 2023).

The effectiveness of vaccination providers' recommendations depends on how much they are trusted by a community (Williamson et al., 2022). This trust could be particularly low among groups that have historically and contemporarily faced substantial discrimination in healthcare settings (Batelaan, 2022). For example, in a study from summer 2021, 82% of White Detroiters but only 56% of Black Detroiters had received a COVID-19 vaccine. Moreover, 90% of White Detroiters viewed a vaccine recommendation from a healthcare provider as important, whereas only 67% of Black Detroiters did. From a mediation analysis, 23% of the differences in COVID-19 vaccine uptake by race could be eliminated if Black Detroiters had similar trust in healthcare providers as their White counterparts (Wagner et al., 2021). This lack of trust has had real consequences. The 2017 measles outbreak among Somali Minnesotans was driven in part by a community distrustful of the medical and scientific establishment, which was fertile ground for advocacy from antivaccine voices (Dyer, 2017). Ways for vaccination providers to earn trust from various communities include distributing timely and transparent information about the vaccine; increasing participation from the community in vaccine development, distribution, and monitoring; including the community in clinical trials; and showing up for the community over time and not just in emergency settings (Batelaan, 2022).

Vaccine recommendations are also predicated on the healthcare provider being willing to provide such a recommendation. Not all healthcare providers, even those formally trained in science and Western medicine, have positive attitudes toward vaccines (Karlsson et al., 2019). In many settings, healthcare providers with higher levels of education, like physicians, have less vaccine hesitancy than nurses (Leigh et al., 2022). Recent research has also examined vaccine attitudes among practitioners of complementary and alternative medicine (CAM), including chiropractic, homeopathy, and naturopathy. There is a broad spectrum of vaccination beliefs among CAM practitioners, although many CAM professional organizations stress that vaccination is out of scope of their practice (Filice et al., 2020). Parents who are vaccine-hesitant are more likely to visit and trust CAM practitioners than medical doctors (Wardle et al., 2016). Regardless, CAM providers could be a source of positive vaccination recommendations, particularly for families less trusting of Western medicine (Wardle et al., 2016).

Still, healthcare providers trained in Western medicine may espouse views counter to the provaccination consensus, including advocating for "alternative schedules," which delay or limit some vaccines (Offit & Moser, 2009), improperly promoting medical exemptions for vaccine mandates (Mohanty et al., 2018), or making targeted decisions for vaccination instead of universally recommending vaccines (Khamisy-Farah et al., 2019). However, most healthcare providers are strongly supportive of vaccines, and low vaccine uptake results, in part, from how healthcare providers issue recommendations.

HOW CAN NUDGES BE USED TO PROMOTE VACCINES?

Healthcare providers are an important source of information on vaccines (Shen & Dubey, 2019) and can substantially influence vaccination uptake through nudges. Nudges, which derive from the field of behavioral economics (Thaler, 2016), are a way to alter behaviors without expressly forbidding the less desired behavior. Nudges include such things as signing new employees for opt-out savings accounts, making generic medications the default in electronic systems, and listing health insurance plans by quality (Ubel & Rosenthal, 2019). Vaccination providers can leverage nudges in how they talk to patients and parents, particularly through the use of a presumptive format (Table 10.1). Because there is a lack of clinical equipoise in routinely recommended vaccines, and by preserving choice and limiting coercion, vaccination nudges can be an ethical way (Navin, 2017) to substantially improve the likelihood of vaccination (Opel, Heritage et al., 2013).

In recent years, many healthcare providers have noticed families coming into appointments with strongly held antivaccine beliefs. Using nudges and starting with a presumptive format can still be effective for these parents (Opel, Heritage et al., 2013). However, the healthcare provider may also have to use a motivational interviewing approach (Figure 10.1).

TABLE 10.1 Example Statements and Questions From Vaccination Providers, Contrasting Between Presumptive and Participatory Formats

PRESUMPTIVE FORMAT (NUDGES)	PARTICIPATORY FORMAT
Your child is due for the chickenpox and hepatitis A vaccines. We will administer those today.	Your child is due for a chickenpox vaccine. We could also give them a hepatitis A vaccine? Would you like the hepatitis A vaccine as well?
I strongly recommend your child gets these vaccines today; we can draw up the shots by the end of the visit.	Looks like in your last visit you didn't want any vaccines for your child. Are you still declining vaccines?
We have to do some shots today. We will have them ready after I check over your child.	What vaccines would you like for your child today?
(Patient receives a text the day before an appointment, indicating that the office has reserved a flu vaccine for them at their appointment.)	Would you like to receive a flu vaccine?

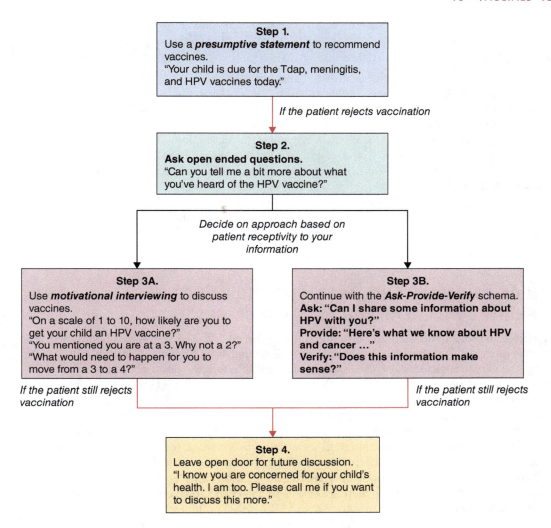

FIGURE 10.1 Example of using the motivational interviewing or Ask-Provide-Verify approach to simulate discussions about vaccination.
HPV, human papillomavirus; Tdap, tetanus, diptheria, acellular pertussis.
Source: Adapted from British Columbia Immunization Committee. (2021). *Immunization communication tool.* http://www.bccdc.ca/resource-gallery/Documents/Guidelines%20and%20Forms/Guidelines%20and%20Manuals/Immunization/Vaccine%20Safety/ICT-2021.pdf; Centers for Disease Control and Prevention. (2011). Ten great public health achievements–Worldwide, 2001–2010. *MMWR. Morbidity and Mortality Weekly Report, 60*(24), 814–818.

CASE STUDY 10.1: ISSUES FACING ADOLESCENT VACCINATION PROGRAMS

Anita is a 45-year-old woman with a 14-year-old son, Anton. Because she had switched jobs several times in the past few years, she has enrolled in different health insurance plans and switched pediatricians. She has been, in general, indifferent about vaccines and has gotten for Anton the minimum number required for school, although many of them have been delayed relative to recommended ages of vaccination.

When Anton turned 11, Anita took him to the doctor for a physical. The doctor was an hour late, was only able to spend about 10 minutes with them, and hastily put in an order for two adolescent vaccines—the Tdap and meningococcal vaccines—that are required for school in their location.

(continued)

CASE STUDY 10.1: ISSUES FACING ADOLESCENT VACCINATION PROGRAMS (*continued*)

At 14, they went to another doctor for another routine checkup for Anton. The nurse practitioner pulled up Anton's records from the government immunization information system. She asked Anita, "It looks like Anton hasn't received the HPV vaccines yet. Would you like to start that series today?" Anita declined, mentioning that she is sure her son does not need a vaccine for a sexually transmitted infection.

This story documents many issues facing adolescent vaccination programs. Adolescents may not have a stable medical home and, in most jurisdictions, require permission from parents to be vaccinated, and the importance of the HPV vaccination may be overlooked by the provider and the parent alike. In this example, the nurse practitioner could have used the presumptive format, talked more personally about the necessity of vaccines, or explored Anita's viewpoints in more depth through an open-ended approach (Figure 10.1).

HOW CAN MOTIVATIONAL INTERVIEWING BE USED TO SHAPE CONVERSATIONS ABOUT VACCINES?

The objective of motivational interviewing is not to directly change someone's behavior, but to have the individual explore inconsistencies in their thoughts and beliefs. Through reflective listening, the clinician can lead, or shape, the individual into talking aloud about the information, experiences, and other processes that influence their behaviors. Early clinical trials for motivational interviewing focused on substance use (Noonan & Moyers, 1997), but it has now been applied to other issues, including vaccination (Gagneur, 2020). In motivational interviewing, individuals may proceed through several stages of behavior change, including precontemplation (no intention of changing), contemplation (of action), preparation (of action), and action itself. The theory behind these stages is delineated through the transtheoretical model (Sutton, 2001).

There are several hypotheses of how motivational interviewing works to affect behavior change. It could be based on the technical skills of the clinician to engage in open questions, affirmations, reflections, and summaries (or OARS)—this is the *technical hypothesis*. The *relational hypothesis* suggests that the potential of motivational interviewing to move individuals across stages of behavior change is predicated on the clinician's empathy and the overall cooperation between the clinician and the individual. Another hypothesis (the *conflict resolution hypothesis*) is that behaviors change as the individual explores and resolves ambivalence in their beliefs (Magill & Hallgren, 2019).

Figure 10.1 shows how motivational interviewing might be used for vaccination in a clinical practice (British Columbia Immunization Committee, 2021; CDC, 2021). Best practice would be for the vaccination provider to presumptively recommend vaccines (Step 1). If the parent or the patient pushes back, the clinician should switch to asking open-ended questions and using reflective listening techniques (Step 2). Under a motivational interviewing paradigm, the clinician could start with a question about how likely the individual would be to get vaccinated on a scale of 1 to 10 (Step 3A). If the individual says 1, they would be considered in the precontemplation stage, according to the motivational interviewing paradigm. In this case, the clinician could exit the conversation, and reopen it later (Step 4). If the individual mentions anything above 1, the clinician can instead move into a motivational interviewing paradigm. Using OARS, the clinician can iteratively ask why the individual is not one point lower and what it would take to make them one point higher. It is possible, although not completely likely, that motivational interviewing will result in the individual deciding to vaccinate themselves or their child in a single visit, but over time their acceptance of vaccines could increase by degrees.

A complementary, but different approach, is the Ask-Provide-Verify schema. In this process, the clinician clarifies what concerns or issues the patient or the parent has, and then asks if they, the clinician, could provide more information on this point to the patient or the parent. Ask-Provide-Verify differs from motivational interviewing in that the clinician is directly providing information to the individual, whereas for motivational interviewing the process is for the individual to clarify ambiguities in their beliefs of vaccines (i.e., not being at a "1" in acceptance) through their own values. Which approach makes most sense may depend on the clinician–patient relationship and the clinician's intuition on how receptive the patient would be to outside, scientific information.

As clinicians learn about what cognitive style their patients have and what kind of information their patients prefer, they can tailor their conversations (Poland & Poland, 2011). One strategy that vaccine providers should avoid, however, is to directly address misinformation and myths. Correcting misinformation can reinforce these beliefs and reduce vaccine intentions (Limaye et al., 2021). A better strategy for clinicians is to *pivot* the conversation to discussing the threat of the disease and the effectiveness of the vaccine (Limaye et al., 2021).

CASE STUDY 10.2: VACCINES AND RELATIONSHIPS

Reese and Sam are next-door neighbors. Reese's child, Rory, and Sam's child, Sawyer, are both 4 years old and often play together. Reese and Sam have a cordial relationship but have different parenting styles and political preferences. These differences have seemed to be exacerbated in recent years in line with the increasing political polarization in their area.

Reese has always kept Rory up-to-date on vaccines, whereas Sam has not. Sam spends a lot of time on social media and participates in many forums that contain stories from parents deciding to not vaccinate their children. Reese hears of a measles outbreak in a nearby town, and wants to make sure Rory stays safe, knowing that no vaccine is 100% effective. Reese and Sam have talked about vaccines previously but have left the conversation with neither changing their stances.

Could motivational interviewing be appropriate in this circumstance? This could be a way for Reese to prompt Sam to more concretely discuss what they know of vaccines and the extent and limitations of their understanding. Motivational interviewing could come off as very forceful, especially between two individuals with opposing beliefs in many areas of their lives. A soft approach might be for Reese to start with the question: "I know we have talked about vaccines previously. Would this be a good time to continue this conversation?" And if given consent, continue with a scaling question: "So how confident are you in not getting Sawyer a measles vaccine, with 1 being not confident at all, and 10 being very confident?"

This situation raises other considerations. Many of Sam's social interactions concern political stances that are opposed to vaccination. By vaccinating Sawyer, Sam may lose these close relationships.

Other strategies that Reese could do would be to highlight the benefits of vaccination. For example, when Sam brings up concerns about vaccines, Reese could mention feeling relieved that Rory is protected after receiving a shot or happy that Rory has antibodies to a serious disease. Reese could also talk about the ongoing outbreaks of vaccine-preventable disease that are in the news. Engaging in these conversations is also a way of normalizing vaccination.

CASE STUDY 10.3: BELIEFS ABOUT VACCINES AND AUTISM

Carrie is bringing her grandchild to the doctor for a 12-month wellness checkup. Carrie's friend has an autistic child, and this friend is highly concerned about vaccines. Carrie brings up this concern to the doctor. The doctor firmly and repeatedly states that "vaccines do not cause autism," but Carrie still defers getting a measles vaccine.

Again, at the 15-month visit, Carrie raises her concerns about the measles vaccine and autism. This time, the doctor prints off a systematic review for Carrie and explains how the scientific establishment knows that vaccines do not cause autism. Carrie did not have much time to talk about her specific concerns and left the appointment without a measles vaccine.

This circumstance illustrates a disconnect between the information that the doctor was offering and the information that Carrie wanted. Repeating over and over that vaccines do not cause autism could actually solidify the connection between these two issues for Carrie, and this might be particularly true if she has other concerns about the medical establishment. Much of the information she receives from friends and families and from more vaccine-questioning websites may be easier to digest and highlight compelling antiauthorities.

A more effective approach would be the doctor firmly recommending the measles vaccine and bringing up the benefits of the measles vaccine. Through a motivational interviewing approach, the doctor could have leveraged positive thoughts that Carrie had about vaccines.

Alternatively, in an Ask-Provide-Verify approach, the doctor would first ask Carrie if Carrie was open to receiving information about vaccines. Although this may include information about autism as well, the doctor would leave space to have Carrie repeat back what she had learned from the conversation.

WHY DO INDIVIDUALS GET VACCINATED?

Worldwide, millions of children do not receive any vaccines, and countless more are partially vaccinated (Muhoza et al., 2021). It is difficult to overstate the role that structural barriers and social processes play in whether an individual is vaccinated or not (Brewer et al., 2017). Nonetheless, vaccination decisions operate on an individual level, and an individual or their child may not be vaccinated because of these individual-level issues. Table 10.2 lists reasons why an individual may get a vaccine for themselves or for a child, as summed up in the 5A mnemonic (Thomson et al., 2016).

Other models of vaccine uptake include the "increasing vaccination model," which separates vaccination antecedents into practical issues (availability, access, cost), social processes (vaccination provider recommendations, social norms), and individual thoughts and feelings (Brewer et al., 2017). Another assonant list of vaccination reasons includes confidence, convenience, and complacency (MacDonald & SAGE Working Group on Vaccine Hesitancy, 2015).

Several behavior change models were developed or have been applied to describe why individuals get vaccinated. The health belief model (HBM) and the theory of planned behavior (TPB) are by far the most popular historically (Corace et al., 2016), but have also been used recently to understand behaviors during the COVID-19 pandemic (Anagaw et al., 2023). Other models (Table 10.3), like the protection motivation theory, self-efficacy theory, and theory of reasoned action, have similar inputs (Sutton, 2001).

In its original formulation, the HBM explained that individuals will change their lifestyle or engage in a certain behavior in response to perceived threats to one's health and the belief that a certain action would be beneficial in reducing the perceived threat at an acceptable cost. As shown in Figure 10.2, using vaccination as an example, perceived threat

10 • VACCINES 201

TABLE 10.2 Factors Associated With Vaccine Uptake

FACTOR	DEFINITION	EXAMPLE
Access	Contact with healthcare systems and convenience of access	Compared with those who lived within 2 km, families who lived more than 4 km from a vaccination center were much less likely to have fully vaccinated children in southern Pakistan (Riaz et al., 2018).
Affordability	Financial and time costs	Adults in the United States were more likely to accept a COVID-19 vaccine for themselves or for a child if there was less waiting time (Prosser et al., 2023).
Awareness	Knowledge of vaccines and details about availability	Parents in India with greater knowledge of HPV and the vaccine were more likely to intend to get it for their child (Shah et al., 2022).
Activation	Prompts, reminders, nudges, and other policies	Individuals in Australia who received an SMS-based nudge were more likely to be vaccinated against influenza and to receive the vaccine in an optimal delivery period (Tuckerman et al., 2023).
Acceptance	Perceptions of vaccines and disease, social norms, and vaccine hesitancy	U.S. adults with hesitancy toward vaccines in general and less perceived risk of infection in the near future were more likely to reject a COVID-19 vaccine (Shih et al., 2021).

HPV, human papillomavirus; SMS, short messaging services.

Source: Modified from Thomson, A., Robinson, K., & Vallée-Tourangeau, G. (2016). The 5As: A practical taxonomy for the determinants of vaccine uptake. *Vaccine, 34*(8), 1018–1024. https://doi.org/10.1016/j.vaccine.2015.11.065.

TABLE 10.3 Health Behavior Models and Their Proximal Determinants of Behavior

MODEL NAME	VACCINATION ANTECEDENTS	SEPARATES OUT INTENTION AND BEHAVIOR?
Health belief model	Perceived susceptibility Perceived severity Benefits Barriers	No
Protection motivation theory	Vulnerability Severity Response efficacy Self-efficacy	Yes
Self-efficacy theory	Outcome expectancies Perceived self-efficacy	No
Theory of reasoned action	Attitude toward the behavior Subjective norm	Yes

(continued)

TABLE 10.3 Health Behavior Models and Their Proximal Determinants of Behavior (*continued*)

MODEL NAME	VACCINATION ANTECEDENTS	SEPARATES OUT INTENTION AND BEHAVIOR?
Theory of planned behavior	Attitude toward the behavior Subjective norm Perceived behavioral control	Yes
Social cognitive theory	Reciprocal interaction of: • Cognition • Environment • Behavioral factors	No

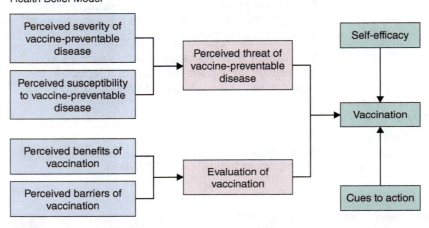

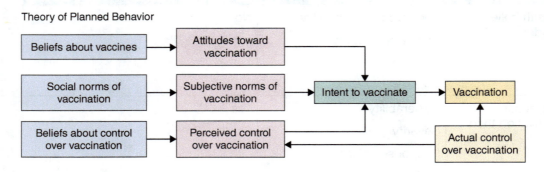

FIGURE 10.2 Diagrams of applications of the health behavior model and the theory of planned behavior to vaccination.

of vaccine-preventable disease comprises perceived severity of vaccine-preventable disease (e.g., perceived risk of hospitalization or likelihood of death if one acquired the disease) and perceived susceptibility (e.g., likelihood of being infected). In evaluating the intervention, the individual would weigh the benefits (e.g., perceived effectiveness of the vaccine) as well as barriers (e.g., perceived safety of the vaccine or time or financial costs in obtaining it). Influenced by other developments in psychology, including the social cognitive theory, the HBM now includes self-efficacy (i.e., the belief that one can make the behavior change and get a vaccine; Rosenstock et al., 1988) and cues to action, which could incorporate notifications from vaccination providers and presumptive messaging.

Although it has several similarities to the HBM, the TPB differs in its incorporation of norms and its distinction between intent to vaccinate and actual vaccination (Ajzen, 1991). Social norms of vaccination influence an individual's subjective norms, or to what extent an individual believes that others approve or disapprove of them being vaccinated. The TPB splits out vaccination intent and actual vaccination, and in this way incorporates measures of self-efficacy, or perceived control over vaccination, which can influence intent, as well as other more objective measures of how much control an individual has over being vaccinated.

These models have had some limitations in their use to explain vaccination and other health behaviors. For one, although the relationship between an individual factor and vaccination is often significant, an early systematic review found that overall effect sizes were small and the models had limited ability to explain most variation in the outcome behavior (Harrison et al., 1992). Moreover, there are inherent difficulties in measuring the constructs, operationalizing them in quantitative models, and building interventions with them. As one example, there could be nonlinear relationships between perceived risk and vaccination intent or behaviors (Shih et al., 2021).

Although there is a clear theoretical basis for these models, how they can inform clinical practice or the development of interventions is less clear (Evans, 2008). These models seem to suppose some sort of knowledge deficit. However, experimental studies that have tried to rectify that deficit, for example, by providing information on disease risk, did not increase vaccination intent (Nyhan et al., 2014). In summary, models like the HBM and the TPB can work well to explain observed vaccination patterns in a population. In contrast, research focusing on nudges may have more promise in developing clinically useful interventions to improve vaccination (Reñosa et al., 2021).

WHAT IS VACCINE HESITANCY?

What we would now name as vaccine hesitancy predates the first smallpox vaccine. In the English colonies in North America, Cotton Mather's promotion of smallpox variolation ran counter to popular narratives that diseases like smallpox were part of God's will and that the inoculation procedure was unnatural (Plotkin & Plotkin, 2024).

Times of innovation and newness in scientific advances are also times when misinformation spreads. The rollout of the smallpox vaccine based actually on the cowpox virus concomitantly saw the rise of antivaccine societies, which put together antivaccine pamphlets highlighting suspected adverse events (**Figure 10.3**).

Yet there does seem to be a qualitative difference between the antivaccine movements of the past and those seen today. For example, the rapid rollout of the DTP, polio, and measles vaccines in the United States—all introduced in a 40-year period between 1923 and 1963 (Plotkin & Plotkin, 2024)—was popular and well-tolerated. Even with notable safety incidents, like improperly prepared vaccine from the Cutter Laboratories leading to cases of paralytic polio, there was not widespread opposition to vaccination (Plotkin & Plotkin, 2024). One hypothesis for why there was no large vaccine boycott was that these were very well-known, and highly feared, diseases.

Vaccine hesitancy in the late 20th and early 21st century has had a different flavor, and perhaps part of this has arisen from the success of the vaccine program. As vaccination programs have sequentially controlled and then eliminated diseases in numerous settings, the populace loses familiarity with these devastating diseases and begins to protest against vaccination.

By the mid-1990s, measles incidence in the United States and in the United Kingdom was exceedingly low. Measles vaccination coverage varied in these countries, but low pockets of vaccination were often tied to structural issues like low public funding and difficulties

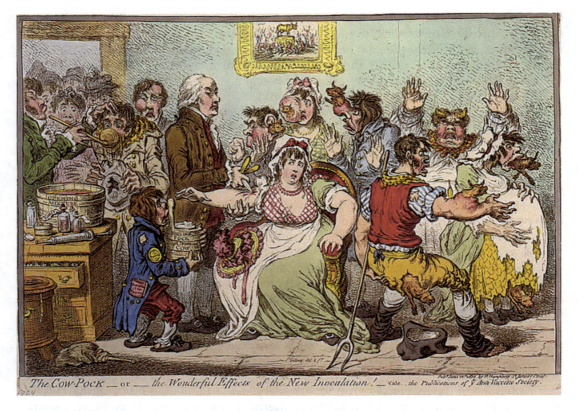

FIGURE 10.3 The cow-pock or the wonderful effects of the new inoculation.
Source: Gillray, J. (1802). *The cow-pock–Or–The wonderful effects of the new inoculation / Js. Gillray, del. & ft.* Library of Congress Prints and Photographs Division Washington, D.C., USA. https://www.loc.gov/resource/cph.3g03147/

accessing healthcare. At this time, Andrew Wakefield, then a licensed physician in the United Kingdom, was involved in several lawsuits suggesting safety issues involving the trivalent measles–mumps–rubella shot, and he submitted a patent for a single-valent measles vaccine (Deer, 2020). He also published a paper in *The Lancet* describing intestinal abnormalities and developmental disorders in 12 children and suggested a linkage to measles vaccination. Subsequent investigations found his research was not ethically cleared, that he failed to mention his conflict of interest, and that the study population included children at his son's birthday party. Although most coauthors had disavowed the paper by 2004, it was not formally retracted by *The Lancet* until 2010 (Eggertson, 2010). In the aftermath of the Wakefield study, vaccination coverage decreased (and has continued to potentiate measles outbreaks decades later; Dyer, 2017) and vaccine skepticism increased (Motta & Stecula, 2021; Torracinta et al., 2021). A systematic review of over a million children in cohort and case–control studies has shown no relationship between MMR vaccination and autism (Taylor et al., 2014). This misinformation persists because of the activity of antivaccine groups, substantial distrust between the medical community and certain segments of the population, and no known consistent strategy to correct misinformation (Limaye et al., 2021).

In our current world, misinformation and concerns about vaccines spread quickly online and through social media. The exact concern or type of misinformation varies and often changes over time. Common concerns include exposure to harmful chemicals in the vaccine and immune "overload" due to multiple vaccines being coadministered at the same visit or administered over a short time during the child's early life (Offit et al., 2002). Parents may also believe that they are able to keep their own children healthy through specific nutrition and "natural living" practices (Reich, 2014).

Thimerosal in vaccines is one example of the difficulties responding to these concerns. Due to public pressure, the U.S. ACIP recommended that vaccine manufacturers remove thimerosal, a mercury-based preservative, from routine pediatric vaccines, despite no evidence of adverse events (CDC, 1999a). Subsequent meta-analyses have also found no evidence of a link between thimerosal and autism (Taylor et al., 2014). However, continued concerns over "mercury poisoning" remain in antivaccine circles. This situation also illustrates problems in trying to respond to or correct vaccine misinformation. Individuals who hold these beliefs may not be in a space to change their thoughts or beliefs, and so anyone else trying to change these individuals' vaccination behaviors would be better served by pivoting the conversation to the benefits of vaccination (Limaye et al., 2021).

Everyone is vaccine-hesitant to a degree. Injections elicit feelings of disgust and parents rightfully have concerns over what chemicals and pharmaceutical products their children are being exposed to. Studying vaccine hesitancy therefore becomes an exercise in measurement and judgment about what boundaries in hesitancy are clinically important. As a term, *vaccine hesitancy* was first used in the 1990s to describe physicians not wanting to prescribe a vaccine, and only applied to individuals making decisions about themselves or a child around 2004 (Bedford et al., 2017).

An early definition of vaccine hesitancy from the WHO Strategic Advisory Group of Experts on Immunization (SAGE) Working Group on Vaccine Hesitancy states that "vaccine hesitancy refers to delay in acceptance or refusal of vaccination despite availability of vaccination services. Vaccine hesitancy is complex and context specific, varying across time, place, and vaccines. It is influenced by factors such as complacency, convenience and confidence" (MacDonald & SAGE Working Group on Vaccine Hesitancy, 2015, p. 4163). Subsequent researchers have advocated for a more precise definition that removes "convenience" from this definition and that distinguishes the psychological state of vaccine hesitancy from the behavior or state of nonvaccination (Bedford et al., 2017). This distinction is important because the lack of vaccination does not necessarily imply hesitancy (see Table 10.2). Another issue brought up is that the word *hesitancy* seems to imply some degree of indecision, whereas there are individuals who are vaccine refusers, with no history of variation in their opinion (Bedford et al., 2017).

With these limitations to the term *vaccine hesitancy*, some, including the CDC, have preferred to use the term *vaccine confidence* (CDC, 2022). Vaccine hesitancy and confidence are not completely opposite. They could coexist, for instance, in an individual who has some concerns about some vaccines, but also who accepts with confidence other vaccines (Dubé et al., 2013). This difference in terminology might also reflect a difference in emphasis: Those in public health or clinical practice may be motivated to increase vaccine confidence, whereas a researcher might be interested in exploring reasoning behind vaccine hesitancy.

Several survey instruments are available to measure vaccine hesitancy. One widely used scale is the 15-item Parent Attitudes about Childhood Vaccine (PACV). This scale includes subdomains of behavior, general attitudes, and safety and efficacy, and can be used to dichotomize individuals into those "hesitant" and those not (Opel, Taylor et al., 2013). The WHO SAGE Working Group on Vaccine Hesitancy has also developed a 10-item scale (Larson et al., 2015), which has also been modified for use in adult vaccinations (Akel et al., 2021). In the original formulation of the SAGE scale, there was not clear guidance on how to use the scale to categorize individuals by hesitancy, and it has been operationalized into multiple subdomains based on a continuous score sum (Wagner et al., 2019), a dichotomous variable (Akel et al., 2021), or a latent class analysis (Wagner et al., 2022).

CONCLUSION

Vaccines are among the most impactful, cost-effective, and safe interventions in public health. In the centuries since vaccines were first used, billions have been immunized and protected from infection, substantial clinical disease, and death. Despite these benefits, antivaccine organizations have grown up alongside vaccines, and vaccine-hesitant individuals struggle to make decisions for themselves or for their children. Clinicians can use presumptive messaging and motivational interviewing to increase vaccine uptake in their patient population, and vaccine mandates can improve vaccination coverage over a large geographic scale. Yet many vaccine-preventable diseases are highly infectious. To eliminate vaccine-preventable diseases, researchers, clinicians, and public health practitioners need to have a better understanding of the population's potential push back against mandates, how best to use behavior change models, and new innovations that can increase vaccine uptake.

SUMMARY KEY POINTS

- Vaccines, and the smallpox inoculation precursor, have been used for hundreds of years to mitigate burden of infectious diseases. Across this time, many individuals have not been vaccinated, mostly due to social or structural issues. However, vaccine hesitancy and antivaccine movements have also existed throughout this time.

- On a societal level, governmental vaccine mandates can increase vaccination coverage. However, they might not be evenly applied geographically, and there still could be clusters of low vaccination coverage that could potentiate outbreaks of vaccine-preventable disease.

- Clinicians can use presumptive messaging to improve vaccination uptake in their practice. Also known as nudges, presumptive messaging is a way to indicate a strong recommendation for vaccination while still preserving the right of the patient to refuse vaccination.

- Clinicians can use motivational interviewing with patients who are skeptical about vaccines. In motivational interviewing, the vaccine provider shapes the direction of the conversation by asking the patient to talk about why they are as confident about vaccines as they are and what it would take to make them more motivated to be vaccinated.

- Behavior change models, like the HBM and the TPB, are often used in observational studies to explain why individuals have not been vaccinated. They have less use in constructing interventions to improve vaccine uptake.

DISCUSSION QUESTIONS

1. What concerns about vaccines do you have, and what have you heard from friends, family members, and colleagues?

2. How would approaches to increase vaccination coverage vary by political group, racial or ethnic background, or other markers of sociodemographic status?

3. Does a vaccine protecting against disease but not infection influence whether it should be mandated or whether we should focus on increasing its uptake in the community?

4. When are mechanisms to increase vaccination uptake too coercive? Do you see nudges from physicians or government mandates as paternalistic or infringing on autonomy?

5. Of the mechanisms to increase vaccine uptake listed in this chapter, which ones would seem to work best with vaccine-hesitant individuals you know in your life?

A robust set of instructor resources designed to supplement this text is located at http://connect.springerpub.com/content/book/978-0-8261-4265-8. Qualifying instructors may request access by emailing textbook@springerpub.com.

REFERENCES

Ajzen, I. (1991). The theory of planned behavior. *Organizational Behavior and Human Decision Processes, 50,* 179–211. https://doi.org/10.1016/0749-5978(91)90020-T

Akel, K. B., Masters, N. B., Shih, S.-F., Lu, Y., & Wagner, A. L. (2021). Modification of a vaccine hesitancy scale for use in adult vaccinations in the United States and China. *Human Vaccines & Immunotherapeutics, 17*(8), 2639–2646. https://doi.org/10.1080/21645515.2021.1884476

Anagaw, T. F., Tiruneh, M. G., & Fenta, E. T. (2023). Application of behavioral change theory and models on COVID-19 preventive behaviors, worldwide: A systematic review. *SAGE Open Medicine, 11,* 20503121231159750. https://doi.org/10.1177/20503121231159750

Andreae, M. C., Freed, G. L., & Katz, S. L. (2004). Safety concerns regarding combination vaccines: The experience in Japan. *Vaccine, 22*(29–30), 3911–3916. https://doi.org/10.1016/j.vaccine.2004.04.013

Bardosh, K., de Figueiredo, A., Gur-Arie, R., Jamrozik, E., Doidge, J., Lemmens, T., Keshavjee, S., Graham, J. E., & Baral, S. (2022). The unintended consequences of COVID-19 vaccine policy: Why mandates, passports and restrictions may cause more harm than good. *BMJ Global Health, 7*(5), e008684. https://doi.org/10.1136/bmjgh-2022-008684

Batelaan, K. (2022). 'It's not the science we distrust; it's the scientists': Reframing the anti-vaccination movement within Black communities. *Global Public Health, 17*(6), 1099–1112. https://doi.org/10.1080/17441692.2021.1912809

Bedford, H., Attwell, K., Danchin, M., Marshall, H., Corben, P., & Leask, J. (2017). Vaccine hesitancy, refusal and access barriers: The need for clarity in terminology. *Vaccine, 36*(44), 6556–6558. https://doi.org/10.1016/j.vaccine.2017.08.004

Bednarczyk, R. A., King, A. R., Lahijani, A., & Omer, S. B. (2019). Current landscape of nonmedical vaccination exemptions in the United States: Impact of policy changes. *Expert Review of Vaccines, 18*(2), 175–190. https://doi.org/10.1080/14760584.2019.1562344

Bowling, A. M. (2018). Immunizations–Nursing interventions to enhance vaccination rates. *Journal of Pediatric Nursing: Nursing Care of Children and Families, 42,* 126–128. https://doi.org/10.1016/j.pedn.2018.06.009

Brewer, N. T., Chapman, G. B., Rothman, A. J., Leask, J., & Kempe, A. (2017). Increasing vaccination: Putting psychological science into action. *Psychological Science in the Public Interest, 18*(3), 149–207. https://doi.org/10.1177/1529100618760521

British Columbia Immunization Committee. (2021). *Immunization communication tool.* http://www.bccdc.ca/resource-gallery/Documents/Guidelines%20and%20Forms/Guidelines%20and%20Manuals/Immunization/Vaccine%20Safety/ICT-2021.pdf

Centers for Disease Control and Prevention. (1999a). Recommendations regarding the use of vaccines that contain thimerosal as a preservative. *MMWR. Morbidity and Mortality Weekly Report, 48*(43), 996–998.

Centers for Disease Control and Prevention. (1999b). Ten great public health achievements, 1900–1999: Impact of vaccines universally recommended for children. *MMWR. Morbidity Mortality Weekly Report, 48*(12), 243–248.

Centers for Disease Control and Prevention. (2011). Ten great public health achievements–Worldwide, 2001–2010. *MMWR. Morbidity and Mortality Weekly Report, 60*(24), 814–818.

Centers for Disease Control and Prevention. (2021, November 3). *Talking with patients about COVID-19 vaccination.* https://www.cdc.gov/vaccines/covid-19/hcp/engaging-patients.html

Centers for Disease Control and Prevention. (2022, February 7). *How to build COVID-19 vaccine confidence.* https://www.cdc.gov/vaccines/covid-19/vaccinate-with-confidence/building-trust.html

Christianson, B., Sharif-Mohamed, F., Heath, J., Roddy, M., Bahta, L., Omar, H., Rockwood, T., & Kenyon, C. (2020). Parental attitudes and decisions regarding MMR vaccination during an outbreak of measles among an undervaccinated Somali community in Minnesota. *Vaccine, 38*(45), 6979–6984. https://doi.org/10.1016/j.vaccine.2020.09.022

Corace, K. M., Srigley, J. A., Hargadon, D. P., Yu, D., MacDonald, T. K., Fabrigar, L. R., & Garber, G. E. (2016). Using behavior change frameworks to improve healthcare worker influenza vaccination rates: A systematic review. *Vaccine, 34*(28), 3235–3242. https://doi.org/10.1016/j.vaccine.2016.04.071

Deer, B. (2020). *The doctor who fooled the world: Science, deception, and the war on vaccines.* Johns Hopkins University Press.

Dimitrova, A., Carrasco-Escobar, G., Richardson, R., & Benmarhnia, T. (2023). Essential childhood immunization in 43 low- and middle-income countries: Analysis of spatial trends and socioeconomic inequalities in vaccine coverage. *PLoS Medicine, 20*(1), e1004166. https://doi.org/10.1371/journal.pmed.1004166

Dixon, M. G., Ferrari, M., Antoni, S., Li, X., Portnoy, A., Lambert, B., Hauryski, S., Hatcher, C., Nedelec, Y., Patel, M., Alexander, J. P., Steulet, C., Gacic-Dobo, M., Rota, P. A., Mulders, M. N., Bose, A. S., Rosewell, A., Kretsinger, K., & Crowcroft, N. S. (2021). Progress toward regional measles elimination–Worldwide, 2000–2020. *MMWR. Morbidity and Mortality Weekly Report, 70*(45), 1563–1569. https://doi.org/10.15585/mmwr.mm7045a1

Dubé, E., Laberge, C., Guay, M., Bramadat, P., Roy, R., & Bettinger, J. (2013). Vaccine hesitancy: An overview. *Human Vaccines and Immunotherapeutics, 9*(8), 1763–1773. https://doi.org/10.4161/hv.24657

Dyer, O. (2017). Measles outbreak in Somali American community follows anti-vaccine talks. *BMJ, 357*, j2378. https://doi.org/10.1136/bmj.j2378

Eggertson, L. (2010). Lancet retracts 12-year-old article linking autism to MMR vaccines. *CMAJ : Canadian Medical Association Journal, 182*(4), 199–200. https://doi.org/10.1503/cmaj.109-3179

Eshun-Wilson, I., Mody, A., Tram, K. H., Bradley, C., Sheve, A., Fox, B., Thompson, V., & Geng, E. H. (2021). Preferences for COVID-19 vaccine distribution strategies in the US: A discrete choice survey. *PLoS One, 16*(8), e0256394. https://doi.org/10.1371/JOURNAL.PONE.0256394

Evans, D. (2008). Chapter 25–Teaching patients to manage their asthma. In M. Castro & M. Kraft (Eds.), *Clinical asthma* (pp. 221–228). Mosby. https://doi.org/10.1016/B978-032304289-5.10025-6

Filice, E., Dubé, E., Graham, J. E., MacDonald, N. E., Bettinger, J. A., Greyson, D., MacDonald, S., Driedger, S. M., Kawchuk, G., & Meyer, S. B. (2020). Vaccination discourses among chiropractors, naturopaths and homeopaths: A qualitative content analysis of academic literature and Canadian organizational webpages. *PLoS One, 15*(8), e0236691. https://doi.org/10.1371/journal.pone.0236691

Gagneur, A. (2020). Motivational interviewing: A powerful tool to address vaccine hesitancy. *Canada Communicable Disease Report, 46*(4), 93–97. https://doi.org/10.14745/ccdr.v46i04a06

Garnier, R., Nedell, E. R., Omer, S. B., & Bansal, S. (2020). Getting personal: How childhood vaccination policies shape the landscape of vaccine exemptions. *Open Forum Infectious Diseases, 7*(3), ofaa088. https://doi.org/10.1093/ofid/ofaa088

Guzman-Cottrill, J. A., Lancioni, C., Eriksson, C., Cho, Y.-J., & Liko, J. (2019). Notes from the Field: Tetanus in an Unvaccinated Child–Oregon, 2017. *MMWR. Morbidity and Mortality Weekly Report, 68*(9), 231–232. https://doi.org/10.15585/mmwr.mm6809a3

Hall, V., Banerjee, E., Kenyon, C., Strain, A., Griffith, J., Como-sabetti, K., Heath, J., Bahta, L., Martin, K., Mcmahon, M., Johnson, D., & Roddy, M. (2017). Measles outbreak–Minnesota April – May 2017. *MMWR. Morbidity and Mortality Weekly Report, 66*(27), 713–717. https://doi.org/10.15585/mmwr.mm6627a1

Halsey, N. A., & Salmon, D. A. (2015). Measles at Disneyland, a problem for all ages. *Annals of Internal Medicine, 162*(9), 655. https://doi.org/10.7326/M15-0447

Harrison, J. A., Mullen, P. D., & Green, L. W. (1992). A meta-analysis of studies of the Health Belief Model with adults. *Health Education Research, 7*(1), 107–116. https://doi.org/10.1093/her/7.1.107

Haruyama, R., Obara, H., & Fujita, N. (2022). Japan resumes active recommendations of HPV vaccine after 8·5 years of suspension. *The Lancet. Oncology, 23*(2), 197–198. https://doi.org/10.1016/S1470-2045(22)00002-X

Jamrozik, E. (2022). Public health ethics: Critiques of the "new normal." *Monash Bioethics Review, 40*, 1–16. https://doi.org/10.1007/s40592-022-00163-7

Kaiser Family Foundation. (2021). *1 in 4 workers say their employer required them to get a COVID-19 vaccine, up since june; 5% of unvaccinated adults say they left a job due to a vaccine requirement.* https://www.kff.org/coronavirus-covid-19/press-release/1-in-4-workers-say-their-employer-required-them-to-get-a-covid-19-vaccine-up-since-june-5-of-unvaccinated-adults-say-they-left-a-job-due-to-a-vaccine-requirement/

Karlsson, L. C., Lewandowsky, S., Antfolk, J., Salo, P., Lindfelt, M., Oksanen, T., Kivimäki, M., & Soveri, A. (2019). The association between vaccination confidence, vaccination behavior, and willingness to recommend vaccines among Finnish healthcare workers. *PLoS One, 14*(10), e0224330. https://doi.org/10.1371/journal.pone.0224330

Khamisy-Farah, R., Adawi, M., Jeries-Ghantous, H., Bornstein, J., Farah, R., Bragazzi, N. L., & Odeh, M. (2019). Knowledge of Human Papillomavirus (HPV), attitudes and practices towards anti-HPV vaccination among Israeli pediatricians, gynecologists, and internal medicine doctors: Development and validation of an Ad Hoc questionnaire. *Vaccines, 7*(4), 157. https://doi.org/10.3390/vaccines7040157

Larson, H. J., Jarrett, C., Schulz, W., Chaudhuri, M., Zhou, Y., Dube, E., Schuster, M., MacDonald, N. E., & Wilson, R. (2015). Measuring vaccine hesitancy: The development of a survey tool. *Vaccine, 33*, 4165–4175. https://doi.org/10.1016/j.vaccine.2015.04.037

Leigh, J. P., Moss, S. J., White, T. M., Picchio, C. A., Rabin, K. H., Ratzan, S. C., Wyka, K., El-Mohandes, A., & Lazarus, J. V. (2022). Factors affecting COVID-19 vaccine hesitancy among healthcare providers in 23 countries. *Vaccine, 40*(31), 4081–4089. https://doi.org/10.1016/j.vaccine.2022.04.097

Leslie, T. F., Delamater, P. L., & Yang, Y. T. (2018). It could have been much worse: The Minnesota measles outbreak of 2017. *Vaccine, 36*(14), 1808–1810. https://doi.org/10.1016/j.vaccine.2018.02.086

Limaye, R. J., Opel, D. J., Dempsey, A., Ellingson, M., Spina, C., Omer, S. B., Dudley, M. Z., Salmon, D. A., & O'Leary, S. T. (2021). Communicating with vaccine-hesitant parents: A narrative review. *Academic Pediatrics, 21*(Suppl. 4), S24–S29. https://doi.org/10.1016/j.acap.2021.01.018

Lytras, T., Kopsachilis, F., Mouratidou, E., Papamichail, D., & Bonovas, S. (2016). Interventions to increase seasonal influenza vaccine coverage in healthcare workers: A systematic review and meta-regression analysis. *Human Vaccines & Immunotherapeutics, 12*(3), 671–681. https://doi.org/10.1080/21645515.2015.1106656

MacDonald, N. E., & SAGE Working Group on Vaccine Hesitancy. (2015). Vaccine hesitancy: Definition, scope, and determinants. *Vaccine, 33*, 4161–4164. https://doi.org/10.1016/j.vaccine.2015.04.036

Magill, M., & Hallgren, K. A. (2019). Mechanisms of behavior change in motivational interviewing: Do we understand how MI works? *Current Opinion in Psychology, 30*, 1–5. https://doi.org/10.1016/j.copsyc.2018.12.010

Mashinini, D. P., Fogarty, K. J., Potter, R. C., & Berles, J. D. (2020). Geographic hot spot analysis of vaccine exemption clustering patterns in Michigan from 2008 to 2017. *Vaccine, 38*(51), 8116–8120. https://doi.org/10.1016/j.vaccine.2020.10.091

Masters, N. B., Eisenberg, M. C., Delamater, P. L., Kay, M., Boulton, M. L., & Zelner, J. (2020). Fine-scale spatial clustering of measles nonvaccination that increases outbreak potential is obscured by aggregated reporting data. *Proceedings of the National Academy of Sciences of the United States of America, 117*(45), 28506–28514. https://doi.org/10.1073/pnas.2011529117

Mohanty, S., Buttenheim, A. M., Joyce, C. M., Howa, A. C., Salmon, D., & Omer, S. B. (2018). Experiences with medical exemptions after a change in vaccine exemption policy in California. *Pediatrics, 142*(5), e20181051. https://doi.org/10.1542/peds.2018-1051

Motta, M., & Stecula, D. (2021). Quantifying the effect of Wakefield et al. (1998) on skepticism about MMR vaccine safety in the U.S. *PLoS One, 16*(8), e0256395. https://doi.org/10.1371/journal.pone.0256395

Muhoza, P., Danovaro-Holliday, M. C., Diallo, M. S., Murphy, P., Sodha, S. V., Requejo, J. H., & Wallace, A. S. (2021). Routine vaccination coverage–Worldwide, 2020. *MMWR. Morbidity and Mortality Weekly Report, 70*(43), 1495–1500. https://doi.org/10.15585/MMWR.MM7043A1

Murray, E., Bieniek, K., Del Aguila, M., Egodage, S., Litzinger, S., Mazouz, A., Mills, H., & Liska, J. (2021). Impact of pharmacy intervention on influenza vaccination acceptance: A systematic literature review and meta-analysis. *International Journal of Clinical Pharmacy, 43*(5), 1163–1172. https://doi.org/10.1007/s11096-021-01250-1

Navin, M. C. (2017). The ethics of vaccination nudges in pediatric practice. *HEC Forum: An Interdisciplinary Journal on Hospitals' Ethical and Legal Issues, 29*, 43–57. https://doi.org/10.1007/s10730-016-9311-2

Newman, P. A., Logie, C. H., Lacombe-Duncan, A., Baiden, P., Tepjan, S., Rubincam, C., Doukas, N., & Asey, F. (2018). Parents' uptake of human papillomavirus vaccines for their children: A systematic review and meta-analysis of observational studies. *BMJ Open, 8*(4), e019206. https://doi.org/10.1136/BMJOPEN-2017-019206

Noonan, W. C., & Moyers, T. B. (1997). Motivational interviewing. *Journal of Substance Misuse, 2*(1), 8–16. https://doi.org/10.3109/14659899709084610

Nyhan, B., Reifler, J., Richey, S., & Freed, G. L. (2014). Effective messages in vaccine promotion: A randomized trial. *Pediatrics, 133*(4), e835–e842. https://doi.org/10.1542/peds.2013-2365

Offit, P. A., & Moser, C. A. (2009). The problem with Dr Bob's alternative vaccine schedule. *Pediatrics, 123*(1), e164–e169. https://doi.org/10.1542/peds.2008-2189

Offit, P. A., Quarles, J., Gerber, M. A., Hackett, Ch. J., Marcuse, E. K., Kollman, T. R., Gellin, B. G., & Landry, S. (2002). Addressing parents' concerns: Do multiple vaccines overwhelm or weaken the infant's immune system? *Pediatrics, 109*(1), 124–129. https://doi.org/10.1542/peds.109.1.124

Opel, D. J., Heritage, J., Taylor, J. A., Mangione-Smith, R., Salas, H. S., DeVere, V., Zhou, C., & Robinson, J. D. (2013). The architecture of provider-parent vaccine discussions at health supervision visits. *Pediatrics, 132*(6), 1037–1046. https://doi.org/10.1542/peds.2013-2037

Opel, D. J., Taylor, J. A., Zhou, C., Catz, S., Myaing, M., & Mangione-Smith, R. (2013). The relationship between parent attitudes about childhood vaccines survey scores and future child immunization status: A validation study. *JAMA Pediatrics, 167*(11), 1065–1071. https://doi.org/10.1001/jamapediatrics.2013.2483

Parmet, W. E., Goodman, R. A., & Farber, A. (2005). Individual rights versus the public's health–100 years after Jacobson v. Massachusetts. *New England Journal of Medicine, 352*(7), 652–654. https://doi.org/10.1056/nejmp048209

Plotkin, S. L., & Plotkin, S. A. (2024). A short history of vaccination. In W. A. Orenstein, P. A. Offit, K. M. Edwards, & S. A. Plotkin (Eds.), *Plotkin's vaccines* (8th ed., pp. 1–16). Elsevier. https://www.us .elsevierhealth.com/plotkins-vaccines-9780323790581.html

Poland, C. M., & Poland, G. A. (2011). Vaccine education spectrum disorder: The importance of incorporating psychological and cognitive models into vaccine education. *Vaccine, 29*(37), 6145–6148. https://doi.org/10.1016/j.vaccine.2011.07.131

Prosser, L. A., Wagner, A. L., Wittenberg, E., Zikmund-Fisher, B. J., Rose, A. M., & Pike, J. (2023). A discrete choice analysis comparing COVID-19 vaccination decisions for children and adults. *JAMA Network Open, 6*(1), e2253582. https://doi.org/10.1001/jamanetworkopen.2022.53582

Rachlin, A., Patel, J., Burns, C. C., Jorba, J., Tallis, G., O'Leary, A., Wassilak, S. G. F., & Vertefeuille, J. F. (2022). Progress toward polio eradication–Worldwide, January 2020–April 2022. *MMWR. Morbidity and Mortality Weekly Report, 71*(19), 517–522. https://doi.org/10.15585/mmwr.mm7219a3

Reich, J. A. (2014). Neoliberal mothering and vaccine refusal: Imagined gated communities and the privilege of choice. *Gender and Society, 28*(5), 679–704. https://doi.org/10.1177/0891243214532711

Reñosa, M. D. C., Landicho, J., Wachinger, J., Dalglish, S. L., Bärnighausen, K., Bärnighausen, T., & McMahon, S. A. (2021). Nudging toward vaccination: A systematic review. *BMJ Global Health, 6*(9), e006237. https://doi.org/10.1136/bmjgh-2021-006237

Riaz, A., Husain, S., Yousafzai, M. T., Nisar, I., Shaheen, F., Mahesar, W., Dal, S. M., Omer, S. B., Zaidi, S., & Ali, A. (2018). Reasons for non-vaccination and incomplete vaccinations among children in Pakistan. *Vaccine, 36*(35), 5288–5293. https://doi.org/10.1016/j.vaccine.2018.07.024

Rosenstock, I. M., Strecher, V. J., & Becker, M. H. (1988). Social learning theory and the Health Belief Model. *Health Education Quarterly, 15*(2), 175–183. https://doi.org/10.1177/109019818801500203

Roush, S. W., Murphy, T. V., & the Vaccine-Preventable Disease Table Working Group. (2007). Historical comparisons of morbidity and mortality for vaccine-preventable diseases in the United States. *JAMA, 298*(18), 2155–2163. https://doi.org/10.1001/jama.298.18.2155

Salmon, D. A., & Siegel, A. W. (2001). Religious and philosophical exemptions from vaccination requirements and lessons learned from conscientious objectors from conscription. *Public Health Reports, 116*(4), 289–295. https://doi.org/10.1093/phr/116.4.289

Sargent, R. H., Laurie, S., Moncada, L., Weakland, L. F., Lavery, J. V., Salmon, D. A., Orenstein, W. A., & Breiman, R. F. (2022). Masks, money, and mandates: A national survey on efforts to increase COVID-19 vaccination intentions in the United States. *PLoS One, 17*(4). https://doi.org/10.1371 /journal.pone.0267154

Shah, P. M., Ngamasana, E., Shetty, V., Ganesh, M., & Shetty, A. K. (2022). Knowledge, attitudes and HPV vaccine intention among women in India. *Journal of Community Health, 47*(3), 484–494. https:// doi.org/10.1007/s10900-022-01072-w

Shen, A. K., Browne, S., Srivastava, T., Kornides, M. L., & Tan, A. S. L. (2023). Trusted messengers and trusted messages: The role for community-based organizations in promoting COVID-19 and routine immunizations. *Vaccine, 41*(12), 1994–2002. https://doi.org/10.1016/j.vaccine.2023.02.045

Shen, S. (Cindy), & Dubey, V. (2019). Addressing vaccine hesitancy: Clinical guidance for primary care physicians working with parents. *Canadian Family Physician, 65*(3), 175–181. https://www.cfp.ca /content/65/3/175

Shih, S.-F., Wagner, A. L., Masters, N. B., Prosser, L. A., Lu, Y., & Zikmund-Fisher, B. J. (2021). Vaccine hesitancy and rejection of a vaccine for the novel coronavirus in the United States. *Frontiers in Immunology, 12*, 558270. https://doi.org/10.3389/fimmu.2021.558270

Steffen, C. A., Henaff, L., Durupt, A., Omeiri, N. E., Ndiaye, S., Batmunkh, N., Liyanage, J. B. L., Hasan, Q., Mosina, L., Jones, I., O'Brien, K., & Hombach, J. (2021). Evidence-informed vaccination decision-making in countries: Progress, challenges and opportunities. *Vaccine, 39*(15), 2146–2152. https://doi.org/10.1016/j.vaccine.2021.02.055

Sutton, S. (2001). Health behavior: Psychosocial theories. In N. J. Smelser & P. B. Baltes (Eds.), *International encyclopedia of the social & behavioral sciences* (pp. 6499–6506). Pergamon. https://doi .org/10.1016/B0-08-043076-7/03872-9

Szarke, M. (2022). Textual "Piqûres": Vaccination in the hands of nineteenth-century French writers. *Nineteenth-Century French Studies, 51*(1–2), 1–19. https://doi.org/10.1353/ncf.2022.0011

Taylor, L. E., Swerdfeger, A. L., & Eslick, G. D. (2014). Vaccines are not associated with autism: An evidence-based meta-analysis of case-control and cohort studies. *Vaccine, 32*(29), 3623–3629. https://doi.org/10.1016/j.vaccine.2014.04.085

Thaler, R. H. (2016). Behavioral economics: Past, present, and future. *American Economic Review, 106*(7), 1577–1600. https://doi.org/10.1257/aer.106.7.1577

Thomson, A., Robinson, K., & Vallée-Tourangeau, G. (2016). The 5As: A practical taxonomy for the determinants of vaccine uptake. *Vaccine, 34*(8), 1018–1024. https://doi.org/10.1016/j.vaccine .2015.11.065

Torracinta, L., Tanner, R., & Vanderslott, S. (2021). MMR vaccine attitude and uptake research in the United Kingdom: A critical review. *Vaccines, 9*(4), Article 4. https://doi.org/10.3390/vaccines9040402

Tuckerman, J., Harper, K., Sullivan, T. R., Cuthbert, A. R., Fereday, J., Couper, J., Smith, N., Tai, A., Kelly, A., Couper, R., Friswell, M., Flood, L., Blyth, C. C., Danchin, M., & Marshall, H. S. (2023). Short message service reminder nudge for parents and influenza vaccination uptake in children and adolescents with special risk medical conditions: The flutext-4U randomized clinical trial. *JAMA Pediatrics, 177*(4), 337–344. https://doi.org/10.1001/jamapediatrics.2022.6145

Ubel, P. A., & Rosenthal, M. B. (2019). Beyond nudges–When improving health calls for greater assertiveness. *New England Journal of Medicine, 380*(4), 309–311. https://doi.org/10.1056/NEJMp1806371

Ulrich, A. K., Sundaram, M. E., & Basta, N. E. (2022). Supporting individual vaccine decision-making: A role for vaccination counselors. *Vaccine, 40*(14), 2123–2125. https://doi.org/10.1016/J.VACCINE.2022.02.012

Wagner, A. L., Masters, N. B., Domek, G. J., Mathew, J. L., Sun, X., Asturias, E. J., Ren, J., Huang, Z., Contreras-Roldan, I. L., Gebremeskel, B., & Boulton, M. L. (2019). Comparisons of vaccine hesitancy across five low- and middle-income countries. *Vaccines (Basel), 7*(4), 155. https://doi.org/10.3390/vaccines7040155

Wagner, A. L., Porth, J. M., Wu, Z., Boulton, M. L., Finlay, J. M., & Kobayashi, L. C. (2022). Vaccine hesitancy during the COVID-19 pandemic: A latent class analysis of middle-aged and older US adults. *Journal of Community Health, 47*(3), 408–415. https://doi.org/10.1007/s10900-022-01064-w

Wagner, A. L., Wileden, L., Shanks, T. R., Goold, S. D., Morenoff, J. D., & Sheinfeld Gorin, S. N. (2021). Mediators of racial differences in COVID-19 vaccine acceptance and uptake: A cohort study in Detroit, MI. *Vaccines, 10*(1), 36. https://doi.org/10.3390/vaccines10010036

Wardle, J., Frawley, J., Steel, A., & Sullivan, E. (2016). Complementary medicine and childhood immunisation: A critical review. *Vaccine, 34*(38), 4484–4500. https://doi.org/10.1016/j.vaccine.2016.07.026

Williamson, L. D., Thompson, K. M., & Ledford, C. J. W. (2022). Trust Takes Two . . . . *Journal of the American Board of Family Medicine: JABFM, 35*(6), 1179–1182. https://doi.org/10.3122/jabfm.2022.220126R1

Wodi, A. P., & Morelli, V. (2021). Principles of vaccination. In E. Hall, A. P. Wodi, J. Hamborsky, & V. M. S. Schillie (Eds.), *Epidemiology and prevention of vaccine-preventable diseases* (14th ed., pp. 1–7). Public Health Foundation. https://www.cdc.gov/vaccines/pubs/pinkbook/downloads/table-of-contents.pdf

World Health Organization. (2017). *Summary of WHO Position Papers–Recommendations for Routine Immunization*. https://www.who.int/publications/m/item/table1-summary-of-who-position-papers-recommendations-for-routine-immunization

Zipprich, J., Winter, K., Hacker, J., Xia, D., Watt, J., & Harriman, K. (2015). Measles outbreak–California, December 2014–February 2015. *MMWR. Morbidity Mortality Weekly Report, 64*(6), 153–154.

CHAPTER 11

SEXUAL AND REPRODUCTIVE HEALTH

JEWEL GAUSMAN, KATHRYN BARKER, MAHESH KARRA, AND ANA LANGER

LEARNING OBJECTIVES

- Apply the social-ecological model to identify key determinants of sexual and reproductive health (SRH).
- Describe SRH challenges faced by marginalized and underserved populations globally.
- Recognize different approaches to measuring demand for family planning and the limitations of current measurement approaches.
- Identify a range of intervention pathways to promote social and behavior change to overcome key SRH challenges globally.
- Draw upon social and behavior change theories to identify opportunities for intervention across a range of SRH challenges.

INTRODUCTION: A HISTORICAL PERSPECTIVE

The 1994 International Conference on Population and Development (ICPD) in Cairo, Egypt changed the field of sexual and reproductive health (SRH). This conference reframed SRH within a framework of reproductive rights, gender equity, and women's empowerment, representing a critical shift away from the field's origins in demography and population policy. The Programme of Action that emanated from the ICPD was adopted by over 170 countries and emphasized the link between SRH and sustainable development. Specifically highlighted are the need for universal access to safe, affordable, and effective reproductive healthcare and services, including those for young people, and the need for a gender perspective in providing a comprehensive package of information and services, including family planning and contraception, skilled care at pregnancy and childbirth, safe abortion services where legal, and treatment and management of sexually transmitted infections (STIs) and HIV/AIDS (Langer, 2006).

Over the last 30 years since the Cairo Conference, the field has made substantial progress. Technological advances have meant that HIV/AIDS can be treated as a chronic condition by way of antiretroviral therapies (ARTs), cervical cancer can be prevented through a safe and effective vaccine against human papillomavirus (HPV), and declines in the global fertility rate have led to safer pregnancy and childbearing while being coupled with increases in contraceptive use that enables women and men to achieve their fertility goals.

Despite this progress, important challenges remain. The field of SRH has struggled to gain a foothold in the global agenda. In fact, SRH was initially omitted from the Millennium Development Goals in 2000 as a result of concerns that its inclusion would put the adoption of the Millennium Declaration at risk (Starrs et al., 2018). The subsequent set of goals adopted in 2015, known as the Sustainable Development Goals (SDGs), includes only one target focused on achieving universal access to SRH.

DEFINING SEXUAL AND REPRODUCTIVE HEALTH

The most widely used definition of SRH is based on the World Health Organization's (WHO) definition of reproductive health, which defines it as a "state of complete physical, mental and social well-being and not merely the absence of disease or infirmity, in all matters related to the reproductive health system and to its functions and processes" (WHO, 1995). The definition of SRH recognizes its complex and multidimensional nature and refers to positive health, not just the absence of disease, dysfunction, or disability. In addition, sexual health is an important element within this definition that encompasses physical, psychological, individual, and relational health, as well as pleasure and self-esteem.

While much of the field tends to focus specifically on women's SRH and rights, men's needs are often overlooked as both the sexual and intimate partners of women and as individuals who have their own SRH needs. Moreover, there are a range of sex and gender categories along with gender identities and sexual orientations, and their diverse needs are only now beginning to be recognized by mainstream SRH policies and programs. Globally, laws and policies are often still focused on the traditional binary categories of male and female.

While the vision that evolved from the Cairo Conference has largely become mainstreamed within the field of SRH, it too continues to evolve. Rights-based definitions have emerged to define SRH as a critical component of social justice, highlighting the needs of underrepresented and underserved populations such as sexual minority populations, adolescents, migrants, people living with disabilities, and other marginalized groups. Furthermore, some definitions have included language that calls for states to guarantee access to safe abortion care, a critical component of comprehensive SRH services, but also a most polarizing issue in the United States and globally.

The inclusion of rights as an inherent aspect of SRH makes this field distinct from many other areas of health (**Box 11.1**). A rights-based perspective is essential to understanding social and behavior change within the context of SRH. What does it mean to say "sexual and reproductive rights?" Rights were first mentioned in the Programme of Action of the

---

BOX 11.1 WHAT DOES IT MEAN TO EMPHASIZE RIGHTS IN THE CONTEXT OF SEXUAL AND REPRODUCTIVE HEALTH?

The Guttmacher-Lancet Commission emphasized the intersection between an individual's behavior and the underlying social systems and infrastructure that influence whether individuals (Starrs et al., 2018):

- Have their bodily integrity, privacy, and personal autonomy respected
- Freely define their own sexuality, including sexual orientation and gender identity and expression
- Decide whether and when to be sexually active
- Choose their own sexual partners

What impact does this idea have on people's lives? In very tangible ways, it means that all people should be able to:

- Have safe and pleasurable sexual experiences
- Decide whether, when, and whom to marry
- Decide whether, when, and by what means to have a child or children, and how many to have
- Have access over their lifetimes to the information, resources, services, and support necessary to achieve all the above, free from discrimination, coercion, exploitation, and violence.

ICPD Beijing Conference in 1995 and are generally taken to mean that all individuals have a right to make decisions governing their bodies and to access services that support that right (WHO, 1995).

The Cairo and Beijing Conferences have been instrumental in shifting the field toward a rights-based focus to include a broader range of services within the domain of SRH, from contraception and maternal health to sexual education and gender equality, with the aim of promoting healthier families and contributing to sustainable development.

SEXUAL AND REPRODUCTIVE HEALTH FROM A SOCIAL-ECOLOGICAL PERSPECTIVE

Many factors influence SRH (Figure 11.1). Achieving SRH from a rights-based perspective requires access to appropriate, timely, and quality healthcare services, often combined with support from other sectors, such as education, labor, and transportation. For example, young people have a right to sexual education in schools, as they need information to keep themselves safe. The role of transportation is also important. All women in childbirth have the right to get to a hospital during an emergency, but because of a lack of timely transport in many countries around the world they are unable to do so.

Persistent gender inequality adversely influences SRH and rights. Beyond the biological reasons for the observed differences in men's and women's health (determined by sex), power dynamics, distribution of resources, entitlements, norms, and values place women at a disadvantage in fulfilling their reproductive intentions and meeting other health needs (Mumtaz & Salway, 2009). Sexual relationships are often between individuals with unequal power in the relationship because of gender norms, age, access to resources, and social position (Pulerwitz et al., 2000). In some settings, social expectations undermine a woman's ability to negotiate safer sexual behavior with their sexual partner(s). National health policy also often reflects and reinforces the normative power structures within relationships. For example, some countries require male partner permission in order for a woman to receive a contraceptive method, reinforcing male dominance (Blanc, 2001). Hence, addressing gender inequality is critical to improving SRH and access to healthcare, and reducing disparities in health outcomes.

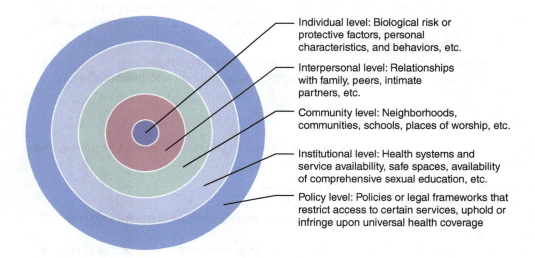

FIGURE 11.1 Adapted version of the social-ecological model as it applies to sexual and reproductive health.

Gender Equality Versus Gender Equity

Gender equality and gender equity are key concepts to keep in mind when thinking about SRH and rights through a gender lens. *Gender equality* recognizes differences and unique needs determined by biological sex while ensuring the same outcomes for all. *Gender equity* refers to addressing differences that are unnecessary, avoidable, and not rooted in biological differences between the sexes—differences in access to services, educational attainment, economic assets and control over them, and so forth. While traditionally applied to men and women, these terms also apply to people who are sexually and gender diverse.

Differences that undermine gender equity are considered "unfair and unjust." *Empowerment* is a term related to gender equity. To achieve equality and equity, people need to be empowered. In relationships between men and women, enabling women to achieve their SRH goals requires male involvement. However, it may be challenging to identify ways to encourage men to be involved in women's SRH in ways that uphold women's autonomy and do not reinforce harmful gender norms and practices. Gender-based violence is one way in which individual's autonomy may be limited (Heidari & Moreno, 2016). Violence not only disproportionally affects women and can cause physical injury, death, and severe mental health implications, but it can also make it so women cannot access needed health services. Some studies have found that nonbinary people may be at increased risk of experiencing intimate partner violence (IPV; Closson et al., 2023). Ensuring gender equity within the context of SRH also requires that the health system as well as the larger cultural and legal environments are supportive and enable autonomy (Yaya et al., 2018). For example, gender-based misconceptions among providers affect women's access to care (Gausman et al., 2021; Langer et al., 2015). Making positive change within this domain is sometimes slow, variable, and impermanent, but without an enabling social environment making progress is extremely difficult.

Other challenges limit individuals' autonomy to seek quality reproductive health services even when they are available. Bronfenbrenner's Ecological Systems Theory posits that an individual is surrounded by nested levels of context, ranging from the most narrow microsystem consisting of the immediate context surrounding one's life to the macrosystem, which captures the broadest attributes of place (Bronfenbrenner, 1994).

Intertwined across all levels is the complex influence of social and gender norms. The levels of the social-ecological model interact: Women's relative economic vulnerability, potential lower education level, reduced social status, and gender discrimination combine to increase their exposure to the hazards of unsafe sex, risky working and housing conditions, poverty, and violence. Women and girls in vulnerable subpopulations such as migrants, those living with disabilities, and ethnic minorities face additional challenges in accessing health services as a result of factors such as language barriers, cultural attitudes, perceptions of service availability, provider bias, and discrimination (Adanu & Johnson, 2009). Further, there remain tremendous disparities in SRH and rights between people in high-income and low- and middle-income countries (LMICs). Many of the barriers that limit choice and access are exacerbated in places with weak health systems and resource scarcity.

Ensuring everyone's ability to attain SRH and exercise their rights is fundamental to sustainable development. Opportunity exists to influence social and behavior change at all levels of the social-ecological framework to help support SRH and rights globally.

CONTRACEPTION AND FAMILY PLANNING

A History of Global Family Planning Programs

While family planning, as a means to manage fertility and promote reproductive health, has existed for centuries, the origins of modern family planning programs can be traced to the early 20th century (Robinson & Ross, 2007). One of the earliest initiatives in the United States was the birth control movement led by Margaret Sanger, who opened the first birth control clinic in 1916 and played a pivotal role in advocating for family planning as a key driver of women's reproductive rights (Hufnagel, 2010). In the decades that followed, and particularly after the Second World War, family planning programs gained momentum and expanded to various countries and nongovernmental organizations. In the decades that followed, private funders and international agencies began to allocate large-scale funding to specifically support population programs in these settings, which gave rise to the modern family planning movement.

Several governments in LMICs recognized the role of family planning to promote a broader social and economic development agenda, particularly within a context of global demographic transition and population growth. The earliest national family planning programs were launched in South Asia (India, Pakistan, and Bangladesh) and East Asia (Taiwan, Singapore, and South Korea; Mason, 2001), almost concurrently with the introduction of new modern contraceptive methods such as the intrauterine device (IUD) and the oral contraceptive pill (Potts & Campbell, 2002). These programs adopted a range of approaches to implementing family planning and population policy, with some ascribing more rigorously to the principles of voluntarism and reproductive rights than others. Indonesia and Taiwan have achieved notable success in national family programs. In addition, Bangladesh's community-based family planning program, implemented in the 1980s, has been recognized for its success in promoting access to contraception and reproductive health services through grassroots-level education and outreach (Robinson & Ross, 2007).

ROLE OF COERCION
In contrast, the role of coercion in family planning programs has been, and continues to be, a serious source of concern and debate. Coercion in these programs has manifested in various forms, ranging from subtle pressures to more explicit and forceful measures. Over the last century, several instances of coercive practices have been documented in a range of settings.

India's family planning program, launched in the 1950s, initially emphasized voluntarism and informed choice. However, during the 1970s, forced sterilizations and sterilization targets were embedded into the country's fifth 5-year development plan that was implemented by Indira Gandhi, India's prime minister who declared a national "Emergency" that suspended civil liberties between 1975 and 1977 (Bansal & Dwivedi, 2020). This led to allegations of coercion and human rights abuses, particularly through the targeting of minority and vulnerable populations. This period of the program was marked by controversy, and while it has since shifted toward a more rights-based approach, outstanding concerns remain. China's one-child policy, implemented in 1979, is one of the most well-known and controversial state-led family planning programs (Wang, 2012). By setting birth quotas and enforcing punitive measures to ensure compliance, including forced sterilizations, forced abortions, and economic fines, the program has come under wide criticism for being coercive, violating human rights, reinforcing gender imbalances, and contributing to adverse social outcomes.

Other countries have also seen coercion in family planning programs. Under the Fujimori administration, Peru's government implemented aggressive sterilization programs in the 1990s that targeted women from Indigenous and impoverished communities (López, 2014). In the United States, forced sterilizations were carried out as part of eugenics programs, disproportionately affecting marginalized communities, racial minorities, and other individuals who were deemed "unfit" to reproduce (Reilly, 2015). Indigenous communities in Canada and Australia also were subject to coerced sterilizations as part of assimilation and population control policies (Dyck, 2013).

Coercion in family planning programs is not limited to state-led initiatives. Numerous studies have documented evidence of healthcare provider bias where individuals or communities have been pressured to conform to certain family planning practices, often in violation of rights and autonomy (Solo & Festin, 2019). Such practices have undermined trust in reproductive health services and have hindered efforts to improve access to voluntary and rights-based family planning.

DEMAND FOR FAMILY PLANNING AND CONTRACEPTION

In spite of significant improvements in access to family planning and reproductive health services, more than 99 million pregnancies each year are unintended either because they were mistimed or were unwanted at the time of conception (Bearak et al., 2018). Moreover, more than four out of five unintended pregnancies occur among sexually active women of reproductive age who are not using a contraceptive method even when they say that they do not want to become pregnant (Darroch, 2017).

A central objective of a family planning program is not only to help women and couples achieve good reproductive outcomes, but to help them navigate and maximize a complex set of preferences around future fertility, health, and well-being. Moreover, the patient's central role is distinct in family planning from many other contexts in health decision-making where providers play a leading (or even exclusive) role in determining the type of care that a patient receives. For these reasons, identifying an individual's demand for family planning differs from most other health services.

Measuring Contraceptive Demand: Current Approaches and Limitations

Since the Cairo Conference, the global family planning community has made it a priority to effectively quantify and meet demand. This commitment is reflected in several development agendas, most recently as a target in the 2030 SDGs, whereby the proportion of family planning demand satisfied, calculated as the proportion of women of reproductive age (ages 15–49) who have their need for family planning satisfied through the use of modern methods of contraception, was added as a key indicator of progress (Table 11.1).

Over the years, numerous methodological and empirical critiques have highlighted the need for alternative approaches to conceptualizing and measuring contraceptive demand and reproductive well-being. These critiques have argued that conventional measures such

TABLE 11.1 Common Indicators to Measure Demand for Contraception			
MEASURE	**DEFINITION**	**STRENGTHS**	**KEY CHALLENGES**
Contraceptive prevalence	Proportion of women of reproductive age who are using a contraceptive method	• Straightforward to calculate • Most commonly used measure	• May not accurately measure demand in the context of coercion
Unmet need for family planning	Proportion of sexually active women of reproductive age who want to delay or stop childbearing but are not using contraception	• Quantifies the gap between the demand for contraception and actual contraceptive use	• Assumes that family planning users have had their needs met through quality services
Total demand for family planning	Proportion of sexually active women of reproductive age who want to delay or stop childbearing but are not using contraception	• Provides an estimation of need	• Assumes all women who want to delay or stop childbearing want to use contraception

as unmet need do not capture the reasons that drive contraceptive use and nonuse. Moreover, they argue that the measures, although convenient for programmatic use, are not reflective of welfare outcomes (e.g., health, sexual well-being, and rights) that are essential to and relevant to individuals who demand contraception (Senderowicz, 2020). Recent calls for innovations in family planning and reproductive health measurement have underscored a need to develop and adopt rights-based and person-centered (as opposed to program-centered) indicators that capture the diversity of motivations and experiences related to contraceptive use, which will promote reproductive autonomy and well-being (Bingenheimer et al., 2023; Gausman et al., 2023).

DRIVERS OF CONTRACEPTIVE DEMAND

There are various motivations for individuals to demand and use contraception. Perhaps unsurprisingly, the most commonly expressed reasons for demanding contraception are linked to fertility—the desire to limit childbearing and to space births (Bongaarts, 1978; Cleland, 2009; Stover, 1998). These factors are often intertwined with and driven by individuals' life goals, social and economic considerations, and personal preferences. Fertility, both desired and realized, acts as a dominant mediating channel to shape contraceptive preferences and behavior. However, the reasons for contraceptive use are diverse and may extend beyond family planning. For example, individuals may demand and rely on contraception to address health conditions that may be alleviated with the use of certain hormonal methods (e.g., acne, endometriosis, heavy menstruation, and anemia). Relatedly, the use of barrier methods such as condoms serve as a means of dual protection against pregnancy as well as HIV and other STIs. More broadly, contraception may also be demanded to improve an individual's sexual functioning and well-being (Fennell, 2014). A body of evidence on the changing nature of sexual partnerships has shown that changes in sexual behavior, reshaped in the face of economic development and social secularization, may lead to changes in demand for contraception (Kaa, 1988). Taken together, the motivations behind contraceptive demand can vary significantly from one person to another, highlighting the need for a nuanced understanding of this phenomenon.

INHIBITORS OF CONTRACEPTIVE DEMAND

Conversely, there is an equal (or perhaps greater) number of reasons, spanning various levels of influence, for individuals to not demand contraception (Casterline & Sinding, 2000; Gahungu et al., 2021). At the individual level, concerns about potential side effects from hormonal contraceptive use; worries about the impact of contraception on future fertility, sexual functioning, and health; lack of or occasional sexual activity; and concerns over the impact of contraception on the health of future children are common factors that contribute to reluctance, nonuse, and lack of demand for contraception. In addition, religious beliefs, financial constraints, lack of knowledge about contraceptive options and where to obtain them, and lack of access to service providers are also frequently reported. Interpersonal dynamics play a pivotal role, particularly if a woman's partner, family members, or others in their community do not approve of their contraceptive use. Relatedly, a fear of backlash or violence if any contraceptive use is discovered can also contribute to hesitancy. Institutional factors, such as erratic or limited supply options and frequent stockouts, coupled with poor quality of care and provider bias toward particular methods, may further constrain an individual from realizing their contraceptive preferences. At the community level, societal norms and expectations also exert a powerful influence whereby women and couples face considerable societal pressure to have a first child soon after marriage. Concerns over partner perceptions and fear that contraceptive use may be misconstrued as infidelity may further act as barriers to demand and use. In this intricate landscape, it is crucial to recognize that contraceptive choices, and the ability to choose, significantly impact sexual behavior and reproductive well-being. Addressing these multifaceted

INTERVENTIONS TO ADDRESS, MEET, AND GENERATE CONTRACEPTIVE DEMAND

barriers is essential to support individuals making informed and autonomous decisions about their own reproductive health.

Interventions that aim to influence SRH behaviors, inform women and couples about the benefits of family planning, and improve access to contraceptives have become increasingly common in developing countries. Since the 1970s, numerous family planning program evaluations at varying scales have been undertaken to demonstrate the impact of "demand generation" and service-delivery improvements on contraceptive use (Gahungu et al., 2021). These interventions have targeted key populations in a variety of ways, from education and awareness programs, to mass media communications efforts, to multicomponent, community-based, or provider-oriented campaigns. Studies of both demand-side and supply-side interventions have shown improvements in attitudes toward and knowledge of family planning and sexuality from exposure to these programs. However, evidence of program effects on outcomes related to downstream health and well-being is limited. Most evaluations of family planning to date have been limited to small-scale interventions that have been implemented over relatively brief periods of time. There is little evidence that assesses the long-term behavioral effects of such interventions, and inference on the differential impact of such programs on high-risk populations is limited. This lack of evidence restricts the extent to which policy makers and practitioners are able to successfully channel resources to target these vulnerable groups.

Spousal and familial preferences for family planning are key determinants of women's access to and use of family planning. Studies have shown that in many contexts men are not actively engaged in most issues of maternal and child health, particularly in issues concerning reproductive health (Sharma et al., 2018). Men's limited involvement in and reluctance to support family planning might be explained by (a) perceived side effects of both male and female contraceptive methods, which may disrupt sexual activity and in some cases functioning; (b) the limited choice of available male contraceptives; (c) general perceptions that reproductive health is considered to be "a woman's domain" and is of little relevance or concern for men; (d) discordance in preferences for children; and (e) concerns that women's contraceptive use may lead to promiscuity and extramarital sexual relations (Adelekan et al., 2014; Kabagenyi et al., 2014).

A number of studies have shown that including men in family planning counseling may increase women's use of family planning services through two potential channels (El-Khoury et al., 2015; Sternberg & Hubley, 2004). First, counseling provides men with information on methods or services, including services that women may desire (Lundgren et al., 2005; Shattuck et al., 2011), making them more accepting of such methods. In addition, counseling husbands and wives together provides a platform for increased spousal communication and offers couples the opportunity to discuss their fertility and contraception method preferences (Hartmann et al., 2012). These findings are also confirmed in a series of cross-sectional studies that find a positive link between spousal communication and contraceptive use (Jejeebhoy et al., 2015). To date, however, experimental evidence on spousal concordance and the role of men in family planning decision-making remains mixed, particularly in low- and middle-income settings.

Most conventional measures of contraceptive demand do not account for husband or partner preferences for contraception. Even if such preferences could be accounted for empirically, it is not clear as to how women's demand for contraception should account for partner preferences, particularly in the case where there is discordance in preferences between men and women (Karra & Zhang, 2021). Would a couple have an unmet need for contraception if women want to use contraception but their male partners do not? What about the converse? The (lack of) inclusion of male preferences in the measurement of demand speaks to the field's ongoing tension and debate between women's reproductive rights over contraceptive choice and male involvement in contraceptive decision-making.

CASE STUDY 11.1: ENGAGING MEN IN FAMILY PLANNING: THE MALAWI MALE MOTIVATORS PROJECT

Adolescent women in Malawi face high rates of child marriage and pregnancy, with more than a quarter of married women between the ages of 15 and 19 years having an unmet need for family planning. Healthcare decisions for these women are often gatekept by their male partners, making it difficult to reach these women with interventions geared to improve their SRH. Following the priorities of ICPD, the Malawi Male Motivators Project was designed to meet the reproductive health needs of these young women by engaging their male partners in family planning programming. The intervention was based on the information–motivation–behavioral skills model (IMB), which had primarily previously been used in HIV/AIDs-related behavior change efforts (Fisher & Fisher, 1992). At the core of the intervention, male motivators were selected from within communities to serve as information resources for other men. The motivators were married men aged 30 years or older, which gave them additional social standing and respect based on community norms, and had high enthusiasm for modern contraceptives. The motivators were tasked with engaging younger men in discussions about family planning, the harmful consequences of rigid gender roles, and by challenging notions about virility that were dominant in the community. Motivators were trained to provide information and help build skills but not pressure anyone into using contraceptives. The intervention was highly effective at increasing contraceptive use, and qualitative data suggested that the intervention improved partner communication (Shattuck et al., 2011).

HUMAN PAPILLOMAVIRUS, CANCER, AND VACCINATION

Human Papillomavirus and Health Across the Life Course

HPV is the most common STI in the United States and one of the most common globally. In middle-aged women between 35 and 50 years of age, HPV prevalence is estimated to be 20% in Africa and the Americas and 15% in the rest of the world (Smith et al.,2008). Most infections are acquired during adolescence. Women who begin having sex at an early age or who have had multiple sexual partners are at increased risk for HPV and cervical cancer. However, as with any STI, a woman can be infected with HPV even if they have had only one sexual partner. HPV infection is also common in men, with a recent study estimating the global prevalence among men to be 31% (95% CI: 27–35; Bruni et al., 2023). As with women, HPV prevalence is high in young adults, reaching a maximum between the ages of 25 and 29 years.

Some strains of HPV cause the two most common types of cervical cancer worldwide: squamous cell carcinoma, and less commonly adenocarcinoma. Cervical cancer is the fourth most common cancer globally in women, with an estimated 530,000 new cases annually, with 270,000 deaths (Small et al., 2017). An estimated 85% of deaths from cervical cancer occur in LMICs, with studies estimating that cervical cancer death rates being up to 20 times higher in some parts of Africa compared with wealthier countries (Singh et al., 2023). HPV also causes other cancers. Men who have sex with men (MSM) are estimated to be up to 20 times more likely to develop anal cancer than men who have sex only with women (Machalek et al., 2012). Recent research also suggests that the incidence is increasing for cancers of the oropharynx among both women and men, which is associated with the transmission of HPV during oral sexual contact.

General wisdom is that prevention is better than treatment and the lack of curative treatments for HPV infection emphasizes the importance of prevention. While cryotherapy and surgical interventions like loop electrosurgical excision procedure (LEEP) are effective in treating the health problems that the virus can cause, they do not eliminate the underlying virus from the body. There are six licensed vaccines that are highly effective in preventing infection with virus types responsible for 70% of cervical cancer cases (WHO, 2022). WHO has recently updated its recommended vaccination schedule to recommend a one- or two-dose schedule for girls aged 9 to 14 years and 15 to 20 years, and two doses with a 6-month interval for women older than age 21 (2022). The revised guidelines may make it easier for individuals to achieve full vaccination status. The Centers for Disease Control and Prevention (CDC) recommends routine vaccination for all adolescents, including boys (CDC, 2016). While it is optimal to administer the vaccine prior to sexual debut, sexually experienced individuals may also benefit from the vaccine (Meites et al., 2016).

Disparities in Vaccination Coverage

WHO has issued a call to action to eliminate cervical cancer as a public health problem (Gültekin et al., 2020). Fundamental to this goal is to ensure universal vaccine coverage. While HPV vaccination rates are not optimal in the United States, the percentage of women aged 18 and 21 years who received at least one dose increased from 32% in 2010 to 55% in 2018. Among men in the same age range, the percentage increased from 2% in 2010 to 34% in 2018 (Chen et al., 2021).

Research has found lower HPV vaccination rates among sexual minority populations in the United States. One study found that girls and women with only female past-year sexual partners had a lower prevalence of HPV vaccine awareness and initiation than those with only male past-year sexual partners (Agénor et al., 2016). Worldwide, full HPV vaccination coverage for women is estimated at 1.4%, with 33.6% of females aged 10 to 20 years having received the full course of vaccine in high-income countries, compared with only 2.7% in less developed regions (Bruni et al., 2016). Less than 30% of LMICs have introduced HPV vaccination compared with more than 85% of high-income countries (PATH, 2020).

Opportunities for Intervention at Different Levels of the Social-Ecological Model

Weak health systems and cost are some of the factors that have stalled progress in resource-poor countries; however, creating demand from the public is a critical aspect of efforts to increase vaccination coverage. Like other vaccines, vaccine hesitancy is central to the lack of HPV uptake; however, some of the challenges related to the HPV vaccine are inherent to its sensitivity as being linked to sexual behavior. Applying a social-ecological perspective to understand vaccine hesitancy related to the unique factors related to the HPV vaccine helps identify some important areas to target in behavior change interventions. At the individual level, a primary driver of vaccine hesitancy in general is concern over side effects, which is the same in relation to the HPV vaccine (Karafillakis et al., 2019). As adolescents, however, are the main targets of HPV vaccination programs, their parents often serve as gatekeepers to their healthcare. Parents have expressed concern that vaccinating their children might lead them to engage in sexual activity (Forster et al., 2010), and many parents who oppose the HPV vaccine for their children thought their children to be at low behavioral risk of infection (Zimet & Rosenthal, 2010). Leveraging social contacts through an individual's social network may be an effective intervention strategy to address vaccine hesitancy and increase uptake among parents. A study conducted among African American parents in the United States found that those with social contacts who tended to express negative viewpoints toward the HPV vaccine were more likely to have similar views and refuse the vaccine for their children (Fu et al., 2019). Other intervention attempts have shown success in changing parents' minds about knowledge, attitudes, and practices related to the HPV vaccine. Using radio *novelas* (short stories) have been shown to be a culturally appropriate platform to deliver health messaging to low literacy, Spanish-speaking Latinx communities in the United States. Through a participatory design process, formative research was conducted among Latinx parents to better understand how they perceive barriers and facilitators in the decision-making process relating to vaccinating their daughters against HPV. Specific barriers were identified about knowledge related to HPV, although health service providers were seen as a trusted source of information. With their findings, researchers developed several prototypes of radionovela scenarios to address the barriers identified in their formative research. Finally, members of the target community decided which among the prototypes was the most influential. Results from a randomized control trial showed that the radio *novela* had a positive impact on increasing knowledge related to the HPV vaccine and to develop more favorable attitudes toward vaccinating their daughters (Kepka et al., 2011).

At the institutional level, there are policy restrictions that limit vaccine availability. According to the United Nations Population Fund (UNFPA) country data, approximately 40% of 102 countries that provide data have no enabling law or policy in place relating to HPV vaccination (UNFPA, 2020). In terms of availability, there are cost and supply-side considerations that may impact demand. During the COVID-19 pandemic, the HPV vaccination was one of the most disrupted vaccines as it is often delivered through a mixture of activities and strategies using schools, health facilities, and community outreach, most of which were shut down during the pandemic. This resulted in up to a 20% drop in coverage rates (UNICEF, 2020). Vaccine affordability is also a concern, with cost having been cited as the most prominent factor limiting HPV vaccine availability worldwide (Gupta et al., 2017). Finally, at the level of social norms, efforts to increase vaccine uptake among girls and women have led to a "feminization" of HPV, resulting in lower vaccine uptake among boys and men, and gender biases for HPV-related diseases (Gupta et al., 2017). There have been recent calls for gender-neutral expansion of HPV vaccination programs (Chido-Amajuoyi et al., 2019). Some evidence suggests that male HPV vaccine uptake can be improved by programs emphasizing altruistic motivations, such as focusing on the health benefits conferred for their sexual partners while still focusing on the personal health benefits they themselves may experience (Bonafide & Vanable, 2015). Such efforts may not only alleviate the burden of HPV-related cancers among men, but increase men's sense of responsibility over HPV prevention by reframing it as not being just a woman's issue.

Interventions using institutional platforms to promote HPV vaccine uptake have shown promise, both in the United States and globally, especially where there is either no existing vaccination program, or in areas where vaccination programs have limited reach. School-based programs are a common intervention point given the ease at which they provide access to the target population for vaccine uptake (Escoffery et al., 2023). These programs may target many different aspects related to vaccine uptake, for example, by reducing supply-side barriers, improving vaccine knowledge and demand among students, or reaching parents. Intervention strategies may also address multiple challenges in HPV vaccine uptake simultaneously. Programs offering both information combined with vaccination services have shown considerable progress in increasing vaccine uptake. One intervention targeting a rural, underserved community in Texas found that combining school-based on-site vaccination events with community-based education had a higher impact on adolescent HPV vaccination rate compared with schools that received community-based education only (Kaul et al., 2019). Another school-based intervention that resulted in increased vaccination rates engaged students and school nurses in a face-to-face educational session based on the health belief model that provided basic information about HPV, the vaccine, and where students could get the vaccine free of charge (Grandahl et al., 2016).

HIV/AIDS: TREATMENT AND PREVENTION

Global Evolution of the Epidemic

In 2014, the Joint United Nations Programme on HIV/AIDS (UNAIDS) set a global goal to diagnose 90% of people living with HIV, provide treatment to 90% of people diagnosed, and achieve viral suppression in 90% of people being treated by 2020 (Sidibé et al., 2016). However, global progress toward meeting this goal was uneven. As a result, a subsequent 95-95-95 goal has been set for 2030 (Frescura et al., 2022). In 2019, an estimated 37 million people were living with HIV worldwide, with 15% more women than men (Jahagirdar et al., 2021).

The global evolution of the HIV epidemic has led to new disparities and new challenges regarding social and behavior change interventions. Advances in medical treatments have improved the outcomes for most persons with HIV who are able to access ART and medical care. Dramatic improvements in HIV treatment came in 1996, when combination ART became available. The advent of ART changed the lives of many of those with HIV in the United States, turning HIV from a uniformly fatal disease into a chronic disease for which strict adherence to a drug regimen is necessary.

Prevention efforts have also evolved with new medical technologies as well as behavioral intervention strategies to reduce risk of transmission. While HIV continues to be primarily transmitted via sexual activity, injection drug use remains an important risk factor. In addition to blood, HIV can be transmitted through semen, vaginal fluids, and breast milk of a person infected with HIV. Unfortunately, a vaccine or cure for HIV remains far from being available.

The evolution of the HIV epidemic in the United States highlights important health disparities. Recent data show that the epidemic is largely concentrated in the Southern United States, and among specific minority populations, including MSM and Black and Latinx populations (Grandahl et al., 2016). Gay, bisexual, and other MSM carry a disproportionate burden of HIV infection in the United States and the incidence has been increasing within this group since the mid-1990s. This disparity is driven primarily by increases among African American and Hispanic/Latinx MSM (McCree et al., 2019) Risk factors also overlap, putting individuals with intersecting identities at increased risk. Black women have 17 times the lifetime risk of contracting HIV than that of White women. Some projections suggest that 50% of Black MSM will acquire HIV during their lifetime (Hess et al., 2017).

Globally, while sub-Saharan Africa continues to have the highest HIV burden, it has also made the greatest progress between 1990 and 2019 (Jahagirdar et al., 2021). Elsewhere in the world, the HIV incidence has remained relatively stable or even increased; however, the prevalence of people living with HIV has also simultaneously increased, suggesting that more people are living longer with the disease.

New Challenges and Opportunities in Social and Behavior Change to Improve Treatment and Prevention

Along with greatly improving morbidity and mortality, ART's viral suppression is currently considered the single most effective intervention to prevent HIV-positive individuals from transmitting HIV to their sexual partners. A multicountry trial of primarily heterosexual couples (HIV Prevention Trials Network 052 study [HPTN 052]) demonstrated that ART was associated with a 96% reduction in HIV transmission (Cohen et al., 2016). These findings further emphasize the importance of routine testing, linkage to HIV care, and early institution of ART.

Compared with other medicines, ART requires a high degree of adherence to achieve maximum benefit. The goal of ART is to achieve viral suppression with an undetectable viral load. The level of adherence required may vary at an individual level based on factors such as medication pharmacokinetics and potency, drug interactions, and viral and host characteristics. In general, the goal is perfect or near-perfect adherence, defined as 95% or more of doses taken (Paterson et al., 2000). Unfortunately, suboptimal adherence to ART is common and associated with poor outcomes, including therapeutic failure and loss of future treatment options. Treatment interruption is associated with rebound viremia, worsening of immune function, and poor health outcomes (Strategies for Management of Antiretroviral Therapy Study Group, 2006). In the United States, 10% of those who have been prescribed ART have not achieved viral suppression. Disparities exist in ART adherence as well. For example, Black women in the United States are more likely to miss a dose of ART medication than White or Latinx women (Geter et al., 2019). The continued advent of novel strategies to support individuals on ART adhere to their treatment regimen can help them live longer, healthier lives and prevent the spread of HIV to others.

New approaches to promote adherence have been grounded in behavior change theory and have taken advantage of new technologies (Whiteley et al., 2021). A wide range of mobile phone and digital interventions have been found to be effective at improving ART adherence, especially when combined with behavior change theory to improve knowledge, reduce barriers, or increase self-efficacy and confidence. Some interventions provide personalized, real-time messages when missed doses were detected by smart pill dispensers (Sabin et al., 2015). Interactive text message interventions guided by the social cognitive theory have been thought to improve adherence by building knowledge, motivation, and skills to maintain the treatment regimen (Garofalo et al., 2016). Interventions involving digital games designed to be goal-oriented, motivating, and immersive, with the goal of influencing learning or behavior change, are currently under development within the sphere of ART (Whiteley et al., 2021). In LMICs, simple short messaging service (SMS) has also shown promise in adherence (Kanters et al., 2017). More research is needed to demonstrate effectiveness in youth and adolescent populations (Mehra et al., 2021).

Promoting safer sex is another strategy to prevent transmission of HIV from an infected partner to another partner during sexual intercourse. Safer sex refers to sexual intercourse that prevents the exchange of infectious bodily fluids (i.e., semen, vaginal secretions, breast milk, and blood). One of the most common ways of preventing transmission of HIV and some other STIs during sexual intercourse is the use of latex condoms. Despite the high level of knowledge in the United States about HIV and STI transmission, condom use remains low. Although the prevalence of sexual risk behavior generally declines following HIV diagnosis, a substantial proportion of HIV-positive persons continue to engage in unprotected intercourse. In the United States, condom use tends to be low among college students. A study of new sexually active female college students found that condoms were used in only one-third of intercourse events with male partners (Fairfortune et al., 2020). Barriers to condom use among college students include low perceived risk of contracting an STI, low self-efficacy for using a condom or negotiating condom use, embarrassment in purchasing condoms, and perceived social norms that are unsupportive of condom use (Whiting et al., 2019). Interventions that address information, motivation, skills and self-efficacy have been effective at changing attitudes toward condom use and improving behavioral intentions to use condoms, with some interventions showing evidence of increased condom use (Whiting et al., 2019).

Recently, strong evidence has emerged regarding the protective benefits of voluntary medical male circumcision (VMMC) on HIV transmission. Randomized trials have found that VMMC can reduce the risk of HIV acquisition by approximately 50% to 60%, while also providing other benefits, such as linking men and boys to other HIV prevention and treatment services (Gray et al., 2007). Substantial global investments have been made in improving the uptake of VMMC, especially in sub-Saharan Africa where HIV prevalence is high and circumcision rates tend to be low (US Agency for International Development, 2023). Demand creation interventions have been a cornerstone to improving the uptake of VMMC. Several barriers to VMMC have been identified, including that it is believed to be a practice linked to foreign cultures or religions, fear of the pain caused by the procedure, and that VMMC was not necessary due to low risk perception of HIV transmission (Carrasco et al., 2019). Facilitating factors that have been identified include beliefs that VMMC improves hygiene, that family and peers are in support of VMMC, and that it leads to enhanced sexual performance and satisfaction. Addressing social norms and cultural influences has been an effective strategy to improve uptake, and interventions have been found to be more impactful when careful attention is paid to ensure that they are deemed both appropriate and acceptable by the population that they intend to reach (Ensor et al., 2019).

Engaging religious leaders has been identified as an effective strategy to combat concerns about VMMC being fueled by an external agenda. In Tanzania, an intervention that equipped religious leaders with improved knowledge to engage their communities, while allowing the religious leaders to develop culturally appropriate ways to encourage uptake of VMMC, was shown to increase VMMC by more than 23% compared with the control group (Downs et al., 2017). In general, interventions consisting of food or transport vouchers as well as conditional cash transfers to mitigate lost wages were most effective at increasing uptake of VMMC; however, some interventions have been found to raise suspicions (Kennedy et al., 2020). In Tanzania, an intervention whereby men who underwent VMMC were enrolled in a lottery to obtain a smartphone was found to be largely ineffective. Focus group data revealed that some men grew suspicious of the intervention because they felt the smartphone was too expensive and out of touch with the community needs, and an older phone model or food/transport vouchers would have been better (Bazant et al., 2016).

SEXUAL AND GENDER-BASED VIOLENCE

Sexual and gender-based violence (SGBV) is an umbrella term for harmful acts of abuse directed against a person because of their gender and ranges from street-based harassment to forced early marriage, to sexual violence. SGBV is a fundamental and widespread violation of human rights. This form of violence, including threats of such acts, coercion, or arbitrary deprivation of liberty, results in, or is likely to result in, physical, sexual or psychological harm or suffering (Pandey, 2023). Although people of all genders experience SGBV, globally it is women and girls who are most likely to be subjected to it in one or all its many forms in their lifetime: physical, sexual, psychological, or economic harm or suffering caused by either an intimate partner or nonpartner.

In part since SBGV encompasses multiple types of violence, global estimates range substantially. Global estimates indicate that 27% of ever-partnered women aged 15 to 49 years have experienced physical, sexual, or both forms of violence by an intimate partner in their lifetime (Sardinha et al., 2022). These estimates do not account for incidence of sexual harassment, nonpartner violence, nor femicide—when a woman is killed by her partner or family member—which occurs on average to one woman every 11 minutes globally (United Nations Office on Drugs and Crime [UNODC], 2021).

Although the prevalence of violence against women and girls remains high globally, regional variations in prevalence estimates exist. In the United States, nearly one in two women report having experienced IPV at some point in their lifetime (as compared with two in five men; Leemis et al., 2022). This is in contrast to less than one in five (16%) women in Central Europe who report lifetime experience of IPV (Sardinha et al., 2022). This variation in prevalence of violence against women and girls is evidence that this form of SGBV is not inevitable; societal and structural differences across populations and time modify prevalence rates.

Ecological Perspectives to Understand and Prevent Sexual and Gender-Based Violence

A number of theories from a range of disciplines have been used to understand the factors that contribute to SBGV, from criminology to sociology, and more recently public health (Meyer et al., 2023). Using an ecological approach to organize these theories, we see a complex interplay of contributing factors across various levels of analysis (Heise, 1998). These factors at the individual level, for example, include witnessing or experiencing violence as a child; at a relationship level, problem alcohol use or male dominance in family decision-making; at the community level, poverty levels or crime rates; and at the societal level, rigid gender and social norms that see violence as an acceptable and useful way to control intimate partners (Heise, 1998).

This complex causal architecture that contributes to the incidence of SBGV requires an equally comprehensive set of strategies to reduce and prevent this widespread form of violence, and many prevention efforts have been implemented and proposed. However, a common characteristic across effective interventions is a focus on addressing the power imbalances between women and men stemming from inequitable gender norms and practices (Michau & Namy, 2021).

CASE STUDY 11.2: SASA!: A COMMUNITY-BASED INITIATIVE TO PREVENT VIOLENCE AGAINST WOMEN

SASA! is grounded in the transtheoretical (stages of change) model (Prochaska & DiClemente, 1983; Prochaska et al., 1997). The intervention engages community members in discussion and action across a four-phase process to transform power imbalances between men and women (Michau & Namy, 2021):

- *Start (precontemplation):* involves learning about the community through a baseline survey, relationship building, and selection and training of women and men who live and work in the community to connect with their *power within*

- *Awareness (contemplation):* introduces (or deepens) a feminist analysis of men's *power over* women as the root cause of IPV and the community's silence about this injustice as key drivers that enable violence to continue

- *Support (preparation for action):* builds momentum as more and more community members learn skills around balancing power and join their *power with* others to support women experiencing violence, couples trying to change, and community activists speaking out and holding men who use violence accountable

- *Action (action and maintenance):* cultivates the *power to* act and formalize mechanisms that sustain new norms that reject violence and encourage balanced power between women and men

Program evaluation results from a randomized controlled trial showed that *SASA!* had community-level impacts on reducing women's risk of physical IPV by 52% and reducing social acceptability of violence (76% of women and men in *SASA!* communities rejected men's use of violence against women, compared with only 26% in the control communities; Abramsky et al., 2014). The steady progress and innovation in violence prevention programs seen in the past two decades provides a sense of optimism that change can be made to address the inequitable gender norms and practices that underlie violence against women and girls (Raising Voices, 2023).

Child, Early, and Forced Marriages and Unions

Child, early, and forced marriages and unions (CEFMU) are another form of SBGV that is rooted in gender inequality and defined by the United Nations as a marriage or informal union under age 18 years (Malhotra & Elnakib, 2021). Compared with those who marry as adults, women who marry as children are more likely to experience physical, sexual, and psychological/emotional violence (Tenkorang, 2019). Gender norms, household autonomy, and socioeconomic status help explain the relationship between child marriage and physical and sexual IPV (Tenkorang, 2019). Further, child marriage is linked to rates of early pregnancy and adverse maternal health outcomes (Raj, 2010), mental distress (John et al., 2019), as well as having a negative impact on child health (Anjorin & Yaya, 2021).

SDG Target 5.3 aims to end girl-child marriage by 2030 as part of a global commitment to "eliminate all harmful practices, such as child, early and forced marriage and female genital mutilation." While CEFMU is most commonly practiced among women, young men and boys are also at risk, although the prevalence is less understood. Globally, 20% of girls are married as children annually, and 650 million women and girls currently alive were married prior to the age of 18. LMICs have the highest burden of CEFMU, with the highest prevalence observed in sub-Saharan Africa (37%) and South Asia (30%; (Malhotra & Elnakib, 2021). In the United States, the prevalence of child marriage has been found to vary from 10 per 1,000 children in West Virginia, Hawaii, and North Dakota, to less than 4 per 1,000 in Maine, Rhode Island, and Wyoming (Koski & Heymann, 2018). Marriage before the age of 18 is legal in the majority of U.S. states (Reiss, 2021).

The underlying drivers of child marriage exist across the socioecological system. Poverty and socioeconomic inequality may drive child marriage in some settings, especially when girls are given for economic benefit, while other drivers such as religion, gender inequality, and cultural norms also drive the continuation of the practice (Tenkorang, 2019). Humanitarian crises, especially those characterized by conflict-driven displacement (Leigh, 2020), are thought to be behind increases in CEFMU. While many of the same drivers may also be behind the uptick in child marriage observed in humanitarian settings, other upstream factors that contribute to the ongoing practice of child marriage, such as economic vulnerabilities and safety concerns, may also play a role (Gausman et al., 2019; Leigh, 2020). Social pressure has an important influence on decisions relating to CEFM within humanitarian contexts, with some families fearing social ostracization and punishment if they do not conform to perceived behavioral norms (Presler-Marshall et al., 2020). Ensuring that humanitarian programs address the underlying drivers of CEFM by addressing gender inequality through transformative programming has been identified as a global priority, but there continue to be important intervention gaps in this domain (Gausman et al., 2022).

The increased global attention to ending child marriage has seen many countries attempt to pass legislation to ban this practice. Closing the legal loopholes that continue to allow children to be married has been an important target for policy-level intervention as one way to promote social and behavior change (Gausman et al., 2019). The evidence of the effectiveness of legal change has been mixed. While some research points to the positive impact that these laws have had in reducing the prevalence of child marriage (Maswikwa et al., 2015), such laws are difficult to enforce, especially in rural and hard-to-reach areas, or in countries where there may be authorities outside of the formal system of governance, such as religious institutions, that can grant marriages (Batyra & Pesando, 2021).

Other interventions have attempted to address other upstream drivers of child marriage to encourage social and behavior change. A systematic review of over 20 years of what works to prevent child marriage indicates that the enhancement of girls' own human capital and opportunities is the most compelling pathway to delay marriage (Malhotra & Elnakib, 2021). The types of programs that show the clearest pattern of success in delaying CEFMU include interventions that support girls' schooling through cash or in-kind transfers (Malhotra & Elnakib, 2021); however, there are still several studies that have shown no impact (Dake et al., 2018; Handa et al., 2015). Critics of cash transfer programs argue that as child marriage is a multidimensional problem a more holistic programmatic approach is needed to fully address the multiplicity of underlying drivers (Amin et al., 2017).

CONCLUSION

The field of SRHR covers a wide range of issues, but similar underlying determinants drive disparities around the world. Interventions have evolved over time to prioritize those embedded in a rights-based agenda. The field continues to evolve and there remain critical challenges in improving equity and universal access to SRH services. Social and behavior change interventions occurring at all levels of the social-ecological model have been effective in improving health outcomes globally. Examples of interventions from the domains of family planning, HPV, HIV/AIDS, and SGBV highlight the application of theory to design culturally appropriate social and behavior change interventions at the individual, peer, community, and policy levels.

SUMMARY KEY POINTS

- The 1994 ICPD reframed SRH within a framework of reproductive rights, gender equity, and women's empowerment.
- Achieving SRH from a rights-based perspective requires access to appropriate, timely, and quality healthcare services, often combined with support from other sectors, such as education, labor, and transportation. Persistent gender inequality adversely influences SRH and rights.
- Government family planning programs can promote a broad social and economic development agenda. These programs can empower women and families, but can also use coercive practices that strip citizens of reproductive autonomy.
- In spite of significant improvements in access to family planning and reproductive health services, there are more than 99 million unintended pregnancies each year.
- Drivers of contraception demand include the desire to have control over one's own fertility, address health conditions, and protect against HIV and other STIs.
- Inhibitors of contraception include fears about side effects, religious beliefs, financial restraints, lack of knowledge and access, and interpersonal and community dynamics and beliefs.
- Interventions that aim to influence SRH behaviors, inform women and couples about the benefits of family planning, and improve access to contraceptives have become increasingly common in developing countries.
- HPV is one of the most common STIs globally and causes the two most common types of cervical cancer. While there is a vaccine that can prevent HPV infection, its implementation has been hindered by vaccine hesitancy, lack of access or knowledge, and specific concerns about the disease being linked to sexual behavior. Applying a social-ecological perspective to understand vaccine hesitancy related to the unique factors related to the HPV vaccine helps identify some important areas to target in behavior change interventions.
- While ART has shifted HIV from a fatal disease into a chronic disease, disparities persist in ART adherence. Technological approaches grounded in behavior change theory have been found effective in improving ART adherence. Strategies to prevent HIV infection include ART adherence, safer sex practices, and voluntary male circumcision.
- Although people of all genders experience SGBV, women and girls are most likely to be subjected to it in one or all its many forms in their lifetime globally. A common characteristic of effective SGBV interventions is a focus on addressing the power imbalances between women and men stemming from inequitable gender norms and practices.

DISCUSSION QUESTIONS

1. What do you think are the most important priorities in social and behavior change in SRHR for the next 10 years from a social-ecological perspective?
2. Thinking about your own community, what are some of the challenges that interventions seeking to engage men in family planning might face?
3. How would you use the social-ecological model to design a technology-based intervention to improve adherence to HIV medication?
4. What might be some ethical challenges in using cash transfer interventions in the field of SRHR? How can those challenges be mitigated?
5. What are some challenges that might limit the impact of a policy-only focused intervention to address child marriage? Do you think policy or legal change is a necessary component?

A robust set of instructor resources designed to supplement this text is located at http://connect.springerpub.com/content/book/978-0-8261-4265-8. Qualifying instructors may request access by emailing textbook@springerpub.com.

REFERENCES

Abramsky, T., Devries, K., Kiss, L., Nakuti, J., Kyegombe, N., Starmann, E., Cundill, B., Francisco, L., Kaye, D., Musuya, T., Michau, L., & Watts, C. (2014). Findings from the SASA! Study: A cluster randomized controlled trial to assess the impact of a community mobilization intervention to prevent violence against women and reduce HIV risk in Kampala, Uganda. *BMC Medicine, 12*(1), 1–17. https://doi.org/10.1186/s12916-014-0122-5

Adanu, R. M., & Johnson, T. R. (2009). Migration and women's health. *International Journal of Gynecology & Obstetrics, 106*(2), 179–181. https://doi.org/10.1016/j.ijgo.2009.03.036

Adelekan, A., Omoregie, P., & Edoni, E. (2014). Male involvement in family planning: Challenges and way forward. *International Journal of Population Research, 2014*(3), 1–9. http://doi.org/10.1155/2014/416457

Agénor, M., McCauley, H. L., Peitzmeier, S. M., Haneuse, S., Gordon, A. R., Potter, J., & Austin, S. B. (2016). Sex of sexual partners and human papillomavirus vaccination among US girls and women. *American Journal of Preventive Medicine, 50*(3), 318–327. https://doi.org/10.1016/j.amepre.2015.08.025

Amin, S., Asadullah, N., Hossain, S., & Wahhaj, Z. (2017). Can conditional transfers eradicate child marriage? *Economic and Political Weekly, 52*(6), 20–22.

Anjorin, S., & Yaya, S. (2021). Anaemia among under-five children: Is maternal marriage at 18th birthday and above protective? Evidence from 15 countries in Sub-Saharan Africa. *Maternal & Child Nutrition, 17*(4), e13226. https://doi.org/10.1111/mcn.13226

Bansal, A., & Dwivedi, L. K. (2020). Sterilization regret in India: Is quality of care a matter of concern? *Contraception and Reproductive Medicine, 5*, 1–12. https://doi.org/10.1186/s40834-020-00115-8

Batyra, E., & Pesando, L. M. (2021). Trends in child marriage and new evidence on the selective impact of changes in age-at-marriage laws on early marriage. *SSM-Population Health, 14*, 100811. https://doi.org/10.1016/j.ssmph.2021.100811

Bazant, E., Mahler, H., Machaku, M., Lemwayi, R., Kulindwa, Y., Lija, J. G., Mpora, B., Ochola, D., Sarkar, S., Williams, E., Plotkin, M., & Juma, J. (2016). A randomized evaluation of a demand creation lottery for voluntary medical male circumcision among adults in Tanzania. *Journal of Acquired Immune Deficiency Syndromes (1999), 72*(Suppl. 4), S285–S292. https://doi.org/10.1097/QAI.0000000000001042

Bearak, J., Popinchalk, A., Alkema, L., & Sedgh, G. (2018). Global, regional, and subregional trends in unintended pregnancy and its outcomes from 1990 to 2014: Estimates from a Bayesian hierarchical model. *The Lancet Global Health, 6*(4), e380–e389. https://doi.org/10.1016/S2214-109X(18)30029-9

Bingenheimer, J. B., Hardee, K., Hindin, M., Jain, A., Mumah, J., & Dam, J. V. (2023). Introduction to the special issue: Indicators in sexual and reproductive health and rights. *Studies in Family Planning, 54*(1), 9–16. https://doi.org/10.1111/sifp.12239

Blanc, A. K. (2001). The effect of power in sexual relationships on sexual and reproductive health: An examination of the evidence. *Studies in Family Planning, 32*(3), 189–213. https://doi.org/10.1111/j.1728-4465.2001.00189.x

Bonafide, K. E., & Vanable, P. A. (2015). Male human papillomavirus vaccine acceptance is enhanced by a brief intervention that emphasizes both male-specific vaccine benefits and altruistic motives. *Sexually Transmitted Diseases, 42*(2), 76–80. https://doi.org/10.1097/olq.0000000000000226

Bongaarts, J. (1978). A framework for analyzing the proximate determinants of fertility. *Population and Development Review, 4*, 105–132. https://doi.org/10.2307/1972149

Bronfenbrenner, U. (1994). Ecological models of human development. *International Encyclopedia of Education, 3*(2), 37–43.

Bruni, L., Albero, G., Rowley, J., Alemany, L., Arbyn, M., Giuliano, A. R., Markowitz, L. E., Broutet, N., & Taylor, M. (2023). Global and regional estimates of genital human papillomavirus prevalence among men: A systematic review and meta-analysis. *The Lancet Global Health, 11*(9), e1345–e1362. https://doi.org/10.1016/s2214-109x(23)00305-4

Bruni, L., Diaz, M., Barrionuevo-Rosas, L., Herrero, R., Bray, F., Bosch, F. X., de Sanjose, S., & Castellsagué, X. (2016). Global estimates of human papillomavirus vaccination coverage by region and income level: A pooled analysis. *The Lancet Global Health, 4*(7), e453–e463. https://doi.org/10.1016/s2214-109x(16)30099-7

Carrasco, M. A., Wilkinson, J., Kasdan, B., & Fleming, P. (2019). Systematic review of barriers and facilitators to voluntary medical male circumcision in priority countries and programmatic implications for service uptake. *Global Public Health, 14*(1), 91–111. https://doi.org/10.1080/17441692.2018.1465108

Casterline, J. B., & Sinding, S. W. (2000). Unmet need for family planning in developing countries and implications for population policy. *Population and Development Review, 26*(4), 691–723. https://doi.org/10.1111/j.1728-4457.2000.00691.x

Centers for Disease Control and Prevention. (2016). *Human papillomavirus (HPV) ACIP vaccine recommendations.* https://www.cdc.gov/vaccines/hcp/acip-recs/vacc-specific/hpv.Html

Chen, M. M., Mott, N., Clark, S. J., Harper, D. M., Shuman, A. G., Prince, M. E., & Dossett, L. A. (2021). HPV vaccination among young adults in the US. *JAMA, 325*(16), 1673–1674. https://doi.org/10.1001/jama.2021.0725

Chido-Amajuoyi, O. G., Domgue, J. F., Obi-Jeff, C., Schmeler, K., & Shete, S. (2019). A call for the introduction of gender-neutral HPV vaccination to national immunisation programmes in Africa. *The Lancet Global Health, 7*(1), e20–e21. https://doi.org/10.1001/jama.2021.0725

Cleland, J. (2009). Contraception in historical and global perspective. *Best Practice & Research Clinical Obstetrics & Gynaecology, 23*(2), 165–176. https://doi.org/10.1016/j.bpobgyn.2008.11.002

Closson, K., Nemutambwe, T., Osborne, Z., Lee, G. Y., Hangle, C., Stephenson, S., Magagula, P., Leonce, I., Raj, A., Nicholson, V., & Kaida, A. (2023). Relationship and gender equity measurement among gender-inclusive young women and non-binary youth in British Columbia (RE-IMAGYN BC): Planning a youth-led, community-based, qualitative research study. *International Journal of Qualitative Methods, 22*, 16094069221148415. http://doi.org/10.1177/16094069221148415

Cohen, M. S., Chen, Y. Q., McCauley, M., Gamble, T., Hosseinipour, M. C., Kumarasamy, N., Hakim, J. G., Kumwenda, J., Grinsztejn, B., Pilotto, J. H., Godbole, S. V., Chariyalertsak, S., Santos, B. R., Mayer, K. H., Hoffman, I. F., Eshleman, S. H., Piwowar-Manning, E., Cottle, L., Zhang, X. C., . . . Fleming, T. R. (2016). Antiretroviral therapy for the prevention of HIV-1 transmission. *New England Journal of Medicine, 375*(9), 830–839. https://doi.org/10.1056/nejmoa1600693

Dake, F., Natali, L., Angeles, G., de Hoop, J., Handa, S., Peterman, A., Malawi Cash Transfer Evaluation Team, & the Zambia Cash Transfer Evaluation Team. (2018). Cash transfers, early marriage, and fertility in Malawi and Zambia. *Studies in Family Planning, 49*(4), 295–317. https://doi.org/10.1111/sifp.12073

Darroch, J. E. (2017). Adding it up: Investing in contraception and maternal and newborn health, 2017—Estimation Methodology, New York: Guttmacher Institute, 2018. https://www.guttmacher.org/report/adding-it-up-investing-in-contraception-maternalnewborn-health-2017-methodology

Downs, J. A., Mwakisole, A. H., Chandika, A. B., Lugoba, S., Kassim, R., Laizer, E., Magambo, K. A., Lee, M. H., Kalluvya, S. E., Downs, D. J., & Fitzgerald, D. W. (2017). Educating religious leaders to promote uptake of male circumcision in Tanzania: A cluster randomised trial. *The Lancet, 389*(10074), 1124–1132. https://doi.org/10.1016/s0140-6736(16)32055-4

Dyck, E. (2013). *Facing eugenics: Reproduction, sterilization, and the politics of choice.* University of Toronto Press.

El-Khoury, M., Thornton, R., Chatterji, M., & Choi, S. K. (2015). Effectiveness of evidence-based medicine on knowledge, attitudes, and practices of family planning providers: A randomized experiment in Jordan. *BMC Health Services Research, 15*, 1–9. https://doi.org/10.1186/s12913-015-1101-z

Ensor, S., Davies, B., Rai, T., & Ward, H. (2019). The effectiveness of demand creation interventions for voluntary male medical circumcision for HIV prevention in sub-Saharan Africa: A mixed methods systematic review. *Journal of the International AIDS Society, 22*, e25299. https://doi.org/10.1002/jia2.25299

Escoffery, C., Petagna, C., Agnone, C., Perez, S., Saber, L. B., Ryan, G., Dhir, M., Sekar, S., Yeager, K. A., Biddell, C. B., Madhivanan, P., Lee, S., English, A. S., Savas, L., Daly, E., Vu, T., & Fernandez, M. E. (2023). A systematic review of interventions to promote HPV vaccination globally. *BMC Public Health, 23*(1), 1262. https://doi.org/10.1186/s12889-023-15876-5

Fairfortune, T. S., Stern, J. E., Richardson, B. A., Koutsky, L. A., & Winer, R. L. (2020). Sexual behavior patterns and condom use in newly sexually active female university students. *Archives of Sexual Behavior, 49*, 1053–1065. https://doi.org/10.1007/s10508-019-1411-z

Fennell, J. (2014). "And Isn't that the point?": Pleasure and contraceptive decisions. *Contraception, 89*(4), 264–270. https://doi.org/10.1016/j.contraception.2013.11.012

Fisher, J. D., & Fisher, W. A. (1992). Changing AIDS-risk behavior. *Psychological Bulletin, 111*(3), 455. https://doi.org/10.1037/0033-2909.111.3.455

Forster, A., Wardle, J., Stephenson, J., & Waller, J. (2010). Passport to promiscuity or lifesaver: Press coverage of HPV vaccination and risky sexual behavior. *Journal of Health Communication, 15*(2), 205–217. https://doi.org/10.1080/10810730903528066

Frescura, L., Godfrey-Faussett, P., Feizzadeh, A. A., El-Sadr, W., Syarif, O., & Ghys, P. D. (2022). Achieving the 95 95 95 targets for all: A pathway to ending AIDS. *PLoS One, 17*(8), e0272405. https://doi.org/10.1371/journal.pone.0272405

Fu, L. Y., Zimet, G. D., Latkin, C. A., & Joseph, J. G. (2019). Social networks for human papillomavirus vaccine advice among African American parents. *Journal of Adolescent Health, 65*(1), 124–129. https://doi.org/10.1016/j.jadohealth.2019.01.029

Gahungu, J., Vahdaninia, M., & Regmi, P. R. (2021). The unmet needs for modern family planning methods among postpartum women in Sub-Saharan Africa: A systematic review of the literature. *Reproductive Health, 18*, 1–15. https://doi.org/10.1186/s12978-021-01089-9

Garofalo, R., Kuhns, L. M., Hotton, A., Johnson, A., Muldoon, A., & Rice, D. (2016). A randomized controlled trial of personalized text message reminders to promote medication adherence among HIV-positive adolescents and young adults. *AIDS and Behavior, 20*, 1049–1059. https://doi.org/10.1007/s10461-015-1192-x

Gausman, J., Huda, F. A., Othman, A., Al Atoom, M., Shaheen, A., Hamad, I., Dabobe, M., Mahmood, H. R., Ibnat, R., & Langer, A. (2022). Girl child marriage and the social context of displacement: A qualitative comparative exploration of Syrian refugees in Jordan and Rohingya refugees in Bangladesh. *BMC Public Health, 22*(1), 1–12. https://doi.org/10.1186/s12889-022-14832-z

Gausman, J., Othman, A., Al-Qotob, R., Shaheen, A., Abu Sabbah, E., Aldiqs, M., Hamad, I., Dabobe, M., & Langer, A. (2021). Health care professionals' attitudes towards youth-friendly sexual and reproductive health services in Jordan: A cross-sectional study of physicians, midwives and nurses. *Reproductive Health, 18*, 1–12. https://doi.org/10.1186/s12978-021-01137-4

Gausman, J., Othman, A., Amawi, A., & Langer, A. (2019). Child marriage in the Arab world. *The Lancet, 394*(10201), 825–826. https://doi.org/10.1016/s0140-6736(19)31287-5

Gausman, J., Saggurti, N., Adanu, R., Bandoh, D. A., Berrueta, M., Chakraborty, S., Kenu, E., Khan, N., Langer, A., Nigri, C., Odikro, M. A., Pingray, V., Ramesh, S., Vázquez, P., Williams, C. R., & Jolivet, R. R. (2023). Validation of a measure to assess decision-making autonomy in family planning services in three low-and middle-income countries: The Family Planning Autonomous Decision-Making scale (FP-ADM). *PLoS One, 18*(11), e0293586. https://doi.org/10.1371/journal.pone.0293586

Geter, A., Sutton, M. Y., Armon, C., Buchacz, K., & the HIV Outpatient Study Investigators. (2019). Disparities in viral suppression and medication adherence among women in the USA, 2011–2016. *AIDS and Behavior, 23*(11), 3015–3023. https://doi.org/10.1007/s10461-019-02494-9

Grandahl, M., Rosenblad, A., Stenhammar, C., Tydén, T., Westerling, R., Larsson, M., Oscarsson, M., Andrae, B., Dalianis, T., & Nevéus, T. (2016). School-based intervention for the prevention of HPV among adolescents: A cluster randomised controlled study. *BMJ Open, 6*(1), e009875. https://doi.org/10.1136/bmjopen-2015-009875

Gray, R. H., Kigozi, G., Serwadda, D., Makumbi, F., Watya, S., Nalugoda, F., Kiwanuka, N., Moulton, L. H., Chaudhary, M. A., Chen, M. Z., Sewankambo, N. K., Wabwire-Mangen, F., Bacon, M. C., Williams, C. F. M., Opendi, P., Reynolds, S. J., Laeyendecker, O., Quinn, T. C., & Wawer, M. J. (2007). Male circumcision for HIV prevention in men in Rakai, Uganda: A randomised trial. *The Lancet, 369*(9562), 657–666. https://doi.org/10.1016/s0140-6736(07)60313-4

Gültekin, M., Ramirez, P., Broutet, N., & Hutubessy, R. (2020). World Health Organization call for action to eliminate cervical cancer globally. *International Journal of Gynecological Cancer, 30*(4), 426–427. https://doi.org/10.1136/ijgc-2020-001285

Gupta, G., Glueck, R., & Patel, P. R. (2017). HPV vaccines: Global perspectives. *Human Vaccine Immunotherapeutics, 13*(6), 1421–1424. https://doi.org/10.1080/21645515.2017.1289301

Handa, S., Peterman, A., Huang, C., Halpern, C., Pettifor, A., & Thirumurthy, H. (2015). Impact of the Kenya cash transfer for orphans and vulnerable children on early pregnancy and marriage of adolescent girls. *Social Science & Medicine, 141*, 36–45. https://doi.org/10.1016/j.socscimed.2015.07.024

Hartmann, M., Gilles, K., Shattuck, D., Kerner, B., & Guest, G. (2012). Changes in couples' communication as a result of a male-involvement family planning intervention. *Journal of Health Communication, 17*(7), 802–819. https://doi.org/10.1080/10810730.2011.650825

Heidari, S., & Moreno, C. G. (2016). Gender-based violence: A barrier to sexual and reproductive health and rights. *Reproductive Health Matters, 24*(47), 1–4. https://doi.org/10.1016/j.rhm.2016.07.001

Heise, L. L. (1998). Violence against women: An integrated, ecological framework. *Violence Against Women, 4*(3), 262–290. https://doi.org/10.1177/1077801298004003002

Hess, K. L., Hu, X., Lansky, A., Mermin, J., & Hall, H. I. (2017). Lifetime risk of a diagnosis of HIV infection in the United States. *Annals of Epidemiology, 27*(4), 238–243. https://doi.org/10.1016/j.annepidem.2017.02.003

Hufnagel, G. L. (2010). Margaret Sanger and the origin of the birth control movement, 1910–1930: The concept of women's sexual autonomy, and: Our bodies, our crimes: The policing of women's reproduction in America, and: The infertility treadmill: Feminist ethics, personal choice, and the use of reproductive technologies. *Feminist Formations, 22*(2), 195–201.

Jahagirdar, D., Walters, M. K., Novotney, A., Brewer, E. D., Frank, T. D., Carter, A., Biehl, M. H., Abbastabar, H., Abhilash, E. S., Abu-Gharbieh, E., Abu-Raddad, L. J., Adekanmbi, V., Adeyinka,

D. A., Adnani, Q. E. S., Afzal, S., Aghababaei, S., Ahinkorah, B. O., Ahmad, S., Ahmadi, K., . . . Kyu, H. H. (2021). Global, regional, and national sex-specific burden and control of the HIV epidemic, 1990–2019, for 204 countries and territories: The Global Burden of Diseases Study 2019. *The Lancet HIV, 8*(10), e633–e651. https://doi.org/10.1016/s2352-3018(21)00152-1

Jejeebhoy, S. J., Prakash, R., Acharya, R., Singh, S. K., & Daniel, E. (2015). Meeting contraceptive needs: Long-term associations of the PRACHAR project with married women's awareness and behavior in Bihar. *International Perspectives on Sexual and Reproductive Health, 41*(3), 115–125. https://doi.org/10.1363/4111515

John, N. A., Edmeades, J., & Murithi, L. (2019). Child marriage and psychological well-being in Niger and Ethiopia. *BMC Public Health, 19*(1), 1–12. https://doi.org/10.1186/s12889-019-7314-z

Kaa, D. J. (1988). *The second demographic transition revisited: Theories and expectations.* Universiteit van Amsterdam.

Kabagenyi, A., Jennings, L., Reid, A., Nalwadda, G., Ntozi, J., & Atuyambe, L. (2014). Barriers to male involvement in contraceptive uptake and reproductive health services: A qualitative study of men and women's perceptions in two rural districts in Uganda. *Reproductive Health, 11*(1), 1–9. https://doi.org/10.1186/1742-4755-11-21

Kanters, S., Park, J. J., Chan, K., Socias, M. E., Ford, N., Forrest, J. I., Thorlund, K., Nachega, J. B., & Mills, E. J. (2017). Interventions to improve adherence to antiretroviral therapy: A systematic review and network meta-analysis. *The Lancet HIV, 4*(1), e31–e40. https://doi.org/10.1016/s2352-3018(16)30206-5

Karafillakis, E., Simas, C., Jarrett, C., Verger, P., Peretti-Watel, P., Dib, F., Angelis, S. D., Takacs, J., Ali, K. A., Celentano, L. P., & Larson, H. (2019). HPV vaccination in a context of public mistrust and uncertainty: A systematic literature review of determinants of HPV vaccine hesitancy in Europe. *Human Vaccines & Immunotherapeutics, 15*(7–8), 1615–1627. https://doi.org/10.1080/21645515.2018.1564436

Karra, M., & Zhang, K. (2021). User-centered counseling and male involvement in contraceptive decision making: Protocol for a randomized controlled trial. *JMIR Research Protocols, 10*(4), e24884. https://doi.org/10.2196/24884

Kaul, S., Do, T. Q. N., Hsu, E., Schmeler, K. M., Montealegre, J. R., & Rodriguez, A. M. (2019). School-based human papillomavirus vaccination program for increasing vaccine uptake in an underserved area in Texas. *Papillomavirus Research, 8*, 100189. https://doi.org/10.1016/j.pvr.2019.100189

Kennedy, C. E., Yeh, P. T., Atkins, K., Fonner, V. A., Sweat, M. D., O'Reilly, K. R., Rutherford, G. W., Baggaley, R., & Samuelson, J. (2020). Economic compensation interventions to increase uptake of voluntary medical male circumcision for HIV prevention: A systematic review and meta-analysis. *PLoS One, 15*(1), e0227623. https://doi.org/10.1371/journal.pone.0227623

Kepka, D., Coronado, G. D., Rodriguez, H. P., & Thompson, B. (2011). Evaluation of a radionovela to promote HPV vaccine awareness and knowledge among Hispanic parents. *Journal of Community Health, 36*, 957–965. https://doi.org/10.1007/s10900-011-9395-1

Koski, A., & Heymann, J. (2018). Child marriage in the United States: How common is the practice, and which children are at greatest risk? *Perspectives on Sexual and Reproductive Health, 50*(2), 59–65. https://doi.org/10.1363/psrh.12055

Langer, A. (2006). Cairo after 12 years: Successes, setbacks, and challenges. *The Lancet, 368*(9547), 1552–1554. https://doi.org/10.1016/S0140-6736(06)69486-5

Langer, A., Meleis, A., Knaul, F. M., Atun, R., Aran, M., Arreola-Ornelas, H., Bhutta, Z. A., Binagwaho, A., Bonita, R., Caglia, J. M., Claeson, M., Davies, J., Donnay, F. A., Gausman, J. M., Glickman, C., Kearns, A. D., Kendall, T., Lozano, R., Seboni, N., . . . Frenk, J. (2015). Women and health: The key for sustainable development. *The Lancet, 386*(9999), 1165–1210. https://doi.org/10.1016/s0140-6736(15)60497-4

Leemis, R. W., Friar, N., Khatiwada, S., Chen, M. S., Kresnow, M.-j., Smith, S. G., Caslin, S., & Basile, K. C. (2022). *The national intimate partner and sexual violence survey: 2016/2017 report on intimate partner violence.* https://stacks.cdc.gov/view/cdc/124646

Leigh, J. (2020). *Child marriage in humanitarian settings in South Asia: Study results from Bangladesh and Nepal.* UNFPA Asia Pacific Regional Office (APRO) and UNICEF. https://www.unicef.org/rosa/reports/child-marriage-humanitarian-settings-south-asia

López, R. N. (2014). *A history of family planning in twentieth-century Peru.* UNC Press Books.

Lundgren, R. I., Gribble, J. N., Greene, M. E., Emrick, G. E., & De Monroy, M. (2005). Cultivating men's interest in family planning in rural El Salvador. *Studies in Family Planning, 36*(3), 173–188. https://doi.org/10.1111/j.1728-4465.2005.00060.x

Machalek, D. A., Poynten, M., Jin, F., Fairley, C. K., Farnsworth, A., Garland, S. M., Hillman, R. J., Petoumenos, K., Roberts, J., Tabrizi, S. N. Templeton, D. J., & Grulich, E. A. (2012). Anal human papillomavirus infection and associated neoplastic lesions in men who have sex with men: A systematic review and meta-analysis. *The Lancet Oncology, 13*(5), 487–500. https://doi.org/10.1016/s1470-2045(12)70080-3

Malhotra, A., & Elnakib, S. (2021). 20 years of the evidence base on what works to prevent child marriage: A systematic review. *Journal of Adolescent Health, 68*(5), 847–862. https://doi.org/10.1016/j.jadohealth.2020.11.017

Mason, A. (2001). *Population change and economic development in East Asia: Challenges met, opportunities seized*. Stanford University Press.

Maswikwa, B., Richter, L., Kaufman, J., & Nandi, A. (2015). Minimum marriage age laws and the prevalence of child marriage and adolescent birth: Evidence from Sub-Saharan Africa. *International Perspectives on Sexual and Reproductive Health, 41*(2), 58–68. https://doi.org/10.1363/4105815

McCree, D. H., Williams, A. M., Chesson, H. W., Beer, L., Jeffries IV, W. L., Lemons, A., Prather, C., Sutton, M. Y., & McCray, E. (2019). Changes in disparities in estimated HIV incidence rates among black, Hispanic/Latino, and white men who have sex with men (MSM) in the United States, 2010–2015. *JAIDS Journal of Acquired Immune Deficiency Syndromes, 81*(1), 57–62. https://doi.org/10.1097/qai.0000000000001977

Mehra, N., Tunje, A., Hallström, I. K., & Jerene, D. (2021). Effectiveness of mobile phone text message reminder interventions to improve adherence to antiretroviral therapy among adolescents living with HIV: A systematic review and meta-analysis. *PLoS One, 16*(7), e0254890. https://doi.org/10.1371/journal.pone.0254890

Meites, E., Kempe, A., & Markowitz, L. E. (2016). Use of a 2-dose schedule for human papillomavirus vaccination—Updated recommendations of the advisory committee on immunization practices. *MMWR. Morbidity and Mortality Weekly Report, 65*(49), 1405–1408. https://doi.org/10.15585/mmwr.mm6549a5

Meyer, S. R., Hardt, S., Brambilla, R., Shukla, S., & Stöckl, H. (2023). Sociological theories to explain intimate partner violence: A systematic review and narrative synthesis. *Trauma Violence Abuse, 25*(3), 15248380231210939. https://doi.org/10.1177/15248380231210939

Michau, L., & Namy, S. (2021). SASA! together: An evolution of the SASA! approach to prevent violence against women. *Eval Program Plann, 86*, 101918. https://doi.org/10.1016/j.evalprogplan.2021.101918

Mumtaz, Z., & Salway, S. (2009). Understanding gendered influences on women's reproductive health in Pakistan: Moving beyond the autonomy paradigm. *Social Science & Medicine, 68*(7), 1349–1356. https://doi.org/10.1016/j.socscimed.2009.01.025

Pandey, M. (2023). Introduction: Combatting gender-based violence: A multi-approach call to action. In M. Pandey (Ed.), *International perspectives on gender-based violence* (pp. 1–11). Springer International Publishing.

Paterson, D. L., Swindells, S., Mohr, J., Brester, M., Vergis, E. N., Squier, C., Wagener, M. M., & Singh, N. (2000). Adherence to protease inhibitor therapy and outcomes in patients with HIV infection. *Ann Intern Med, 133*(1), 21–30. https://doi.org/10.7326/0003-4819-133-1-200007040-00004. Erratum in: *Ann Intern Med* 2002 Feb 5;136(3), 253.

PATH. (2020). Global HPV vaccine introduction overview: Projected and current national introductions, demonstration/pilot projects, gender-neutral vaccination programs, and global HPV vaccine introduction maps (2006–2023). https://media.path.org/documents/Global_Vaccine_Intro_Overview_Slides_Final_PATHwebsite_MAR_2022_qT92Wwh.pdf

Potts, M., & Campbell, M. (2002). The history of contraception. *Gynecology and Obstetrics, 6*(8).

Presler-Marshall, E., Jones, N., Alheiwidi, S., Youssef, S., Hamad, B. A., Odeh, K. B., Baird, S., Oakley, E., Guglielmi, S., & Małachowska, A. (2020). *Exploring the complex drivers of child marriage in humanitarian contexts*. https://www.gage.odi.org/wp-content/uploads/2020/12/Child-marriage-report-final.pdf

Prochaska, J. O., & DiClemente, C. C. (1983). Stages and processes of self-change of smoking: Toward an integrative model of change. *Journal of Consulting and Clinical Psychology, 51*(3), 390–395. https://doi.org/10.1037//0022-006x.51.3.390

Prochaska, J. O., DiClemente, C. C., & Norcross, J. C. (1997). In search of how people change: Applications to addictive behaviors. *The American Psychologist, 47*(9), 1102–1114. https://doi.org/10.1037//0003-066x.47.9.1102

Pulerwitz, J., Gortmaker, S. L., & DeJong, W. (2000). Measuring sexual relationship power in HIV/STD research. *Sex Roles, 42*, 637–660. http://doi.org/10.1023/A:1007051506972

Raising Voices. (2023). *The SASA! story*. https://raisingvoices.org/women/sasa-approach/

Raj, A. (2010). When the mother is a child: The impact of child marriage on the health and human rights of girls. *Archives of Disease in Childhood, 95*(11), 931–935. https://doi.org/10.1136/adc.2009.178707

Reilly, P. R. (2015). Eugenics and involuntary sterilization: 1907–2015. *Annual Review of Genomics and Human Genetics, 16*(1), 351–368. https://doi.org/10.1146/annurev-genom-090314-024930

Reiss, F. (2021). Child marriage in the United States: Prevalence and implications. *Journal of Adolescent Health, 69*(6S), S8–S10. https://doi.org/10.1016/j.jadohealth.2021.07.001

Robinson, W. C., & Ross, J. A. (2007). *The global family planning revolution: Three decades of population policies and programs*. World Bank Publications.

Sabin, L. L., DeSilva, M. B., Gill, C. J., Zhong, L., Vian, T., Xie, W., Cheng, F., Xu, K., Lan, G., Haberer, J. E., Bangsberg, D. R., Li, Y., Lu, H., & Gifford, A. L. (2015). Improving adherence to antiretroviral therapy with triggered real-time text message reminders: The China adherence through technology study. *JAIDS Journal of Acquired Immune Deficiency Syndromes, 69*(5), 551–559. https://doi.org/10.1097/qai.0000000000000651

Sardinha, L., Maheu-Giroux, M., Stöckl, H., Meyer, S. R., & García-Moreno, C. (2022). Global, regional, and national prevalence estimates of physical or sexual, or both, intimate partner violence against women in 2018. *The Lancet, 399*(10327), 803–813. https://doi.org/10.1016/s0140-6736(21)02664-7

Senderowicz, L. (2020). Contraceptive autonomy: Conceptions and measurement of a novel family planning indicator. *Studies in Family Planning, 51*(2), 161–176. https://doi.org/10.1111/sifp.12114

Sharma, S., Kc, B., & Khatri, A. (2018). Factors influencing male participation in reproductive health: A qualitative study. *Journal of Multidisciplinary Healthcare, 11*, 601–608. https://doi.org/10.2147/jmdh.s176267

Shattuck, D., Kerner, B., Gilles, K., Hartmann, M., Ng'ombe, T., & Guest, G. (2011). Encouraging contraceptive uptake by motivating men to communicate about family planning: The malawi male motivator project. *American Journal of Public Health, 101*(6), 1089–1095. https://doi.org/10.2105/ajph.2010.300091

Sidibé, M., Loures, L., & Samb, B. (2016). The UNAIDS 90–90–90 target: A clear choice for ending AIDS and for sustainable health and development. *Journal of the International AIDS Society, 19*(1), 21133. https://doi.org/10.7448/IAS.19.1.21133

Singh, D., Vignat, J., Lorenzoni, V., Eslahi, M., Ginsburg, O., Lauby-Secretan, B., Arbyn, M., Basu, P., Bray, F., & Vaccarella, S. (2023). Global estimates of incidence and mortality of cervical cancer in 2020: A baseline analysis of the WHO global cervical cancer elimination initiative. *The Lancet Global Health, 11*(2), e197–e206. https://doi.org/10.1016/s2214-109x(22)00501-0

Small, W., Jr., Bacon, M. A., Bajaj, A., Chuang, L. T., Fisher, B. J., Harkenrider, M. M., Jhingran, A., Kitchener, H. C., Mileshkin, L. R., Viswanathan, A. N., & Gaffney, D. K. (2017). Cervical cancer: A global health crisis. *Cancer, 123*(13), 2404–2412. https://doi.org/10.1002/cncr.30667

Smith, J. S., Melendy, A., Rana, R. K., & Pimenta, J. M. (2008). Age-specific prevalence of infection with human papillomavirus in females: A global review. *Journal of Adolescent Health, 43*(Suppl. 4), S5.e1–S5. e62. https://doi.org/10.1016/j.jadohealth.2008.07.009

Solo, J., & Festin, M. (2019). Provider bias in family planning services: A review of its meaning and manifestations. *Global Health: Science and Practice, 7*(3), 371–385. https://doi.org/10.9745/GHSP-D-19-00130

Starrs, A. M., Ezeh, A. C., Barker, G., Basu, A., Bertrand, J. T., Blum, R., Coll-Seck, A. M., Grover, A., Laski, L., Roa, M., Sathar, Z. A., Say, L., Serour, G. I., Singh, S., Stenberg, K., Temmerman, M., Biddlecom, A., Popinchalk, A., Summers, C., & Ashford, L. S. (2018). Accelerate progress—sexual and reproductive health and rights for all: Report of the Guttmacher–Lancet Commission. *The Lancet, 391*(10140), 2642–2692. https://doi.org/10.1016/s0140-6736(18)30293-9

Sternberg, P., & Hubley, J. (2004). Evaluating men's involvement as a strategy in sexual and reproductive health promotion. *Health Promotion International, 19*(3), 389–396. https://doi.org/10.1093/heapro/dah312

Stover, J. (1998). Revising the proximate determinants of fertility framework: What have we learned in the past 20 years? *Studies in Family Planning, 29*(3), 255–267.

Strategies for Management of Antiretroviral Therapy Study Group. (2006). CD4+ count–guided interruption of antiretroviral treatment. *New England Journal of Medicine, 355*(22), 2283–2296. https://doi.org/10.1056/nejmoa062360

Tenkorang, E. Y. (2019). Explaining the links between child marriage and intimate partner violence: Evidence from Ghana. *Child Abuse & Neglect, 89*, 48–57. https://doi.org/10.1016/j.chiabu.2019.01.004

UNICEF. (2020). *Human papillomavirus vaccine: Supply and demand update*. https://www.unicef.org/supply/media/5406/file/Human-Papillomavirus-Vaccine-Market-Update-October2020.pdf

United Nations Office on Drugs and Crime. (2021). *Killings of women and girls by their intimate partner or other family members*. https://www.unodc.org/documents/data-and-analysis/statistics/crime/UN_BriefFem_251121.pdf

United Nations Population Fund. (2020). *Sexual and reproductive health and reproductive rights country profil*. https://www.unfpa.org/resources/sexual-and-reproductive-health-and-reproductive-rights-country-profile

US Agency for International Development. (2023). *Voluntary medical male circumcision*. https://www.usaid.gov/global-health/health-areas/hiv-and-aids/technical-areas/accelerating-scale-voluntary-medical-male

Wang, C. (2012). History of the Chinese family planning program: 1970–2010. *Contraception, 85*(6), 563–569. https://doi.org/10.1016/j.contraception.2011.10.013

Whiteley, L. B., Olsen, E. M., Haubrick, K. K., Odoom, E., Tarantino, N., & Brown, L. K. (2021). A review of interventions to enhance HIV medication adherence. *Current HIV/AIDS Reports, 18*(5), 443–457. https://doi.org/10.1007/s11904-021-00568-9

Whiting, W., Pharr, J. R., Buttner, M. P., & Lough, N. L. (2019). Behavioral interventions to increase condom use among college students in the United States: A systematic review. *Health Education & Behavior, 46*(5), 877–888. https://doi.org/10.1177/1090198119853008

World Health Organization. (1995). *Constitution of the world health organization.* https://apps.who.int/gb/gov/assets/constitution-en.pdf

World Health Organization. (2022). Human papillomavirus vaccines: WHO position paper (2022 update). *Weekly Epidemiological Record, 97*(50), 645–672.

Yaya, S., Uthman, O. A., Ekholuenetale, M., & Bishwajit, G. (2018). Women empowerment as an enabling factor of contraceptive use in sub-Saharan Africa: A multilevel analysis of cross-sectional surveys of 32 countries. *Reproductive Health, 15*(1), 1–12. https://doi.org/10.1186/s12978-018-0658-5

Zimet, G. D., & Rosenthal, S. L. (2010). HPV vaccine and males: Issues and challenges. *Gynecologic Oncology, 117*(Suppl. 2), S26–S31. https://doi.org/10.1016/j.ygyno.2010.01.028

CHAPTER 12

BEHAVIOR CHANGE APPROACHES TO PREVENTING UNINTENTIONAL INJURIES

DAVID A. SLEET AND ANDREA C. GIELEN

LEARNING OBJECTIVES

- Describe the public health burden of unintentional injuries in the United States.
- Explain how the burden of injury differs by social and demographic characteristics.
- Identify examples of successful efforts to reduce injuries.
- Describe the difference between an injury and an accident.
- Explore the application of behavioral science theory and models to injury prevention.
- Describe future innovations and challenges in injury prevention research and how their applications can contribute to health behavior change.

INTRODUCTION

In 1966, a historic publication from the National Research Council defined injury as the "Disease of Modern Society" (National Research Council, 1966). Even today, injury ranks as one of the nation's most pressing health problems, causing more years of potential life lost than a disease and has remained as the leading cause of death in young people for decades (Centers for Disease Control and Prevention [CDC], 2021b).

Injuries result from different types of events: accidental or intentional. Whereas the word *accident* implies an unexpected and often random event (Girasek, 2023), the word *injury* refers to the medical consequences of the event. Injuries are caused by acute exposure to (and release of) energy in amounts that exceed human tolerance, such as the kinetic energy released in a car crash or a fall, or exposure to excessive heat or cold, electricity, or ionizing radiation. It may also be caused by the sudden absence of essentials, such as heat in the case of hypothermia, or oxygen in the case of drowning or suffocation (Institute of Medicine, Committee on Trauma Research [IOM], 1985). Injury may be either unintentional—in the case of a fall, motor vehicle crash, drowning, suffocation, poisoning (including drug overdose and carbon monoxide exposure), fire and burns, or sports and recreation-related injuries—or they may be intentional and deliberate, as in the case of assault, sexual violence, abuse, homicide, self-harm, or suicide. This chapter focuses on unintentional injuries.

12 • BEHAVIOR CHANGE APPROACHES TO PREVENTING UNINTENTIONAL INJURIES 237

The use of behavioral and social science theories and methods in injury prevention has not developed on pace with their use in disease prevention and health promotion, yet their application to preventing unintentional injury is equally important. Unintentional injuries are largely predictable and preventable when using evidence-based prevention measures. Behavioral, psychosocial, and sociocultural factors are known contributors to injuries and can be modified using sound theoretical frameworks. While structural and environmental approaches have traditionally been associated with the greatest potential to prevent injuries, it is rarely feasible to achieve injury reduction without some element of behavior change. For practitioners, the use of behavioral theory can both improve the effectiveness of interventions and accelerate the diffusion process. Much can be done to address the behavioral and psychosocial factors that give rise to injury—whether it be by reducing behavioral risk factors to implementing behavioral interventions. Ecological approaches that consider the dynamic interaction between behavior and the environment hold the most promise for reducing injury.

The CDC's National Center for Injury Prevention and Control, the lead federal agency for nonoccupational injury, has a mission to prevent injuries through science and action with a focus on improving lives by stopping injuries before they happen (Sleet et al., 2012). In this context, the disciplines of social and behavioral science (including human factors), epidemiology, biomechanics, environmental sciences, and others, are key elements of prevention. Maximum impact requires coordinated efforts among these specialties.

Psychologists often limit their involvement in injury and trauma to the postinjury phase of assessment, treatment, and rehabilitation, and neglect psychology's role in prevention (Agarwal et al, 2020; Hickling & Blanchard, 2000; Spielberger & Frank, 1992). However, for decades, the discipline of psychology and the social and behavioral sciences have generally made important contributions to the prevention of injuries for decades (Frank et al., 1992; Gibson, 1964; Margolis & Kroes, 1975; O'Brien et al., 2019; Roberts et al., 1987; Sleet & Hopkins, 2004;). Behavioral and social sciences are needed in efforts to document behavioral and social risk factors, and to develop interventions that influence social norms and shape individual and community preventive behaviors (Gielen et al., 2012; Hilliard et al., 2018; Sleet et al., 2004). As DiLillo et al. (2002) notes " . . . more people are beginning to recognize that, for injury control to be effective, behavior must change among some groups, such as children, parents, legislators, manufacturers, and educators. Furthermore, many of the constructs with which psychologists are most conversant (e.g. motivation, perception, learning) are thought by many to be the key determinants of injury-related behaviors. . ." (p. 565).

PUBLIC HEALTH BURDEN OF UNINTENTIONAL INJURIES

The health burden of injury is felt by all Americans, regardless of their age or demographic characteristics. Americans under age 45 die more frequently from injuries than from any other cause, including heart disease and cancer. Additionally, the annual number of total deaths due to unintentional injury among those under 45 years rose steeply between 2019 and 2021, from 63,000 to 89,700. This is compared with approximately 24,000 deaths each in 2021 due to the next two leading causes of death—suicide and COVID-19—among this age group (CDC, 2023).

Unintentional injuries are both costly and preventable. Using data from the CDC's Web-Based Injury Statistics Query and Reporting System, researchers estimate that the U.S. economic cost of injuries topped $4 trillion in 2019, with more than half of this cost ($2.4 trillion) occurring among adults of working ages between 25 and 64 years (Peterson et al., 2021). In addition to being costly, nonfatal injuries often result in lifelong disabilities, chronic pain, and dramatic changes in an individual's lifestyle, including the ability to be gainfully employed. These costs and public health burdens highlight the primary importance of understanding and preventing injury as a public health priority (CDC, 2021a).

Fatal Injuries

In 2021, unintentional injuries were the fourth leading cause of death in the United States, behind heart disease, cancers, and COVID-19, accounting for around 6% of all deaths. An estimated 224,935 people died from unintentional injuries at a crude rate of 67.8 per 100,000 population. The highest death rates from unintentional injuries were found among older adults. There were more unintentional injury deaths that year than there were from influenza and pneumonia, respiratory diseases, diabetes, and hypertension, making unintentional injuries a significant public health problem (CDC WONDER, 2021). Unintentional injuries figure prominently as one of the 10 leading causes in every age group. Groups at the highest risk are children, adolescents, and young adults (**Figure 12.1**).

In 2020, unintentional injuries were also a leading cause of years of potential life lost before age 65, meaning more than any other cause of death these injuries led to the largest decreases in the average number of years that people could have lived (**Figure 12.2**).

Nonfatal Injuries

Deaths are only the tip of the iceberg when it comes to unintentional injury burdens. In 2021, there were over 23 million visits to the ED for unintentional injuries (age-adjusted rate = 7,063; Cairns & Kang, 2021; CDC, 2021b) and 24.8 million visits to a physician's office in 2018 for an unintentional injury (Santo & Okeyode, 2018).

	≤1	1–4	5–9	10–14	15–24	25–34	35–44	45–54	55–64	65+	All Ages
1	Congenital Anomalies 3,963	Unintentional Injury 1,299	Unintentional Injury 827	Unintentional Injury 915	Unintentional Injury 15,792	Unintentional Injury 34,452	Unintentional Injury 36,444	Covid-19 36,881	Malignant Neoplasms 108,023	Heart Disease 553,214	Heart Disease 695,547
2	Short Gestation 2,946	Congenital Anomalies 412	Malignant Neoplasms 347	Suicide 598	Homicide 6,635	Suicide 8,862	Covid-19 16,006	Heart Disease 34,535	Heart Disease 89,342	Malignant Neoplasms 446,354	Malignant Neoplasms 605,213
3	Sids 1,459	Homicide 309	Homicide 188	Malignant Neoplasms 449	Suicide 6,528	Homicide 7,571	Heart Disease 12,754	Malignant Neoplasms 33,567	Covid-19 73,725	Covid-19 282,457	Covid-19 416,893
4	Unintentional Injury 1,306	Malignant Neoplasms 282	Congenital Anomalies 171	Homicide 298	Covid-19 1,401	Covid-19 6,133	Malignant Neoplasms 11,194	Unintentional Injury 31,407	Unintentional Injury 33,471	Cerebrovascular 139,257	Unintentional Injury 224,935
5	Maternal Pregnancy Comp. 1,113	Heart Disease 116	Heart Disease 66	Congenital Anomalies 179	Malignant Neoplasms 1,323	Heart Disease 4,155	Suicide 7,862	Liver Disease 10,501	Diabetes Mellitus 18,603	Chronic Low. Respiratory Disease 120,152	Cerebrovascular 162,890
6	Placenta Cord Membranes 672	Perinatal Period 68	Covid-19 63	Heart Disease 132	Heart Disease 944	Malignant Neoplasms 3,615	Liver Disease 5,833	Diabetes Mellitus 7,597	Liver Disease 17,664	Alzheimer's Disease 117,922	Chronic Low. Respiratory Disease 142,342
7	Bacterial Sepsis 557	Cerebrovascular 55	Chronic Low. Respiratory Disease 54	Covid-19 79	Congenital Anomalies 419	Liver Disease 1,833	Homicide 4,863	Suicide 7,401	Chronic Low. Respiratory Disease 17,620	Diabetes Mellitus 72,451	Alzheimer's Disease 119,399
8	Respiratory Distress 414	Covid-19 54	Cerebrovascular 35	Cerebrovascular 53	Diabetes Mellitus 345	Diabetes Mellitus 1,285	Diabetes Mellitus 2,961	Cerebrovascular 5,755	Cerebrovascular 14,634	Unintentional Injury 69,003	Diabetes Mellitus 103,294
9	Circulatory System Disease 402	Influenza & Pneumonia 47	Septicemia 28	Chronic Low. Respiratory Disease 45	Complicated Pregnancy 214	Complicated Pregnancy 797	Cerebrovascular 2,189	Chronic Low. Respiratory Disease 3,174	Suicide 7,267	Nephritis 44,013	Liver Disease 56,585
10	Intrauterine Hypoxia 358	Benign Neoplasms 37	Influenza & Pneumonia 27	Diabetes Mellitus 39	Cerebrovascular 190	Cerebrovascular 624	Septicemia 1,108	Homicide 2,768	Septicemia 6,477	Parkinson's Disease 37,568	Nephritis 54,358

FIGURE 12.1 Ten leading causes of death, by age group, race/ethnicity, and sex, United States, 2021.

Source: From Centers for Disease Control and Prevention, National Center for Injury Prevention and Control. (2024). *Web-based Injury Statistics Query and Reporting System (WISQARS)* [online]) [2024 JAN 31]. Available from www.wisqars.cdc.gov

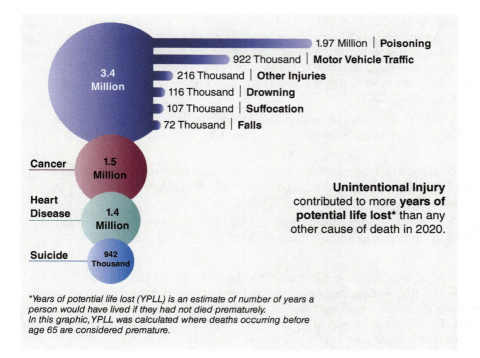

FIGURE 12.2 Years of potential life lost due to the four leading causes of death in the United States, 2020.
Source: Adapted from 2020 NCHS Vital Statistics System produced by CDC WISQARS (www.cdc.gov/injury/wisqars/fatal.html).

INJURY DISPARITIES

The Latin origin of the word *injury* is *iniuria*, which refers to a wrong or an injustice. The Latin word for *disparity* is *disparitatem* (nominative *disparitas*) or *not equal* (from *dis-* "not" + *paritas* "parity"). It is well-known that injuries are disparate and not distributed evenly throughout the population. Children, adolescents, males, older adults, people living in poverty, certain racial and ethnic groups, and people with lower socioeconomic status are at elevated risk of injury (Moore et al., 2019). Injury epidemiology, particularly when practiced in a frame that includes the social determinants of health, can be an important tool to help explain these variations, identify groups at higher risk for injury, and focus the implementation of specific interventions within an ethical framework to reduce the burden (Ameratunga et al., 2019).

- *Age:* Unintentional injury death rates vary by age, with the lowest rate among those 5 to 14 years old (3.8 per 100,000 population in 2020) and the highest rate among those 75 years of age and older (191.2 per 100,000 population; CDC, 2021b). Traffic injuries are the leading cause of death for children and adolescents in the United States (Mokdad et al, 2020).
- *Sex:* Males are 2.3 times more likely to die from an unintentional injury than females (age-adjusted death rates: 80.4 vs. 35.6, respectively; CDC, 2021b). Females in traffic crashes are 73% more likely to suffer serious injury and 9% to 28% more likely to die in a crash than men. The main culprit for these discrepancies is thought to be outdated crash (dummy) test standards, which do not accurately reflect female bodies (VERITY Now, 2023).
- *Race and ethnicity:* Unintentional injury death rates also vary by race and ethnicity. The highest death rates are among people who are non-Latinx Native

American and Alaska Natives (99.8) and non-Latinx Black (66.9), while non-Latinx Asian Americans and Latinx people of all other races have the lowest rates (18.2 and 41.2, respectively; CDC, 2021b). Disparities by race and ethnicity may also vary by specific injury cause. For example, suicide death rates are highest among non-Latinx Native American and Alaska Natives (23.9) and non-Latinx Whites (16.8; CDC, 2021b).

- *Urbanization level:* Death rates for unintentional injuries in nonmetro areas are 1.2 times higher than rates in metro areas (68.8 vs. 55.7, respectively; CDC, 2021b).

- *Community-level poverty:* Unintentional injury death rates for counties with >20% poverty are 79% higher compared with counties with <5% poverty, and this gap has been widening over time (Karb et al., 2016).

- *Disability:* The risk of unintentional injury is two to three times higher among youth with a disability than among those with no disability (Francescutti et al., 2019).

More research is needed to better understand the key drivers of these disparities and how policy and tailored prevention strategies can be used to address injury and lessen the gap in injury burden by these social and demographic factors (Ameratunga et al., 2019; Nesbit et al., 2022). These efforts to elevate science-based equity research should conform to the latest best practices for health equity science in public health as outlined by Burton et al. (2024).

PREVENTING INJURIES: APPLYING THEORIES FROM BEHAVIORAL SCIENCE

The development and applications of sound theory are critical to intervention planning and implementation in injury prevention (Gielen & Sleet, 2003). Over 20 years ago, Smedley and Syme (2000) declared in an Institute of Medicine report that "[p]erhaps the most significant contribution of behavioral and social sciences to health research is the development of strong theoretical models for interventions" (p. 9).

Behavioral theory is relevant to a wide variety of injury topics, such as installing and maintaining working smoke alarms; reducing occupational injuries; preventing falls and sports injuries; reducing fires, burns, and scalds; improving road safety; or reducing child injuries (Guerin & Sleet, 2020; Lakhan et al., 2020; McGlashan, & Finch, 2010; Schwebel et al, 2014; Sleet & Dellinger, 2020; Vankov, 2021).

Theories and models are being used in injury prevention with increasing frequency, including theories such as the theory of planned behavior, the social cognitive theory, the social learning theory, and the theory of reasoned action, among others. Models such as the social ecological model, the PRECEDE-PROCEED model, the health belief model, the transtheoretical model (stages of change), and others are applied to many injury problems (Allegrante et al., 2006; Gielen et al., 2014). Some of the most widely used models and theories in unintentional injury prevention include the PRECEDE-PROCEED model, the theory of planned behavior, and the health belief model (Gabriel et al., 2019; Lakhan et al., 2020; McGlashan & Finch, 2010; Trifiletti et al., 2005).

Theories can help us understand behavioral determinants and can uncover underlying principles about how people change behaviors and how changing environments, both physical and social, play an important role in the process (Michielsen et al., 2012). The interventions that drive these improvements may not only change behavior but may also change environments in ways that predispose and reinforce safe behaviors (Sleet et al., 2013). The use of behavioral theory can improve and speed up this process. For these reasons, injury prevention efforts based on theory are more likely to succeed than those developed without it.

In implementing efforts to change high-risk behaviors, the temptation is to recite facts, prescribe needed change, and emphasize changes in behavior that will lead to improvements in health and reductions in injury. On the surface, this is a sensible approach; however, education alone is often not enough to change behavior. The underlying assumption is that when individuals are provided sound advice, they will act on the advice, but reality is not that straightforward. Peterson and Roberts (1992) made the point that "[t]hose interventions that attempt behavior change at a population wide level through simple provision of information with weak contingencies between behavior and potential reward seem doomed to failure. On the other hand, those interventions that yield clear, positive consequences for the involved participants, provide individualized attention, and mandate the opportunity to rehearse and receive feedback on the desired behavior are the most successful" (p. 1043).

CASE STUDY 12.1: EDUCATION FOR BEHAVIOR CHANGE: SPEEDING BEHAVIOR

A report by Brainbox Research and the University of Leeds in the United Kingdom on the components of interventions that are most likely to change drivers' speeding behavior led to the conclusion that theory-based interventions can be successfully used to prevent or reduce driver speeding (Fylan et al, 2006). They concluded that several intervention approaches map onto models of health-related behaviors that could be applied to reducing driver speeding, including the following:

- *Information and education* (cognitive strategies) are included in a number of speeding interventions, including facts about speeding risks and hazard perception. Labeling is used in some interventions, such as labeling 35 mph as the "killing speed."

- *Enforcement messages* that focus on the consequences of speeding (e.g., fines, speed cameras) are often used and may include presentations by police officers.

- *Instruction, modeling, and skill rehearsal* are practical ways to increase driving competency and involve driving sessions with an instructor that focus on situations where maintaining the speed limit can be difficult.

- *Attitudes* are often targeted to focus on participants' perceptions of the acceptability of speeding.

- *Framing* is focused on the negative outcomes of speeding and may include a talk from a paramedic who has attended a roadside collision, a victim, or a relative of someone who has died.

- *Barriers* are tackled by interventions that focus on the excuses provided by individuals regarding their speeding behavior (e.g., "I didn't see a speed limit sign").

- *Attributions* are targeted by interventions that focus on responsibility awareness, for example, awareness that the driver is responsible for the speed at which they drive.

- *Reminders* are provided by some of the speed interventions in the form of booklets or small gifts mailed that serve as reminders after their attendance in a course on speeding.

No studies were identified that expressly compared the effectiveness of different theoretical approaches to reducing speeding. The reviews did provide evidence that effective interventions should target the following:

- Attitudes (beliefs and values) toward speeding

- Assessing drivers' readiness to change and increasing motivation not to speed

- Beliefs about the acceptability and ubiquity of speeding (norms)

- Perceptions of responsibility for each driver's choice of speed (attributions)

(continued)

CASE STUDY 12.1: EDUCATION FOR BEHAVIOR CHANGE: SPEEDING BEHAVIOR (*continued*)

- Perceptions of the benefits of speeding (response costs)
- Perceptions of the likelihood of drivers being detected if they speed (susceptibility)
- Negative consequences of crashing or being caught speeding (anticipated regret)
- Perceived barriers to driving at an appropriate speed (perceived behavioral control)
- Drivers' perceptions of their ability to drive at an appropriate speed (self-efficacy)
- When and where drivers will reduce their speed (implementation intentions)

The reviews indicated that self-efficacy (and perceived behavioral control) may be a particularly important target because of its strong association with behavior and the fact that there is good evidence about how to intervene effectively. Persuasive messages should be paired with strategies that promote elaboration (e.g., group discussion), and there should be interactive sessions on joint problem-solving to help individuals identify and adhere to appropriate speeds.

While educating the public about preventing unintentional injuries may reinforce safer behaviors, other social, ecological, and individual factors clearly shape behaviors as well (Mack et al., 2015). To be effective, interventions to prevent injuries should consider people's motives, cultural context, lifestyle, and specific needs—in an ecological context (Allegrante et al., 2006; Mercy et al., 2007). According to Fishbein (2006) ". . . even more than most behavioral scientists, injury prevention scientists have taken an ecological perspective that has led them to pay important attention to the interaction between people and their environment" (p. x). This emphasis (sometimes referred to as "reciprocal determinism" by behavioral scientists) has had a major effect on our thinking about the causes and prevention of injuries. For example, to reduce drinking and driving, policies that increase enforcement, reduce permissible blood alcohol levels, reduce alcohol outlet density, and change social norms, attitudes, and beliefs around drinking and driving will, together, support efforts to change individual and population behaviors (National Academies of Sciences, Engineering, and Medicine [NAS], 2018).

Ecological Models

Unintentional injuries are frequently multicausal. While legislation has been an important tool in preventing injuries, it is usually insufficient when behaviors are involved or causally related. For example, passenger safety legislation has saved many lives, but only because parents were educated about the mandate and learned how to install and use car seats correctly. Legislation can be important in incentivizing safe behaviors, such as driving without distractions, obeying legal speed limits, changing batteries in smoke alarms, or closing and locking gates to four-sided residential swimming pools—but only if the public is educated and willing to comply. These are examples of the need for ecological approaches that consider the interaction between behavior and the policy environment (Sleet & Gielen, 2015).

CASE STUDY 12.2: LEGISLATION FOR BEHAVIOR CHANGE: ALCOHOL-IMPAIRED DRIVING

On average, from 2012 to 2021, about 10,850 people died every year in drunk-driving crashes. In every state, it is illegal to drive with a blood alcohol content (BAC) at or above 0.08%, yet one person was killed in an alcohol-related crash every 39 minutes in the United States in 2021.

(continued)

CASE STUDY 12.2: LEGISLATION FOR BEHAVIOR CHANGE: ALCOHOL-IMPAIRED DRIVING (*continued*)

The BAC has a direct and dose—response effect on driving performance. In 1950, many states set their BAC standard at 0.15%. By the 1960s, states began lowering their BAC limit from 0.15% to 0.10% as scientific evidence mounted on the relationship between drivers' BAC and fatal crashes. It was not until 1980 that the first state, Utah, lowered its limit to 0.08%.

By 1992, the National Highway Traffic Safety Administration had proposed that all states adopt 0.08% BAC laws, and in 1998 a legislative proposal was introduced in Congress that would have required states to enact and enforce 0.08% BAC laws or face cuts in highway funding. The proposal failed, and instead grants were offered to states that lowered their BAC limits to 0.08%, but only three states did so. At the time, there were only four published studies that demonstrated the effectiveness of 0.08% BAC laws in reducing traffic fatalities.

Subsequently, the CDC and the Community Preventive Services Task Force conducted a systematic review of the effectiveness of 0.08% BAC laws. The results demonstrated a median of 7% decline in fatalities in states with 0.08% BAC laws, estimating that if all states had 0.08% BAC laws, 400 to 600 lives could be saved annually. The Task Force concluded that 0.08% BAC laws were effective in reducing alcohol-related traffic fatalities and recommended enactment of these laws based on strong evidence. Shortly afterward, a 0.08% BAC bill was approved and subsequently signed into law on October 23, 2000. It included cuts in highway funds for states without 0.08% BAC laws (Sleet et al., 2011).

By 2004, all U.S. states had enacted 0.08% BAC legislation. Changes in behavior and the impact on reduced fatalities were not realized until several years later. Self-reported episodes of drinking and driving declined from 161 million per year in 2006 to 112 million in 2010. Death rates from alcohol-impaired driving showed similar declines, with steep reductions since 2005.

Similar efforts are currently underway to reduce driver BACs even further—to 0.05%. Utah became the first state to enact 0.05% BAC legislation in 2017. Evaluation of its impact in 2019 showed a 20% decline in Utah's fatal crash rate. Of the drinkers, 22% indicated they had changed their behaviors once the law went into effect. The most common behavior change reported was making sure transportation was available when drinking away from home (Thomas et al., 2022).

Behavior change is still necessary even when structural changes or policies and legislation are in place (Allegrante et al., 2006). Mack et al. (2015) point out that we can study the influence of cultural norms, socialization, social capital, concentration of poverty, and economic inequalities on injury and its prevention—independent of individual risk and protective factors. However, they go on to say "we must also be cognizant of the potential that structural and environmental change in the lower tiers of the Health Impact Pyramid may ignore or de-empower individuals and communities" (p. 119S), and they cite Lieberman et al. (2013, p. 522) as saying "efforts to tweak physical, social, economic, or political conditions in order to produce behavior change, without the active engagement of the individual affected, reflect a decision to prioritize certain choices over others."

To help reduce the gap between policy and behavior using behavioral economics strategies, the National Academy of Sciences' recent book, *Behavioral Economics: Policy Impact and Future Directions* (NAS, 2023), presents evidence of how behavioral economics is being used effectively in areas of health promotion, such as smoking and HIV prevention. Focusing on ways of making the preferred alternatives easy, attractive, aligned with social norms, and providing timely feedback can potentially be important features of approaches to encourage healthier behaviors (Hallsworth & Kirkman, 2020), potentially including injury-related

Social Norms

"Where there is behavior, there are social norms" (Bicchieri et al, 2023, p. A4). Social norms can have positive or negative effects on injury-related behavior. *Social norms* are defined as those values, beliefs, attitudes, and behaviors shared by a group of people or a population. Norms are what most people value, believe, and do. Positive social norms can establish an expectation and acceptance of attitudes, behaviors, programs, and policies that affect injuries. Momentum for behavior change grows when more people recognize that the norms in the community and of people around them support injury prevention.

Perceptions of injury-related norms can also be strong predictors of behavior. Research has shown that perceived norms influence a wide variety of injury-related behaviors, including high-risk drinking (Neighbors et al., 2004), impaired driving (Perkins et al., 2010), bullying (Perkins et al., 2011), and the use of sunscreen (Kulik et al., 2008). Focusing on the problem of dangerous driving, Shaer (2024) points out that "bad driving behavior tends to be contagious –the more of it we come in regular contact with the more likely we are to drive badly ourselves, and the more likely we are to accept bad driving as the status quo" (the norm).

Several psychosocial theories predicting individual behavior recognize that perceived norms can influence the decisions of individuals and groups (Bicchieri et al., 2023). Promoting positive community norms to support safety behaviors includes correcting misperceptions of norms. Normative misperceptions can influence a wide variety of both risk and protective factors. Promoting positive community norms that support injury prevention requires an understanding of the roles of accurate perceptions and inaccurate misperceptions of norms on behavior (Schultz et al., 2007). A critical analysis of social norms affecting health-related behavior can be found in Dempsey et al. (2018).

Another approach that is gaining support in the traffic safety community is the concept of "safety culture" (Jared, 2024). As states and localities struggle with ways to reduce traffic fatalities, greater attention is being given to cultural factors related to communication, collaboration, leveraging resources, and applying a systemic approach to traffic safety. The approach is rooted in a change in the "culture" of road users and traffic safety agencies. "This change in culture is tied to education, engineering, enforcement, and emergency services . . . the goal is to develop a process for changing values and attitudes so that safety is part of every transportation decision, individual or organizational, for all users of the roadway transportation system" (Jared, 2024, p. ix). The claim is that promoting a positive traffic safety culture would support traffic safety goals by reducing risky behaviors and increasing protective behaviors.

CASE STUDY 12.3: HEALTH COMMUNICATIONS FOR BEHAVIOR CHANGE: SUNSMART

Australia has one of the highest rates of skin cancer in the world. Each year over 2,000 Australians die from skin cancer. More than two in three Australians will be diagnosed with skin cancer in their lifetime and it can be almost entirely prevented with good sun protection.

Established in 1988, SunSmart is one of the longest running—and most successful—skin cancer prevention programs in the world. Their work has resulted in melanoma rates declining or stabilizing in all age groups under 60 in Victoria, Australia.

The SunSmart program is dedicated to reducing skin cancer incidence, morbidity, and mortality through a targeted health communication/prevention and early detection

(continued)

CASE STUDY 12.3: HEALTH COMMUNICATIONS FOR BEHAVIOR CHANGE: SUNSMART (*continued*)

program. They use a combination of grassroots tactics, mass media campaigns, health communications, and advocacy to influence skin cancer knowledge, attitudes, and behaviors in sun protection. Programs operate in each state and territory of Australia.

SunSmart is supported by the Centre for Behavioural Research in Cancer (CBRC), whose mission is research and evaluation focusing on finding the best ways to prevent or reduce behaviors that increase cancer risk.

The SunSmart campaigns (SunSmart, 2017) have resulted in changes to sun protection-related behaviors, social norms, and health outcomes, including the following:

- Significant improvements in sun-protective behaviors were seen at a population level, such as using sunscreen and hats.

- It is estimated to have prevented more than 43,000 skin cancers and 1,400 deaths from the disease in Victoria between 1988 and 2011.

- While melanoma incidence in Victoria continues to rise, incidence rates in Victorians younger than 60 years are now stabilizing or falling, consistent with the positive effect of the SunSmart program on behavior change.

- In contrast to the pre-SunSmart "baby boomers," the number of basal and squamous cell carcinoma skin cancer treatments among those aged under 45 years is also decreasing relative to population growth.

- SunSmart is extremely cost-effective, with a $2.22 return for every dollar spent in the program in Victoria, Australia.

- A related impact was that Victoria was one of the first states in Australia to legislate solariums in 2008 and ban commercial solariums entirely in 2015.

Integrative Models

Health behavior change theory and its application can often benefit from a focus on integrative models that examine the interplay of individual, interpersonal, social, cultural, and environmental factors (Gielen & Girasek, 2001; Sleet & Dellinger, 2020). A theorists' workshop at the National Institutes of Health (NIH) in 1991 (Fishbein et al., 1991) brought together creators of behavioral theory to develop a unifying framework to facilitate health behavior change. Their discussions led to the enumeration of five theories that, taken together, contain virtually all the variables that have been used in attempts to understand and change human behaviors: the health belief model, the social cognitive theory, the theory of reasoned action, the theory of self-regulation and self-control (Kanfer & Kanfer, 1991), and the theory of subjective culture and interpersonal relations (Triandis, 1980).

Considering all five theories and their many variables, eight variables appear to account for most of the variations in health-related behaviors: (a) intentions, (b) environmental barriers, (c) skills, (d) outcome expectancies (or attitude), (e) social norms, (f) self-standards, (g) emotional reactions, and (h) self-efficacy. Likely, these same eight variables might also regulate and predict changes in injury risk behavior (Dr. Martin Fishbein, personal communication, January 23, 2003). Translating this guidance to action, Fishbein et al. (2001) concluded that for a person to perform a given behavior, they must be able to do one or more of the following:

- Form a strong positive intention or make a commitment to perform the behavior

- Have no environmental barriers that make it *impossible* to perform the behavior

246 II • PRIORITIZED BEHAVIORS FOR PRIMARY PREVENTION OF DISEASE

- Possess the skills necessary to perform the behavior
- Believe that the advantages of the behavior outweigh the disadvantages
- Perceive more normative pressure to perform than not to perform the behavior
- Perceive that performance of the behavior is consistent with their self-image or values
- Have an emotional reaction to performing the behavior that is more positive than negative
- Perceive that they have the capabilities to perform the behavior under different circumstances

The first three factors are viewed as necessary and sufficient for producing any behavior, while the remaining five are viewed as modifying variables, influencing the strength and direction of intentions.

By way of a hypothetical example, we can apply these notions to the injury control behavior of testing the functionality of a residential smoke alarm. If a homeowner is committed to testing the smoke alarm every month, has access to the alarms in the home, and has the skills necessary to successfully test the alarm, we would predict that there is a high probability they will perform the behavior. The probability that the individual will test their smoke alarm monthly would be predicted to increase even more if the homeowner also believes that testing is worth the time and trouble, knows that neighbors all test their alarms, believes that testing is consistent with their values as a responsible homeowner, has no negative emotional reaction to testing, and can test the alarms under different conditions in the home. According to this notion, the probability of testing monthly would be predicted to reach nearly 100% under these conditions. In practice, this integrated model has not been applied to this or any other injury-related behavior, but could hold promise as an innovative approach to program development until sufficient research is available to suggest otherwise.

It is encouraging to learn that various attempts are being made to develop new theories, modify existing ones, and tailor applications of theories in developing injury interventions (NAS, 2023; Sleet & Gielen, 2007).

CASE STUDY 12.4: FALL PREVENTION

The CDC produced a pocket guide for healthcare providers that uses the stages of change model to help tailor fall prevention messages for patients based on their readiness to change. The model recognizes that patients will be at different stages of readiness, from the precontemplation stage (not on the patient's radar) to the action stage (ready for change). Tailoring the message to fit the patient's stage will garner the most effective response. For example, a patient in the precontemplation stage may not attend to a message from their provider to optimize their medications to help reduce their risk of falling because they do not see themselves at risk for a fall. Alternatively, a patient who asks about fall prevention strategies is in the action stage and ready for change. Table 12.1 in this case study shows the advice provided in the CDC pocket guide for talking with patients about falls using the stages of change model (Haddad et al., 2018; Sleet & Dellinger, 2020).

The pocket guide and other provider resources from the CDC STEADI (Stopping Elderly Accidents, Deaths, and Injuries) initiative can be found at www.cdc.gov/steadi/materials.html.

(continued)

CASE STUDY 12.4: FALL PREVENTION (*continued*)

TABLE 12.1 Using the Tenets of the Transtheoretical Model (Stages of Change) in a Healthcare Conversation About Preventing Older Adult Falls

If you hear this from a patient:	You can respond with:
PRECONTEMPLATION STAGE	
Falling is just a matter of bad luck.	As we age, falls are more likely for many reasons, including changes in our balance and how we walk.
CONTEMPLATION STAGE	
My friend down the street fell and ended up in a nursing home.	Preventing falls can prevent broken hips and help you stay independent.
PREPARATION STAGE	
I'm worried about falling. Do you think there's anything I can do to keep from falling?	Let's look at some factors that may make you likely to fall and talk about what you could do about one or two of them.
ACTION STAGE	
I know a fall can be serious. What can I do to keep from falling and stay independent?	I'm going to refer you to a specialist who can help you improve your vision, balance, and optimize your medications.

Source: From Centers for Disease Control and Prevention. See the STEADI (Stopping Elderly Accidents, Deaths, and Injuries) brochure at https://www.cdc.gov/steadi/pdf/STEADI-FactSheet-TalkingWPatients-508.pdf.

CONCLUSION

While many people accept unintentional injuries as "part of life," random, or beyond their control, events resulting in injury, death, or disability are often predictable and therefore preventable. It is difficult to prevent all injuries by policy, education, environmental change, product improvements, or technology alone since each has an element that affects any given injury risk and can prompt behavior to change—and they can work synergistically. Each preventive intervention builds on the strength of every other one. As can be seen from other chapters in this book, behavioral interventions have been critical to improving many areas of public health and can also be effectively applied to prevent injuries.

Behavioral interventions can be used to complement structural and environmental approaches but can also be used to facilitate changing the behavior of those who make laws and design products, such as legislators and engineers, in ways that can ultimately protect whole populations. Implementing behavior change strategies may sometimes be the only solution to prevent an injury when environmental, structural, or technological solutions are unavailable, or worse yet when they fail to protect, as in the case of airbag-related deaths to children (CDC, 1995).

In some ways, efforts to prevent injuries face more challenges than efforts to prevent diseases. There are no vaccines, drugs, or treatment protocols to prevent injuries. When injury risks are reduced, patients feel no relief, no reduction in pain, and generally receive no reinforcement when an injury is prevented. Although the behavioral science applications to injury prevention outlined here were modeled mostly from a disease prevention perspective, it remains challenging to identify the right combination of policies, education, environmental change, and technology that will encourage and reward safe behaviors.

Lack of dissemination, implementation failure, and adoption hesitancy are sometimes mentioned as barriers to preventing injuries (Haegerich et al., 2014; Pollack et al., 2010; Sogolow et al., 2007). While products, practices, and programs to prevent injuries exist and can save lives, many people have either not heard about them or have not accepted or adopted them. Individuals may not perceive themselves to be at risk of injury, do not believe the risks are serious or relevant to themselves, or do not have access to affordable safety products or programs that could save their lives. Behavioral scientists can help overcome these barriers. An important contemporary challenge in injury prevention is the need to make the best use of technologies that can prevent injuries at the individual and population levels while mitigating the potentially hazardous effects of technology such as those contributing to distracted driving.

Because of the wide range of injury types, preventive behaviors, and group- and community-related differences in injury, additional research could focus on behavioral risk and protective factors, and the relevance of disparities, and consider the role of developmental factors especially for children and youth. Efficacy and effectiveness trials are needed to establish evidence-based recommendations. We need to ensure that practice informs research, much as research informs practice (CDC, 2014). Training more health researchers, practitioners, and providers in the science of injury prevention is an urgent priority to ensure we are growing and educating the next generation. Furthermore, fostering collaborations with those in behavioral medicine may contribute to efforts to reduce unintentional injuries (Sleet et al., 2010). We believe these are important steps for strengthening the application of behavioral and social science to injury control, which in turn can contribute to changing individual behaviors, environmental conditions, and social structures in ways that protect everyone.

SUMMARY KEY POINTS

- Unintentional injuries contribute substantially to the leading causes of death and years of potential life lost in the United States.
- Injuries are not distributed evenly throughout the population.
- It is rarely feasible to achieve injury reduction without some element of behavior change.
- Theory-based behavioral strategies can be effective in reducing injuries.
- Future injury prevention research can benefit from studying the interaction among environments, products, and human behavior in an ecological framework.

DISCUSSION QUESTIONS

1. What if any social norms around safety have you seen grow or change in your lifetime?

2. What are risk factors for injury in your community? Do you feel like they are being addressed adequately? How could they be addressed more thoroughly?

3. What messages have you heard in your life about alcohol-impaired driving? Have the social norms of your community reflected those messages?

4. What attempts toward behavior change have you seen fail? How could the messaging been more effective?

5. How have unintentional injuries affected your life or the life of your loved ones?

A robust set of instructor resources designed to supplement this text is located at http://connect.springerpub.com/content/book/978-0-8261-4265-8. Qualifying instructors may request access by emailing textbook@springerpub.com.

REFERENCES

Agarwal, T. M., Muneer, M., Asim, M., Awad, M., Afzal, Y., Al-Thani, H., Alhassan, A., Mollazehi, M., & El-Menyar, A. (2020). Psychological trauma in different mechanisms of traumatic injury: A hospital-based cross-sectional study. *PLoS One, 15*(11), e0242849. https://doi.org/10.1371/journal.pone.0242849

Allegrante, J. P., Sleet, D. W., Marks, R., & Hanson, D. W. (2006). Ecological models for the prevention and control of unintentional injury. In A. C. Gielen, D. A. Sleet, & R. DiClemente (Eds.), *Injury and violence prevention: Behavior change theories, methods and applications*. Jossey-Bass.

Ameratunga, S., Jones, M., & Blank, D. (2019). Preventing unintentional injuries: Ethical considerations in public health. In A. Mastroianni, J. P. Kahn, & N. E. Kass (Eds.), *The Oxford handbook of public health ethics*. Oxford University Press. ISBN-13:9780190245191.

Bicchieri, C., Dimant, E., Gelfand, M., & Sonderegger, S. (2023). Social norms and behavior change. *The Interdisciplinary Research Frontier, 205*, A4–A7. http://doi.org/10.1016/j.jebo.2022.11.007

Burton, D. C., Kelly, A., Cardo, D., Daskalakis. D., Huang, D.T., Penman-Aguilar, A., Raghunathan, P. L., Zhu, B. P., & Bunnell, R. (2024). Principles of health equity science for public health action. *Public Health Rep. 139*(3), 277–283. https://doi.org/10.1177/00333549231213162

Cairns, C., & Kang, K. (2021). *National hospital ambulatory medical care survey: 2021 emergency department summary tables (table 15)*. https://ftp.cdc.gov/pub/Health_Statistics/NCHS/ Dataset Documentation /NHAMCS/doc21-ed-508.pdf

CDC WONDER. (2021). National Center for Health Statistics. National Vital Statistics System, Mortality 2018-2021, WONDER Online Database, released in 2021. Accessed February 2, 2024. http://wonder.cdc.gov/ucd-icd10-expanded.html

Centers for Disease Control and Prevention. (1995). Air-bag-associated fatal injuries to infants and children riding in front passenger seats–United States. *MMWR. Morbidity and Mortality Weekly Report, 44*(45), 845–847.

Centers for Disease Control and Prevention. (2014). CDC grand rounds: Evidence-based injury prevention. *MMWR. Morbidity Mortality Weekly Report, 62*(51–52), 1048–1050.

Centers for Disease Control and Prevention. (2021a). *Number of injuries and associated costs*. National Center for Injury Prevention and Control. WISQARS database. https://wisqars.cdc.gov/cost/

Centers for Disease Control and Prevention. (2021b). *Web-based Injury Statistics Query and Reporting System (WISQARS)*. Centers for Disease Control and Prevention, National Center for Injury Prevention and Control, Atlanta. https://www.cdc.gov/injury/wisqars

Centers for Disease Control and Prevention. (2023, October 25). *Unintentional injury deaths in the U.S. for ages 1–44 from 1981–2021*. https://www.cdc.gov/injury/wisqars/animated-leading-causes.html

Dempsey, R. C., McAlaney, J., & Bewick, B. M. (2018). A critical appraisal of the social norms approach as an interventional strategy for health-related behavior and attitude change. *Frontiers in Psychology, 9*, 2180. https://doi.org/10.3389/fpsyg.2018.02180

Dilillo, D., Peterson, L., & Farmer, J. E. (2002). Injury and poisoning. In T. Boll (Ed.), *Handbook of clinical health psychology* (pp. 555–582). American Psychological Association.

Fishbein, M. (2006). Foreword. In D. A. Sleet, A. C. Gielen, & R. J. DiClement (Eds.), *Injury and violence prevention: Behavioral science theories, methods and applications*. Jossey Bass.

Fishbein, M., Bandura, A., Triandis, H. C., Kanfer, F. H., Becker, M. H., & Middlestadt, S. E. (1991). *Factors influencing behavior and behavior change. Final report – Theorists workshop*. National Institute of Mental Health.

Fishbein, M., Triandis, H. C., Kanfer, F. H., Becker, M., Middlestadt, S. E., & Eichler, A. (2001). Factors influencing behavior and behavior change. In A. Baum, T. A. Tevenson, & J. E. Singer (Eds.), *Handbook of health psychology* (pp. 3–17). Lawrence Erlbaum Associates.

Francescutti, L. H., Sleet, D. A., Hill, L., & Xiang, H. (2019). Unintentional injuries to disabled persons: An unrecognized preventable problem. In J. Rippe (Ed.), *Lifestyle medicine* (3rd ed., pp. 1349–1354). Taylor & Francis CRC Press.

Frank, R. G., Bouman, D. E., Cain, K., & Watts, C. (1992). Primary prevention of injury. *American Psychologist, 47*, 1045–1049.

Fylan, F., Hempel, S., Grunfeld, B., Conner, M., & Lawton, R. (2006). *Effective interventions for speeding motorists*. Final Report (Contract Number PPAD 9/031/133). Brainbox Research Ltd and University of Leeds (N.D).

Gabriel, E. H., McCann, R. S., & Hoch, M. C. (2019). Use of social or behavioral theories in exercise-related injury prevention program research: A systematic review. *Sports Medicine, 49*(10), 1515–1528. https://doi.org/10.1007/s40279-019-01127-4

Gibson, J. J. (1964). The contribution of experimental psychology to the formulation of the problem of safety–A brief for basic research. In W. Haddon, E. A. Suchman, & D. Klein (Eds.), *Accident research: Methods and approaches.* Harper & Row.

Gielen, A., Sleet, D. A., & Parker, E. (2014). Unintentional injury and behavior change. In S. Kahan, A. C. Gielen, P. J. Fagan, & L.W. Green (Eds.), *Health behavior change in populations* (pp. 294–314). Johns Hopkins University Press.

Gielen, A. C., & Girasek, D. C. (2001). Integrating perspectives on the prevention of unintentional injuries. In N. Schneiderman, M. A. Speers, J. M. Silva, H. Tomes, & J. H. Gentry (Eds.), *Integrating behavioral and social sciences with public health* (pp. 203–230). American Psychological Association.

Gielen, A. C., McDonald, E. M., & McKenzie, L. B. (2012). Behavioral approach. In G. Li & S. P. Baker (Eds.), *Injury research: Theories, methods, and approaches.* Springer.

Gielen, A. C., & Sleet, D. A. (2003). Application of behavior-change theories and methods to injury prevention. *Epidemiologic Reviews, 25*, 65–76. https://doi.org/10.1093/epirev/mxg004

Girasek, D. C. (2023). Does scientific evidence support a ban on using the word "accident"? *American Journal of Lifestyle Medicine.* https://doi.org/10.1177/15598276231198048

Guerin, R. J, & Sleet, D. A. (2020). Using behavioral theory to enhance occupational safety and health: Applications to healthcare workers. *American Journal of Lifestyle Medicine, 15*(3), 269–278. https://doi.org/10.1177/1559827619896979

Haddad, Y. K., Bergen, G., & Luo, F. (2018). Reducing fall risk in older adults. *The American Journal of Nursing, 118*(7), 21–22. https://doi.org/10.1097/01.NAJ.0000541429.36218.2d

Hallsworth, M., & Kirkman, E. (2020). *Behavioral insights.* MIT Press.

Haegerich, T. M., Dahlberg, L. L., Simon, T. R., Greenspan, L., Sleet, D. A., Baldwin, G., & Degutis, L. (2014). Advancing injury and violence prevention in the United States. *Lancet, 384*(9937), 64–74.

Hickling, E. J., & Blanchard, E. B. (2000). *The International handbook of road traffic accidents and psychological trauma: Current understanding, treatment and law.* Elsevier Science.

Hilliard, M. E., Riekert, K. A., & Ockene, K. A. (2018). *The handbook of health behavior change* (5th ed.). Springer.

Institute of Medicine, Committee on Trauma Research. (1985). *Injury in America: A continuing public health problem.* National Academy Press.

Jared, D. M. F. (2024). Traffic safety culture research roadmap. In W. Kumfer, S. LaJeunesse, & S. Heiny, et al. (Eds.), National Academies of Sciences, Engineering, and Medicine. 2024. *Traffic Safety Culture Research Roadmap.* Washington, DC: The National Academies Press. https://doi.org/10.17226/27488.

Kanfer, R., & Kanfer, F. H. (1991). Goals and self-regulation: Applications of theory to work settings. In M. L. Machr & P. R. Pintrich (Eds.), *Advances in motivation and achievement* (Vol. 7, pp. 287–326). JAI Press.

Karb, R. A., Subramanian, S. V., & Fleegler, E. W. (2016). County poverty concentration and disparities in unintentional injury deaths: A fourteen-year analysis of 1.6 million US fatalities. *PLoS One, 11*(5), e0153516. https://doi.org/10.1371/journal.pone.0153516

Kulik, J. A., Butler, H. A., Gerrard, M., Gibbons, F. X., & Mahler, H. (2008). Social norms information enhances the efficacy of an appearance-based sun protection intervention. *Social Science & Medicine, 67*(2), 321–329. https://doi.org/10.1016/j.socscimed.2008.03.037

Lakhan, R., Ranabir, P., Baluja, A., Moscote-Salazar, L. R., & Agrawal, A. (2020). Important aspects of human behavior in road traffic accidents. *Indian Journal of Neurotrauma, 17*, 85–89. https://doi.org/10.1055/s-0040-1713079 ISSN 2277-954X

Lieberman, L., Golden, S. D., Earp, J. A. (2013). Structural approaches to health promotion: What do we need to know about policy and environmental change? *Health Education & Behavior, 40*, 520–525. http://doi.org/10.1177/1090198113503342

Mack, K., Liller, K. D., Baldwin, G. T., & Sleet, D. A. (2015). Preventing unintentional injuries in the home using the health impact pyramid. *Health Education and Behavior, 42*(1S), 115S–122S. https://doi.org/10.1177/1090198114568306

Margolis, B. L., & Kroes, W. H. (Eds.). (1975). *The human side of accident prevention: Psychological concepts and principles which bear on industrial safety.* Charles C Thomas Publishers.

McGlashan, A. J., & Finch, C. F. (2010). The extent to which behavioural and social sciences theories and models are used in sport injury prevention research. *Sports Medicine, 40*, 841–858. https://doi.org/10.2165/11534960-000000000-00000

Mercy, J. A., Mack, K. A., & Steenkamp, M. (2007). Changing the social environment to prevent injuries. In L. Doll, S. Bonze, J. Mercy, & D. Sleet (Eds.), *Handbook of injury and violence prevention.* Springer.

Michielsen, K., Chersich, M., Temmerman, M., Dooms, T., & Van Rossem, R. (2012). Nothing as practical as a good theory? The theoretical basis of HIV prevention interventions for young people in Sub-Saharan Africa: A systematic review. *AIDS Research and Treatment, 2012*, Article 345327. https://doi.org/10.1155/2012/345327

Mokdad, A. A., Wolf, L. L., Pandya, S., Ryan, M., & Qureshi, F. G. (2020). Road traffic accidents and disparities in child mortality. *Pediatrics, 146*(5), e20193009. https://doi.org/10.1542/peds.2019-3009

Moore, M., Conrick, K. M., Fuentes, M., Rowhani-Rahbar, A., Graves, J. M., Patil, D., Herrenkohl, M., Mills, B., Rivara, F. P., Ebel, B., & Vavilala, M. S. (2019). Research on injury disparities: A scoping review. *Health Equity, 3*(1), 504–511. https://doi.org/10.1089/heq.2019.0044

National Academies of Sciences, Engineering, and Medicine. (2018). *Getting to zero alcohol-impaired driving fatalities: A comprehensive approach to a persistent problem*. The National Academies Press. https://doi.org/10.17226/24951

National Academies of Sciences, Engineering, and Medicine. (2023). *Behavioral economics: Policy impact and future directions*. The National Academies Press. https://doi.org/10.17226/26874

National Research Council. Division of Medical Sciences, Committee on Trauma and Committee on Shock. (1966). *Accidental death and disability: The neglected disease of modern society*. National Academy of Sciences.

Neighbors, C., Larimer, M. E., & Lewis, M. A. (2004). Targeting misperceptions of descriptive drinking norms: Efficacy of a computer-delivered personalized normative feedback intervention. *Journal of Consulting and Clinical Psychology, 72*(3), 434–447. https://doi.org/10.1037/0022-006x.72.3.434

Nesbit, B., Robinson, I., & Bryan, S. (2022). A national landscape: Injury and violence prevention health equity scan findings and implications for the field of practice. *Journal of Safety Research, 80*, 457–462. https://doi.org/10.1016/j.jsr.2021.12.026

O'Brien, J., Finch, C. F., Pruna, R., & McCall, A. (2019). A new model for injury prevention in team sports: The Team-sport Injury Prevention (TIP) cycle. *Science and Medicine in Football, 3*(1), 77–80. http://doi.org/10.1080/24733938.2018.1512752

Perkins, H. W., Craig, D. W., & Perkins, J. M. (2011). Using social norms to reduce bullying: A research intervention among adolescents in five middle schools. *Group Processes & Intergroup Relations, 14*(5), 703–722. https://doi.org/10.1177/1368430210398004

Perkins, H. W., Linkenbach, J. W., Lewis, M. A., & Neighbors, C. (2010). Effectiveness of social norms media marketing in reducing drinking and driving: A statewide campaign. *Addictive Behaviors, 35*(10), 866–874. https://doi.org/10.1016/j.addbeh.2010.05.004

Peterson, C., Miller, G. F., Barnett, S. B. L., & Florence, C. (2021). Economic Cost of Injury–United States, 2019. *MMWR. Morbidity Mortality Weekly Report, 70*(48), 1655–1659. https://doi.org/10.15585/mmwr.mm7048a1

Peterson, L., & Roberts, M. C. (1992). Complacency, misdirection, and effective prevention of children's injuries. *American Psychologist, 47*(8), 1040–1044.

Pollack, K., Samuels, A., Frattaroli, S., & Gielen, A. C. (2010). The translation imperative: Moving research into policy. *Injury Prevention, 16*, 141–142. https://doi.org/10.1136/ip.2010.026740

Roberts, M. C., Fanurik, D., & Layfield, D. A. (1987). Behavioral approaches to preventing childhood injuries. *Journal of Social Issues, 43*, 105–108. https://doi.org/10.1111/j.1540-4560.1987.tb01298.x

Santo, L., & Okeyode, T. (2018). *National ambulatory medical care survey: 2018 national summary tables (table 16)*. https://www.cdc.gov/nchs/data/ahcd/namcs_summary/2018-namcs-web-tables-508.pdf

Schultz, P. W., Nolan, J. M, Cialdini, R. B., Goldstein, N. J., & Griskevicius, V. (2007). The constructive, destructive, and reconstructive power of social norms. *Psychological Science, 18*(5), 429–434. https://doi.org/10.1111/j.1467-9280.2007.01917.x

Schwebel, D. C., Barton, B. K., Shen, J., Wells, H. L., Bogar, A., Heath, G., & McCullough, D. (2014). Systematic review and meta-analysis of behavioral interventions to improve child pedestrian safety. *Journal of Pediatric Psychology, 39*(8), 826–845. https://doi.org/10.1093/jpepsy/jsu024

Shaer, M. (2024, January 10). Why are American drivers so deadly? *New York Times Magazine*. https://www.nytimes.com/2024/01/10/magazine/dangerous-driving.html [accessed 2024 JUN 14]

Sleet, D., & Hopkins, K. (Eds.). (2004). *Bibliography on behavioral science research in unintentional injury prevention* [CD-ROM]. Centers for Disease Control and Prevention.

Sleet, D. A., Ballesteros, M., & Baldwin, G. (2013). Injuries and lifestyle medicine. In J. M. Rippe (Ed.), *Lifestyle medicine* (2nd ed., pp. 1447–1456). CRC Press.

Sleet, D. A., Baldwin, G., Marr, A., Spivak, H., Patterson, S., Morrison, C., Holmes, W., Peeples, A. B., & Degutis, L. C. (2012). History of injury and violence as public health problems and emergence of the National Center for Injury Prevention and Control at CDC. *Journal of Safety Research, 43*(4), 233–247. https://doi.org/10.1016/j.jsr.2012.09.002

Sleet, D. A., & Dellinger, A. (2020). Using behavioral theory to enhance public health nursing. *Public Health Nursing, 37*(6), 895–899. https://doi.org/10.1111/phn.12795

Sleet, D. A, & Gielen, A. (2007). Behavioral interventions for injury and violence prevention. In L. Doll, S. Bonzo, J. Mercy, & D. Sleet (Eds.), *Handbook of injury and violence prevention* (pp. 397–410). Springer.

Sleet, D. A., & Gielen, A. (2015, May). Injury prevention and behavioral science: Opportunities to impact population health. In R. M. Kaplan, M. Spittel, & D. David (Eds.), *Population health: Behavioral and social science insights*. AHRQ Publication No. 15-0002. Agency for Healthcare Research and Quality and Office of Behavioral and Social Sciences Research, National Institutes of Health.

Sleet, D. A., Gielen, A. C., Diekman, S., & Ikeda, R. (2010). Preventing unintentional injury: A review of behavior change theories for primary care. *American Journal of Lifestyle Medicine, 4*(1), 25–31. https://doi.org/10.1177/1559827609349573

Sleet, D. A., Hammond, W. R., Jones, R. T., Thomas, N., & Whitt, B. (2004). Using psychology for injury and violence prevention in the community. In R. H. Rozensky, N. G. Johnson, C. D. Goodheart, & W. R. Hammond (Eds.), *Psychology builds a healthy world: Opportunities for research and practice* (pp. 185–216). American Psychological Association. https://doi.org/10.1037/10678-007

Sleet, D. A., Mercer, S., Cole, K. H., Shults, R., Elder, R., & Nichols, J. (2011). Scientific evidence and policy change: Lowering the legal limit to 0.08 % in the USA. *Global Health Promotion, 18*(1), 23–26. https://doi.org/10.1177/1757975910393707

Smedley, B. D., & Syme, S. L. (Eds.). (2000). *Promoting health: Intervention strategies from social and behavioral research*. National Academy Press.

Sogolow, E. S., Sleet, D. A., & Saul, J. (2007). Dissemination, implementation and widespread use of injury prevention interventions. In L. Doll, S. Bonzo, J. Mercy, & D. Sleet (Eds.), *Handbook of injury and violence prevention* (pp. 493–510). Springer.

Spielberger, C. D., & Frank, R. G. (1992). Injury control: A promising field for psychologists. *American Psychologist, 47*(8), 1029–1030. https://doi.org/10.1037//0003-066x.47.8.1029

SunSmart. (2017). *Prevent skin cancer & sunburn this summer – SunSmart*. https://www.sunsmart.com.au/

Thomas, F. D., Blomberg R., Darrah, J., Graham, L., Southcott, T., Dennert, R., Taylor, E., Treffers, R., Tippetts, S., McKnight, S., & Berning, A. (2022). *Evaluation of Utah's .05 BAC per se law* (Report No. DOT HS 813 233). National Highway Traffic Safety Administration, Washington, DC.

Triandis, H. C. (1980). Values, attitudes and interpersonal behavior. In H. E. Howe, & M. M. Page (Eds.), *Nebraska symposium on motivation 1979* (pp. 197–259). University of Nebraska Press.

Trifiletti, L. B., Gielen, A. C., Sleet, D. A., & Hopkins, K. (2005). Behavioral and social sciences theories and models: Are they used in unintentional injury prevention research? *Health Education Research, 20*(3), 298–307. https://doi.org/10.1093/her/cyg126

Vankov, D. (2021). Beyond user experience and technology acceptance: Criteria to select a technology for a road safety behavioural change intervention. *Transactions on Transport Sciences, 12*(2), 53–61. http://doi.org/10.5507/tots.2021.017

VERITY Now. (2023, November 9). *A Coalition for vehicle equity rules in transportation. VERITY Now Statement on Notice of Proposed Rulemaking on the THOR 50th Percentile Adult Male Test Dummy*. https://www.veritynow.org/press/verity-now-statement-on-notice-of-proposed-rulemaking-on-thethor-50th-percentile-adult-male-test-

PART III: PRIORITIZED BEHAVIORS FOR SECONDARY PREVENTION

CHAPTER 13

SCREENING FOR CANCER

KIRSTEN NGUYEN AND JENNIFER RICHMOND

LEARNING OBJECTIVES

- Identify factors contributing to cancer burden and cancer screening use.
- Understand potential benefits and harms of cancer screening.
- Describe recommended cancer screening types and their current eligibility criteria.
- Identify evidence-based interventions with potential to increase appropriate cancer screening use.
- Denote considerations and challenges that remain for equitably improving cancer screening outcomes

OVERVIEW OF CANCER AND CANCER SCREENING IN THE UNITED STATES

After heart disease, cancer is the leading cause of death in the United States (Siegel et al., 2023). The most common cancers diagnosed in men are prostate, lung, and colorectal cancer, accounting for about 48% of all new diagnoses. In women, the most common cancers diagnosed are breast, lung, and colorectal cancer, which account for about 52% of new diagnoses (Siegel et al., 2023). In terms of mortality, the largest number of cancer deaths occurs from lung, prostate, and colorectal cancer in men, and from lung, breast, and colorectal cancer in women. For men and women, lung cancer is the leading cause of cancer deaths, accounting for about one in five cancer deaths in the United States (Siegel et al., 2023).

It is important to know that cancer incidence and mortality rates vary widely across different populations. For example, while overall cancer incidence is highest among the White population, Black men have the highest sex-specific incidence of cancer (Siegel et al., 2023). Among women, cancer incidence is highest among White and American Indian and Alaska Native populations. In terms of cancer deaths, the highest mortality rates occur among American Indian and Alaska Native and Black people in the United States. Such racial inequities in cancer incidence and mortality largely stem from structural racism that disempowers and marginalizes people of color (Siegel et al., 2023).

Structural racism operates through the United States' long-standing history of racially discriminatory laws and policies in housing, criminal justice, healthcare, employment, and other sectors, thereby limiting access to health-promoting resources (e.g., wealth and health insurance; Bailey et al., 2017; Yearby et al., 2022). Although cancer incidence and mortality rates are commonly compared across racial and ethnic groups, there are also widespread inequities across other groups (e.g., sex, geography, age, sexual orientation, and socioeconomic status; Figures 13.1 and 13.2; Islami et al., 2023; Siegel et al., 2023; Singh & Jemal, 2017).

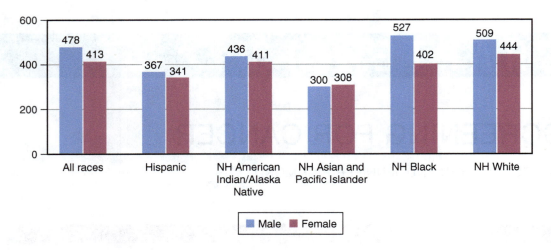

FIGURE 13.1 Cancer diagnoses in the United States by sex and race/ethnicity.
NH, non-Hispanic.
Note: Age-adjusted rates per 100,000 derived from 2016 to 2020.
Source: Data from National Cancer Institute. (n.d.). *Cancer stat facts: Cancer disparities*. https://seer.cancer.gov/statfacts/html/disparities.html

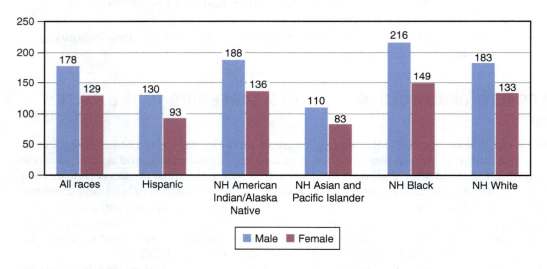

FIGURE 13.2 Cancer deaths in the United States by sex and race/ethnicity.
NH, non-Hispanic.
Note: Age-adjusted rates per 100,000 derived from 2016 to 2020.
Source: Data from National Cancer Institute. (n.d.). *Cancer stat facts: Cancer disparities*. https://seer.cancer.gov/statfacts/html/disparities.html

ROUTINE SCREENING OF COMMON CANCERS: POTENTIAL BENEFITS AND HARMS

Cancer screening is an important tool that can help reduce the population-level burden of cancer (Loud & Murphy, 2017). Screening tests help healthcare providers find cancer at an early stage before it has spread throughout the body and before symptoms typically appear (National Cancer Institute, 2023). If cancer is diagnosed at an early stage, it is generally more treatable through options like curative surgery. Screening for breast, cervical, lung, and colorectal cancer is largely considered effective and is recommended by many expert groups in the United States (National Cancer Institute, 2022). These cancer types are relatively common, can often be detected with a test, and grow slowly enough that early disease can be detected before advanced disease progresses (Loud & Murphy, 2017). As such, these screening tests may decrease one's chance of dying from breast, cervical, lung, or colorectal cancer.

However, screening a large population with no symptoms of cancer can also cause significant harms and incur costs. Screening can detect lesions that are not cancer (a false positive result) and lead to unnecessary follow-up tests, treatment, and stress for patients (Kamineni et al., 2022). Potential drawbacks of cancer screening can be summarized using a taxonomy of the harms of screening (Harris et al., 2014). This taxonomy includes four domains: physical harms, psychological harms, financial strain, and opportunity costs. As examples, some cancer screening tests can cause physical harm from radiation exposure, psychological harm from worrying about test results, and financial strain from paying out of pocket for screening if one does not have health insurance coverage. Screening also has opportunity costs—opportunities given up to participate in cancer screening—such as using paid time off from work to go to a screening facility instead of spending it with family and friends (Harris et al., 2014). Expert groups weigh evidence about benefits and harms when making cancer screening recommendations. Importantly, there are many types of cancer other than breast, cervical, colorectal, and lung that cause significant cancer mortality (e.g., prostate), but screening is not consistently recommended for other cancer types because potential harms may outweigh benefits (National Cancer Institute, 2022). The potential benefits and harms of cancer screening are summarized in **Box 13.1**.

Although screening can help reduce mortality for many cancer types, it is often underused. In 2021, about 76% of adults were up-to-date on breast cancer screening, 75% were up-to-date on cervical cancer screening, and 72% were up-to-date on colorectal cancer screening (Sabatino et al., 2023). In other words, about one in four U.S. adults are not up-to-date on breast, cervical, and colorectal cancer screening. Even fewer adults are up-to-date on lung cancer screening. Recent studies estimate that only between 5% and 21% of screening-eligible U.S. adults have ever received lung cancer screening, which is recommended for adults 50 to 80 years of age with at least a 20 pack-year history of smoking (Fedewa et al., 2020; Lopez-Olivo et al., 2020; Maki et al., 2023; Zahnd & Eberth, 2019). Screening rates are often lower among populations that bear a disproportionate burden of cancer incidence and mortality. Indeed, cancer screening rates are generally lower among people of color, those without health insurance, and people with lower socioeconomic status (Islami et al., 2023). As an example, about 78% of people with a college degree are up-to-date on colorectal cancer screening, but only 58% of people without a high school diploma are up-to-date on this screening type (Islami et

BOX 13.1 POTENTIAL BENEFITS AND HARMS OF CANCER SCREENING

Potential Benefits
- Early detection of cancer
- Cancer detection before symptoms appear
- More treatment options
- Decreased chance of dying from cancer

Potential Harms
- Physical harms (e.g., exposure to radiation)
- Psychological harms (e.g., stress and anxiety from a false positive result)
- Financial strain (e.g., costs of screening and follow-up tests)
- Opportunity costs (e.g., time off work spent at a healthcare facility instead of spent with family)

al., 2023). Furthermore, populations living in rural areas may have more difficulty accessing healthcare facilities that offer cancer screening than those in urban areas due to longer travel times (Islami et al., 2023). Collectively, there remains a critical need to help all eligible patients access and benefit from cancer screening.

In this chapter, we describe the current evidence on cancer screening. We provide an overview of common cancer screening test recommendations and evidence-based interventions to increase appropriate use of cancer screening. We also outline how screening has the potential to affect equity in cancer outcomes across populations. For brevity, we focus on cancer screening in the United States. However, cancer ranks as a leading cause of death in every country in the world (Sung et al., 2021). Accordingly, cancer is an important global concern that warrants public health attention.

COMMON CANCER SCREENING TEST RECOMMENDATIONS

Currently, there is sufficient evidence suggesting that screening for breast, cervical, colorectal, and lung cancer can reduce mortality rates (National Cancer Institute, 2022). Therefore, several expert groups recommend routine screening for these cancer types. In this section, we discuss how cancer screening recommendations are made and provide an overview of current guidelines for breast, cervical, colorectal, and lung cancer screening. Of note, we focus on cancer types that have sufficient evidence suggesting benefits outweigh harms, but there is ongoing research to generate more evidence and create new technological advances in cancer screening. For example, there is growing interest in multicancer early detection tests that might one day allow universal screening by detecting multiple cancer types through a single test (Hubbell et al., 2021).

How Cancer Screening Recommendations Are Made

The U.S. Preventive Services Task Force (USPSTF) is one of the most widely known expert groups that make cancer screening recommendations. The USPSTF is an independent national group that provides evidence-based recommendations about preventive health services, such as cancer screening (USPSTF, 2021c). They follow a rigorous process when developing recommendations that includes conducting a review of the scientific evidence about the topic at hand. The USPSTF weighs the resulting evidence about screening benefits and harms before making a recommendation. They also solicit and consider public input throughout the process (USPSTF, 2021c). In 2010, a provision of the Affordable Care Act mandated that U.S. commercial health insurers cover preventive health services, without patient cost sharing, if they are recommended by the USPSTF (Curfman & Bibbins-Domingo, 2023).

In the United States, there are several other important expert groups that make recommendations for cancer screening. For example, the American Cancer Society develops guidelines by commissioning independent systematic reviews of evidence and evaluating the benefits, limitations, and harms associated with cancer screening tests (Brawley et al., 2011). The National Comprehensive Cancer Network is another panel of experts that reviews available evidence to make recommendations (National Comprehensive Cancer Network, 2023). These are only a few examples of expert groups that provide cancer screening guidelines.

Expert groups also provide cancer screening recommendations in many countries other than the United States. Examples of other national expert groups include the UK National Screening Committee, Canadian Task Force on Preventive Health Care, and Switzerland League Against Cancer (Ebell et al., 2018). In contrast to opportunistic screening in the United States, where the healthcare provider or patient needs to initiate screening, many countries like the Netherlands and Denmark utilize organized screening. In the organized screening method, cancer screening invitations are distributed to all eligible individuals using resources like population registers or national health insurance lists (Sivaram et al., 2018). Low- and middle-income countries vary in access to and use of cancer screening guidelines, although the World Health Organization (WHO) offers cancer screening guidance that can be applied. However, low- and middle-income countries often experience limited healthcare infrastructure and resources, making implementation of cancer screening programs challenging (Sivaram et al., 2018).

Because expert groups comprise different decision-makers and create cancer screening recommendations using different internal processes, recommendations are often inconsistent across groups. For example, different groups sometimes recommend that individuals start or stop screening for cancer at different ages. Experts often have different opinions about the implications of research evidence. Additionally, these groups regularly review new cancer screening evidence, causing their recommendations to change over time. Because commercial health insurers in the United States are mandated to cover cancer screenings recommended by the USPSTF, we provide an overview of USPSTF recommendations in this chapter and note examples of key differences in other expert group recommendations (Table 13.1).

TABLE 13.1 Simplified Summary of the U.S. Preventive Services Task Force Guidelines for Breast, Cervical, Colorectal, and Lung Cancer Screening					
CANCER TYPE	SCREENING TEST(S)	POPULATION OF FOCUS	AGE TO START SCREENING	AGE TO STOP SCREENING	RECOMMENDED FREQUENCY
Breast	Mammography	Women	40 years	74 years	Screening should occur every 2 years.
Cervical	Pap test, high-risk HPV test, or Pap and HPV cotest	Women	21 years	65 years	Depends on screening test. Pap testing should occur every 3 years. HPV testing and Pap/HPV cotesting should occur every 5 years.
Colorectal	Various stool-based (e.g., FIT) and direct observation (e.g., colonoscopy) tests	Adults	45 years	75 years	Depends on screening test. For example, FIT screening should occur every year, whereas colonoscopy should occur every 10 years.
Lung	Low-dose CT scan	Adults with at least a 20 pack-year history of smoking	50 years	80 years	Screening should occur annually.

FIT, fecal immunochemical test; HPV, human papillomavirus.

Note: This table is a simplified summary of recommendations that are current as of December 2023. Screening guidelines change often with the emergence of new evidence. Also, the U.S. Preventive Services Task Force is only one expert group that makes cancer screening recommendations. Other expert groups have different guidelines.

Breast Cancer Screening

Recommendations for breast cancer screening, primarily through mammography, have varied over time in the United States and caused controversy along the way (Nagler et al., 2019). In 2023, the USPSTF released an updated draft statement for breast cancer screening, recommending that women (persons assigned female at birth) aged 40 to 74 years receive a mammogram (an x-ray of the breast) every 2 years (USPSTF, 2023). The USPSTF guidelines have changed several times over the years. For example, in 2002, the USPSTF recommended that women aged 40 and older get breast cancer screening every 1 to 2 years. In 2009, the USPSTF recommended that women aged 50 to 74 receive breast cancer screening every 2 years, and they maintained this recommendation in their 2016 statement (USPSTF, 2016). Clinical and self-breast examinations are generally no longer recommended for breast cancer screening due to lack of evidence of benefit and high risk of false positives (Oeffinger et al., 2015; USPSTF, 2016).

The controversy surrounding these recommendations has largely centered on changes in the ages to start and stop mammography, as well as the recommendation to screen every 2 years instead of every year. Changes in recommended breast cancer screening age and frequency have generally occurred because of emerging research and different interpretations of evidence regarding the net benefit of annual screening for women aged 40 to 49 and for age 75 and older (Monticciolo, 2020). For example, annual breast cancer screening may increase the risk of false positive results, and the ratio of potential screening benefits to harms differs across age groups (Canelo-Aybar et al., 2022). Due to the complex evidence about breast cancer screening, the American Cancer Society, along with several other expert groups, has different recommendations than the USPSTF. The 2015 American Cancer Society guideline recommends that women of average risk for breast cancer ages 40 to 44 *can* have an annual mammogram, women ages 45 to 54 *should* have an annual mammogram, and women ages 55 and older can have an annual mammogram or transition to screening every 2 years (Oeffinger et al., 2015). The American Cancer Society also recommends that women continue screening for breast cancer if their overall health is good and their life expectancy is 10 years or more. With so many conflicting and changing breast cancer screening guidelines, it is perhaps unsurprising that the public may be confused and/or mistrustful about the motives for these changes (Housten et al., 2022).

Another breast cancer screening controversy has centered on the diversity of populations included in research studies that make up the collective evidence about screening. Historically, recommendations for breast cancer screening (and other cancer screening types) have been based on evidence from studies of predominantly White populations (Monticciolo, 2020). However, Black women experience higher breast cancer risk and death rates than White women (Monticciolo, 2020). Furthermore, Black, Hispanic, and Asian women have a younger median age at breast cancer diagnosis than White women (Stapleton et al., 2018). Therefore, guidelines recommending that women wait until later ages to start screening for breast cancer may disproportionately reduce screening benefits among women in minoritized racial and ethnic groups. The USPSTF referenced these inequities when they released their 2023 draft statement, which recommends that women start screening for breast cancer at age 40 rather than at age 50 as they previously recommended (USPSTF, 2023). In this recent statement, the USPSTF noted that screening beginning at age 40 is an important step to improve breast cancer inequities for Black women, but more evidence is needed to understand ways to ensure equity in screening outcomes for all women.

Cervical Cancer Screening

Screening is a powerful tool in cervical cancer prevention and control because more than half of cervical cancers are diagnosed in women who have not had regular screening (Perkins et al., 2021). The USPSTF recommends that women aged 21 to 29 years receive a Pap test (also called cervical cytology) every 3 years (USPSTF, 2018). For women aged 30 to 65 years, the USPSTF recommends screening every 3 years with Pap testing, every 5 years with high-risk human papillomavirus (HPV) testing, or every 5 years with cotesting consisting of a combined Pap test and HPV test.

During a Pap test, a healthcare provider collects a sample of cells from a patient's cervix so that a lab can check for abnormal cells that may lead to cancer (National Cancer Institute, 2022). HPV is a group of viruses that can infect cells in some parts of the body, such as the cervix, and potentially cause cancer (Perkins et al., 2023). Most cervical cancer cases are caused by HPV, and many of these cases can be prevented by receiving the HPV vaccine (Perkins et al., 2023). However, HPV vaccination cannot prevent all cases of cervical cancer, and uptake of HPV vaccination in the United States is suboptimal (Perkins et al., 2023). Therefore, screening continues to play an important role in cervical cancer prevention.

There are also several expert groups that provide cervical cancer screening guidelines (e.g., the USPSTF, American College of Obstetricians and Gynecologists, and American Cancer Society). Again, recommendations vary across expert groups and change over time. However, for the most part, expert groups agree that women aged 25 to 65 should receive regular testing with either a Pap test, HPV test, or an HPV and Pap cotest (Perkins et al., 2021). Cervical cancer screening recommendations have also caused controversy through the years as, for example, experts have disagreed on the ages to start and stop screening (Bus-Kwofie et al., 2019). Additionally, past guidelines from some expert groups, including the USPSTF, recommended that women start screening for cervical cancer after becoming sexually active (USPSTF, 2003). Such recommendations linking screening to sexual activity, along with the association between cervical cancer and HPV (a sexually transmitted infection), can result in stigma and inaccurate beliefs that cervical cancer develops when individuals have multiple sexual partners and/or do not take responsibility for their health (Peterson et al., 2021).

Colorectal Cancer Screening

The USPSTF recommends that adults of average colorectal cancer risk aged 45 to 75 years get screened for colorectal cancer (USPSTF, 2021a). The recommended frequency for colorectal cancer screening varies by the screening method chosen. Some recommended screening methods involve direct observation tests, including colonoscopy, CT colonography, and flexible sigmoidoscopy. These three methods use varying approaches (either a camera or x-ray) to visualize the colon and rectum and check for signs of cancer (USPSTF, 2021a). The USPSTF recommends that colonoscopies be repeated every 10 years, whereas CT colonography and flexible sigmoidoscopy be repeated every 5. Other recommended colorectal cancer screening methods involve stool-based tests, including the high-sensitivity guaiac fecal occult blood test (gFOBT), fecal immunochemical test (FIT), and stool DNA test. The gFOBT and FIT detect blood in the stool that may be indicative of cancer; patients using these screening methods should be screened every year (USPSTF, 2021a). Stool DNA tests can detect biomarkers for cancer in cells that shed into stool. The only currently recommended stool DNA test should be repeated for patients every 1 to 3 years.

When stool-based tests, CT colonography, or flexible sigmoidoscopy suggest abnormal results, follow-up testing with a colonoscopy is needed (USPSTF, 2021a). Colonoscopies use a flexible tube that is inserted into the rectum. This tube has a camera to help healthcare providers check for and potentially remove abnormal tissue during the colonoscopy (Pluta et al., 2011). Because colonoscopy is invasive, requires bowel preparation to ensure the colon and rectum are empty, and uses anesthesia, many patients prefer to use another recommended screening test even though colonoscopies are still needed if abnormal results are found (Hyams et al., 2021; Makaroff et al., 2023).

Most countries that offer colorectal cancer screening recommend that screening start at age 50 (Kanth & Inadomi, 2021). However, there is currently an alarming increase in colorectal cancer incidence among individuals age 20 to 49 years (Kanth & Inadomi, 2021). Accordingly, the USPSTF began recommending colorectal cancer screening starting at age 45 instead of age 50 in 2021 (USPSTF, 2021a). Similar to other cancer screening guidelines, expert groups have different recommendations for colorectal cancer screening (Kanth & Inadomi, 2021). Of note, expert groups generally avoid recommending any one colorectal cancer screening test in favor of tests consistent with patient values and preferences.

Lung Cancer Screening

Until somewhat recently, there was no recommended test for lung cancer screening. Lung cancer screening using low-dose CT scans received its first recommendation from the USPSTF in 2013 (Moyer, 2014). Historically, there had been insufficient evidence to recommend a lung cancer screening test, but this evidence changed when the National Lung Screening Trial results were published suggesting that low-dose CT testing significantly reduces lung cancer-specific mortality (National Lung Screening Trial Research Team, 2011). Healthcare providers can use low-dose CT devices to scan the lungs and look at the images for signs of cancer (Boiselle et al., 2013). This test is described as low-dose because it uses a lower radiation dose than regular diagnostic CT scans.

Currently, the USPSTF recommends annual lung cancer screening using low-dose CT scans for patients age 50 to 80 years who have at least a 20 pack-year smoking history and either currently smoke or have quit smoking within the past 15 years (USPSTF, 2021b). Unlike other guidelines that generally recommend cancer screening based on age and sex, lung cancer screening is only recommended for individuals who have at least a 20 pack-year history of cigarette smoking. A pack-year is a way to measure how much someone has smoked over time and is calculated by multiplying the average number of cigarette packs someone has smoked per day by the number of years someone has smoked. For example, someone who has smoked two packs of cigarettes per day for 10 years has a 20 pack-year smoking history. Because smoking and older age are strongly associated with lung cancer risk, lung cancer screening guidelines include age and pack-year smoking history requirements to help identify individuals who would likely receive the greatest net benefit from screening (USPSTF, 2021b).

The age and pack-year smoking history requirements for lung cancer screening have also been controversial and frequently critiqued. The initial 2013 USPSTF guidelines recommended low-dose CT screening for individuals aged 55 to 80 years with at least a 30 pack-year smoking history who either currently smoke or have quit within the past 15 years (Moyer, 2014). However, this recommendation was critiqued for possibly being too conservative, especially for Black men who experience a higher risk of lung cancer than White men despite having lower average pack-year smoking histories (Aldrich et al., 2019; Richmond et al., 2018). Landmark research found that, compared with White individuals, a larger percentage of Black individuals diagnosed with lung cancer would not have been eligible for lung cancer screening per the 2013 guidelines (Aldrich et al., 2019). This research suggested that lowering the minimum screening age from 55 to 50 years and reducing the 30 pack-year smoking history requirement to 20 pack-years for Black and African American individuals could potentially result in more equitable lung cancer screening outcomes. In response to this and other emerging evidence, the USPSTF revised their guidelines in 2021, lowering the minimum screening age to 50 years and the minimum smoking history to 20 pack-years for all adults (USPSTF, 2021b). Although these changes may help increase the number of Black adults who are eligible for lung cancer screening, the 2021 guidelines are still heavily critiqued for potentially perpetuating racial, sex, and other inequities in lung cancer outcomes (Aredo et al., 2022; Lozier et al., 2021; Potter et al., 2023). Similar to other cancer screening types, expert groups also have different recommendations for lung cancer screening (Ramaswamy, 2022; Wolf et al., 2023). Overall, much work is needed to optimize lung cancer screening recommendations.

CANCER SCREENING INTERVENTIONS

Despite the potential for reduced cancer-specific mortality, cancer screening is often underused. As noted previously, only about 76% of screening-eligible adults are up-to-date on breast cancer screening, 75% are up-to-date on cervical cancer screening, 72% are up-to-date on colorectal cancer screening, and 5 to 21% have ever received lung cancer screening (Fedewa et al., 2020; Lopez-Olivo et al., 2020; Maki et al., 2023; Sabatino et al., 2023; Zahnd & Eberth, 2019). Accordingly, public health interventions often aim to help address this challenge. Health interventions are actions taken with the goal of improving human health and/or preventing disease (Box 13.2; Rychetnik et al., 2002).

Increasing Cancer Screening Use

Because screening recommendations for breast, colorectal, and cervical cancer have been in place for many years, there is a considerable amount of evidence about interventions in these areas. In terms of patient-focused interventions, prior evidence suggests that reminders (e.g., calling patients or sending mailed letters to remind them they are due for screening) increase breast, cervical, and colorectal cancer screening uptake (Brouwers et al., 2011; Community Preventive Services Task Force, 2023). Evidence also suggests that small media (e.g., mailing patients education booklets or videos) and one-on-one education interventions increase uptake of these three cancer screening types (Figure 13.3) At the provider level, reminding providers that a patient is overdue for screening and using audit and feedback approaches can increase breast, colorectal, and cervical cancer screening rates (Brouwers et al., 2011; Community Preventive Services Task Force, 2023). In audit and feedback approaches, health systems often assess the percentage of a provider's patients who are up-to-date with screening and offer specific feedback about how one provider compares with another provider. Interventions that support providers may be particularly effective because receiving a provider recommendation is a strong predictor of cancer screening receipt (Peterson et al., 2016).

Emerging evidence also suggests that community health workers and patient navigators play an important role in cancer screening interventions (Community Preventive Services Task Force, 2023). Community health workers are individuals who are usually from the

---

BOX 13.2 OVERVIEW OF CANCER SCREENING INTERVENTION EVIDENCE

Examples of Potential Approaches to Increase Cancer Screening Use
- Send patients reminders when due for screening.
- Disseminate patient education materials.
- Remind healthcare providers when their patients are due for screening.
- Offer feedback to healthcare providers about the percentage of their patients who are up-to-date with screening.
- Engage community health workers and patient navigators to provide education and help patients navigate barriers to screening.
- Combine multiple approaches (e.g., patient and provider reminders).

Needs for Future Cancer Screening Interventions
- Investigate approaches to reduce cancer screening overuse (i.e., screening individuals when the harms likely outweigh benefits) as research is limited in this area.
- Focus on upstream social determinants of health (e.g., racism).
- Design interventions in partnership with local communities.

FIGURE 13.3 Example material from a direct mail campaign intervention to promote breast cancer screening.
Source: From National Cancer Institute. (2008). *Using direct mail to increase screening mammography–Program materials.* https://ebccp.cancercontrol.cancer.gov/productDownloads.do?programId=294617

community an intervention wishes to serve (Adams et al., 2021). They are typically trained as part of an intervention or program to deliver health promotion services (i.e., education) to their community. Patient navigators are often trained professionals (e.g., nurses) who help patients overcome barriers to healthcare (Mosquera et al., 2023). For example, patient navigators might help patients access transportation to an appointment or obtain low- or no-cost care. Interventions that focus on engaging community health workers and providing patient navigation can help increase breast, cervical, and colorectal cancer screening rates (Community Preventive Services Task Force, 2023). Furthermore, interventions may be most successful when they are multicomponent (i.e., when they contain two or more effective intervention approaches; Community Preventive Services Task Force, 2023). Pairing a patient with a navigator to help them access cancer screening after receiving a reminder may be a more effective approach than only providing reminders.

Importantly, research studies have evaluated other cancer screening intervention approaches, such as mass media campaigns, offering patients and providers incentives for screening, and group education, but evidence on their effectiveness is mixed (Brouwers et al., 2011). Additionally, there is less evidence available about lung cancer screening interventions because it received its first-ever USPSTF recommendation somewhat recently in 2013 (Moyer, 2014). However, a scoping review found that the most effective lung cancer screening interventions had key features such as raising community-level awareness, tailoring intervention materials for sociocultural appropriateness, and proactively considering costs (Sayani et al., 2023).

Reducing Overuse of Cancer Screening

Most cancer screening interventions focus on increasing cancer screening rates. However, overuse of screening is another important but understudied, area. As described earlier, cancer screening guidelines often include recommendations to stop routine screening if evidence suggests harms outweigh benefits, such as when patients reach an upper age limit. Yet over

45% of older U.S. adults report being screened for breast, colorectal, or cervical cancer after recommended age limits (Moss et al., 2020).

Despite the potential harms of screening overuse, interventions focused on reducing inappropriate cancer screening use are scarce. A systematic review about overuse of cervical cancer screening identified only five interventions in this area (Alber et al., 2018). Often, these cervical cancer screening overuse interventions involved updating electronic health records to alert providers if they requested a screening test that was not consistent with guideline recommendations. All five interventions in the systematic review reported reductions in overuse of cervical cancer screening (Alber et al., 2018). Another recently published study tested an intervention that provided a booklet with personalized information on screening benefits and harms combined with provider education and other health system modifications (Saini et al., 2023). Results suggest the intervention helped align provider screening orders with screening benefit and reduce the overall use of screening (Saini et al., 2023). Collectively, there is a critical need for more evidence about high-quality interventions to ensure appropriate use of cancer screening.

CASE STUDY 13.1: LUNG CANCER SCREENING

Mary is a 55-year-old woman who received a recommendation for lung cancer screening at a routine checkup with her primary care provider. She had smoked a pack of cigarettes a day for 25 years before quitting 5 years ago. She had never been screened for lung cancer. Her provider mentioned lung cancer screening multiple times starting at age 50 but the screening would require another appointment at a different location, forcing Mary to take another day off work that she could not afford to miss. At her latest routine checkup, Mary did agree to get screened for lung cancer using a CT scan. A few hours after her scan, she received a call notifying her that she had a suspicious nodule that her healthcare providers would like to sample to make sure it was not cancer. She scheduled an appointment for a transthoracic fine needle aspiration biopsy a week later. Although she understood that the suspicious nodule might not be cancer, she spent the week stressed and worried that she could have cancer. During her biopsy, she experienced sharp, stabbing shortness of breath due to a small pneumothorax (a collapsed lung), which is a known minor complication of the procedure. She was sent home and recovered in a week. Her biopsy results came back as atypical adenomatous hyperplasia, which is not cancerous. She was instructed to follow up with her primary care provider for the next steps.

Mary's story is not uncommon for those who undergo lung cancer screening. If a suspicious nodule is found during lung cancer screening, a biopsy is needed to determine if it is cancerous. Lung biopsy complication rates are about 24% to 40% for minor complications (Mary's small pneumothorax) and 5% for major complications (e.g., blood pooling between the lungs and rib cage; Heerink et al., 2017). Unfortunately, patients like Mary might experience harm and psychological distress from a lung biopsy when their suspicious nodules are not cancer. Therefore, it is important that patients and healthcare providers thoroughly discuss potential benefits and harms of cancer screening before deciding.

Example Resources for Finding Evidence-Based Cancer Screening Interventions

Finding information about cancer screening interventions can be challenging given how rapidly new evidence emerges. To help with this challenge, the National Cancer Institute houses a website that provides a searchable database of evidence-based cancer control programs (EBCCP) and interventions (National Cancer Institute, 2020). This database, called the EBCCP website, helps public health practitioners quickly find cancer-related interventions that have been tested and evaluated in research studies. EBCCP allows users to search for interventions across categories, such as population or community of focus. The website also links to intervention materials that practitioners can use when implementing an intervention in their own community (i.e., education materials).

Another key resource is the Community Preventive Services Task Force's list of intervention approaches for breast, cervical, and colorectal cancer screening (Community Preventive Services Task Force, 2023). The Community Preventive Services Task Force is an independent panel of public health and prevention experts who provide recommendations on programs and interventions based on systematic reviews of evidence. In one area of focus, this group summarizes evidence for specific cancer screening intervention approaches (like reminding patients to get screened, providing one-on-one patient education, and reminding healthcare providers that their patients are due for cancer screening). Their Findings for Cancer Prevention and Control website provides an easy to understand summary of the evidence regarding each approach (Community Preventive Services Task Force, 2023). As the evidence about cancer screening rapidly evolves, reviewing recent peer-reviewed publications and other literature is another way to stay up-to-date about interventions in this field.

Gaps and Future Needs for Cancer Screening Interventions

Despite ongoing new research about cancer screening, there are still several knowledge gaps in terms of effective interventions. Many interventions focus on downstream factors that affect cancer screening, such as patient knowledge and attitudes about screening (Community Preventive Services Task Force, 2023). However, upstream social determinants of health are also critical factors to consider in interventions. Upstream social determinants of health are conditions in environments that affect a wide range of health outcomes, such as neighborhoods and the built environment (Braveman et al., 2011). As an example, structural racism that causes inadequately resourced schools in communities with large populations of Black residents is one pathway by which upstream factors may reduce access to knowledge about cancer prevention. Highlighting the importance of social determinants, a recent systematic review found that breast, cervical, colorectal, and lung cancer screening interventions that focused on social determinants of health increased screening rates by a median of 8.4 percentage points (Korn et al., 2023). Some of the greatest screening rate improvements occurred in interventions that focused on addressing transportation-related barriers to screening. Importantly, even social determinants of health interventions largely focused on the individual level, like designing cancer screening education materials for individuals with lower health literacy, and ignored structural factors that drive cancer screening inequities, like racism and poverty (Korn et al., 2023).

Another major limitation of the existing evidence base is that cancer screening interventions are typically not designed in partnership with the populations they intend to help (Richardson-Parry et al., 2023). Instead, they are often designed by academic researchers who have scientific expertise about cancer screening but do not understand the lived experience of the population they wish to serve. As such, there is a critical need for cancer screening interventions that are designed in partnership with local communities and focus on upstream social determinants driving screening inequities. Focusing on social determinants and community partnership are two key needs for the future cancer screening interventions.

EQUITY IN CANCER SCREENING

Cancer screening has the potential to reduce cancer deaths, but only if populations have equitable access to screening tests (**Box 13.3**).

BOX 13.3 POTENTIAL WAYS CANCER SCREENING CAN REDUCE OR WIDEN INEQUITIES

Example Ways Screening Can Reduce Cancer Inequities
- Populations with higher cancer mortality rates may receive an early-stage cancer diagnosis after screening, when curative treatment is available.
- When access to and receipt of screening is equitable, the population-level burden of cancer may decline.

Example Ways Screening Can Widen Cancer Inequities
- Populations with greater access to resources (e.g., money, health insurance, transportation) can use those resources to get screened and reduce their risk of cancer death, leaving populations without these resources behind.
- Poorer access to screening among populations with the highest cancer burden may widen existing inequities in cancer mortality.
- Without equitable access to follow-up care after cancer screening (e.g., treatment after a cancer diagnosis), inequities in cancer mortality will persist.

CASE STUDY 13.2: INEQUITIES IN COLORECTAL CANCER SCREENING

There are widespread inequities in colorectal cancer screening in the United States. Limited knowledge about screening options, limited English proficiency, low health literacy and educational attainment, and difficulties navigating the healthcare system are only a few of the barriers to colorectal cancer screening that many patients face (Reuland et al., 2017). Due to these barriers, colorectal cancer screening rates are lower among populations that have been historically marginalized and made vulnerable, such as individuals with limited English proficiency, with low educational attainment, and with Medicaid or no health insurance (Reuland et al., 2017).

One randomized control trial aimed to study potential interventions to increase colorectal screening rates in populations who have historically been made vulnerable (Reuland et al., 2017). This study enrolled participants from two community health center sites that primarily served low-income, racially/ethnically diverse patients. At baseline, the sites had colorectal cancer screening rates of about 35%. The investigators tested the combined effect of a colorectal cancer screening decision aid and patient navigation intervention. Decision aids can help increase patient awareness about screening, promote patient–provider communication, and help patients clarify their screening preferences (Reuland et al., 2017). Decision aid videos of about 15 minutes were developed in English and Spanish and designed to be viewed before a primary care visit. The decision aids included narration, vignettes, graphics, and animations that aimed to deliver information about screening options, addressing barriers in health literacy and clinic time constraints. Patient navigation was facilitated by trained bilingual staff members who contacted patients after their primary care visits. Navigators supported patients to address screening barriers and help patients follow through with colorectal cancer screening. Intervention participants received the decision aid before a primary care visit and patient navigation support after their visit; participants in the control group viewed a food safety video before their visit and received usual care. Study results suggested that participants in the intervention group were more likely to complete colorectal cancer screening within 6 months than participants in the control group (Reuland et al., 2017). Ultimately, the intervention led to a 40% point increase in colorectal cancer screening completion.

Potential for Cancer Screening to Reduce or Widen Cancer-Related Inequities

Many populations bear a disproportionate burden of cancer mortality, and cancer screening represents one potential approach to reduce these inequities. Because screening for cancer can lead to early diagnosis of cancer when curative treatments like surgery are available, screening is a powerful tool that can help reduce cancer mortality across populations (Richardson-Parry et al., 2023). Ensuring that populations with the most need can access and receive screening is a key mechanism by which medical and public health practitioners can reduce cancer-related inequities. Additionally, new screening technologies may eventually become available that reduce screening barriers. For example, less expensive screening tests that can be completed at home and mailed to healthcare providers may become more widely available, thus reducing barriers for populations that do not have transportation, health insurance, or other resources. Additionally, new research may emerge that helps expert groups ensure their eligibility recommendations equitably identify populations that have the greatest net benefit from screening.

Cancer screening also has the potential to widen cancer-related inequities when screening is not received equitably across populations and communities. For example, Black men experience one of the highest lung cancer mortality rates, but Black screening-eligible patients are less likely than White screening-eligible patients to receive lung cancer screening (Kunitomo et al., 2022; Siegel et al., 2023). Therefore, the already existing inequity in lung cancer mortality may widen if Black patients continue receiving lung cancer screening at suboptimal rates (Richmond et al., 2018). Similarly, overall cancer mortality rates are higher in nonmetropolitan areas than in large metropolitan areas, but cancer screening can be harder to access in nonmetropolitan areas where there are fewer healthcare facilities (Islami et al., 2023). Even when cancer mortality rates are similar across populations, inequitable receipt of cancer screening can create inequities in cancer mortality over time. Additionally, screening cannot reduce cancer mortality rates unless patients who have abnormal screening results also receive follow up care and treatment (e.g., biopsies and treatment after a cancer diagnosis). Without equitable access to follow-up care after screening, inequities in cancer mortality will persist.

Furthermore, overuse of cancer screening may also result in inequities, although there is a paucity of research in this area. People who receive screening outside of recommended guidelines are potentially exposed to increased screening harms in exchange for little benefit. Meanwhile, healthcare resources that are spent over screening some patients might be better used by screening patients who fall within the recommended screening guidelines who are at high risk for developing cancer. It is therefore vital to consider available resources when examining how cancer screening may impact equity in outcomes.

As discussed earlier in this chapter, upstream social determinants are important causes of cancer screening inequities (Braveman et al., 2011). Systems of oppression, such as slavery and segregation, result in the inequitable distribution of resources like knowledge, money, and power (Feagin & Bennefield, 2014). This inequitable distribution of resources is a fundamental driver of health inequities in part because people with more resources have better access to technological innovations like screening tests to reduce their risk of cancer death (Clouston & Link, 2021; Feagin & Bennefield, 2014). Therefore, it is perhaps unsurprising that studies find inequities in cancer outcomes across groups with different levels of resources (Benavidez et al., 2021). For example, women with low incomes and without health insurance are less likely to meet the USPSTF guidelines for breast, cervical, and colorectal cancer screening (Benavidez et al., 2021). Furthermore, because racism is a fundamental cause of the inequitable distribution of resources across racial and ethnic groups, racism is a vital factor to consider when evaluating causes of racial and ethnic cancer screening inequities (Phelan & Link, 2015). Even as new and better cancer screening innovations emerge, inequities in receipt and use of these innovations will persist if inequities in upstream social determinants remain unaddressed.

Key Health Equity Challenges for the Future of Cancer Screening

There is growing acknowledgment of the need to understand and address equity in cancer screening efforts, but several challenges remain. Many landmark studies showing evidence of screening effectiveness recruited mostly White participants and were not representative of the entire population that might benefit from screening. For example, about 91% of participants identified as White in the highly influential National Lung Screening Trial, which found low-dose CT scans reduce lung cancer mortality (National Lung Screening Trial Research Team, 2011). There is growing public awareness of the limited diversity in clinical trials that are the basis for creating evidence-based cancer screening recommendations across all populations (Shelton et al., 2021). This awareness can lead to a rational mistrust and limited embracement of cancer screening recommendations in communities that are historically and contemporarily marginalized (Shelton et al., 2021). The need to diversify cancer screening clinical trials and research is not limited to racial and ethnic diversity. Older adults are often excluded from and/or poorly represented in clinical trials, making it challenging to set recommendations for the age to stop screening (Salzman et al., 2016). Furthermore, transgender individuals are poorly represented in cancer screening research, and expert group recommendations largely provide no guidance about cancer screening for transgender patients (Sterling & Garcia, 2020). Even when specific populations are not explicitly excluded from clinical trials, the United States has a long-standing history of medical exploitation and unethical experimentation on historically and contemporarily marginalized populations that contributes to mistrust of researchers and a rational hesitancy to join research studies (Scharff et al., 2010). Overall, substantial work is needed to increase diversity in cancer screening research and ensure recommendations consider net screening benefits equitably across populations.

Additionally, there is an important need to understand and address stigma in efforts to increase cancer screening equity. Stigma can be defined as the "co-occurrence of labeling, stereotyping, separation, status loss, and discrimination in a context in which power is exercised" (Hatzenbuehler et al., 2013, p. 813). Many populations that experience higher cancer incidence and mortality also belong to groups that society has stigmatized, such as minoritized racial and ethnic groups, minoritized sexual orientation groups, groups with a history of tobacco use, and groups with larger body sizes (Hatzenbuehler et al., 2013; Siegel et al., 2023). Yet stigma leads to discriminatory practices that reduce resources needed to access cancer screening. As an example, employers may discriminate against people with larger body sizes by not hiring them, thereby reducing this population's access to money and health insurance (Puhl & Heuer, 2010). Furthermore, many cancer prevention and control interventions contain educational components designed to raise awareness about behaviors that increase cancer risk, such as smoking, limited fruit and vegetable consumption, and physical inactivity (National Cancer Institute, 2020). These programs may have the unintended consequence of contributing to the larger societal stigmatization and inaccurate labeling of individuals who engage in these behaviors as people who "deserve" to get cancer due to their poor choices and behaviors. Stigma is particularly concerning for lung cancer screening. Indeed, stigma and patient fears of being judged or blamed by healthcare providers can contribute to limited engagement in lung cancer screening (Hamann et al., 2018). Novel research is needed to reduce stigma in cancer screening efforts.

CONCLUSION

Cancer is the second leading cause of death in the United States (Siegel et al., 2023). Cancer screening is a powerful tool that can help reduce the population-level burden of cancer mortality. Screening tests can help diagnose cancer in earlier stages when curative treatment options are available (Loud & Murphy, 2017). As such, cancer screening can help decrease the risk of dying from cancer. However, these benefits must be weighed against potential screening harms. For example, screening can show an abnormal result that is actually not cancer (called a false positive result), which can lead to unnecessary follow-up tests, treatment, and stress for patients who worry they have cancer (Kamineni et al., 2022).

Several expert groups recommend routine screening for breast, cervical, colorectal, and lung cancer because there is sufficient evidence that screening can reduce mortality rates for these cancer types (National Cancer Institute, 2022). There are many different expert groups who make recommendations about who should get screened for cancer and how often people should get screened. The USPSTF is one of the most widely known expert groups because commercial health insurers in the United States are mandated to cover preventive health services (e.g., cancer screening) without patient cost sharing if the USPSTF recommends them (Curfman & Bibbins-Domingo, 2023). Expert groups base their recommendations on scientific evidence, but recommendations are often inconsistent across different expert groups. Cancer screening recommendations also change frequently over time as new evidence emerges.

Although cancer screening can save lives, it is underused. Only about three-fourths of eligible patients are up-to-date on breast, cervical, and colorectal cancer screening, and fewer than one-fourth of eligible patients have ever received lung cancer screening (Fedewa et al., 2020; Lopez-Olivo et al., 2020; Maki et al., 2023; Sabatino et al., 2023; Zahnd & Eberth, 2019). Accordingly, many intervention studies aim to increase cancer screening rates. Some key evidence-based interventions for increasing breast, cervical, and colorectal cancer screening rates include sending reminders to patients and providers, providing one-on-one patient education, and engaging community health workers and patient navigators to help patients navigate barriers to screening (Brouwers et al., 2011; Community Preventive Services Task Force, 2023). Importantly, screening overuse also occurs when individuals receive cancer screening outside of recommended guidelines, but there is limited research about interventions to reduce screening overuse (Alber et al., 2018).

Cancer screening also has the potential to reduce inequities in cancer outcomes, such as mortality rates, if it is implemented and received equitably across eligible populations. However, many populations that bear a disproportionate burden of cancer also have poorer access to and receipt of screening for various cancer types. In these situations, pre-existing inequities in cancer mortality rates may widen. Such inequities in cancer screening receipt largely stem from upstream social determinants of health and the inequitable distribution of resources (e.g., knowledge and money), making it harder for populations with fewer resources to access health-promoting services like screening (Clouston & Link, 2021; Feagin & Bennefield, 2014). Overall, substantial work is needed to address the upstream social determinants of cancer inequities and promote the appropriate use of cancer screening.

SUMMARY KEY POINTS

- Cancer screening can help save lives by identifying cancer at earlier stages when curative treatments are available.
- Screening benefits must be weighed against potential harms, such as the risk of receiving a false positive result.
- Screening for breast, cervical, colorectal, and lung cancer is widely recommended by different expert groups because there is sufficient evidence of their effectiveness.
- Cancer screening can be underused (when too few eligible people get screened) or overused (when people who do not meet eligibility guidelines continue receiving screening).
- There are widespread inequities in use of cancer screening as, for example, populations with lower income and without health insurance often have lower screening rates.
- A fundamental cause of cancer screening inequities is the inequitable distribution of resources (e.g., money and health insurance) across society, which makes it easier for individuals with greater resources to access screening, but much harder for individuals with fewer resources.
- Cancer screening has the potential to reduce cancer mortality rates, but this potential can only be reached if screening is implemented equitably across eligible populations.

DISCUSSION QUESTIONS

1. Prior to reading this chapter, what have you heard about cancer screening from sources like the media, family, or friends?
2. How are inequities in cancer screening similar to or different from inequities in other health behaviors, such as physical activity, tobacco use, and vaccine receipt?
3. How should potential harms influence individuals' decisions about whether to get screened for cancer? What advice would you give a loved one trying to weigh the potential benefits and harms of a specific cancer screening test?
4. What controversies and tensions in the cancer screening literature surprised you most? Why?
5. What new interventions or future research should be conducted to reduce inequities in cancer screening outcomes?

A robust set of instructor resources designed to supplement this text is located at http://connect.springerpub.com/content/book/978-0-8261-4265-8. Qualifying instructors may request access by emailing textbook@springerpub.com.

REFERENCES

Adams, L. B., Richmond, J., Watson, S. N., Cené, C. W., Urrutia, R., Ataga, O., Dunlap, P., & Corbie-Smith, G. (2021). Community health worker training curricula and intervention outcomes in african american and latinx communities: A systematic review. *Health Education & Behavior, 48*(4), 516–531. https://doi.org/10.1177/1090198120959326

Alber, J. M., Brewer, N. T., Melvin, C., Yackle, A., Smith, J. S., Ko, L. K., Crawford, A., & Glanz, K. (2018). Reducing overuse of cervical cancer screening: A systematic review. *Preventive Medicine, 116*, 51–59. https://doi.org/10.1016/j.ypmed.2018.08.027

Aldrich, M. C., Mercaldo, S. F., Sandler, K. L., Blot, W. J., Grogan, E. L., & Blume, J. D. (2019). Evaluation of USPSTF lung cancer screening guidelines among African American adult smokers. *JAMA Oncology, 5*(9), 1318–1324. https://doi.org/10.1001/jamaoncol.2019.1402

Aredo, J. V., Choi, E., Ding, V. Y., Tammemägi, M. C., Ten Haaf, K., Luo, S. J., Freedman, N. D., Wilkens, L. R., Marchand, L. L., Wakelee, H. A., Meza, R., Park, S.-S. L., Cheng, I., & Han, S. S. (2022). Racial and ethnic disparities in lung cancer screening by the 2021 USPSTF guidelines versus risk-based criteria: The multiethnic cohort study. *JNCI Cancer Spectrum, 6*(3). https://doi.org/10.1093/jncics/pkac033

Bailey, Z. D., Krieger, N., Agenor, M., Graves, J., Linos, N., & Bassett, M. T. (2017). Structural racism and health inequities in the USA: Evidence and interventions. *Lancet, 389*(10077), 1453–1463. https://doi.org/10.1016/s0140-6736(17)30569-x

Benavidez, G. A., Zgodic, A., Zahnd, W. E., & Eberth, J. M. (2021). Disparities in meeting USPSTF breast, cervical, and colorectal cancer screening guidelines among women in the United States. *Preventing Chronic Disease, 18*, E37. https://doi.org/10.5888/pcd18.200315

Boiselle, P. M., Lynm, C., & Livingston, E. H. (2013). Lung cancer screening. *JAMA, 309*(18), 1948–1948. https://doi.org/10.1001/jama.2013.4324

Braveman, P., Egerter, S., & Williams, D. R. (2011). The social determinants of health: Coming of age. *Annual Review of Public Health, 32*, 381–398. https://doi.org/10.1146/annurev-publhealth-031210-101218

Brawley, O., Byers, T., Chen, A., Pignone, M., Ransohoff, D., Schenk, M., Smith, R., Sox, H., Thorson, A. G., & Wender, R. (2011). New American cancer society process for creating trustworthy cancer screening guidelines. *JAMA, 306*(22), 2495–2499. https://doi.org/10.1001/jama.2011.1800

Brouwers, M. C., De Vito, C., Bahirathan, L., Carol, A., Carroll, J. C., Cotterchio, M., Dobbins, M., Lent, B., Levitt, C., Lewis, N., McGregor, S. E., Paszat, L., Rand, C., & Wathen, N. (2011). What implementation interventions increase cancer screening rates? A systematic review. *Implementation Science, 6*(1), 111. https://doi.org/10.1186/1748-5908-6-111

Bus-Kwofie, A., Chan, C., Kahn, R., & Holcomb, K. (2019). Clinical controversies in cervical cancer screening. *Clinical Obstetrics Gynecology, 62*(4), 644–655. https://doi.org/10.1097/grf.0000000000000478

Canelo-Aybar, C., Posso, M., Montero, N., Solà, I., Saz-Parkinson, Z., Duffy, S. W., Follmann, M., Gräwingholt, A., Rossi, P. G., & Alonso-Coello, P. (2022). Benefits and harms of annual, biennial, or triennial breast cancer mammography screening for women at average risk of breast cancer: A systematic review for the European Commission Initiative on Breast Cancer (ECIBC). *British Journal of Cancer, 126*(4), 673–688. https://doi.org/10.1038/s41416-021-01521-8

Clouston, S. A. P., & Link, B. G. (2021). A retrospective on fundamental cause theory: State of the literature and goals for the future. *Annual Review of Sociology, 47*(1), 134–156. https://doi.org/10.1146/annurev-soc-090320-094912

Community Preventive Services Task Force. (2023). *Findings for cancer prevention and control.* https://www.thecommunityguide.org/pages/task-force-findings-cancer-prevention-and-control.html#cancerscreening

Curfman, G., & Bibbins-Domingo, K. (2023). US preventive services task force challenged in federal court. *JAMA, 329*(20), 1743–1744. https://doi.org/10.1001/jama.2023.6605

Ebell, M. H., Thai, T. N., & Royalty, K. J. (2018). Cancer screening recommendations: An international comparison of high income countries. *Public Health Review, 39,* 7. https://doi.org/10.1186/s40985-018-0080-0

Feagin, J., & Bennefield, Z. (2014). Systemic racism and U.S. health care. *Social Science & Medicine, 103,* 7–14. https://doi.org/10.1016/j.socscimed.2013.09.006

Fedewa, S. A., Kazerooni, E. A., Studts, J. L., Smith, R., Bandi, P., Sauer, A. G., Cotter, M., Sineshaw, H. M., Jemal, A., & Silvestri, G. A. (2020). State variation in low-dose CT scanning for lung cancer screening in the United States. *Journal of the National Cancer Institute, 113*(8), 1044–1052. https://doi.org/10.1093/jnci/djaa170

Hamann, H. A., Ver Hoeve, E. S., Carter-Harris, L., Studts, J. L., & Ostroff, J. S. (2018). Multilevel opportunities to address lung cancer stigma across the cancer control continuum. *Journal Thoracic Oncology, 13*(8), 1062–1075. https://doi.org/10.1016/j.jtho.2018.05.014

Harris, R. P., Sheridan, S. L., Lewis, C. L., Barclay, C., Vu, M. B., Kistler, C. E., Golin, C. E., DeFrank, J. T., & Brewer, N. T. (2014). The harms of screening: A proposed taxonomy and application to lung cancer screening. *JAMA Internal Medicine, 174*(2), 286. https://doi.org/10.1001/jamainternmed.2013.12745

Hatzenbuehler, M. L., Phelan, J. C., & Link, B. G. (2013). Stigma as a fundamental cause of population health inequalities. *American Journal of Public Health, 103*(5), 813–821. https://doi.org/10.2105/ajph.2012.301069

Heerink, W. J., de Bock, G. H., de Jonge, G. J., Groen, H. J. M., Vliegenthart, R., & Oudkerk, M. (2017). Complication rates of CT-guided transthoracic lung biopsy: Meta-analysis. *European Radiology, 27*(1), 138–148. https://doi.org/10.1007/s00330-016-4357-8

Housten, A. J., Hoover, D. S., Britton, M., Bevers, T. B., Street, R. L., McNeill, L. H., Strong, L. L., Hersch, J., McCaffery, K., & Volk, R. J. (2022). Perceptions of conflicting breast cancer screening recommendations among racially/ethnically diverse women: A multimethod study. *Journal of General Internal Medicine, 37*(5), 1145–1154. https://doi.org/10.1007/s11606-021-07336-w

Hubbell, E., Clarke, C. A., Aravanis, A. M., & Berg, C. D. (2021). Modeled reductions in late-stage cancer with a multi-cancer early detection test. *Cancer Epidemiology, Biomarkers & Prevention, 30*(3), 460–468. https://doi.org/10.1158/1055-9965.EPI-20-1134

Hyams, T., Golden, B., Sammarco, J., Sultan, S., King-Marshall, E., Wang, M. Q., & Curbow, B. (2021). Evaluating preferences for colorectal cancer screening in individuals under age 50 using the Analytic Hierarchy Process. *BMC Health Services Research, 21*(1), 754. https://doi.org/10.1186/s12913-021-06705-9

Islami, F., Baeker Bispo, J., Lee, H., Wiese, D., Yabroff, K. R., Bandi, P., Sloan, K., Patel, A. V., Daniels, E. C., Kamal, A. H., Guerra, C. E., Dahut, W. L., & Jemal, A. (2023). American Cancer Society's report on the status of cancer disparities in the United States, 2023. *CA: A Cancer Journal for Clinicians, 74*(2), 136–166. https://doi.org/10.3322/caac.21812

Kamineni, A., Doria-Rose, V. P., Chubak, J., Inadomi, J. M., Corley, D. A., Haas, J. S., Kobrin, S. C., Winer, R. L., Lafata, J. E., Beaber, E. F., Yudkin, J. S., Zheng, Y., Skinner, C. S., Schottinger, J. E., Ritzwoller, D. P., Croswell, J. M., & Burnett-Hartman, A. N. (2022). Evaluation of harms reporting in U.S. cancer screening guidelines. *Annals of Internal Medicine, 175*(11), 1582–1590. https://doi.org/10.7326/M22-1139

Kanth, P., & Inadomi, J. M. (2021). Screening and prevention of colorectal cancer. *BMJ, 374,* n1855. https://doi.org/10.1136/bmj.n1855

Korn, A. R., Walsh-Bailey, C., Correa-Mendez, M., DelNero, P., Pilar, M., Sandler, B., Brownson, R. C., Emmons, K. M., & Oh, A. Y. (2023). Social determinants of health and US cancer screening interventions: A systematic review. *CA: A Cancer Journal for Clinicians, 73*(5), 461–479. https://doi.org/10.3322/caac.21801

Kunitomo, Y., Bade, B., Gunderson, C. G., Akgün, K. M., Brackett, A., Cain, H., Tanoue, L., & Bastian, L. A. (2022). Racial differences in adherence to lung cancer screening follow-up: A systematic review and meta-analysis. *Chest, 161*(1), 266–275. https://doi.org/10.1016/j.chest.2021.07.2172

Lopez-Olivo, M. A., Maki, K. G., Choi, N. J., Hoffman, R. M., Shih, Y.-C. T., Lowenstein, L. M., Hicklen, R. S., & Volk, R. J. (2020). Patient adherence to screening for lung cancer in the US: A systematic review and meta-analysis. *JAMA Network Open, 3*(11), e2025102. https://doi.org/10.1001/jamanetworkopen.2020.25102

Loud, J. T., & Murphy, J. (2017). Cancer screening and early detection in the 21(st) century. *Seminars in Oncology Nursing, 33*(2), 121–128. https://doi.org/10.1016/j.soncn.2017.02.002

Lozier, J. W., Fedewa, S. A., Smith, R. A., & Silvestri, G. A. (2021). Lung cancer screening eligibility and screening patterns among Black and White adults in the United States. *JAMA Network Open, 4*(10), e2130350. https://doi.org/10.1001/jamanetworkopen.2021.30350

Makaroff, K. E., Shergill, J., Lauzon, M., Khalil, C., Ahluwalia, S. C., Spiegel, B. M. R., & Almario, C. V. (2023). Patient preferences for colorectal cancer screening tests in light of lowering the screening age to 45 years. *Clinical Gastroenterology Hepatology, 21*(2), 520–531.e510. https://doi.org/10.1016/j.cgh.2022.07.012

Maki, K. G., Tan, N. Q. P., Toumazis, I., & Volk, R. J. (2023). Prevalence of lung cancer screening among eligible adults in 4 US states in 2021. *JAMA Network Open, 6*(6), e2319172. https://doi.org/10.1001/jamanetworkopen.2023.19172

Monticciolo, D. L. (2020). Current guidelines and gaps in breast cancer screening. *Journal of the American College of Radiology, 17*(10), 1269–1275. https://doi.org/10.1016/j.jacr.2020.05.002

Mosquera, I., Todd, A., Balaj, M., Zhang, L., Benitez Majano, S., Mensah, K., Eikemo T. A., Basu, P., & Carvalho, A. L. (2023). Components and effectiveness of patient navigation programmes to increase participation to breast, cervical and colorectal cancer screening: A systematic review. *Cancer Medicine, 12*(13), 14584–14611. https://doi.org/10.1002/cam4.6050

Moss, J. L., Roy, S., Shen, C., Cooper, J. D., Lennon, R. P., Lengerich, E. J., Adelman, A., Curry, W., & Ruffin, M. T. T. (2020). Geographic variation in overscreening for colorectal, cervical, and breast cancer among older adults. *JAMA Network Open, 3*(7), e2011645. https://doi.org/10.1001/jamanetworkopen.2020.11645

Moyer, V. A. (2014). Screening for lung cancer: U.S. Preventive Services Task Force recommendation statement. *Annals Internal Medicine, 160*(5), 330–338. https://doi.org/10.7326/m13-2771

Nagler, R. H., Fowler, E. F., Marino, N. M., Mentzer, K. M., & Gollust, S. E. (2019). The evolution of mammography controversy in the news media: A content analysis of four publicized screening recommendations, 2009 to 2016. *Women's Health Issues, 29*(1), 87–95. https://doi.org/10.1016/j.whi.2018.09.005

National Cancer Institute. (2008). *Using direct mail to increase screening mammography–Program materials*. https://ebccp.cancercontrol.cancer.gov/productDownloads.do?programId=294617

National Cancer Institute. (2020). *Evidence-Based Cancer Control Programs (EBCCP)*. https://ebccp.cancercontrol.cancer.gov/index.do

National Cancer Institute. (2022). *Screening tests*. https://www.cancer.gov/about-cancer/screening/screening-tests

National Cancer Institute. (2023). *Cancer screening overview (PDQ®)–Patient version*. https://www.cancer.gov/about-cancer/screening/patient-screening-overview-pdq

National Comprehensive Cancer Network. (2023). *Development and update of guidelines*. https://www.nccn.org/guidelines/guidelines-process/development-and-update-of-guidelines

National Lung Screening Trial Research Team. (2011). Reduced lung-cancer mortality with low-dose computed tomographic screening. *New England Journal of Medicine, 365*(5), 395–409. https://doi.org/10.1056/NEJMoa1102873

Oeffinger, K. C., Fontham, E. T., Etzioni, R., Herzig, A., Michaelson, J. S., Shih, Y. C., Walter, L. C., Church, T. R., Flowers, C. R., LaMonte, S. J., Wolf, A. M. D., DeSantis, C., Lortet-Tieulent, J., Andrews, K., Manassaram-Baptiste, D., Saslow, D., Smith, R. A., Brawley, O. W., & Wender, R. (2015). Breast cancer screening for women at average risk: 2015 guideline update from the American Cancer Society. *JAMA, 314*(15), 1599–1614. https://doi.org/10.1001/jama.2015.12783

Perkins, R. B., Guido, R. L., Saraiya, M., Sawaya, G. F., Wentzensen, N., Schiffman, M., & Feldman, S. (2021). Summary of current guidelines for cervical cancer screening and management of abnormal test results: 2016–2020. *Journal of Women's Health (Larchmt), 30*(1), 5–13. https://doi.org/10.1089/jwh.2020.8918

Perkins, R. B., Wentzensen, N., Guido, R. S., & Schiffman, M. (2023). Cervical cancer screening: A review. *JAMA, 330*(6), 547–558. https://doi.org/10.1001/jama.2023.13174

Peterson, C. E., Silva, A., Goben, A. H., Ongtengco, N. P., Hu, E. Z., Khanna, D., Nussbaum, E. R., Jasenof, I. G., Kim, S. J., & Dykens, J. A. (2021). Stigma and cervical cancer prevention: A scoping review of the U.S. literature. *Preventive Medicine, 153*, 106849. https://doi.org/10.1016/j.ypmed.2021.106849

Peterson, E. B., Ostroff, J. S., DuHamel, K. N., D'Agostino, T. A., Hernandez, M., Canzona, M. R., & Bylund, C. L. (2016). Impact of provider-patient communication on cancer screening adherence:

A systematic review. *Preventive Medicine, 93,* 96–105. https://doi.org/10.1016/j.ypmed.2016.09.034

Phelan, J. C., & Link, B. G. (2015). Is racism a fundamental cause of inequalities in health? *Annual Review of Sociology, 41*(1), 311–330. https://doi.org/10.1146/annurev-soc-073014-112305

Pluta, R. M., Lynm, C., & Golub, R. M. (2011). Colonoscopy. *JAMA, 305*(11), 1154. https://doi.org/10.1001/jama.305.16.1154

Potter, A. L., Senthil, P., Srinivasan, D., Raman, V., Kumar, A., Haridas, C., Mathey-Andrews, C., Zheng, W., & Jeffrey Yang, C. F. (2023). Persistent racial and sex-based disparities in lung cancer screening eligibility. *Journal of Thoracic and Cardiovascular Surgery*, S0022-5223(23)00981-9. https://doi.org/10.1016/j.jtcvs.2023.10.025

Puhl, R. M., & Heuer, C. A. (2010). Obesity stigma: Important considerations for public health. *American Journal of Public Health, 100*(6), 1019–1028. https://doi.org/10.2105/ajph.2009.159491

Ramaswamy, A. (2022). Lung cancer screening: Review and 2021 update. *Current Pulmonology Report, 11*(1), 15–28. https://doi.org/10.1007/s13665-021-00283-1

Reuland, D. S., Brenner, A. T., Hoffman, R., McWilliams, A., Rhyne, R. L., Getrich, C., Tapp, H., Weaver, M. A., Callan, D., Cubillos, L., de Hernandez, B. U., & Pignone, M. P. (2017). Effect of combined patient decision aid and patient navigation vs usual care for colorectal cancer screening in a vulnerable patient population: A randomized clinical trial. *JAMA Internal Medicine, 177*(7), 967–974. https://doi.org/10.1001/jamainternmed.2017.1294

Richardson-Parry, A., Baas, C., Donde, S., Ferraiolo, B., Karmo, M., Maravic, Z., Münter, L., Ricci-Cabello, I., Silva, M., Tinianov, S., Valderas, J. M., Woodruff, S., & van Vugt, J. (2023). Interventions to reduce cancer screening inequities: The perspective and role of patients, advocacy groups, and empowerment organizations. *International Journal for Equity in Health, 22*(1), 19. https://doi.org/10.1186/s12939-023-01841-6

Richmond, J., Mbah, O. M., Dard, S. Z., Jordan, L. C., Cools, K. S., Samuel, C. A., Khan, J. M., & Manning, M. A. (2018). Preempting racial inequities in lung cancer screening. *American Journal of Preventive Medicine, 55*(6), 908–912. https://doi.org/10.1016/j.amepre.2018.07.023

Rychetnik, L., Frommer, M., Hawe, P., & Shiell, A. (2002). Criteria for evaluating evidence on public health interventions. *Journal of Epidemiology Community Health, 56*(2), 119–127. https://doi.org/10.1136/jech.56.2.119

Sabatino, S. A., Thompson, T. D., White, M. C., Villarroel, M. A., Shapiro, J. A., Croswell, J. M., & Richardson, L. C. (2023). Up-to-date breast, cervical, and colorectal cancer screening test use in the United States, 2021. *Preventing Chronic Disease, 20,* E94. https://doi.org/10.5888/pcd20.230071

Saini, S. D., Lewis, C. L., Kerr, E. A., Zikmund-Fisher, B. J., Hawley, S. T., Forman, J. H., Zauber, A. G., Lansdorp-Vogelaar, I., van Hees, F., Saffar, D., Myers, A., Gauntlett, L. E., Lipson, R., Kim, H. M., & Vijan, S. (2023). Personalized multilevel intervention for improving appropriate use of colorectal cancer screening in older adults: A cluster randomized clinical trial. *JAMA Internal Medicine, 183*(12), 1334–1342. https://doi.org/10.1001/jamainternmed.2023.5656

Salzman, B., Beldowski, K., & de la Paz, A. (2016). Cancer screening in older patients. *American Family Physician, 93*(8), 659–667.

Sayani, A., Ali, M. A., Dey, P., Corrado, A. M., Ziegler, C., Nicholson, E., & Lofters, A. (2023). Interventions designed to increase the uptake of lung cancer screening: An equity-oriented scoping review. *JTO Clinical and Research Reports, 4*(3), 100469. https://doi.org/10.1016/j.jtocrr.2023.100469

Scharff, D. P., Mathews, K. J., Jackson, P., Hoffsuemmer, J., Martin, E., & Edwards, D. (2010). More than Tuskegee: Understanding mistrust about research participation. *Journal of Health Care for Poor and Underserved, 21*(3), 879–897. https://doi.org/10.1353/hpu.0.0323

Shelton, R. C., Brotzman, L. E., Johnson, D., & Erwin, D. (2021). Trust and mistrust in shaping adaptation and de-implementation in the context of changing screening guidelines. *Ethnicity & Disease, 31*(1), 119–132. https://doi.org/10.18865/ed.31.1.119

Siegel, R. L., Miller, K. D., Wagle, N. S., & Jemal, A. (2023). Cancer statistics, 2023. *CA: A Cancer Journal for Clinicians, 73*(1), 17–48. https://doi.org/10.3322/caac.21763

Singh, G. K., & Jemal, A. (2017). Socioeconomic and racial/ethnic disparities in cancer mortality, incidence, and survival in the United States, 1950–2014: Over six decades of changing patterns and widening inequalities. *Journal of Environmental and Public Health, 2017,* 2819372. https://doi.org/10.1155/2017/2819372

Sivaram, S., Majumdar, G., Perin, D., Nessa, A., Broeders, M., Lynge, E., Saraiya, M., Segnan, N., Sankaranarayanan, R., Rajaraman, P., Trimble, E., Taplin, S., Rath, G. K., & Mehrotra, R. (2018). Population-based cancer screening programmes in low-income and middle-income countries: Regional consultation of the International Cancer Screening Network in India. *The Lancet Oncology, 19*(2), e113–e122. https://doi.org/10.1016/s1470-2045(18)30003-2

Stapleton, S. M., Oseni, T. O., Bababekov, Y. J., Hung, Y.-C., & Chang, D. C. (2018). Race/ethnicity and age distribution of breast cancer diagnosis in the United States. *JAMA Surgery, 153*(6), 594–595. https://doi.org/10.1001/jamasurg.2018.0035

Sterling, J., & Garcia, M. M. (2020). Cancer screening in the transgender population: A review of current guidelines, best practices, and a proposed care model. *Translational Andrology and Urology, 9*(6), 2771–2785. https://doi.org/10.21037/tau-20-954

Sung, H., Ferlay, J., Siegel, R. L., Laversanne, M., Soerjomataram, I., Jemal, A., & Bray, F. (2021). Global cancer statistics 2020: GLOBOCAN estimates of incidence and mortality worldwide for 36 cancers in 185 countries. *CA: A Cancer Journal for Clinicians, 71*(3), 209–249. https://doi.org/10.3322/caac.21660

United States Preventive Services Task Force. (2003). Screening for cervical cancer: Recommendations and rationale. *AJN The American Journal of Nursing, 103*(11), 101–109. https://journals.lww.com/ajnonline/fulltext/2003/11000/screening_for_cervical_cancer__recommendations_and.38.aspx

United States Preventive Services Task Force. (2016). *Final recommendation statement, Breast Cancer: Screening.* https://www.uspreventiveservicestaskforce.org/uspstf/recommendation/breast-cancer-screening

United States Preventive Services Task Force. (2018). Screening for cervical cancer: US preventive services task force recommendation statement. *JAMA, 320*(7), 674–686. https://doi.org/10.1001/jama.2018.10897

United States Preventive Services Task Force. (2021a). Screening for colorectal cancer: US preventive services task force recommendation statement. *JAMA, 325*(19), 1965–1977. https://doi.org/10.1001/jama.2021.6238

United States Preventive Services Task Force. (2021b). Screening for lung cancer: US preventive services task force recommendation statement. *JAMA, 325*(10), 962–970. https://doi.org/10.1001/jama.2021.1117

United States Preventive Services Task Force. (2021c). *USPSTF recommendations development process.* https://www.uspreventiveservicestaskforce.org/uspstf/about-uspstf/task-force-resources/uspstf-recommendations-development-process

United States Preventive Services Task Force. (2023). *Draft recommendation statement: Breast cancer screening.* https://www.uspreventiveservicestaskforce.org/uspstf/draft-recommendation/breast-cancer-screening-adults

Wolf, A. M. D., Oeffinger, K. C., Shih, T. Y.-C., Walter, L. C., Church, T. R., Fontham, E. T. H., Elkin, E. B., Etzioni, R. D., Guerra, C. E., Perkins, R. B., Kondo, K. K., Kratzer, T. B., Manassaram-Baptiste, D., Dahut, W. L., & Smith, R. A. (2023). Screening for lung cancer: 2023 guideline update from the American Cancer Society. *CA: A Cancer Journal for Clinicians, 74*(1), 50–81 https://doi.org/10.3322/caac.21811

Yearby, R., Clark, B., & Figueroa, J. F. (2022). Structural racism in historical and modern US health care policy. *Health Affairs, 41*(2), 187–194. https://doi.org/10.1377/hlthaff.2021.01466

Zahnd, W. E., & Eberth, J. M. (2019). Lung cancer screening utilization: A behavioral risk factor surveillance system analysis. *American Journal of Preventive Medicine, 57*(2), 250–255. https://doi.org/10.1016/j.amepre.2019.03.015

CHAPTER 14

CARDIOVASCULAR DISEASE: A FOCUS ON PRIMARY AND SECONDARY PREVENTION

KRUPAL JAY HARI, YASHASHWI POKHAREL, AND JUSTIN B. MOORE

LEARNING OBJECTIVES

- Describe the patterns, trends, and disparities in the prevalence of cardiovascular disease (CVD) in the United States.
- Identify and discuss three strategies for changing CVD-related health behaviors in individuals with or at risk for CVD.
- Explain the benefits of cardiac rehabilitation (CR) programs for individuals with CVD.
- Describe two implications for future research designed to enhance behavior change in individuals with CVD.

EPIDEMIOLOGY AND SIGNIFICANCE OF CARDIOVASCULAR DISEASE

Cardiovascular disease (CVD) remains the number one cause of death in the United States and resulted in approximately 700,000 deaths in 2020, with an annual healthcare cost of $229 billion (Centers for Disease Control and Prevention [CDC], 2022). While CVD-related deaths have been steadily trending down with medical advances in treatment and promotion of primary and secondary CVD prevention (Mensah et al., 2017), the prevalence of CVD continues to rise (Mohebi et al., 2022). For instance, by year 2060, it is projected that the prevalence of ischemic heart disease, heart failure, myocardial infarction, and stroke will increase by 31.1%, 33%, 30.1%, and 34.3% respectively, compared with year 2025 (Mohebi et al., 2022). This is likely attributed in part to the increasing prevalence of CVD risk factors, most prominently diabetes, hypertension, dyslipidemia, and obesity, with estimated increases by 39.3% (15.4 million), 27.2% (34.7 million), 27.5% (27.1 million), and 18.3% (19.4 million), respectively, by year 2060 (Mohebi et al., 2022). Other factors implicated in the rise of CVD include the aging population with substantial increases in chronic conditions along with adverse behavioral–lifestyle patterns (Benjamin et al., 2017). This is superimposed on the background of healthcare disparities by race and ethnicity (Mohebi et al., 2022), income level (Abdalla et al., 2020), and gender (Gao et al., 2019). For instance, according to the CDC data from 1999 through 2018, Black Americans had a 30% greater CVD and 45% greater stroke mortality compared with White Americans (CDC, 2020). A study looking at the United States-based Atherosclerosis Risk in Communities (ARIC) cohort of 13,688 patients plus the Finnish FINRISK cohort consisting of 8,816 patients found low income to be associated with increased risk of sudden cardiac death in both cohorts (incidence rate of sudden cardiac death per 10,000 [95% CI] low income vs. high income: ARIC cohort 21 [16.5–25.5] vs. 6.5 [4.6–8.3]; FINRISK cohort 22.6 [17.1–28] vs. 8.1 [4.9–11.3]; Kucharska-Newton et al., 2011). Similarly, gender disparity is common. For example, in the Patient and Provider Assessment of Lipid Management national registry, among those who qualify for statin therapy, women compared with men were less likely to receive statin therapy and treated at lower intensities than recommended (36.7% vs. 45.2%, $p < .001$; Virani et al., 2021). Despite advancement in technology such as genomics, a lack of Black population-specific genomic samples poses risk for further CVD disparities (Scott et al., 2022). Racial and ethnic disparities in prevalence and trends of risk factors and lifestyle behaviors known to accelerate CVD processes are well-documented and have led to a call to action by the American Heart Association (AHA; Churchwell et al., 2020). Recent attention has focused on factors that operate beyond the individual level to alter life-course trajectories that result in excess risk and burden of CVD. Examples include social determinants of health (Havranek et al., 2015), role of structural racism in health (Churchwell et al., 2020), and commercial determinants of health. Consistent with the World Health Organization's (WHO) definition of social determinants (Kickbusch et al., 2016), the AHA considers socioeconomic position (SEP; encompassing wealth and income, education, employment/occupational status), race and ethnicity, social support (including social networks), culture (including language), access to healthcare, and residential environments as important factors in cardiovascular health (Havranek et al., 2015). Lifestyle behaviors are central to both prevention and treatment of CVD and are influenced by the structural determinants across the life course (Churchwell et al., 2020; Havranek et al., 2015).

IMPORTANCE OF LIFE-COURSE APPROACHES TO PREVENTION AND MANAGEMENT OF CARDIOVASCULAR DISEASE

Substantial evidence has accumulated over the past several decades indicating that atherosclerotic and hypertensive processes begin early in life and are influenced over time by the interaction of potentially modifiable behaviors and environmental exposures (Hayman et al., 2011). For instance, data show that adverse childhood and adolescent experiences, which encompass childhood maltreatment, household and environmental dysfunction, and violence, among others, are associated with the development of cardiometabolic diseases such as obesity, hypertension, diabetes, and CVD (Suglia et al., 2018). Autopsy studies have demonstrated associations between established risk factors for CVD, including hypertension, dyslipidemia, and obesity, and atherosclerotic changes in coronary arteries in adolescence and young adulthood (Berenson et al., 1998; McGill et al., 2000). These potentially modifiable risk factors track into adulthood (Chen & Wang, 2008; Freedman et al., 2007; Lauer & Clarke, 1990). Importantly, the presence of these risk factors in childhood is associated with vascular changes known to predict cardiovascular events in adulthood (Vlachopoulos et al., 2010). Adding to the evidence in support of life-course approaches to prevention are longitudinal data demonstrating that preservation of ideal cardiovascular health by maintaining healthy lifestyle behaviors is associated with less subclinical atherosclerosis in adulthood (Laitinen et al., 2012). Highlighting the importance of promoting cardiovascular health across the life course, the AHA defined national goals for children and adults with emphasis on potentially modifiable health behaviors and health factors (Lloyd-Jones et al., 2010). Based on accumulated evidence, health behaviors and factors targeted for both prevention and management of CVD include smoking, physical activity, dietary intake, weight management, cholesterol, blood pressure, sleep, and fasting plasma glucose (Lloyd-Jones et al., 2022). These health behaviors and health factors were also recommended as targets for intervention in evidence-based guidelines issued for secondary prevention of CVD (Cardoso et al., 2022; Grundy et al., 2019; Visseren et al., 2021). The longitudinal Special Turku Coronary Risk Factor Intervention Project (STRIP) and the Cardiovascular Risk in Young Finns Study (YFS) provide convincing evidence on the effects of ideal cardiovascular health in childhood on cardiac structure and function in adulthood (Laitinen et al., 2017). Taken together, accumulated evidence from clinical and population-based studies underscores the importance of life-course approaches to the prevention and management of CVD and the critical role of healthy lifestyle behaviors starting at a young age.

HEALTH BEHAVIORS CENTRAL TO MANAGEMENT OF CARDIOVASCULAR DISEASE

Primary prevention focuses on reducing adverse health behaviors and CVD risk factors with the ultimate goal of preventing incident CVD. The 2019 American College of Cardiology (ACC)/AHA Guideline on Primary Prevention of Cardiovascular Disease: A Report of the American College of Cardiology/American Heart Association Task Force on Clinical Practice Guidelines identifies the promotion of a healthy lifestyle throughout life as the number one take-home message for primary prevention of CVD (Arnett et al., 2019). This healthy lifestyle includes smoking cessation, adherence to heart-healthy patterns of dietary intake, physical activity, maintenance of appropriate body weight, adherence to sex-specific recommendations for alcohol consumption, and adherence to prescribed medications for reduction of established risk factors such as hypertension and dyslipidemia (Smith et al., 2015; Stone, 2014). More specifically, the ACC/AHA considers a healthy diet one that is rich in vegetable, fruit, and nut intake, with appropriate portions of whole grains and lean meats. Red meats, processed foods, fatty foods high in trans-fat, artificially sweetened beverages, and refined carbohydrates should be minimized (Eckel et al., 2014). Early recognition and intervention is critical for those who are overweight and obese, identified as a body mass index of 25 to 29.9 kg/m^2 and ≥30 kg/m^2, respectively. For weight reduction, appropriate diet, caloric restriction, and exercise should be performed. Professional assistance, if needed, should be sought to reach and maintain target body mass index (Jensen et al., 2014). Lastly, the ACC/AHA recommends at least 150 minutes of moderate-intensity or 75 minutes of high-intensity exercise weekly (Arnett et al., 2019). Age-appropriate risk estimation for CVD prevention should be performed regularly with the 10-year atherosclerotic CVD risk estimator (Arnett et al., 2019). Health behaviors (smoke-free lifestyles, physical activity, and heart-healthy patterns of dietary intake) will remain the cornerstone of CVD management irrespective of whether the goal is to prevent incident CVD or prevent complications of CVD. While adherence to therapeutic pharmacological agents will also continue to be emphasized, the specific medications recommended for CVD management continue to change as new evidence becomes available.

Patient adherence to lifestyle and pharmacological recommendations for management of CVD is essential to reduce the risk of recurring vascular events and mortality. *Adherence* is defined as the extent to which an individual's behavior coincides with physician or healthcare provider recommendations. It is well-established that adherence is a complex process influenced by many factors, including but not limited to individual patient, healthcare provider, and healthcare system factors (Castellano et al., 2014). Substantial data from clinical trials show that pharmacological interventions with statins and blood pressure-lowering agents considerably reduce the risk of vascular events and total mortality (Cholesterol Treatment Trialists' Collaboration, 2010; Law et al., 2009). Of note, the AHA and the ACC recommend the use of cholesterol and blood pressure-lowering agents regardless of the initial levels of atherogenic low-density lipoprotein cholesterol (LDL-C) or blood pressure in patients with documented vascular disease (Smith et al., 2015; Stone, 2014). It is well-established, however, that patient adherence is less than optimal for most conditions, but particularly for chronic conditions requiring long-term treatment such as CVD (Haynes et al., 1996; O'Flaherty, 2013). A systematic review of studies of medication adherence among patients with established CVD showed that the overall adherence was 57% over a median of 2 years (Naderi et al., 2012). Substantial research has focused on evaluating the effects of medication adherence on outcomes in patients with established CVD. Results indicate that good adherence (generally defined as >80% adherence) to combined therapy with aspirin, statins, and blood pressure-lowering medications is associated with improvement in various cardiovascular outcomes, including cardiovascular mortality, all-cause-mortality, and reduced healthcare costs (Kim et al., 2016; Ruppar et al., 2016).

Numerous approaches have been suggested to increase patient adherence to preventive and therapeutic regimens. For CVD management, although patient-level responsibility is very important, healthcare providers and systems of care are equally important targets for adherence enhancement efforts. A report from the prospective international Reduction of Atherothrombosis for Continued Health (REACH) Registry provides insights on the predictors of long-term adherence to CVD medications (Rodriguez et al., 2013). A major goal of this REACH analysis was to provide useful information for healthcare providers regarding patient groups that may benefit from targeted interventions to improve adherence to evidence-based CVD medications (Rodriguez et al., 2013). Patients (n = 25,737) with established CVD with complete self-report adherence data at enrollment and at year 4 were included in the analyses. *Adherence* was defined as self-report of taking the guideline-based medications as prescribed, while *nonadherence* was defined as failure to take any of the recommended medications. The results indicated that 48.6% of patients were adherent to guideline-recommended medications over the 4-year study period (Rodriguez et al., 2013). Collective findings are consistent with and complementary to other studies that have documented the importance of both clinical and demographic variables on patient adherence (Kumbhani et al., 2013; Maddox & Ho, 2009). Specifically, age influenced complete guideline adherence, with younger patients reporting greater adherence (Kulkarni et al., 2006). Older adults are more likely to have more total medications prescribed and less likely to live independently, an important predictor of medication nonadherence (Kulkarni et al., 2006). In addition, geographic variation in self-reported adherence to recommended therapies for secondary prevention has been documented in other studies and associated with cost of medications and socioeconomic factors (Gast & Mathes, 2019; Kvarnström et al., 2021).

INTERVENTIONS TO CHANGE BEHAVIORS FOCUSED ON MANAGEMENT AND SECONDARY PREVENTION OF CARDIOVASCULAR DISEASE

Secondary prevention of CVD, the focus of this chapter, emphasizes interventions designed to reduce the likelihood of CVD events and/or mortality in individuals who have established disease. The major potentially modifiable targets in the management of CVD in the setting of secondary prevention include health behaviors and established risk factors that are also part of primary prevention protocols. In this regard, clinicians frequently use the terminology "Guideline Directed Medical Therapy," inferring the use of evidence-based medical therapy informed by clinical practice guidelines. Guideline-directed medical therapy is important to curtail the progression and complications of established CVDs, such as coronary artery disease, heart failure, peripheral artery disease, and stroke. Evidence-based interventions to change behaviors in managing CVD include patient education and counseling, therapeutic patient education (TPE) interventions, behavioral skills training, motivational techniques and strategies such as motivational interviewing (MI), and digital health (eHealth) technologies. Of note, multicomponent interventions that combine these approaches and include eHealth technologies focused on behaviors central to managing CVD, such as smoking cessation, increasing physical activity and decreasing sedentary behaviors, enhancing heart-healthy dietary behaviors, and promoting adherence to therapeutic regimens including cardiac rehabilitation (CR) programs, have shown to be highly effective in preventing recurrent CVD events as well as maintenance of behavior change. These multicomponent interventions are most often provided by multidisciplinary teams of healthcare professionals. As discussed in the next section, more recent multicomponent interventions, including CR programs for CVD patients, incorporate eHealth technologies.

Education and Therapeutic Patient Education Interventions

Patient education and counseling focused on both prevention and management of CVD has been a central component of evidence-based guidelines for secondary prevention of CVD (Smith et al., 2015; Stone, 2014). Recently, attention has focused on TPE interventions with the goal of promoting self-management in patients with CVD (Barnason et al., 2017). Defined as an approach to facilitate patient and family learning about the treatment of disease and the adoption of self-management behaviors and lifestyles to improve physical and psychosocial outcomes, a major goal of TPE is to improve health outcomes by *preventing* avoidable complications (Group WHOW, n.d.). A recent systematic review of TPE research on cardiovascular self-management interventions highlighted evidence-based recommendations for clinical practice applicable in the setting of secondary prevention for patients with CVD (Barnason et al., 2017). The results of the review pointed to the importance of multiple modes of TPE delivery, including face to face, telephone, and telehealth, to individualize the needs of patients. Team-based, multidisciplinary approaches were affirmed as optimal, with the recommendation that a structured protocol for delivery of TPE self-management by various healthcare team members be used to provide a framework for communication among providers, consistent messaging to patients, and a system for tracking the follow-up of patients (Barnason et al., 2017).

Behavior change strategies for managing CVD have and continued to emphasize key elements of the social cognitive theory (SCT), including goal setting, self-monitoring, self-efficacy enhancement, social support, and feedback provided by healthcare providers, including reinforcement for positive behavior change (Bandura, 1997; Bandura & National Inst of Mental Health, 1986). Discussed in detail elsewhere in this book, SCT-based behavior change strategies have been effective in reducing single- and multiple-risk behaviors in the setting of secondary prevention of CVD. SCT has also been used in the development, testing, and implementation of mobile health (mHealth) behavioral interventions for patients with CVD (Park et al., 2016; Pfaeffli Dale et al., 2015). While research to date on maintenance of behavior change over time is more limited, results of selected studies indicate that the key elements of SCT combined with other treatment modalities can be effective in long-term smoking cessation and weight loss maintenance (Orth-Gomér, 2012).

MI is a behavior change counseling strategy that emphasizes patient-centered approaches, including eliciting patient priorities, needs, and values; building rapport (i.e., reflective listening and empathy); and support for self-management (Miller & Rollnick, 2002). MI has been used in conjunction with the transtheoretical model of stages of change (Prochaska et al., 1992) to modify CVD-related health behaviors in patients who have experienced a cardiovascular event (Wood et al., 2008) and for individuals at increased CVD risk (Mochari-Greenberger et al., 2010; Steptoe et al., 1999). In both primary and secondary prevention of CVD, MI has also been widely used as an adjunctive strategy to modify physical activity and dietary behaviors for overweight and obese individuals (Armstrong et al., 2011; Artinian et al., 2010)

Several clinical trials have demonstrated the efficacy of incorporating MI with other behavior change strategies in individuals with or at risk for CVD. In the Family Intervention Trial for Heart Health, a 12-month, single-site, randomized controlled trial (RCT), MI was used (in person and by telephone) with stages of change to modify the intake of saturated fat, cholesterol, and other key nutrients among family members of hospitalized CVD patients (Mosca et al., 2008). In this RCT, the special intervention participants had better adherence to a heart-healthy diet with lower fat and cholesterol consumption indicated by a lower MEDFICTS diet score compared with the control group (-18.4% vs. -5.0%; $p = .04$). In addition, control intervention participants were more likely than special intervention participants to revert to lower levels on the stage of change continuum from baseline to 1 year (17% vs. 7%; $p = .002$). As illustrated in other studies, the results indicate MI combined with stages of change and other behavior change strategies can be effective in modifying CVD health behaviors (Martins & McNeil, 2009). Additional observations from these studies suggest that the effectiveness of a stage of change-matched educational intervention varies by baseline stage of change, is dynamic over time, and is positively influenced by dose and duration of MI interventions (Martins & McNeil, 2009; Mosca et al., 2008).

Provider-Delivered Interventions

Kronish and Ye offer a summary of evidence-based strategies designed to assist providers in promoting patient adherence to therapeutic regimens among CVD patients (Kronish & Ye, 2013). These include keeping adherence to the agenda, asking about it in a nonjudgmental manner at every patient visit, and recalling that there are few definite predictors of who will be nonadherent; thus, it is best to directly ask patients. When healthcare providers identify nonadherence, being mindful of patient-centered communication and exploring patients' concerns about the treatment protocol may be key factors in improving adherence, particularly with medications. Additional suggestions include engaging the patient's social network and social support (e.g., spouse or partner), and simplifying and tailoring the treatment regimen with consideration of the patient's literacy level, sociocultural background, area of residence, preferences, and resources (Kronish & Ye, 2013). As discussed in the following, emerging evidence suggests that incorporation of innovations in health information technology designed to empower individuals to assume a more active role in managing their chronic conditions and therapeutic regimens holds promise and potential as an adherence-enhancing approach for patients with CVD (Park et al., 2016; Winter et al., 2016).

Mobile Health and Digital Health Technology and Behavior Change for Cardiovascular Disease Management

Substantial research efforts have recently focused on the development and application of mobile and digital health technologies with emphasis on health behaviors central to both prevention and management of chronic health conditions, including CVD (Burke et al., 2015).

A recent systematic review and meta-analysis evaluated the efficacy of telemedicine in reducing CVD risk factors (Jaén-Extremera et al., 2023). The review consisted of RCTs published between 2017 and 2022 where telemedicine was used to reduce any of the following cardiovascular risk factors: diabetes, hypertension, obesity, or physical activity. There were 28 articles selected, with 13 focusing on diabetes, 6 on hypertension, 7 on obesity, and 2 on physical activity. This large review showed heterogenous statistical significance for hemoglobin A1c improvement, with only 4 out of 13 studies having clearly statistically significant reductions in hemoglobin A1c (between −0.36% and −0.87% decrease in A1c from 3 months to 2 years of intervention with p value between .001 and .03). Ten articles were able to be included in the meta-analysis and showed a significant but small mean reduction in hemoglobin A1c (g = −0.43 [95% CI: −0.52 to −0.34; $p < .001$]). For hypertension, four out of six studies showed statistically significant reduction in blood pressure (reduction in systolic pressure between −5.28 mmHg and −10.10 mmHg between 3 and 6 months of intervention). The meta-analysis showed a significant lowering of both systolic (g = −0.775 [95% CI: −0.89 to −0.66; $p < .001$]) and diastolic pressures (g = −0.45 [95% CI: −0.57 to −0.32; $p < .001$]). Similarly, out of the seven studies focusing on weight loss in the obese population, five showed statistically significant reduction in weight. The meta-analysis showed a moderate weight loss (g = −0.63 [95% CI: −0.74 to −0.52; $p < .001$]). There was no significant change for physical activity (Jaén-Extremera et al., 2023). This study shows that despite heterogenous results of the RCTs on multiple CVD risk factors, telemedicine remains a promising method for managing and reducing CVD risk factors.

From a secondary prevention standpoint, another recent systemic review and meta-analysis showed that combined remote monitoring and consultation for those with heart failure resulted in statistically significant reductions in short-term CVD-related mortality and hospitalization (Kuan et al., 2022). It should be noted that even though telemedicine use has increased with the onset of the COVID-19 pandemic and its use has shown to be cost-effective (Farabi et al., 2020), caution and care should be used given the risk of a digital divide, which could further exacerbate preexisting health disparities (Eberly et al., 2020).

A quantitative systematic review of mobile phone interventions for secondary prevention of CVD suggests the promise and potential of text messaging, mobile applications, and telemonitoring in improving outcomes of patients with CVD (Park et al., 2016). The review encompassed all study designs, including observational cohort studies as well as RCTs. As such, studies ($n = 28$) that met the inclusion criteria (used text messaging and/or mobile application with mobile phones for secondary prevention of CVD) varied significantly in the characteristics of patients, cardiovascular condition, intervention elements, and measurement of effectiveness. Of note, most studies (79%, $n = 22$) were efficacious in improving behaviors and clinical outcomes, particularly in older patients with CVD. Key factors associated with successful interventions included personalized messages with individually tailored advice, greater engagement (two-way text messaging, higher frequency of messages), and use of multiple modalities (Park et al., 2016). Of note, all studies using text messaging or mobile applications compared with another technology intervention (i.e., web-based or continuous monitoring) found both user adherence and satisfaction to be highest in the text messaging or mobile application intervention groups.

The Text4Heart RCT provides additional insight regarding patient benefits and implementation challenges encountered in the incorporation of mHealth technology for CVD self-management and highlights areas for additional research (Pfaeffli Dale et al., 2015). A major aim of this 6-month, two-arm, parallel RCT was to examine the effectiveness of an mHealth-delivered comprehensive CR program (in addition to usual care) in improving adherence to recommended lifestyle behaviors (smoking cessation, physical activity, healthy diet, and nonharmful alcohol use) for patients with CVD. Of note, intervention participants reported high fidelity to the text messaging component, with 85% (52/61) indicating they read all the messages; 90% (55/61) expressed satisfaction with delivery of the program via text messaging. In contrast, less than half of the participants (43%, 26/61) felt that using a website for delivery of program elements was helpful. Challenges in the delivery of behavior change approaches with mHealth technologies, including methods to ensure text message and internet literacy, were highlighted. Several participants who reported these competencies at baseline indicated challenges in accessing the internet during the intervention. Additional lesson learned in this RCT and supported by other behavior change intervention research that did not include mHealth technology is the need to include relapse prevention strategies. The optimal dose and duration of behavior change counseling for maintenance of single or multiple behavior change remains a fertile area of future research, particularly with mHealth technologies. In addition, socially marginalized populations will probably need additional tailoring of such intervention to make the intervention feasible and acceptable. In a review of the effectiveness of mHealth behavior change interventions for CVD self-management, the authors highlight the potential for this technology to change selected lifestyle behaviors and the need for larger scale, longitudinal studies to gain a better understanding of the effects of mHealth over time and across diverse population groups (Pfaeffli Dale et al., 2016).

Lastly, digital healthcare, if delivered with an equitable approach, has the potential to decrease health disparities and improve healthcare equity. For instance, Black people have a higher prevalence of CVD risk factors, which in turn leads to higher rates of CVD and mortality (Carnethon et al., 2017). To address this, Brewer and colleagues created an educational mobile application with the help of local Black communities that improved CVD health as measured by the AHA Life Simple 7 score (Brewer et al., 2022). A nurse-managed telemonitoring program over a 1-year period in urban Black population showed a statistically significant improvement in systolic blood pressure (13 mmHg vs. 7.5 mmHg; $t = -2.09$, $p = .04$) and nonstatistically significant improvement diastolic blood pressure (6.3 mmHg vs. 4.1 mmHg; $t = -1.56$, $p = 0.12$) compared with usual clinic-based care (Artinian et al., 2007). This shows that telemedicine/mHealth is a promising avenue to provide equity-conscious care to bridge the gaps in health disparities.

Multicomponent Interventions: Integrating Behavior Change Strategies With Evidence-Based Multidisciplinary Case Management

Effective management of CVD, similar to other chronic conditions, is a complex process facilitated by multidisciplinary team approaches, multicomponent interventions, and integrated systems of care. In the setting of secondary prevention, individuals with documented CVD normally present with more than one adverse health behavior and with multiple risk factors (Buddeke et al., 2019). Evidence indicates that a multidisciplinary collaborative care team model that focuses on individually tailored, guideline-based, patient-centered interventions, family and social support, healthcare providers, community-level factors (e.g., access to CR programs), and systems of care that enable coordination of care providers is highly effective in reducing multiple adverse health behaviors and risk factors and preventing recurring events (Berra et al., 2011; Smith et al., 2011).

Substantial research demonstrating the effectiveness of multicomponent interventions and multidisciplinary, team-based care for CVD patients has guided and informed the implementation of such care into mainstream healthcare. The MULTIFIT program (DeBusk et al., 1994) was among the first to demonstrate the effectiveness of an integrated multidisciplinary team approach in changing adverse health behaviors and improving major modifiable risk factors in patients with CVD. Concomitantly, the Stanford Coronary Risk Intervention Program (SCRIP) demonstrated the effectiveness of a multidisciplinary team approach (consisting of physicians, nurses, psychologists, and nutritionists) in reducing total cardiovascular events, angiographically measured atherosclerosis, adverse health behaviors, and cardiovascular risk factors in men and women with documented coronary artery disease (Haskell et al., 1994).

Building on lessons learned in MULTIFIT and SCRIP and incorporating MI and selected eHealth technologies, EUROACTION included patients hospitalized with coronary heart disease (CHD) as well as high-risk patients and their partners drawn from general practices across eight countries in Europe and the United Kingdom (Wood et al., 2008). A major goal was to help patients with established CHD and those with high multifactorial risk factors outside specialist CR centers to achieve lifestyle, risk factor, and therapeutic targets defined in the European Society of Cardiology prevention guidelines. At the end of year 1, EUROACTION intervention participants achieved clinically meaningful reduction in most cardiovascular risk factors. Significant improvements in patterns of dietary intake and physical activity were observed in both patients and their partners (Wood et al., 2008). The authors concluded that behavioral–lifestyle changes were key factors in the CVD risk reductions observed in this trial (Wood et al., 2008).

Other multidisciplinary, physician-directed, nurse-based case management studies have shown reductions in cardiovascular-related morbidity and mortality (Berra, 2011; Fonarow et al., 2001). These multidisciplinary team-based approaches were shown to be effective across settings, including hospitalized and primary care patients, low-income clinics, and in community centers (Allen & Dennison, 2010; Berra, 2011). More recently, research focused on multidisciplinary models for both primary and secondary CVD prevention has placed emphasis on the inclusion of community health workers (CHWs) as key members of the care team (Allen et al., 2011; Kim et al., 2016). Results of several RCTs have demonstrated that CHWs, also called "promotoras" or "health navigators," contribute uniquely to community-based healthcare, including behavioral–lifestyle change for individuals with CVD and other chronic conditions. Prompted in part by the recognized need to reduce healthcare costs while improving outcomes, integration of CHWs in multidisciplinary teams has demonstrated the potential for extended outreach to vulnerable groups with or at risk for CVD (Allen et al., 2011; Landers & Levinson, 2016). Critically important in optimizing CHWs in behavior change and other aspects of the research protocol is training and guidance provided by an experienced team member, who is often a nurse. As implemented in the Community Outreach and Cardiovascular Health (COACH) trial, a nurse practitioner (NP)/CHW team intervention focused on promoting therapeutic lifestyle changes and adherence to medications and appointments can be an effective model for risk reduction in patients with CVD (Allen et al., 2011). The results of the COACH trial supported the effectiveness of the NP/CHW team model using individualized treatment regimens based on treat-to-target algorithms in improving CVD risk factor status as well as perceptions of chronic illness care. High-risk patients in the NP/CHW group had significantly greater 12-month improvement in major CVD risk factors. Importantly, based on collective results, the authors recommended nurse-led, patient-centered medical homes as a viable model to improve the quality of CVD care in high-risk and underserved populations, with acknowledgment of the lack of payment policies for CHWs as a deterrent to adoption in mainstream healthcare (Allen et al., 2011). Nevertheless, the current landscape of payment policies for CHWs is changing and CHWs are increasingly recognized as people who can bridge the health system with the communities and have important roles, including self-management coaching of patients and addressing social determinants of health (Ballard et al., 2022; CDC, 2023; Peretz et al., 2020).

While RCTs have demonstrated efficacy and effectiveness in the processes and outcomes of secondary prevention and have resulted in the adoption of adapted models in selected systems of healthcare, universal adoption and sustainability of community-based healthy lifestyle initiatives have not been achieved (Berra et al., 2017). In addition, as summarized by Allen and Dennison (2010) and reaffirmed by others (Hayman et al., 2007; Orth-Gomér, 2012; Stuart-Shor et al., 2012), the optimal combination of intervention components including specific strategy, mode of delivery, and frequency and duration for modifying individual and/or multiple adverse behaviors in patients with documented CVD remains unknown. Particularly lacking are data relevant to modifying CVD-related health behaviors in the setting of secondary prevention of CVD for individuals from racially and ethnically diverse populations.

EVIDENCE-BASED GUIDELINES FOR SECONDARY PREVENTION AND RISK REDUCTION FOR PATIENTS WITH CARDIOVASCULAR DISEASE: THE IMPORTANCE OF CARDIAC REHABILITATION

While secondary prevention programs (SPPs) like CR have been in existence for several decades and endorsed by the AHA and ACC (Smith et al., 2011) and the American Association of Cardiovascular and Pulmonary Rehabilitation (Balady et al., 2007), the real-world use of formal CR program is very low (Ritchey et al., 2020; Van Iterson et al., 2023). However, CR has received recent, renewed attention within the cardiovascular community (Kachur et al., 2017; Rengo et al., 2018; van Halewijn et al., 2017). Based on accumulated evidence on the efficacy and effectiveness of these programs that include multidisciplinary, multicomponent interventions for behavior change and risk factor modification, these programs focus on reducing recurrent events in patients with CVD (Franklin & Brinks, 2015; Smith et al., 2011). The Centers for Medicare & Medicaid Services covers CR services for patients with CHD, heart failure, and peripheral artery disease. The majority of contemporary programs have three phases: inpatient enrollment, a supervised outpatient program, and individual maintenance. A major goal is to combine education, ongoing medical management, dietary modification, individually tailored lifestyle changes, and structured exercise training (Kachur et al., 2017). Inpatient enrollment, termed *phase I*, normally involves low-level exercise training and is considered a preface to *phase II*, the supervised ambulatory early outpatient program that normally extends for 12 weeks. Viewed as the cornerstone of CR, phase II consists of aggressive risk factor reduction and supervised exercise training, with efficacy enhanced with therapeutic education to emphasize the importance of smoking cessation, cardioprotective lifestyle changes, dietary modification, and management of psychosocial stress (van Halewijn et al., 2017). In contemporary, comprehensive multicomponent CR/SPPS programs, patients acquire skills and competencies in stress management and self-regulation/self-control, with support provided by a multispecialty team including physicians, nurses, exercise physiologists, physical and occupational therapists, dietitians, mental health specialists, and a case manager (Kachur et al., 2017). The major emphasis in phase II is placed on promoting comprehensive lifestyle changes, with the goal of long-term behavior modification central to reducing recurring events and mortality in CVD patients (Hammill et al., 2010). Phase III CR continues outside of a supervised healthcare setting and emphasizes maintenance of behavioral–lifestyle changes with the goal of improving health-related quality of life as well as reducing recurrent events (Kachur et al., 2017).

According to the 2017 AHA Heart Disease and Stroke Statistics report, roughly 2.5 million patients need CR each year. This includes those recently treated for heart attack, either medically, or revascularized percutaneously, or with open heart bypass surgery, and those newly diagnosed with heart failure (Benjamin et al., 2017). A systematic review and meta-analysis of 34 RCTs showed CR can reduce repeat heart attack (odds ratio [OR] 0.53, 95% CI: 0.38–0.76), cardiac mortality (0.64, 95% CI: 0.46–0.88), and all-cause mortality (OR 0.74, 95% CI: 0.58–0.95; Lawler, 2011). The 2018 ACC/AHA Clinical Performance and Quality Measures for Cardiac Rehabilitation: A Report of the American College of Cardiology/American Heart Association Task Force on Performance Measures stresses the importance of identifying and enrolling those who qualify for CR early to improve quality of life (Anderson et al., 2016), decrease morbidity and mortality (Janssen et al., 2013), and facilitate earlier return to work/functional activity. Moreover, multiple systematic reviews and meta-analysis showed equivalent efficacy between home-based and center-based CR (Anderson et al., 2017; Buckingham et al., 2016).

Despite the demonstrated benefits of CR/SPPs, the use of these programs remains low. Referral to CR/SPPs programs continues to be a factor in underutilization, with one report indicating that up to 80% of eligible CVD patients are not referred (Menezes et al., 2014). A recent report from the National Cardiovascular Data Registry suggests improvement in referral patterns for CVD patients undergoing percutaneous coronary intervention (PCI; Aragam et al., 2015). The referral rate (2009–2012) for PCI patients across 1,310 hospitals approximated 60%; however, significant variability in referral patterns was observed among sites, with over 25% referring less than 20% of eligible patients. Trends over time indicate that specific patient populations, including women, older adults, ethnic minorities, those with selected comorbidities, and individuals of low socioeconomic status, have especially low referral rates (Franklin & Brinks, 2015; Leon et al., 2005). Disparities in referral rates have prompted exploration of underlying factors and development of alternative models to enhance utilization of CR/SPPs (Arena et al., 2012; Franklin & Brinks, 2015). While systems of healthcare remain in transition in the United States, to be viable and to increase utilization by all eligible CVD patients, alternative models must address known barriers to referral and participation, including associated costs and ease of access. Thought leaders in this critically important component of secondary prevention suggest innovative strategies that include telemedicine, eHealth, as well as internet-based, home-based, and community-based programs (Franklin & Brinks, 2015; Kachur et al., 2017). Available data suggest the promise and potential of these alternative models with outcomes in CVD patients similar to those for conventional hospital-based programs (Clark et al., 2015). Recent research also supports the effectiveness of eHealth- and mHealth-delivered CR programs in enhancing adherence to recommended lifestyle behaviors (Pfaeffli Dale et al., 2015) and behavioral–lifestyle change in patients with documented CVD (Park et al., 2016).

CONCLUSION

Although substantial progress has been made in reducing CVD mortality over the past several decades, CVD remains a major cause of death and disability in the United States. The burden of CVD morbidity and mortality in the United States is not equally distributed. Many population subgroups, defined by race, sex, ethnicity, socioeconomic status, educational level, and area of residence, demonstrate an excess burden of CVD and its comorbidities (Benjamin et al., 2017; Havranek et al., 2015). Research is needed to guide and inform both clinical and public health efforts as well as multilevel policies designed to reduce disparities in both the prevention and treatment of CVD.

Accumulated evidence supports the importance of life-course approaches to the prevention and management of CVD, the critically important role of healthy lifestyle behaviors, and emphasis on factors that operate beyond the individual level to alter life-course trajectories that result in excess risk and burden of CVD. Similarly, accumulated evidence underscores the essential role of aggressive risk factor management and behavioral–lifestyle modification for patients with CVD. Comprehensive, contemporary CR/SPPs that emphasize maintenance of behavior change and risk factor management improve survival, reduce recurrent events, and improve quality of life for individuals with established heart disease. Adherence to provider recommendations for behavior change and medication regimens is an essential component of achieving treatment goals and preventing recurrent events. Consistent with social-ecological models of health and behavior, evidence supports the need and potential for multilevel approaches to increasing adherence to therapeutic regimens. The incorporation of eHealth technologies in treatment regimens has emerged as an adherence-enhancing strategy. Additional research, however, is needed to guide and inform optimal adherence-enhancing strategies as well as treatment approaches for vulnerable individuals with documented CVD. With the goal of reducing CVD-related disparities and promoting health equity, such research should focus on individuals from racial and ethnic minority populations, as well as those who reside in low-income communities and rural areas.

As highlighted in this chapter, substantial evidence supports the effectiveness of multidisciplinary, multicomponent SPPs in reducing adverse health behaviors and CVD risk factors, recurrent events, and in improving the of quality of life of individuals with CVD. Key elements of successful programs underscore the promise and potential of innovative models and integrated systems of care in reducing morbidity and mortality and improving the quality of life of diverse populations of patients with CVD.

CASE STUDY 14.1: TELEMEDICINE FOR HYPERTENSION MANAGEMENT

A 58-year-old Black man with diabetes and chronic kidney disease has been struggling with uncontrolled blood pressure for the last 2 years. High blood pressure runs in his family and many family members had complications like heart attack, stroke, and need for dialysis. The patient wants to prevent these complications. He was referred to see a cardiologist to control his blood pressure. After an initial visit, the patient's cardiologist enrolled him in a remote patient monitoring program where the patient was provided a home blood pressure monitor. Clinic staff demonstrated use of the blood pressure monitor and the patient was asked to check blood pressure at least three times a week. His cardiologist could see the blood pressure values using a telemonitoring application. However, within 1 week of the program initiation, there were no blood pressure data available. The patient's cardiologist learned that the patient had difficulty in using the blood pressure monitor. His cardiologist contacted a community health worker (CHW), who visited the patient's home. They demonstrated how to use the monitor and assured that the patient could use the monitor following standard procedures. Over the next 2 weeks, the patient's cardiologist learned that his blood pressure is on average lower than prior clinic values, but still markedly elevated. The cardiologist offered initiation of two additional blood pressure medications and a lab test. However, the patient admitted that it would be difficult for him to afford these medications. The cardiologist contacted a clinic social worker, and in coordination with the CHW and the hospital pharmacy the patient was offered the blood pressure medications and lab test without any cost, and the patient would be able to use the medications and lab tests free in the future. In addition, clinic nurses called the patient once every 2 weeks and discussed a comprehensive approach to lifestyle management to enhance the patient's self-care skills in taking his blood pressure. Over the course of 4 months, the patient's blood pressure has been well-controlled, and his confidence in behavioral self-care skills and understanding of blood pressure has

(continued)

14 • CARDIOVASCULAR DISEASE: A FOCUS ON PRIMARY AND SECONDARY PREVENTION 285

CASE STUDY 14.1: TELEMEDICINE FOR HYPERTENSION MANAGEMENT (*continued*)

markedly improved. The patient continues to monitor blood pressure at home and is happy with the remote patient monitoring program.

This case illustrates successful use of a multidimensional, multicomponent, hypertension disease-focused approach with particular equity-conscious adaptation of the remote patient monitoring program so that the intervention was effective, acceptable, and appropriate for the patient's specific needs.

CASE STUDY 14.2: CARDIAC REHABILITATION

The patient is a 49-year-old woman with congestive heart failure from uncontrolled hypertension. Her heart's pumping function, ejection fraction, is 35%, which is markedly diminished. She took "water pill" and several other medications over the last 6 months to make her heart "strong." Six months ago, she could barely walk to her mailbox due to breathlessness, but now she can do her groceries without problem. The patient's doctor referred her to local cardiac rehabilitation (CR) program 3 months ago. She has been using the program for a month now. The patient loves the CR program and wonders if she could have joined it much earlier. She enjoys the encouragement from the people at the program and finds it motivating to hear the success stories of other patients joining the program. The patient believes that the CR program has not only helped her heart and other physical health, but equally her mental health and outlook in life.

SUMMARY KEY POINTS

- Although the incidence of cardiovascular death has steadily trended down with medical advances and aggressive cardiovascular prevention, the prevalence of CVD and its risk factors continue to rise.

- Research and evidence over the past several decades indicate that a life-course approach is effective in the prevention and management of CVD. The promotion of a healthy lifestyle throughout life is the number one method of primary prevention of CVD.

- Secondary prevention of CVD emphasizes interventions designed to reduce the likelihood of CVD events and/or mortality in individuals who have established disease. Major potentially modifiable targets include health behaviors and established risk factors that are also part of primary prevention protocols.

- In both the setting of primary and secondary prevention of CVD, MI has also been widely used as an adjunctive strategy to modify physical activity and dietary behaviors for overweight and obese individuals and for smoking cessation.

- The majority of contemporary CR programs have three phases—inpatient enrollment, a supervised outpatient program, and individual maintenance—with the major goal of combining education, ongoing medical management, dietary modification, individually tailored lifestyle changes, and structured exercise training.

- While systems of healthcare remain in transition in the United States, to be viable and to increase utilization by all eligible CVD patients, alternative models must address known barriers to referral and participation, including associated costs and ease of access.

DISCUSSION QUESTIONS

1. Think of your own personal experience with heart disease. Have you prioritized primary prevention for your own health? If you do not prioritize it, what obstacles are in the way? Consider if these same obstacles face your community population at large and how they can be addressed.

2. Consider the success of the Text4Heart RCT focused on secondary prevention. Would you consider a similar program to be appropriate for primary prevention? Why or why not? If it were appropriate, who would be the targeted population? How would you feel if asked to enroll in such a program?

3. Consider the importance of a life-course approach to heart disease and think back to your childhood and adolescence. How was the subject of heart health discussed by your family, teachers, mentors, and healthcare providers? If it was not discussed, what other concerns took priority?

4. Smoking cessation is a major component of both primary and secondary prevention. Think about smoking in your family and community. What messages about smoking, if any, did you receive growing up? If you have never smoked, what would you say prevented you from starting? If you have smoked in the past, what factors pushed you to quit? If you currently smoke, what messages resonate with you about the increased risk of heart disease?

5. The ACC/AHA recommends at least 150 minutes of moderate-intensity or 75 minutes of high-intensity exercise weekly. Think of your own relationship with exercise. Is it realistic for you to meet these recommendations in your current lifestyle? If not, what are the obstacles? Are these same obstacles present for others in your community? Are there more?

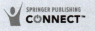

A robust set of instructor resources designed to supplement this text is located at http://connect.springerpub.com/content/book/978-0-8261-4265-8. Qualifying instructors may request access by emailing textbook@springerpub.com.

REFERENCES

Abdalla, S. M., Yu, S., & Galea, S. (2020). Trends in cardiovascular disease prevalence by income level in the United States. *JAMA Network Open, 3*(9), e2018150. https://doi.org/10.1001/jamanetworkopen.2020.18150

Allen, J. K., & Dennison, C. R. (2010). Randomized trials of nursing interventions for secondary prevention in patients with coronary artery disease and heart failure: Systematic review. *The Journal of Cardiovascular Nursing, 25*(3), 207–220. https://doi.org/10.1097/JCN.0b013e3181cc79be

Allen, J. K., Dennison-Himmelfarb, C. R., Szanton, S. L., Bone, L., Hill, M. N., Levine, D. M., West, M., Barlow, A., Lewis-Boyer, L., Donnelly-Strozzo, M., Curtis, C., & Anderson. A. (2011). Community Outreach and Cardiovascular Health (COACH) Trial: A randomized, controlled trial of nurse practitioner/community health worker cardiovascular disease risk reduction in urban community health centers. *Circulation. Cardiovascular Quality and Outcomes, 4*(6), 595–602. https://doi.org/10.1161/CIRCOUTCOMES.111.961573

Anderson, L., Oldridge, N., Thompson, D. R., Zwisler, A.-D., Rees, K., Martin, N., & Taylor, R. S.(2016). Exercise-based cardiac rehabilitation for coronary heart disease: Cochrane systematic review and meta-analysis. *Journal of the American College of Cardiology, 67*(1), 1–12. https://doi.org/10.1016/J.JACC.2015.10.044

Anderson, L., Sharp, G. A., Norton, R. J., Dalal, H., Dean, S. G., Jolly, K., Cowie, A., Zawada, A., & Taylor, R. S. (2017). Home-based versus centre-based cardiac rehabilitation. *The Cochrane Database Systemic Review,* (6), CD007130. https://doi.org/10.1002/14651858.cd007130.pub4

Aragam, K. G., Dai, D., Neely, M. L., Bhatt, D. L., Roe, M. T., Rumsfeld, J. S., & Gurm, H. S. (2015). Gaps in referral to cardiac rehabilitation of patients undergoing percutaneous coronary intervention in the United States. *Journal of American College of Cardiology, 65*(19), 2079–2088. https://doi.org/10.1016/j.jacc.2015.02.063

Arena, R., Williams, M., Forman, D. E., Cahalin, L. P., Coke, L., Myers, J., Hamm, L., Kris-Etherton, P., Humphrey, R., Bittner, V., Lavie, C. J., & American Heart Association Exercise, Cardiac Rehabilitation and Prevention Committee of the Council on Clinical Cardiology, Council on Epidemiology and Prevention, and Council on Nutrition, Physical Activity and Metabolism. (2012). Increasing referral and participation rates to outpatient cardiac rehabilitation: The valuable role of healthcare professionals in the inpatient and home health settings: A science advisory from the American Heart Association. *Circulation, 125*(10), 1321–1329. https://doi.org/10.1161/CIR.0b013e318246b1e5

Armstrong, M. J., Mottershead, T. A., Ronksley, P. E., Sigal, R. J., Campbell, T. S., & Hemmelgarn, B. R. (2011). Motivational interviewing to improve weight loss in overweight and/or obese patients: A systematic review and meta-analysis of randomized controlled trials. *Obesity Reviews, 12*(9), 709–723. https://doi.org/10.1111/j.1467-789X.2011.00892.x

Arnett, D. K., Blumenthal, R. S., Albert, M. A., Buroker, A. B., Goldberger, Z. D., Hahn, E. J., Himmelfarb, C. D., Khera, A., Lloyd-Jones, D., McEvoy, J. W., Michos, E. D., Miedema, M. D., Muñoz, D., Smith, S. C., Jr., Virani, S. S., Williams, K. A., Sr., Yeboah, J., & Ziaeian, B. (2019). 2019 ACC/AHA guideline on the primary prevention of cardiovascular disease: A report of the American College of Cardiology/American Heart Association task force on clinical practice guidelines. *Circulation, 140*(11), e596–e646. https://doi.org/10.1161/CIR.0000000000000678

Artinian, N. T., Flack, J. M., Nordstrom, C. K., Hockman, E. M., Washington, O. G.M., Jen, K.-L. C., & Fathy, M. (2007). Effects of nurse-managed telemonitoring on blood pressure at 12-month follow-up among Urban African Americans. *Nursing Research, 56*(5), 312–322. https://doi.org/10.1097/01.NNR.0000289501.45284.6e

Artinian, N. T., Fletcher, G. F., Mozaffarian, D., Kris-Etherton, P., Van Horn, L., Lichtenstein, A. H., Kumanyika, S., Kraus, W. E., Fleg, J. L., Redeker, N. S., Meininger, J. C., Banks, J., Stuart-Shor, E. M., Fletcher, B. J., Miller, T. D., Hughes, S., Braun, L. T., Kopin, L. A., Berra, K., . . . American Heart Association Prevention Committee of the Council on Cardiovascular Nursing. (2010). Interventions to promote physical activity and dietary lifestyle changes for cardiovascular risk factor reduction in adults: A scientific statement from the American Heart Association. *Circulation, 122*(4), 406–441. https://doi.org/10.1161/CIR.0b013e3181e8edf1

Balady, G. J., Williams, M. A., Ades, P. A., Bittner, V., Comoss, P., Foody, J. M., Franklin, B., Sanderson, B., & Southard, D. (2007). Core components of reha-bilitation/secondary prevention programs: 2007 update: A scientific statement from the American Heart Association and the American Association of Cardiovascular and Pulmonary Rehabilitation. *Circulation, 115*(20), 2675–2682. https://doi.org/10.1161/circulationaha.106.180945

Ballard, M., Odera, M., Bhatt, S., Geoffrey, B., & Westgate, C. (2022). Payment of community health workers. *Lancet Global Health, 10*(9), e1242. https://doi.org/10.1016/S2214-109X(22)00311-4

Bandura, A. (1997). *Self-efficacy: The exercise of control.* W H Freeman/Times Books/ Henry Holt & Co.

Bandura, A., & National Inst of Mental Health. (1986). *Social foundations of thought and action: A social cognitive theory.* Prentice-Hall Inc.

Barnason, S., White-Williams, C., Rossi, L. P., Centeno, M., Crabbe, D. L., Lee, K. S., McCabe, N., Nauser, J., Schulz, P., Stamp, K., & Wood, K. (2017). Evidence for therapeutic patient education interventions to promote cardiovascular patient self-management: A scientific statement for healthcare professionals from the American Heart Association. *Circulation Cardiovascular Quality and Outcomes, 10*(6). https://doi.org/10.1161/HCQ.0000000000000025

Benjamin, E. J., Blaha, M. J., Chiuve, S. E., Cushman, M., Das, S. R., Deo, R., de Ferranti, S. D., Floyd, J., Fornage, M., Gillespie, C., Isasi, C. R., Jiménez, M. C., Jordan, L. C., Judd, S. E., Lackland, D., Lichtman, J. H., Lisabeth, L., Liu, S., Longenecker, C. T., . . . Muntner, P. (2017). Heart disease and stroke statistics—2017 update: A report from the American Heart Association. *Circulation, 135*(10), e146–e603. https://doi.org/10.1161/CIR.0000000000000485

Berenson, G. S., Srinivasan, S. R., Bao, W., Newman, W. P., 3rd., Tracy, R. E., & Wattigney, W. A. (1998). Association between multiple cardiovascular risk factors and atherosclerosis in children and young adults. The Bogalusa Heart Study. *The New England Journal of Medicine, 338*(23), 1650–1656. https://doi.org/10.1056/NEJM199806043382302

Berra, K. (2011). Does nurse case management improve implementation of guidelines for cardiovascular disease risk reduction? *Journal of Cardiovascular Nursing, 26*(2), 145–167. https://doi.org/10.1097/JCN.0b013e3181ec1337

Berra, K., Franklin, B., & Jennings, C. (2017). Community-based healthy living interventions. *Progress in Cardiovascular Diseases, 59*(5), 430–439. https://doi.org/10.1016/j.pcad.2017.01.002

Berra, K., Miller, N. H., & Jennings, C. (2011). Nurse-based models for cardiovascular disease prevention: From research to clinical practice. *Journal of Cardiovascular Nursing, 26*(Suppl. 4), S46–S55. https://doi.org/10.1097/JCN.0b013e318213ef5c

Brewer, L. C., Jenkins, S., Hayes, S. N., Kumbamu, A., Jones, C., Burke, L. E., Cooper, L. A., & Patten, C. A. (2022). Community-based, cluster-randomized pilot trial of a cardiovascular mobile health intervention: Preliminary findings of the FAITH! trial. *Circulation, 146*(3), 175–190. https://doi.org/10.1161/CIRCULATIONAHA.122.059046

Buckingham, S. A., Taylor, R. S., Jolly, K., Zawada, A., Dean, S. G., Cowie, A., Norton, R. J., & Dalal, H. M. (2016). Home-based versus centre-based cardiac rehabilitation: Abridged Cochrane systematic review and meta-analysis. *Open Hear, 3*(2). https://doi.org/10.1136/OPENHRT-2016-000463

Buddeke, J., Bots, M. L., Van Dis, I., Visseren, F. L., Hollander, M., Schellevis, F. G., & Vaartjes, I.(2019). Comorbidity in patients with cardiovascular disease in primary care: A cohort study with routine healthcare data. *The British Journal of General Practice, 69*(683), e398. https://doi.org/10.3399/BJGP19X702725

Burke, L. E., Ma, J., Azar, K. M., Bennett, G. G., Peterson, E. D., Zheng, Y., Riley, W., Stephens, J., Shah, S. H., Suffoletto, B., Turan, T. N., Spring, B., Steinberger, J., Quinn, C. C., & American Heart Association Publications Committee of the Council on Epidemiology and Prevention, Behavior Change Committee of the Council on Cardiometabolic Health, Council on Cardiovascular and Stroke Nursing, Council on Functional Genomics and Translational Biology, Council on Quality of Care and Outcomes Research, and Stroke Council. (2015). Current science on consumer use of mobile health for cardiovascular disease prevention: A scientific statement from the American Heart Association. *Circulation, 132*(12), 1157–1213. https://doi.org/10.1161/CIR.0000000000000232

Cardoso, R., Abovich, A., Boden, W. E., Arbab-zadeh, A., Blankstein, R., & Blumenthal, R. S. (2022). The 2021 AHA/ACC/SCAI coronary artery revascularization recommendations: Need for emphasis on prevention and future considerations. *JACC: Advances, 1*(1), 100006. http://doi.org/10.1016/j.jacadv.2022.100006

Carnethon, M. R., Pu, J., Howard, G., Albert, M. A., Anderson, C. A. M., Bertoni, A. G., Mujahid, M. S., Palaniappan, L., Taylor, H. A., Jr., Willis, M., & Yancy, C. W. (2017). Cardiovascular health in African Americans: A scientific statement from the American Heart Association. *Circulation, 136*(21). https://doi.org/10.1161/CIR.0000000000000534

Castellano, J. M., Sanz, G., Peñalvo, J. L., Bansilal, S., Fernández-Ortiz, A., Alvarez, L., Guzmán, L., Linares, J. C., García, F., D'Aniello, F., Arnáiz, J. A., Varea, S., Martínez, F., Lorenzatti, A., Imaz, I., Sánchez-Gómez, L. M., Roncaglioni, M. C., Baviera, M., Smith, S. C., Jr., . . . Fuster, V. (2014). A polypill strategy to improve adherence: Results from the FOCUS project. *Journal of the American College of Cardiology, 64*(20), 2071–2082. https://doi.org/10.1016/j.jacc.2014.08.021

Centers for Disease Control and Prevention. (2020). *About underlying cause of death, 1999–2020.* https://wonder.cdc.gov/ucd-icd10.html

Centers for Disease Control and Prevention. (2022). *Centers for disease control: Heart disease facts.* http://www.cdc.gov/heartdisease/facts.htm

Centers for Disease Control and Prevention. (2023, July). *CS297214-A policy options for facilitating the use of community health workers in health delivery systems POLICY BRIEF.*

Chen, X., & Wang, Y. (2008). Tracking of blood pressure from childhood to adulthood: A systematic review and meta-regression analysis. *Circulation, 117*(25), 3171–3180. https://doi.org/10.1161/CIRCULATIONAHA.107.730366

Cholesterol Treatment Trialists' (CTT) Collaboration, Baigent, C., Blackwell, L., Emberson, J., Holland, L. E., Reith, C., Bhala, N., Peto, R., Barnes, E. H., Keech, A., Simes, J., & Collins, R. (2010). Efficacy and safety of more intensive lowering of LDL cholesterol: A meta-analysis of data from 170,000 participants in 26 randomised trials. *Lancet, 376*(9753), 1670–1681. https://doi.org/10.1016/S0140-6736(10)61350-5

Churchwell, K., Elkind, M. S.V., Benjamin, R. M., Carson, A. P., Chang, E. K., Lawrence, W., Mills, A., Odom, T. M., Rodriguez, C. J., Rodriguez, F., Sanchez, E., Sharrief, A. Z., Sims, M., Williams, O., & American Heart Association. (2020). Call to action: Structural racism as a fundamental driver of health disparities: A presidential advisory from the American Heart Association. *Circulation, 142*(24), e454–e468. https://doi.org/10.1161/CIR.0000000000000936

Clark, R. A., Conway, A., Poulsen, V., Keech, W., Tirimacco, R., & Tideman, P. (2015). Alternative models of cardiac rehabilitation: A systematic review. *European Journal of Preventive Cardiology, 22*(1), 35–74. https://doi.org/10.1177/2047487313501093

DeBusk, R. F., Miller, N. H., Superko, H. R., Dennis, C. A., Thomas, R. J., Lew, H. T., Berger, W. E., 3rd., Heller, R. S., Rompf, J., Gee, D., Kraemer, H. C., Bandura, A., Ghandour, G., Clark, M., Shah, R. V., Fisher, L., & Taylor, C. B. (1994). A case-management system for coronary risk factor modification after acute myocardial infarction. *Annals of Internal Medicine, 120*(9), 721–729. https://doi.org/10.7326/0003-4819-120-9-199405010-00001

Eberly, L. A., Khatana, S. A. M., Nathan, A. S., Snider, C., Julien, H. M., Deleener, M. E., & Adusumalli, S. (2020). Telemedicine outpatient cardiovascular care during the COVID-19 pandemic. *Circulation, 142*(5), 510–512. https://doi.org/10.1161/CIRCULATIONAHA.120.048185

Eckel, R. H., Jakicic, J. M., Ard, J. D., de Jesus, J. M., Miller, N. H., Hubbard, V. S., Lee, I.-M., H Lichtenstein, A. H., Loria, C. M., Millen, B. E., Nonas, C. A., Sacks, F. M., Smith, S. C. Jr.,

Svetkey, L. P., Wadden, T. A., & Yanovski, S. Z., & American College of Cardiology/American Heart Association Task Force on Practice Guidelines. (2014). 2013 AHA/ACC guideline on lifestyle management to reduce cardiovascular risk: A report of the American College of Cardiology/American Heart Association task force on practice guidelines. *Journal of the American College of Cardiology, 63*(25 Pt B), 2960–2984. https://doi.org/10.1016/J.JACC.2013.11.003

Farabi, H., Rezapour, A., Jahangiri, R., Jafari, A., Rashki Kemmak, A., & Nikjoo, S. (2020). Economic evaluation of the utilization of telemedicine for patients with cardiovascular disease: A systematic review. *Heart Failure Reviews, 25*(6), 1063–1075. https://doi.org/10.1007/S10741-019-09864-4/METRICS

Fonarow, G. C., Gawlinski, A., Moughrabi, S., & Tillisch, J. H. (2001). Improved treatment of coronary heart disease by implementation of a Cardiac Hospitalization Atherosclerosis Management Program (CHAMP). *The American Journal of Cardiology, 87*(7), 819–822. https://doi.org/10.1016/s0002-9149(00)01519-8

Franklin, B. A., & Brinks, J. (2015). Cardiac rehabilitation: Underrecognized/underutilized. *Current Treatment Options Cardiovascular Medicine, 17*(12), 62. https://doi.org/10.1007/s11936-015-0422-x

Freedman, D. S., Mei, Z., Srinivasan, S. R., Berenson, G. S., & Dietz, W. H. (2007). Cardiovascular risk factors and excess adiposity among overweight children and adolescents: The Bogalusa Heart Study. *The Journal of Pediatrics, 150*(1), 12–17.e2. https://doi.org/10.1016/j.jpeds.2006.08.042

Gao, Z., Chen, Z., Sun, A., & Deng, X. (2019). Gender differences in cardiovascular disease. *Medicine in Novel Technology and Devices, 4*(2), 100025. https://doi.org/10.1016/J.MEDNTD.2019.100025

Gast, A., & Mathes, T. (2019). Medication adherence influencing factors–An (updated) overview of systematic reviews. *Systematic Reviews, 8*(1), 1–17. https://doi.org/10.1186/s13643-019-1014-8

Group WHOW. (n.d.). *Therapeutic patient education: Continuing education programmes for health care providers in the field of chronic diseases*. WHO Regional Office for Europe. https://iris.who.int/handle/10665/108151

Grundy, S. M., Stone, N. J., Bailey, A. L., Beam, C., Birtcher, K. K., Blumenthal, R. S., Braun, L. T., de Ferranti, S., Faiella-Tommasino, J., Forman, D. E., Goldberg, R., Heidenreich, P. A., Hlatky, M. A., Jones, D. W., Lloyd-Jones, D., Lopez-Pajares, N., Ndumele, C. E., Orringer, C. E., Peralta, C. A., . . . Yeboah, J. (2019). 2018 AHA/ACC/AACVPR/AAPA/ABC/ACPM/ADA/AGS/APhA/ASPC/NLA/PCNA guideline on the management of blood cholesterol: A report of the American College of Cardiology/American Heart Association task force on clinical practice guidelines. *Circulation, 139*(25), E1082–E1143. https://doi.org/10.1161/CIR.0000000000000625

Hammill, B. G., Curtis, L. H., Schulman, K. A., & Whellan, D. J. (2010). Relationship between cardiac rehabilitation and long-term risks of death and myocardial infarction among elderly Medicare beneficiaries. *Circulation, 121*(1), 63–70. https://doi.org/10.1161/CIRCULATIONAHA.109.876383

Haskell, W. L., Alderman, E. L., Fair, J. M., Maron, D. J., Mackey, S. F., Superko, H. R., Williams, P. T., Johnstone, I. M., Champagne, M. A., & Krauss, R. M. (1994). Effects of intensive multiple risk factor reduction on coronary atherosclerosis and clinical cardiac events in men and women with coronary artery disease. The Stanford Coronary Risk Intervention Project (SCRIP). *Circulation, 89*(3), 975–990. https://doi.org/10.1161/01.cir.89.3.975

Havranek, E. P., Mujahid, M. S., Barr, D. A., Blair, I. V., Cohen, M. S., Cruz-Flores, S., Davey-Smith, G., Dennison-Himmelfarb, C. R., Lauer, M. S., Lockwood, D. W., Rosal, M., Yancy, C. W., & American Heart Association Council on Quality of Care and Outcomes Research, Council on Epidemiology and Prevention, Council on Cardiovascular and Stroke Nursing, Council on Lifestyle and Cardiometabolic Health, and Stroke Council. (2015). Social determinants of risk and outcomes for cardiovascular disease: A scientific statement from the American Heart Association. *Circulation, 132*(9), 873–898. https://doi.org/10.1161/cir.0000000000000228

Hayman, L. L., Helden, L., Chyun, D. A., & Braun, L. T. (2011). A life course approach to cardiovascular disease prevention. *The Journal of Cardiovascular Nursing, 26*(Suppl. 4), 22–34. https://doi.org/10.1097/jcn.0b013e318213ef7f

Hayman, L. L., Meininger, J. C., Daniels, S. R., McCrindle, B. W., Helden, L., Ross, J., Dennison, B. A., Steinberger, J., Williams, C. L., American Heart Association Committee on Atherosclerosis, Hypertension, and Obesity in Youth of the Council on Cardiovascular Disease in the Young; American Heart Association Council on Cardiovascular Nursing; American Heart Association Council on Epidemiology and Prevention, & American Heart Association Council on Nutrition, Physical Activity, and Metabolism. (2007). Primary prevention of cardiovascular disease in nursing practice: Focus on children and youth: A scientific statement from the American Heart Association Committee on Atherosclerosis, Hypertension, and Obesity in Youth of the Council on Cardiovascular Disease in the Young, Council on Cardiovascular Nursing, Council on Epidemiology and Prevention, and Council on Nutrition, Physical Activity, and Metabolism. *Circulation, 116*(3), 344–357. https://doi.org/10.1161/CIRCULATIONAHA.107.184595

Haynes, R. B., McKibbon, K. A., & Kanani, R. (1996). Systematic review of randomised trials of interventions to assist patients to follow prescriptions for medications. *Lancet, 348*(9024), 383–386. https://doi.org/10.1016/s0140-6736(96)01073-2

Jaén-Extremera, J., Afanador-Restrepo, D. F., Rivas-Campo, Y., Gómez-Rodas, A., Aibar-Almazán, A., Hita-Contreras, F., Carcelén-Fraile, M. D. C., Castellote-Caballero, Y., & Ortiz-Quesada, R. (2023). Effectiveness of telemedicine for reducing cardiovascular risk: A systematic review and meta-analysis. *Journal of Clinical Medicine, 12*(3), 841. https://doi.org/10.3390/JCM12030841

Janssen, V., De Gucht, V., Dusseldorp, E., & Maes, S. (2013). Lifestyle modification programmes for patients with coronary heart disease: A systematic review and meta-analysis of randomized controlled trials. *European Journal of Preventive Cardiology, 20*(4), 620–640. https://doi.org/10.1177/2047487312462824

Jensen, M. D., Ryan, D. H., Apovian, C. M., Ard, J. D., Comuzzie, A. G., Donato, K. A., Hu, F. B., Hubbard, V. S., Jakicic, J. M., Kushner, R. F., Loria, C. M., Millen, B. E., Nonas, C. A., Pi-Sunyer, F. X., Stevens, J., Stevens, V. J., Wadden, T. A., Wolfe, B. M., Yanovski, S. Z., . . . Obesity Society. (2014). AHA/ACC/TOS guideline for the management of overweight and obesity in adults: A report of the American College of Cardiology/American Heart Association task force on practice guidelines and the obesity society. *Journal of the American College of Cardiology, 63*(25 Pt B), 2985–3023. https://doi.org/10.1016/J.JACC.2013.11.004

Kachur, S., Chongthammakun, V., Lavie, C. J., De Schutter, A., Arena, R., Milani, R. V., & Franklin, B. A. (2017). Impact of cardiac rehabilitation and exercise training programs in coronary heart disease. *Progress in Cardiovascular Disease, 60*(1), 103–114. https://doi.org/10.1016/j.pcad.2017.07.002

Kickbusch, I., Allen, L., Franz, C. (2016). The commercial determinants of health. *The Lancet Global Health, 4*(12), e895–e896. https://doi.org/10.1016/S2214-109X(16)30217-0

Kim, S., Shin, D. W., Yun, J. M., Hwang, Y., Park, S. K., Ko, Y.-J., & Cho, B. (2016). Medication adherence and the risk of cardiovascular mortality and hospitalization among patients with newly prescribed antihypertensive medications. *Hypertension, 67*(3), 506–512. https://doi.org/10.1161/HYPERTENSIONAHA.115.06731

Kronish, I. M., & Ye, S. (2013). Adherence to cardiovascular medications: Lessons learned and future directions. *Progress in Cardiovascular Diseases, 55*(6), 590–600. https://doi.org/10.1016/j.pcad.2013.02.001

Kuan, P. X., Chan, W. K., Fern Ying, D. K., Rahman, M. A. A., Peariasamy, K. M., Lai, N. M., Mills, N. L., & Anand, A. (2022). Efficacy of telemedicine for the management of cardiovascular disease: A systematic review and meta-analysis. *Lancet Digital Health, 4*(9), e676–e691. https://doi.org/10.1016/S2589-7500(22)00124-8

Kucharska-Newton, A. M., Harald, K., Rosamond, W. D., Rose, K. M., Rea, T. D., & Salomaa, V. (2011). Socioeconomic indicators and the risk of acute coronary heart disease events: Comparison of population-based data from the United States and Finland. *Annals of Epidemiology, 21*(8). https://doi.org/10.1016/j.annepidem.2011.04.006

Kulkarni, S. P., Alexander, K. P., Lytle, B., Heiss, G., & Peterson, E. D. (2006). Long-term adherence with cardiovascular drug regimens. *American Heart Journal, 151*(1), 185–191. https://doi.org/10.1016/j.ahj.2005.02.038

Kumbhani, D. J., Fonarow, G. C., Cannon, C. P., Hernandez, A. F., Peterson, E. D., Peacock, W. F., Laskey, W. K., Pan, W., Schwamm, L. H., Bhatt, D. L., & Get With the Guidelines Steering Committee and Investigators. (2013). Predictors of adherence to performance measures in patients with acute myocardial infarction. *The American Journal of Medicine, 126*(1), 74.e1–9. https://doi.org/10.1016/j.amjmed.2012.02.025

Kvarnström, K., Westerholm, A., Airaksinen, M., & Liira, H. (2021). Factors contributing to medication adherence in patients with a chronic condition: A scoping review of qualitative research. *Pharmaceutics, 13*(7), 1100. https://doi.org/10.3390/PHARMACEUTICS13071100

Laitinen, T. T., Pahkala, K., Magnussen, C. G., Viikari, J. S. A., Oikonen, M., Taittonen, L., Mikkilä, V., Jokinen, E., Hutri-Kähönen, N., Laitinen, T., Kähönen, M., Lehtimäki, T., Raitakari, O. T., & Juonala, M. (2012). Ideal cardiovascular health in childhood and cardiometabolic outcomes in adulthood: The cardiovascular risk in young finns study. *Circulation, 125*(16), 1971–1978. https://doi.org/10.1161/CIRCULATIONAHA.111.073585

Laitinen, T. T., Ruohonen, S., Juonala, M., Magnussen, C. G., Mikkilä, V., Mikola, H., Hutri-Kähönen, N., Laitinen, T., Tossavainen, P., Jokinen, E., Niinikoski, H., Jula, A., Viikari, J. S. A., Rönnemaa, T., Raitakari, O. T., & Pahkala, K. (2017). Ideal cardiovascular health in childhood-Longitudinal associations with cardiac structure and function: The Special Turku Coronary Risk Factor Intervention Project (STRIP) and the Cardiovascular Risk in Young Finns Study (YFS). *International Journal of Cardiology, 230*, 304–309. https://doi.org/10.1016/j.ijcard.2016.12.117

Landers, S., & Levinson, M. (2016). Mounting evidence of the effectiveness and versatility of community health workers. *American Journal of Public Health, 106*(4), 591–592. https://doi.org/10.2105/AJPH.2016.303099

Lauer, R. M., & Clarke, W. R. (1990). Use of cholesterol measurements in childhood for the prediction of adult hypercholesterolemia. The muscatine study. *JAMA, 264*(23), 3034–3038.

Law, M. R., Morris, J. K., & Wald, N. J. (2009). Use of blood pressure lowering drugs in the prevention of cardiovascular disease: Meta-analysis of 147 randomised trials in the context of expectations from prospective epidemiological studies. *BMJ, 338*, b1665. https://doi.org/10.1136/bmj.b1665

Lawler, P. R., Filion, K. B., & Eisenberg, M. J. (2011). Efficacy of exercise-based cardiac rehabilitation post-myocardial infarction: A systematic review and meta-analysis of randomized controlled trials. *American Heart Journal, 162*(4), 571–584.e2. https://doi.org/10.1016/J.AHJ.2011.07.017

Leon, A. S., Franklin, B. A., Costa, F., Balady, G. J., Berra, K. A., Stewart, K. J., Thompson, P. D., Williams, M. A., Lauer, M. S., American Heart Association, Council on Clinical Cardiology (Subcommittee on Exercise, Cardiac Rehabilitation, and Prevention), Council on Nutrition, Physical Activity, and Metabolism (Subcommittee on Physical Activity), & American association of Cardiovascular and Pulmonary Rehabilitation. (2005). Cardiac rehabilitation and secondary prevention of coronary heart disease: An American Heart Association scientific statement from the Council on Clinical Cardiology (Subcommittee on Exercise, Cardiac Rehabilitation, and Prevention) and the Council on Nutrition, Physical Activity, and Metabolism (Subcommittee on Physical Activity), in collaboration with the American association of Cardiovascular and Pulmonary Rehabilitation. *Circulation, 111*(3), 369–376. https://doi.org/10.1161/01.CIR.0000151788.08740.5C

Lloyd-Jones, D. M., Allen, N. B., Anderson, C. A. M., Black, T., Brewer, L. C., Foraker, R. E., Grandner, M. A., Lavretsky, H., Perak, A. M., Sharma, G., & Rosamond, W., & American Heart Association. (2022). Life's essential 8: Updating and enhancing the American Heart Association's construct of cardiovascular health: A presidential advisory from the American Heart Association. *Circulation, 146*(5), e18–e43. https://doi.org/10.1161/CIR.0000000000001078

Lloyd-Jones, D. M., Hong, Y., Labarthe, D., Mozaffarian, D., Appel, L. J., Van Horn, L., Greenlund, K., Daniels, S., Nichol, G., Tomaselli, G. F., Arnett, D. K., Fonarow, G. C., Ho, P. M., Lauer, M. S., Masoudi, F. A., Robertson, R. M., Roger, V., Schwamm, L. H., Sorlie, P., . . . American Heart Association Strategic Planning Task Force and Statistics Committee. (2010). Defining and setting national goals for cardiovascular health promotion and disease reduction: The American Heart Association's strategic Impact Goal through 2020 and beyond. *Circulation, 121*(4), 586–613. https://doi.org/10.1161/CIRCULATIONAHA.109.192703

Maddox, T. M., & Ho, P. M. (2009). Medication adherence and the patient with coronary artery disease: Challenges for the practitioner. *Current Opinion in Cardiology, 24*(5), 468–472. https://doi.org/10.1097/HCO.0b013e32832ed62d

Martins, R. K., & McNeil, D. W. (2009). Review of Motivational Interviewing in promoting health behaviors. *Clinical Psychology Review, 29*(4), 283–293. https://doi.org/10.1016/j.cpr.2009.02.001

McGill, H. C., Jr., McMahan, C. A., Zieske, A. W., Sloop, G. D., Walcott, J. V., Troxclair, D. A., Malcom, G. T., Tracy, R. E., Oalmann, M. C., & Strong, J. P. (2000). Associations of coronary heart disease risk factors with the intermediate lesion of atherosclerosis in youth. The Pathobiological Determinants of Atherosclerosis in Youth (PDAY) research group. *Arteriosclerosis, Thrombosis and Vascular Biology, 20*(8), 1998–2004. https://doi.org/10.1161/01.atv.20.8.1998

Menezes, A. R., Lavie, C. J., Milani, R. V., Forman, D. E., King, M., & Williams, M. A. (2014). Cardiac rehabilitation in the United States. *Progress in Cardiovascular Diseases, 56*(5), 522–529. https://doi.org/10.1016/j.pcad.2013.09.018

Mensah, G. A., Goff, D. C., & Gibbons, G. H. (2017). Cardiovascular mortality differences-place matters. *JAMA, 317*(19), 1955–1957. https://doi.org/10.1001/jama.2017.4168

Miller, W. R., & Rollnick, S. (2002). *Motivational interviewing: Preparing people for change* (2nd ed.). The Guilford Press.

Mochari-Greenberger, H., Terry, M. B., & Mosca, L. (2010). Does stage of change modify the effectiveness of an educational intervention to improve diet among family members of hospitalized cardiovascular disease patients? *Journal of the American Dietetic Association, 110*(7), 1027–1035. https://doi.org/10.1016/j.jada.2010.04.012

Mohebi, R., Chen, C., & Ibrahim, N. (2022). Cardiovascular disease projections in the United States based on the 2020 census estimates. *Journal of American College of Cardiology, 80*(6), 565–578. https://doi.org/10.1016/j.jacc.2022.05.033

Mosca, L., Mochari, H., Liao, M., Christian, A. H., Edelman, D. J., Aggarwal, B., & Oz, M. C. (2008). A novel family-based intervention trial to improve heart health: FIT heart: Results of a randomized controlled trial. *Circulation. Cardiovascular Quality and Outcomes, 1*(2), 98–106. https://doi.org/10.1161/CIRCOUTCOMES.108.825786

Naderi, S. H., Bestwick, J. P., & Wald, D. S. (2012). Adherence to drugs that prevent cardiovascular disease: Meta-analysis on 376,162 patients. *The American Journal of Medicine, 125*(9), 882–7.e1. https://doi.org/10.1016/j.amjmed.2011.12.013

O'Flaherty, M., Buchan, I., & Capewell, S. (2013). Contributions of treatment and lifestyle to declining CVD mortality: Why have CVD mortality rates declined so much since the 1960s? *Heart, 99*(3), 159–162. https://doi.org/10.1136/heartjnl-2012-302300

Orth-Gomér, K. (2012). Behavioral interventions for coronary heart disease patients. *BioPsychoSocial Medicine, 6*(1), 5. https://doi.org/10.1186/1751-0759-6-5

Park, L. G., Beatty, A., Stafford, Z., & Whooley, M. A. (2016). Mobile phone interventions for the secondary prevention of cardiovascular disease. *Progress in Cardiovascular Diseases, 58*(6), 639–650. https://doi.org/10.1016/j.pcad.2016.03.002

Peretz, P. J., Islam, N., & Matiz, L. A. (2020). Community health workers and Covid-19—Addressing social determinants of health in times of crisis and beyond. *The New England Journal of Medicine, 383*(19), e108. https://doi.org/10.1056/NEJMP2022641

Pfaeffli Dale, L., Dobson, R., Whittaker, R., & Maddison, R. (2016). The effectiveness of mobile-health behaviour change interventions for cardiovascular disease self-management: A systematic review. *European Journal of Preventive Cardiology, 23*(8), 801–817. https://doi.org/10.1177/2047487315 613462

Pfaeffli Dale, L, Whittaker, R., Jiang, Y., Stewart, R., Rolleston, A., & Maddison, R. (2015). Text message and internet support for coronary heart disease self-management: Results from the text4heart randomized controlled trial. *Journal of Medical Internet Research, 17*(10), e237. https://doi.org/10.2196/jmir.4944

Prochaska, J. O., DiClemente, C. C., & Norcross, J. C. (1992). In search of how people change. Applications to addictive behaviors. *The American Psychologist, 47*(9), 1102–1114. https://doi.org/10.1037//0003-066x.47.9.1102

Rengo, J. L., Savage, P. D., Barrett, T., & Ades, P. A. (2018). Cardiac rehabilitation participation rates and outcomes for patients with heart failure. *Journal of Cardiopulmonary Rehabilitation and Prevention, 38*(1), 38–42. https://doi.org/10.1097/HCR.0000000000000252

Ritchey, M. D., Maresh, S., McNeely, J., Shaffer, T., Jackson, S. L., Keteyian, S. J., Brawner, C. A., Whooley, M. A., Chang, T., Stolp, H., Schieb, L., & Wright, J. (2020). Tracking cardiac rehabilitation participation and completion among medicare beneficiaries to inform the efforts of a national initiative. *Circulation. Cardiovascular Quality and Outcomes, 13*(1), e005902. https://doi.org/10.1161/CIRCOUTCOMES.119.005902

Rodriguez, F., Cannon, C. P., Steg G, Kumbhani, D. J., Goto, S., Smith, S. C., Eagle, K. A., Ohman, E. M., Umez-Eronini, A. A., Hoffman, E., & Bhatt, D. L., & REACH Registry Investigators. (2013). Predictors of long-term adherence to evidence-based cardiovascular disease medications in outpatients with stable atherothrombotic disease: Findings from the REACH registry. *Clinical Cardiology, 36*(12), 721–727. https://doi.org/10.1002/clc.22217

Ruppar, T. M., Cooper, P. S., Mehr, D. R., Delgado, J. M., & Dunbar-Jacob, J. M. (2016). Medication adherence interventions improve heart failure mortality and readmission rates: Systematic review and meta-analysis of controlled trials. *Journal of the American Heart Association, 5*(6), e002606. https://doi.org/10.1161/JAHA.115.002606

Scott, J., Cousin, L., Woo, J., Gonzalez-Guarda, R., & Simmons, L. A. (2022). Equity in genomics: A brief report on cardiovascular health disparities in African American adults. *The Journal of Cardiovascular Nursing, 37*(1), 58–63. https://doi.org/10.1097/JCN.0000000000000725

Smith, S. C., Jr., Benjamin, E. J., Bonow, R. O., Braun, L. T., Creager, M. A., Franklin, B. A., Gibbons, R. J., Grundy, S. M., Hiratzka, L. F., Jones, D. W., Lloyd-Jones, D. M., Minissian, M., Mosca, L., Peterson, E. D., Sacco, R. L., Spertus, J., Stein, J. H., Taubert, K. A., & World Heart Federation and the Preventive Cardiovascular Nurses Association. (2011). AHA/ACCF secondary prevention and risk reduction therapy for patients with coronary and other atherosclerotic vascular disease: 2011 update: A guideline from the American Heart Association and American College of Cardiology Foundation. *Circulation, 124*(22), 2458–2473. https://doi.org/10.1161/CIR.0b013e318235eb4d

Steptoe, A., Doherty, S., Rink, E., Kerry, S., Kendrick, T., & Hilton, S. (1999). Behavioural counselling in general practice for the promotion of healthy behaviour among adults at increased risk of coronary heart disease: Randomised trial. *BMJ, 319*(7215), 943–947; discussion 947–948. https://doi.org/10.1136/bmj.319.7215.943

Stone, N. J., Robinson, J. G., Lichtenstein, A. H., Merz, C. N. B., Blum, C. B., Eckel, R. H., Goldberg, A. C., Gordon, D., Levy, D., Lloyd-Jones, D. M., McBride, P., Schwartz, J. S., Shero, S. T., Smith, S. C., Jr., Watson, K., Wilson, P. W. F., & American College of Cardiology/American Heart Association Task Force on Practice Guidelines. (2014). 2013 ACC/AHA guideline on the treatment of blood cholesterol to reduce atherosclerotic cardiovascular risk in adults: A report of the American College of Cardiology/American Heart Association task force on practice guidelines. *Journal of the American College of Cardiology, 63*(25 Pt B), 2889–2934. https://doi.org/10.1016/j.jacc.2013.11.002

Stuart-Shor, E. M., Berra, K. A., Kamau, M. W., & Kumanyika, S. K. (2012). Behavioral strategies for cardiovascular risk reduction in diverse and underserved racial/ethnic groups. *Circulation, 125*(1), 171–184. https://doi.org/10.1161/CIRCULATIONAHA.110.968495

Suglia, S. F., Koenen, K. C., Boynton-Jarrett, R., Chan, P. S., Clark, C. J., Danese, A., Faith, M. S., Goldstein, B. I., Hayman, L. L., Isasi, C. R., Pratt, C. A., Slopen, N., Sumner, J. A., Turer, A., Turer, C. B., & Zachariah, J. P., American Heart Association Council on Epidemiology and Prevention, Council on Cardiovascular Disease in the Young, Council on Functional Genomics and Translational Biology, Council on Cardiovascular and Stroke Nursing, & Council on Quality of Care and Outcomes Research. (2018). Childhood and adolescent adversity and cardiometabolic outcomes: A scientific statement from the American Heart Association. *Circulation, 137*(5), e15–e28. https://doi.org/10.1161/CIR.0000000000000536

van Halewijn, G., Deckers, J., Tay, H. Y., van Domburg, R., Kotseva, K., & Wood, D. (2017). Lessons from contemporary trials of cardiovascular prevention and rehabilitation: A systematic review and meta-analysis. *Internaltion Journal of Cardiology, 232*, 294–303. https://doi.org/10.1016/j.ijcard .2016.12.125

Van Iterson, E. H., Laffin, L. J., Bruemmer, D., & Cho, L. (2023). Geographical and urban-rural disparities in cardiac rehabilitation eligibility and center-based use in the US. *JAMA Cardiology, 8*(1), 98–100. https://doi.org/10.1001/JAMACARDIO.2022.4273

Virani, S. S., Alonso, A., Aparicio, H. J., Benjamin, E. J., Bittencourt, M. S., Callaway, C. W., Carson, A. P., Chamberlain, A. M., Cheng, S., Delling, F. N., Elkind, M. S. V., Evenson, K. R., Ferguson, J. F., Gupta, D. K., Khan, S., Kissela, B. M., Knutson, K. L., Lee, C. D., Lewis, T. T., . . . Tsao, C. W. (2021). Heart Disease and Stroke Statistics–2021 update. *Circulation, 143*(8), e254–e743. https://doi .org/10.1161/cir.0000000000000950

Visseren, F. L. J., Mac, H. F., Smulders, Y. M., Carballo, D., Koskinas, K. C., Bäck, M., Benetos, A., Biffi, A., Boavida, J.-M., Capodanno, D., Cosyns, B., Crawford, C., Davos, C. H., Desormais, I., Di Angelantonio, E., Franco, O. H., Halvorsen, S., Richard Hobbs, F. D., Hollander, M., . . . ESC Scientific Document Group. (2021). 2021 ESC Guidelines on cardiovascular disease prevention in clinical practice. *European Heart Journal, 42*(34), 3227–3337. https://doi.org/10.1093/EURHEARTJ /EHAB484

Vlachopoulos, C., Aznaouridis, K., & Stefanadis, C. (2010). Prediction of cardiovascular events and all-cause mortality with arterial stiffness: A systematic review and meta-analysis. *Journal of the American Colloge of Cardiology, 55*(13), 1318–1327. https://doi.org/10.1016/j.jacc.2009.10.061

Winter, S. J., Sheats, J. L., & King, A. C. (2016). The use of behavior change techniques and theory in technologies for cardiovascular disease prevention and treatment in adults: A comprehensive review. *Progress in Cardiovascular Disease, 58*(6), 605–612. https://doi.org/10.1016/j.pcad.2016.02.005

Wood, D. A., Kotseva, K., Connolly, S., Jennings, C., Mead, A., Jones, J., Holden, A., De Bacquer, D., Collier, T., De Backer, G., Faergeman, O., & EUROACTION Study Group. (2008). Nurse-coordinated multidisciplinary, family-based cardiovascular disease prevention programme (EUROACTION) for patients with coronary heart disease and asymptomatic individuals at high risk of cardiovascular disease: A paired, cluster-randomised controlled trial. *Lancet, 371*(9629), 1999–2012. https://doi .org/10.1016/S0140-6736(08)60868-5

CHAPTER 15

DIABETES MANAGEMENT BEHAVIORS: THE KEY TO OPTIMAL HEALTH AND QUALITY OF LIFE OUTCOMES

KOREY K. HOOD AND RYAN D. TWEET

LEARNING OBJECTIVES

- Understand and distinguish between the types of diabetes.
- Understand the public health impact of diabetes.
- Understand how to manage the different types of diabetes and the barriers that prevent effective management.
- Discuss the various methods for facilitating effective management of diabetes.
- Understand the impact of technology on improving the quality of life of people with diabetes.

INTRODUCTION

The landscape of diabetes and its management has changed dramatically since the first results of the landmark Diabetes Control and Complications Trial (DCCT) were published in 1993. The DCCT transformed the notion of intensive diabetes management and fostered a new approach that focuses on performing multiple daily behaviors to optimize short- and long-term health. A host of other seminal studies have been published since documenting new therapeutics and technologies aimed at reducing patient burden and maximizing health outcomes. There is work under way to optimize our models of prevention for all types of diabetes and to produce an artificial pancreas that would relieve the patient of chronic decision-making and problem-solving around diabetes (Herold et al., 2019; Lal et al., 2019). Until these projects and programs are fully realized, the engagement in multiple behaviors to treat diabetes is still the single best method for optimizing health and quality of life outcomes in patients with diabetes. This chapter provides a review of the important background and context of diabetes and highlights the critical nature of health behaviors to diabetes management and outcomes. In addition, barriers to conducting these behaviors and interventions aimed at breaking down these barriers and promoting effective problem-solving and coping skills will be highlighted.

DIABETES 101

Types of Diabetes

Diabetes is a chronic disease caused by a relative deficiency in insulin. This manifests in one of two ways; either the body is unable to produce sufficient insulin (type 1 diabetes), or the body does not respond appropriately to insulin (type 2 diabetes). Acutely, elevated blood sugars can be deadly. Over the long term, chronic elevated blood sugars can result in damage to multiple body systems.

Type 1 diabetes is an autoimmune disease in which the immune system attacks the pancreatic beta cells, which make insulin. A combination of genetic, environmental, and biological factors is hypothesized to lead to the development of type 1 diabetes (Atkinson & Eisenbarth, 2001; Bluestone et al., 2010). Type 2 diabetes had previously been characterized as adult-onset or non–insulin-dependent diabetes; however, these descriptions are no longer appropriate. Children are diagnosed with type 2 diabetes (Liese et al., 2006), and patients with type 2 diabetes may require insulin treatment. Overweight, obesity, sedentary behavior, decreased physical activity, and older age are associated with type 2 diabetes. Type 2 diabetes accounts for 90% to 95% of all cases of diabetes (Centers for Disease Control and Prevention [CDC], 2022).

Public Health Impact of Diabetes

Diabetes is a serious public health issue. More than 37 million people in the United States have diabetes (CDC, 2022). As per the World Health Organization (WHO), 422 million people worldwide have diabetes. The rates of diabetes in U.S. adults vary by location, such that the disease disproportionately affects the "diabetes belt" in Southeastern United States. Additionally, although diabetes affects individuals from all racial, ethnic, and socioeconomic backgrounds, certain groups have historically had higher rates of diabetes and related illness and death. According to the Centers for Disease Control and Prevention's (CDC) National Diabetes Statistics Report (2022), those with the highest diabetes prevalence include Native American or Alaska Native (14.5%), Black, non-Hispanic (12.1%), Hispanic overall (11.8%), and Asian (9.5%). Risk factors for diabetes include age, a family history of diabetes, being a woman with a history of gestational diabetes, lifestyle factors, barriers to optimal diet and physical activity, cultural practices, historical trauma (CDC, 2022; Espinosa et al., 2022), and limited access or barriers to healthcare (Canedo et al., 2018; CDC, 2022).

Diabetes that is poorly controlled, for whatever reasons, can result in significant morbidity and mortality. In 2012, an estimated 3.7 million people in the world died from diabetes complications. The largest number of deaths related to diabetes occurs in upper-middle-income countries around the world, and the lowest number of deaths occurs in low-income countries. WHO (2012) projects that diabetes deaths will increase by 66% between 2008 and 2030. Overall, the risk of death among people with diabetes is about twice the risk in people of similar age without diabetes.

Diabetes can also result in significant morbidity via acute and chronic complications. Uncontrolled diabetes causes increased susceptibility to illness and difficulty overcoming routine infections. Over time, elevated blood glucose levels can be damaging to multiple organ systems and result in such issues as heart and kidney disease, as well as retinopathy and neuropathy. Adults with diabetes have 1.5 to 2 times higher risk of stroke and death from heart disease compared with adults without diabetes. Additionally, diabetes is a leading cause of kidney failure and new cases of blindness among adults (CDC, 2022).

Epidemic of Diabetes: Increasing Prevalence and Incidence

The prevalence (the total number of existing diagnoses) and incidence (the number of new cases diagnosed for a given time period) of diabetes have increased substantially in the

United States and worldwide over the past several decades. Type 1 diabetes is still the most common diagnosis among those under 20 years of age in the United States, but the incidence of type 2 diagnoses in this age group is increasing. In the past several decades, the prevalence of both type 1 and type 2 diabetes has increased in children, adolescents, and adults (Dabelea et al., 2014; Menke et al., 2015). In 2017, approximately 1.3 million new cases of diabetes were diagnosed in people aged 18 years or older in the United States (CDC, 2022). If current trends continue, one in three adults in the United States will have diabetes by 2050 (Imperatore et al., 2012). There are several known factors contributing to the overall rise in type 2 diabetes diagnoses, including an aging population and an increasing number of persons at increased risk of developing diabetes. There are multiple hypotheses regarding the reason for the increased rates of type 1 diabetes, including environmental triggers, in utero and early life exposures, and various infections (Allen et al., 2018; Kostic et al., 2015). However, none of these hypotheses have been able to explain the etiology of the increasing prevalence and incidence of type 1 diabetes.

MANAGEMENT OF DIABETES

Differences and Similarities by Type

The daily management of diabetes will vary between patients across types of diabetes (e.g., type 1 vs. type 2 diabetes); however, within types, there are often many similarities. The required and hallmark component of the daily management of type 1 diabetes is insulin. Insulin is administered by multiple daily injections or continuous subcutaneous insulin infusion (CSII; i.e., insulin pump). Insulin is typically injected or administered through an insulin pump more than four times per day. People with type 1 diabetes are also required to check their blood glucose levels multiple times daily by pricking the end of a finger and applying the blood sample to a glucose meter, or to use continuous glucose monitoring (CGM). It is typically recommended to check at least four times daily, but those in optimal diabetes control can check ten or more times daily. These tasks are demanding enough, but the complexity rises when the individual has to coordinate insulin administration with blood glucose levels, dietary intake, and physical activity. It is a delicate balance and is aimed at preserving short-term health and quality of life, as well as long-term health.

The treatment of type 2 diabetes is more variable and patient-dependent. Traditionally, the first-line treatment is lifestyle modification. These alterations include a balanced diet (e.g., whole grains, lean proteins, vegetables, limited processed and sugary foods), increased physical activity, and weight loss. In addition to required lifestyle changes, oral medications may be used to improve the body's sensitivity to insulin or increase insulin secretion. With the more recent development of highly effective drugs for diabetes treatment, a debate has emerged regarding the order of prescribing lifely versus drugs for individuals with or at risk for type 2 diabetes (Lewis et al., 2023). Despite this debate, lifestyle behavior change remains the frontline treatment for diabetes. If these treatments are ineffective, type 2 diabetes can progress over time to an insulin-deficient state necessitating use of insulin (by injection or insulin pump) or extreme insulin resistance; management then becomes similar to patients with type 1 diabetes.

In both type 1 and type 2 diabetes, glucose, blood pressure, and lipid control are critical. It is recommended that patients with diabetes have thorough evaluations by their endocrinologist three to four times per year. They are also required to have routine screenings for diabetes complications, including close monitoring of their heart, kidneys, eyes, and other systems impacted by elevated blood glucose levels. Of note, prior to becoming pregnant and during their pregnancy, patients with type 1 diabetes must have even tighter control of their diabetes and more intensive management (American Diabetes Association [ADA], 2018).

Adherence to Prescribed Management Regimens

Both type 1 and type 2 represent complex medical regimens that are difficult to follow as prescribed. Behavioral adherence to the type 1 diabetes regimen varies by task (Johnson, 1992; Kutz, 1990; McNabb, 1997). For example, rates of adherence to blood glucose monitoring and the regulation of carbohydrate intake tend to be the lowest (39%), while rates of adherence to insulin administration tend to be the highest (Peyrot et al., 2015). With multiple daily injections of insulin, the method of injection can influence adherence: Switching to an insulin pen rather than syringe has been shown to improve adherence (Davies et al., 2013). Furthermore, patients on insulin pumps tend to experience both a clinical benefit in terms of adherence and control (Phillip et al., 2007), as well as quality of life (Barnard et al., 2007; Ingerski et al., 2010). Greater adherence to a continuous monitoring device (CGM) is linked to greater benefit in glycemic control (Hirsch et al., 2008; Polonsky et al., 2022) and greater treatment satisfaction (Martens et al., 2021). However, many with type 1 diabetes opt to discontinue using their devices for a variety of reasons, including cost, too many alarms, issues with accuracy, and discomfort wearing a device on one's body (Tanenbaum et al., 2016).

A variety of factors have been linked to poor adherence in individuals with type 1 and type 2 diabetes. For example, those with greater depressive symptoms and/or diabetes distress have lower rates of adherence (Gonzalez et al., 2008, 2016). Background contextual factors such as family structure, access to resources and healthcare, and social support are also related to adherence rates (Delamater, 2006; Mayberry et al., 2015).

For type 2 diabetes management, adherence to lifestyle modifications (e.g., increasing physical activity, maintaining a balanced diet) is highly variable (Peyrot et al., 2015). Research on individuals with type 2 diabetes has demonstrated that adherence to the prescribed meal plan is around 37% and adherence to the prescribed physical activity recommendations is 35%. A large study of pharmacy claims, which defined medication adherence as patients having filled their prescriptions 80% of the time, found that 27% of the sample on one oral medication were considered adherent, while only 4.5% of the sample taking two oral medications met the criteria for adherence (Kirkman et al., 2015). This study identified several factors related to adherence, including age, sex, education and income level, total daily pill burden, and length of time being prescribed the medications (Kirkman et al., 2015). For adolescents with type 1 diabetes, adherence has been shown to decrease over time. This is linked to a corresponding decrease in parental involvement (King et al., 2014).

Link Between Adherence and Health Outcomes

After the DCCT was first published in 1993 for patients with type 1 diabetes and similar data were published by the U.K. Prospective Diabetes Study (UKPDS) for patients with type 2 diabetes in 1995, the diabetes world has used a biological measure of a patient's overall level of diabetes control. This measure is the hemoglobin A1c value, which reflects the prior 8 to 12 weeks of glucose "control." The reference range for people without diabetes is 4% to 6%. Treatment target for people with diabetes is at or below 7.0% (ADA, 2023), yet there are considerations for higher targets based on age, support, and type of treatment. However, the majority of patients have this A1c target and most do not meet these targets (McKnight et al., 2015).

There are a number of factors that contribute to A1c values, but the variable assumed to be the largest contributor is adherence to management regimen. Data from pediatric and adult patients, across type 1 and type 2 diabetes, highlight that 30% to 50% of overall control can be attributed to adherence (Hood et al., 2009). The remaining contributors cut across contextual variables such as access to healthcare, family structure, social support, and other psychosocial variables. Further, in youth, growth and puberty play a major role in A1c outcomes (Moreland et al., 2004).

BARRIERS TO EFFECTIVE DIABETES MANAGEMENT

As noted previously, diabetes management includes a set of complex and demanding behaviors that must be carried out multiple times daily. While there are a number of barriers to ongoing chronic disease management covered in other chapters in this text, there are diabetes-specific considerations or variants of those barriers. One set of barriers to carrying out diabetes management tasks cuts across habits and routines and competing needs and priorities.

CASE STUDY 15.1: BARRIERS TO POSITIVE DIABETES MANAGEMENT

Frank, a 49-year-old man, was just diagnosed with type 2 diabetes. He knew for several years that he was at risk for type 2 diabetes given his family history, and he tried to eat a healthier diet and walk for 60 minutes three to four times per week. There were large gaps where he was not able to do these positive lifestyle behaviors because of arriving home late from work and not having them scheduled into his daily plans. He also saw no incentive for walking or eating healthier because he did not physically feel very different and never noticed any weight loss. Frank's diabetes care team decided to put him on an oral medication (metformin) twice daily to help his glucose control. Mindful of the difficulties making lifestyle changes previously, his diabetes care team set up a system of reminders and support around management. For example, the team helped him set reminders in his phone to take his pills. Further, they paired eating breakfast, something he always does at the same time, with checking his blood sugar. They had him leave his blood glucose meter by the breakfast food cabinet in his kitchen. They were able to embed these behaviors into his daily life by combining them with existing and routine events.

The story of Frank is similar to many attempting to engage in positive diabetes management behaviors and not having success, and the need for more structured behaviors. Few are successful at embedding these behaviors into daily life and breaking down this significant behavior without the collaboration with and direction of the team.

Emotional Barriers and Impact on Diabetes Management

DEPRESSION

There are clear data that having diabetes doubles an individual's likelihood of having depression (Anderson et al., 2001) and that having depression can significantly impact a person's ability to manage diabetes (Gonzalez et al., 2008; McGrady et al., 2009). It is also the case that having depression places a person at increased risk for type 2 diabetes, possibly because it impairs an individual's ability to carry out generally healthy behaviors (Golden et al., 2008) or because long-term use of antidepressant medication is associated with increased risk of developing diabetes (Andersohn et al., 2009). Whether depression started before or after the diagnosis of diabetes (see Bergmans et al., 2021), having depression can make the challenging lifestyle modifications and daily management behaviors seem overwhelming. Further, the definition of "depression" in studies is not always similar and often it is more likely diabetes-related emotional distress (described later).

CASE STUDY 15.2: INTERVENTIONS TO ADDRESS BARRIERS

After making progress taking his medications and checking his blood sugar, Frank reported feeling unsupported in his diabetes management during one of his medical visits. His team, mindful of his history of having depression, referred him to a psychosocial group for adults newly diagnosed with diabetes. The aim of the group was to promote coping with diabetes and its management and address emotional barriers.

(continued)

CASE STUDY 15.2: INTERVENTIONS TO ADDRESS BARRIERS (*continued*)

In this group, there was a focus on diabetes problem-solving and cognitive restructuring. Specifically, a four-step method of solving problems related to diabetes was taught along with attempts to challenge irrational beliefs about diabetes (e.g., "I cannot live with this disease" and "it is always getting the best of me"). Frank learned to effectively identify problems related to his diabetes (step 1), come up with possible solutions (step 2), develop a plan to address barriers and work toward resolution of the problem (step 3), and how to evaluate and rework potential solutions if needed (step 4). Frank made significant progress in diabetes-specific problem-solving, felt less stressed about diabetes in general, and was better at integrating diabetes management into his daily life.

Later in this chapter, we will review more details about the components of an intervention like the one Frank participated in to break down behavioral and emotional barriers through problem-solving.

DIABETES DISTRESS AND PSYCHOLOGICAL INSULIN RESISTANCE

A related emotional barrier to effective diabetes management has been termed *diabetes distress* (Polonsky et al., 1995). Diabetes distress is related to the emotional burden of diabetes, including the self-management regimen, interpersonal factors, and physician care (Polonsky et al., 1995). These emotions may be different from having feelings of depression, but because of their diabetes-specific nature they have direct implications for diabetes care.

A phenomenon unique to type 2 diabetes is the patient's resistance to initiate insulin therapy, also known as "psychological insulin resistance" (Polonsky, 2007). Patients with type 2 diabetes often interpret initiating insulin therapy as a failure of the previous regimen. In addition, patients are resistant to initiating insulin therapy because of the belief that their diabetes is not "serious" enough to begin insulin therapy or because starting insulin treatment means they "failed" and are likely to now develop diabetes complications as a result of that "failure" (Stuckey et al., 2019). Polonsky and his associates (2005) demonstrated that of 708 patients with type 2 diabetes, 28% were unwilling to take insulin to treat their diabetes. Of those patients who were unwilling to initiate insulin therapy to treat their diabetes, 55% believed that needing to be on insulin indicated they failed in properly controlling their diabetes with oral agents. Likewise, 56% believed that being on insulin would restrict their lives and 53% believed that once they started insulin therapy it would be a permanent change in their regimen. Research has shown that healthcare providers who treat individuals with type 2 diabetes also have beliefs and attitudes about the initiation of insulin therapy that present obstacles to patients being willing to use insulin to treat their diabetes. For example, the initiation of insulin therapy in patients with type 2 diabetes is often used as a threat to patients in motivating them to adhere more closely to the diabetes regimen despite the limited effectiveness of fear-based motivation techniques for repeated behaviors (Tannenbaum et al., 2015). In addition, healthcare providers believe that insulin therapy for patients with type 2 diabetes is only for those whose diabetes is poorly controlled (Peyrot, et al., 2005). Thus, barriers to the initiation of insulin therapy in patients with type 2 diabetes exist for both patients and healthcare providers and are largely attitudinal.

FEAR OF HYPOGLYCEMIA

Fear of hypoglycemia (low blood glucose) is considered one of the major barriers to optimal glucose control in type 1, and advanced type 2, diabetes. Hypoglycemia is common; studies show that patients with type 1 diabetes experience approximately three episodes of hypoglycemia per month and three severe hypoglycemic episodes per year (UK Hypoglycaemia Study Group, 2007). Cryer (2008) reported that 6% to 10% of all deaths in people with type 1 diabetes were due to hypoglycemia.

A review by Barnard et al. (2010) examining the fear of hypoglycemia in parents with young children (<12 years of age) with type 1 diabetes concluded fear of hypoglycemia impacts parental health and quality of life, although direct effects on regimen adherence and glycemic control are less clear. Barnard and colleagues' review supported the hypothesis that parents' hypoglycemia avoidance adversely impacts glucose control, whereas a newer review by Driscoll et al. (2016) reported no association found in the majority of studies. Studies supporting a relationship between parents' fear of hypoglycemia and glycemic control suggest parents are more likely to underdose insulin when fears of hypoglycemia are present, resulting in higher blood sugar levels. Regarding fear of hypoglycemia among people living with diabetes, reviews by Wild et al. (2007) and Driscoll and colleagues (2016) reveal mixed findings in that some studies report a positive association between fear of hypoglycemia and A1c and others report no association. The authors hypothesized interventions, including blood glucose awareness and cognitive behavioral therapy, may reduce levels of fear and improve diabetes management. Additionally, using certain diabetes technology (e.g., insulin pumps with automatic bolus calculators) may reduce fear of hypoglycemia (Barnard et al., 2012). Wild et al. (2007) recommended addressing the fear of hypoglycemia during clinic visits and education.

PSYCHOSOCIAL GUIDELINES

Given the impact of emotional factors on diabetes management, the American Diabetes Association (ADA) published psychosocial care guidelines to promote optimal care (Young-Hyman et al., 2016). They recommend the integration of psychosocial care into usual care for all people with diabetes, including ongoing assessment of emotional well-being and self-management performance and timely intervention when required. Specifically, regular assessment of depression, diabetes distress, anxiety, and self-management performance is recommended using standardized, validated tools. For those with difficulties in the assessed areas, the ADA recommends addressing the difficulties immediately during their diabetes visit or making a referral to a qualified behavioral healthcare provider.

Family Barriers

Diabetes-specific family barriers include a lack of adequate support around management and conflict and poor communication between patients and their families around the treatment regimen. The interpersonal conflict that emerges around diabetes can and often does result in significant declines in diabetes self-care behaviors, and in turn results in poorer glucose control (Wysocki, 1993).

Of the family factors that impact health behaviors and health status of youths with diabetes, family conflict emerges as a primary issue that needs attention (DiMatteo, 2004; Psihogios et al., 2019). Many of the conflictual interactions between patients and family revolve around how the patient is managing their diabetes. Anderson and Coyne (1991) outlined a process known as "miscarried helping" for understanding how interpersonal conflict emerges in families of individuals with a chronic illness. Anderson and Coyne (1991) highlight how good intentions on the part of caregivers result in interpersonal conflict between the patient with diabetes and other family members, further polarizing the two parties and putting the patient's diabetes at greater risk. There are several reasons why the family is the primary focus for examining miscarried helping. First, those closest to an individual with diabetes are family members who are most likely to assist with day-to-day demands of the treatment regimen. Second, family members are the most likely to advise or influence a patient with diabetes around issues of disease management and general healthcare (DiMatteo, 2004). Finally, the family represents a model for health behaviors including diet, exercise, and interactions with the healthcare team. Thus, family involvement in diabetes management can result in poor health behaviors via a lack of adequate support, increased interpersonal conflict, and poor communication about how best to manage diabetes (Harris et al., 2008; Pierce et al., 1996).

FACILITATING EFFECTIVE MANAGEMENT OF DIABETES

The Evidence Base

Over two decades of research in the behavioral management of diabetes led us to conclude that (a) providing education for diabetes management is important, but not sufficient for optimal outcomes; and (b) breaking down barriers and fostering new skills serve as the most powerful interventions. These two points led to a larger conclusion: Multicomponent interventions that focus on behavior change and the facilitators of those changes will have the most robust effect on quality of life and health outcomes for people with diabetes. These can be carried out in the clinical setting, within families, and in the communities where the patients with diabetes reside. The following section draws on the evidence base to highlight the best ways to facilitate behavior change in the management of diabetes.

Importantly, this evidence base has supported modern standards of care, published by the ADA in 2023. One particularly relevant section of the guidelines focuses on "Facilitating Positive Health Behaviors and Well-Being to Improve Health Outcomes" (ElSayed et al., 2023), with key recommendations around diabetes self-management education (DMSE) including identification of key timepoints in the disease course when such education must be provided (e.g., at diagnosis, when complicating factors develop), suggestion of delivery modalities including digital interventions, and engagement in group or individual settings. The standards of care also note that DSME and support programs must address barriers that exist at multiple levels (e.g., individual, family, community, health system), including identifying and addressing social determinants of health with an ultimate goal of health equity.

Multicomponent Interventions

In a meta-analysis of nearly 1,000 youth and young adults with type 1 diabetes, interventions that directly attempted to increase management behaviors (e.g., blood glucose monitoring) and addressed facilitators of those behaviors (e.g., better communication in the family) were the only interventions that had a positive effect on hemoglobin A1c values (Hood et al., 2010). Those interventions provided direct education and support around management behaviors while promoting better coping and problem-solving skills. The interventions that just focused on one or the other were far less effective in changing A1c values. Other problem-solving interventions not included in that meta-analysis have been shown to change behaviors and A1c values (Mulvaney et al., 2011).

Problem-solving interventions are popular in adults as well and these interventions cut across type 1 and type 2 diabetes. A systematic review by Hill-Briggs and Gremmel (2007) synthesized findings from nearly 40 studies on problem-solving with adults with diabetes. Only about 50% of the adult studies had a significant impact on A1c values, but most did change health behaviors positively. The most effective interventions were those that focused on diabetes-specific problem-solving, not just a general framework for solving everyday problems. Further, those that focused on decision-making utilizing diabetes examples were particularly effective. Potential reasons for not observing as widespread an effect on A1c from these studies included too short of a time to follow up to see whether the behaviors had been embedded in daily lives (to have an effect on A1c values). The results, however, are promising given their relative low intensity and large effects (for about half those sampled).

CASE STUDY 15.3: EVIDENCE-BASED PROBLEM-SOLVING INTERVENTION

An example of an evidence-based problem-solving intervention for adults with diabetes comes from the work of Fisher and colleagues. The major goals of their intervention are to decrease the distress and negative impact associated with diabetes (i.e., diabetes burnout), increase coping skills, and minimize the likelihood of similar problems reoccurring in the future. This problem-solving intervention includes educating patients, via a live diabetes counselor, about the impact of distress and burnout on diabetes (and vice versa), making a list of problems associated with diabetes and distress, prioritizing them, and, over a series of sessions, devising problem-solving strategies to address each. Adults with diabetes participating in this intervention receive two in-person sessions and four live phone calls across 5 months. Then they receive a supplemental in-person booster session and four more live calls across the remaining 6 months. They are taught an eight-step process to identify and define diabetes distress, establish realistic goals, generate ways to meet these goals, weigh the pros and cons of each, choose and evaluate solutions, create a diabetes distress action plan, evaluate outcome, and engage in pleasant activities. Also, summary reports permit ongoing feedback to primary providers to foster doctor–patient communication and facilitate ongoing clinical care.

Motivational Interviewing

Motivational interviewing (MI) offers a brief, practical method for helping patients increase their motivation or readiness to change (Berg-Smith et al., 1999). The steps of MI are establishing a relationship; setting an agenda; assessing importance, confidence, and readiness; exploring importance; helping patients select a plan of action; and building confidence in their ability to change (Rollnick et al., 1999). The main goal of MI is for patients and providers to decide collaboratively on the patient's next steps in a supportive, empathetic way.

Multiple MI interventions have been successful in patients with type 1 and type 2 diabetes. Channon and colleagues (2007) completed a multicenter, 12-month intervention trial investigating MI in teenagers with type 1 diabetes. At the end of the intervention, the mean A1c in the MI group was significantly lower than the control group. At 24 months, the difference between A1c was maintained. The MI group also reported more positive well-being and improved quality of life. A 2012 randomized controlled trial (RCT) by Chen et al. (2012) found MI resulted in improved self-management, psychological outcomes, and glycemic control in patients with type 2 diabetes. These promising results highlight the need for collaborative, empathetic communication between patients and providers to facilitate improvements in diabetes management (Young et al., 2020).

Family-Based Interventions

Involvement from family in diabetes management can result in better metabolic control and increased treatment adherence in individuals with diabetes (Anderson et al., 1989). Many family-based interventions have targeted improving behavioral management of diabetes in youth with diabetes (Feldman et al., 2018). Some research has supported the health benefits of parental involvement in a crisis intervention program upon diagnosis of their child with diabetes (Galatzer et al., 1982). Furthermore, several researchers have tested a clinic-based family intervention that involved collaborative problem-solving ("Teamwork") between adolescents with type 1 diabetes and their parents (Anderson et al., 1999; Auslander, 1993; Laffel et al., 2003). The Teamwork intervention involves family problem-solving around three key areas: (a) examining the multiple causes of high blood sugars during early adolescence, (b) establishing realistic expectations for blood sugar values during adolescence, and (c) ongoing involvement from parents in diabetes management without shaming or blaming the youth. Youth and care providers spent approximately 20 to 30 minutes before or after each routine medical visit discussing these topics. During those meetings, a researcher provided information about the specific topic of focus and encouraged family-based discussion regarding pertinent issues. Also, each family was assisted in the process of developing a responsibility-sharing plan. The intervention proved effective in reducing diabetes-related conflict coupled with significant improvements in glycemic control.

Wysocki and colleagues (2000, 2006, 2007, 2008) conducted a series of RCTs examining the efficacy of a family-based psychosocial intervention (behavioral family systems therapy for diabetes [BFST-D]) for adolescents with type 1 diabetes. BFST-D is a skills-based intervention for families that addresses four primary areas of family functioning—(a) problem-solving, (b) communication, (c) strong beliefs, and (d) family structure—with additional sessions involving parent simulation of diabetes and nurse-directed identification of blood glucose patterns. Results from this series of RCTs have demonstrated that participation in BFST-D can result in significant improvements in glycemic control, treatment adherence, diabetes-related problem-solving, and diabetes-related family conflict. Harris and colleagues (Harris, 2003; Harris et al., 2005) conducted two studies examining a home-based version of BFST-D with adolescents with poorly controlled diabetes. Results from these two studies demonstrated that implementation of BFST-D in the home can result in significant decreases in general family conflict, diabetes-related family conflict, and behavior problems; increases in diabetes treatment adherence; and improvements in glycemic control. **Box 15.1** highlights the components and sets expectations for families as they start this manualized, evidence-based, family-based intervention.

Community-Based Interventions

Many of the multicomponent interventions highlighted in the preceding section were delivered in clinical settings. Community-based interventions are fundamentally different in that they are purposefully carried out away from the clinical setting. Community-based interventions aim to promote generalization of learned skills and new education in the setting where these behaviors are conducted. Often, these interventions incorporate peer support.

Lack of social support has been identified as a risk factor for poor diabetes management and increased morbidity and mortality (Brownson & Heisler, 2009). Peer support can provide the additional understanding and reinforcement individuals need to manage their diabetes. Additionally, peer support interventions are more cost-effective and efficient than traditional diabetes management approaches. Based on a review of peer support interventions by Heisler (2007), five models of peer support have been identified, including (a) face-to-face group self-management programs, (b) peer coaches or mentors, (c) community health workers, (d) telephone-based peer support, and (e) internet or email-based peer support; while no specific peer support intervention was found to be superior to others, peer support interventions were at least as effective, if not more effective, than standard clinical care models. Participant satisfaction was generally positive in all interventions, which may facilitate longer term "buy-in" to the programs.

A large, community-based, peer support program that has successfully decreased the risk of developing diabetes in at-risk patient populations is the Diabetes Prevention Program (DPP, 2002). Results show that intensive lifestyle interventions can result in weight loss and reduce the risk of developing diabetes. The intervention included multiple components: (a) individual case managers or "lifestyle coaches"; (b) frequent behavioral self-management strategies for weight loss and physical activity; (c) a structured, state-of-the-art, 16-session core-curriculum teaching behavioral self-management strategies for weight loss and physical activity; (d) supervised physical activity sessions; (e) a more flexible maintenance intervention combining group and individual approaches, motivational campaigns, and "restarts";

BOX 15.1 WHAT CAN YOU EXPECT DURING BEHAVIORAL FAMILY SYSTEMS THERAPY (BFST) SESSIONS?

Your family will participate in 12 sessions of BFST that will be conducted by a highly trained psychologist or social worker. It will be important that teenagers and parents participate fully in order to learn how to restructure family rules and roles in a way that family members can grow as individuals without disrupting the stability of your family. In addition, the therapist will try to understand how the other parts of your life, such as school, your community, and your medical team can play a role in your ability to take care of your diabetes. The therapists will plan and carry out four components of the BFST approach that will be tailored to your family's specific needs. The following are the four components of the BFST:

- *Problem-solving training:* The therapist will teach your family to use a structured approach to problem-solving. This will help you define problems clearly, brainstorm a variety of possible solutions, and reach an agreement as a family on solutions to problems. You will practice these skills at home as well as in the sessions. You will be asked to monitor your problem-solving plan, evaluate the success of failure of the plan, and redefine the plan as needed. A nurse will be participating in sessions 6 and 7 to teach advanced problem-solving using blood glucose data. The nurse will also train parents to simulate living with diabetes for 1 week. Parents will give themselves injections of sterile saline, test their blood glucose, follow a meal plan, test for ketones, and manage one unexpected simulated episode of hypoglycemia.
- *Communication skills training:* In each of the 12 sessions, the therapist will ask you to talk together as a family about problems you might have at home. The therapist will offer you alternative ways to communicate in order to facilitate good family problem-solving. The therapist will also give you feedback about your communication skills during the sessions to help you express your thoughts and feelings in a more clear and less threatening way. You may be asked to practice new communication skills in your session. In addition, your family will be given "homework assignments" to help you practice at home what you have learned in the sessions.
- *Strong belief restructuring:* Along with communication skills and problem-solving, there is another basic aspect of family interactions that determines how families get along. Sometimes parents and teenagers have strong beliefs, attitudes, and opinions about each other's behaviors and intentions. These beliefs are sometimes so strong that they get in the way of dealing more effectively with conflict. The therapist will help you identify and "soften" strong beliefs to help you communicate and problem-solve better as a family.
- *Family structuring:* The way a family structures itself can determine how well the other components of the BFST are implemented. Every family has specific roles for its member and rules to follow. These are often unspoken, but all family members are aware of them. The therapist will help families vocalize these roles and rules and determine if some of them need to change. The therapist will also explain some of the basic developmental stages of preteens and teens. This will help families understand that some of their child's behavior changes are normal and necessary for growth.

(f) individualization through a "toolbox" of adherence strategies; (g) tailoring of materials and strategies to address ethnic diversity; and (h) an extensive network of training, feedback, and clinical support.

The DPP has been successfully translated into various community settings, some through partnerships with the *Young Men's Christian Association* (YMCA; Ackermann & Marrero,

2007; Boltri et al., 2008). In particular, the YMCA was found to be an inexpensive, effective way to impact the health of the community. A review of 28 community-based programs modeled after the DPP concluded that the programs produced clinically significant weight loss (4%–5%, on average) that was maintained over 9 months (Ali et al., 2012). Programs delivered by lay community staff (as opposed to medical professionals) achieved greater weight loss.

The Novel Interventions in Children's Healthcare (NICH) is a promising program that combines BFST with care coordination and case management to adapt services to the needs of youth and families with diabetes and other chronic conditions, and complex psychosocial and economic needs (Wagner et al., 2015). Recipients of this program have 24/7 access to support from NICH interventionists to assist with practical barriers to self-management, such as transportation to medical appointments or the pharmacy, and connection to psychological or supportive services. Youth had lower A1cs, spent fewer days in the hospital, and had lower healthcare costs after participating in the NICH.

System-Based Interventions

System-based interventions are another example of multicomponent diabetes interventions. System-based interventions have a focus beyond individual patients. These interventions work directly with policy makers, public health officials, medical providers and health centers caring for patients with diabetes, government, and institutions conducting diabetes research, and function at national, state, and institutional levels.

At the national level, the CDC works to reduce the burden of preventable diabetes diagnoses and complications. The CDC addresses their goals through public health leadership, partnerships, research, policies, and programs to translate science into practice. The CDC's Division of Diabetes Translation (DDT) focuses on public health surveillance, research delivery in clinical and public health practices, development and maintenance of effective state-based diabetes prevention and control programs, and closure of health gaps among the population most severely affected by diabetes (CDC, 2015).

South Carolina's Department of Health and Environmental Control has organized a comprehensive, statewide, system-based intervention to address diabetes—the Diabetes Initiative of South Carolina (DSC). The DSC directs efforts toward prevention of diabetes and reduction of diabetes-related complications and hospitalizations. The DSC partners with other diabetes-focused healthcare organizations to ensure evidence-based diabetes prevention, screening, diagnosis, treatment, and control interventions are distributed to the community. This information is disseminated to healthcare providers through professional education sessions, symposia, and support of recognized DMSE programs. In the first 10 years of its existence, the DSC has seen increases in rates of glucose self-monitoring, decreases in preventable hospitalizations, and decreases in amputations (DSC, 2011).

The Michigan Diabetes Research and Training Center (MDRTC) is one example of an institutional, system-based intervention to address the diabetes burden (Michigan Diabetes Research and Training Center, 2017). The MDRTC provides a Behavioral, Clinical, and Health Systems Intervention Research Core (BCHS). It is an avenue for collaboration, training, and tangible resources to support high-quality, diabetes-focused research. The BCHS provides interdisciplinary review and suggestions for research studies. It provides a route for translation of research from bench to bedside, and supports collaboration that will increase the likelihood of successful research efforts.

All of these system-based interventions, and the resultant community-based or direct clinic-based interventions, are aimed at improving outcomes for people with diabetes. Given the complexity of diabetes and its management, and the multiple contributors to quality of life and health outcomes, improvements in mortality and morbidity require a multipronged approach. The core component of all of these interventions and approaches is an attempt to change health behaviors.

Reducing Health Disparities in Diabetes Care

The ADA provided guidance in 2017 on strategies to reduce disparities related to the treatment of diabetes (ADA, 2017). Major recommendations to come from this guidance included three principles. The first was that healthcare providers should assess a patient's social context to understand their unique barriers to care. These might include food insecurity, housing instability, financial barriers, uninsurance or underinsurance, lack of transportation, or poor health literacy (Hill-Briggs & Fitzpatrick, 2023). The ADA recommended that this information, once assessed, be applied to treatment decisions. The second principle was that providers should refer patients to local community resources, such as food assistance, subsidized housing, social workers, transportation assistance, and lay health coaches, when available. Related, the third recommendation was that patients should be connected with health system resources, such as patient navigators or community health workers, who can also address some of the social-contextual factors that might be barriers to care.

Some have argued that the ADA's guidance is not comprehensive enough in its identification of social determinants of health (Hill-Briggs et al., 2022). These authors and others (LeBrón et al., 2019) argue that Latinx and Black adults experience diabetes disparities that stem from where they live that cannot be addressed with a health sector response alone. They argue that systemic racism and socioeconomic discrimination are root causes of disparities in diabetes and other diseases, and that solutions must address these upstream causes. Building on this guidance, other authors have suggested that social cohesion, neighborhood safety, and other social factors also play a role in creating neighborhood environments that in turn influence the development of diabetes (Mujahid et al., 2023). As such, it can be argued that addressing systemic racism and reversing historical inequities should be policy targets to aid in the prevention and treatment in historically marginalized populations (Johnson, 2022).

Role of Technology

As noted earlier in this chapter, insulin pumps and CGMs can improve glycemic control and improve quality of life for people with diabetes. A major advance in diabetes technology has been the development of closed loop automated insulin delivery systems. These systems include an insulin pump, a CGM, and an additional device that employs an algorithm to automate insulin delivery based on CGM data. The first systems to reach consumers (Gordon, 2016) will be hybrid closed loop systems that require mealtime bolusing (Ly & Buckingham, 2015). These systems have demonstrated an ability to keep users' glucose levels in the target range of 70% to 80% of the time (Ly & Buckingham, 2015; Russell et al., 2016), and have the potential to improve quality of life by reducing the burden of diabetes management.

To maximize benefit from these new closed loop systems, users will need to wear an insulin pump and CGM continuously. However, the rates of uptake of these technologies are lagging. Therefore, interventions are needed to address barriers to diabetes device uptake. In particular, attention needs to be paid to human factors related to using these devices. The term *human factors* refers to characteristics related to the design and engineering of a product that promote sustained and optimized use. In the context of diabetes, these characteristics must include the device's safety and reliability, but ideally should also include users' attitudes, beliefs, and feelings about using the devices. Psychologists have an essential role to play in eliciting these human factors and designing interventions that incorporate them to promote uptake and prevent discontinuation of these devices.

Some studies have already begun to elicit human factors related to closed loop systems. For example, one recent qualitative study interviewed individuals about their experience of participating in a hybrid closed loop trial. Participants who expected that they would need to bolus and count carbohydrates had a more positive experience than those who expected a more hands-off role (Iturralde et al., 2017). Other studies of human factors related to closed loop found that users prioritize the system's usability, convenience, and potential benefit to their health in considering whether to use a system in the future (Bevier et al., 2014), and that some users had difficulty trusting the accuracy of the CGM and insulin delivery (Barnard et al., 2014).

In addition to the substantial developments in insulin pumps, CGM systems, and closed loop systems over the past decade, there have been developments in the realm of mobile applications, which can serve as adjunct strategies for improving diabetes management and outcomes. As of 2016, several thousand diabetes-related applications are available (Hartz et al., 2016). Some apps target health behaviors such as physical activity, sleep, and nutrition, while others target blood glucose monitoring, provide diabetes education, and/or enable users to share their diabetes data with others. For example, applications such as *bant* enable users to link their blood glucose meter directly to an application that synthesizes data. Adolescents were shown to increase rates of glucose checking while using bant (Cafazzo et al., 2012), while users of another application that enabled meter syncing experienced improved glycemic control (Rothenberg et al., 2015). Other programs synthesize these important data and connect users to a social media forum where they can communicate about their diabetes with other diabetes patients. Other technologies such as *CareCoach*, developed by Verilogue, Inc., focus on patient–provider communication and help patients know how to phrase questions to their diabetes care providers and set goals based on provider recommendations. A randomized trial of a mobile application that provided behavioral coaching and enabled patient–provider communication demonstrated clinically significant reductions in A1c for patients with type 2 diabetes (Quinn et al., 2011).

Programs that incorporate recommendations and goal setting appear most promising and poised to facilitate diabetes management behaviors. However, research on the effectiveness of these applications in facilitating behavior change lags behind the pace that these applications hit the marketplace. Further, a review of available applications in 2012 found that most did not adhere to standards set by the American Association of Diabetes Educators (Breland et al., 2013). A more recent review of applications as well as wearable technology for diabetes prevention and management noted that these technologies are most successful when incorporated into structured behavioral interventions (Hartz et al., 2016). Mobile phone applications are effective at increasing self-management behaviors (i.e., frequency of them and across aspects of diabetes regimen adherence) and lower hemoglobin A1c in adults with type 2 diabetes (Liang et al., 2011), as well as adolescents and young adults with type 1 diabetes. Mulvaney and colleagues (2010, 2011) have shown the utility of a mobile and web-based program called YourWay to improve the management and glycemic outcomes of adolescents with type 1 diabetes. There are other programs as well, and several recent papers have focused on this topic (Harris et al., 2012; Rizzo et al., 2011). Interestingly, another study found that for adolescents with type 1 diabetes, use of technology (e.g., social networking, websites, pump/glucose meter software) resulted in them being more engaged in diabetes self-management behaviors, while adolescents who used diabetes websites were more likely to have worse glycemic control (Vaala et al., 2015). Evidence appears to demonstrate that technology and applications that provide scaffolding for patients to internalize the salience and routine of specific health behaviors, with clear contingencies in place for positive reinforcement, are most likely to increase and sustain diabetes management behaviors (Castle et al., 2022; Polonsky et al., 2020).

CONCLUSION

The conduct and coordination of multiple management behaviors remains the best way to optimize health outcomes and quality of life in people with diabetes. Given the substantial individual and public health burden of diabetes, and the trajectory toward an even greater burden in the future, a focus on facilitating behavior change in people with diabetes is timely and important. The evidence base indicates that diabetes-specific barriers to effective diabetes management include feeling distressed and burned out about diabetes, fear of hypoglycemia, and family conflict. Each of these directly contributes to the conduct, frequency, and durability of multiple diabetes management behaviors, which have been linked with poorer outcomes. Identification of these barriers is the first step in determining how to best facilitate behavior change. Once identified, there are appropriate and applicable interventions.

The evidence-based interventions that facilitate behavior change in people with diabetes range from individual programs to larger, systems-based interventions. In general, multicomponent interventions are more effective at changing behavior than those that just provide education and support for specific behaviors, or the facilitators of those behaviors. Both components are necessary. Problem-solving interventions that help people with diabetes develop a framework for identifying diabetes-specific problems, solutions to those problems, goal setting, and an ability to evaluate outcomes. MI can also be effective at engaging and facilitating behavior change for diabetes-specific barriers to management. A number of family-based interventions have been shown to be effective at positively changing behaviors, particularly in pediatric diabetes. The most notable family-based interventions combine problem-solving, coping, and the use of a diabetes-specific context for implementation of those newly learned skills. Community- and system-based interventions are also effective, but the specific components that trickle down to individuals are not well-understood. Finally, technologies and applications can serve as scaffolding to and facilitators of behavior change. Their initial uptake and feasibility seem strong, but the sustainability for maintenance of diabetes management has yet to be established.

In sum, current evidence and clinical expertise indicate that diabetes-specific behavior change is most likely to occur when interventions are offered that break down barriers, promote problem-solving, and engage patients in a way that synthesizes data from management. Given the complex and demanding and lifelong nature of diabetes management, efforts to facilitate diabetes management are likely to promote better health and quality of life outcomes for people with diabetes.

SUMMARY KEY POINTS

- The landscape of diabetes and its management has changed dramatically since the first results of the landmark DCCT were published in 1993. The DCCT transformed the notion of intensive diabetes management and fostered a new approach that focuses on performing multiple daily behaviors to optimize short- and long-term health.

- Diabetes manifests in one of two ways: The body is unable to produce sufficient insulin (type 1 diabetes), or the body does not respond appropriately to insulin (type 2 diabetes).

- Diabetes is a serious public health issue. Although diabetes affects individuals from all racial, ethnic, and socioeconomic backgrounds, certain groups have historically had higher rates of diabetes and related illness and death.

- The prevalence and incidence of diabetes have increased substantially in the United States and worldwide over the past several decades.

- The daily management of diabetes will vary between patients across types of diabetes. In type 1, insulin is typically injected or administered through an insulin pump more than four times per day. People with type 1 diabetes are also required to check their blood glucose levels multiple times daily by pricking the end of a finger and applying the blood sample to a glucose meter, or to use CGM. The treatment of type 2 diabetes is more variable and patient-dependent.

- Both type 1 and type 2 represent complex medical regimens that are difficult to follow as prescribed. Diabetes treatment can be impacted by emotional, familial, and societal factors.

(continued)

SUMMARY KEY POINTS (*continued*)

- Providing education for diabetes management is important, but not sufficient for optimal outcomes. Breaking down barriers and fostering new skills serve as the most powerful interventions.
- MI, family involvement, community- and system-based interventions, reducing health disparities, and technology are necessary tools to improving diabetes outcomes.

DISCUSSION QUESTIONS

1. What are some societal messages you have perceived about diabetes from books, movies, television shows, and news headlines, along with perspectives from friends and family? What are the differences between how type 1 and type 2 are portrayed?

2. Imagine you were speaking to someone who has a history of suicidal ideation and has taken prescription drugs to successfully manage symptoms of depression for several years. They have read that long-term use of antidepressants may increase the risk of developing type 2 diabetes and now want to go off their medication. How would you respond to their decision? What further information would be helpful in forming a plan going forward?

3. Review the concept of "miscarried helping" by Anderson and Coyne mentioned in the "Family Barriers" section of this chapter. If you have observed this in your own life or in the lives of others, regarding diabetes or another illness, how did the family's good intentions conflict with the patient's needs? What if any resources could have been a help in this situation? If you have not observed this, put yourself in the shoes of the family members involved in the miscarried helping. What factors in their lives may lead to them being unable to or unwilling to be a positive resource for their loved one's illness?

4. Consider the role of technology in diabetes management. Could you imagine any concerns potential users may have about an app that stores personal health information such as glucose monitoring? What factors in a potential user's life would you expect would increase or decrease their likelihood of using such an app? Would you be willing to use one yourself? Why or why not?

5. Consider the role that food plays in culture and family. Describe the potential emotional impact a diabetes diagnosis could have on a patient who is being told they must avoid or limit certain foods that are staples of family gatherings or celebrations. How would you feel in their situation? How would your family or loved ones react to you suddenly not eating a shared family meal? What if anything would help mitigate these unpleasant feelings?

A robust set of instructor resources designed to supplement this text is located at http://connect.springerpub.com/content/book/978-0-8261-4265-8. Qualifying instructors may request access by emailing textbook@springerpub.com.

REFERENCES

Ackermann, R. T., & Marrero, D. G. (2007). Adapting the diabetes prevention program lifestyle intervention for delivery in the community: The YMCA model. *The Diabetes Educator, 33*(1), 69, 74–65, 77–68. https://doi.org/10.1177/0145721706297743

Ali, M. K., Echouffo-Tcheugui, J. B., & Williamson, D. F. (2012). How effective were lifestyle interventions in real-world settings that were modeled on the Diabetes Prevention Program? *Health Affairs, 31*(1), 67–75. https://doi.org/10.1377/hlthaff.2011.1009

Allen, D. W., Kim, K. W., Rawlinson, W. D., & Craig, M. E. (2018). Maternal virus infections in pregnancy and type 1 diabetes in their offspring: Systematic review and meta-analysis of observational studies. *Reviews in Medical Virology, 28*(3), e1974. https://doi.org/10.1002/rmv.1974

American Diabetes Association. (2017). 1. Promoting health and reducing disparities in populations. *Diabetes Care, 40*(Suppl. 1), S6–S10. https://doi.org/10.2337/dc17-S004

American Diabetes Association. (2018). Management of diabetes in pregnancy: Standards of medical care in diabetes–2018. *Diabetes Care, 41*(Suppl. 1), S137–S43. https://doi.org/10.2337/dc18-s013

American Diabetes Association. (2023). Standards of care in diabetes–2023. *Diabetes Care, 46*(Suppl. 1), S1–S284.

Andersohn, F., Schade, R., Suissa, S., & Garbe, E. (2009). Long-term use of antidepressants for depressive disorders and the risk of diabetes mellitus. *The American Journal of Psychiatry, 166*(5), 591–598. https://doi.org/10.1176/appi.ajp.2008.08071065

Anderson, B. J., Brackett, J., Ho, J., & Laffel, L. (1999). An office-based intervention to maintain parent-adolescent teamwork in diabetes management: Impact on parent involvement, family conflict, and subsequent glycemic control. *Diabetes Care, 22*(5), 713–721. https://doi.org/10.2337/diacare.22.5.713

Anderson, B. J., & Coyne, J. C. (1991). "Miscarried helping" in families of children and adolescents with chronic diseases. In J. H. Johnson & S. B. Johnson (Eds.), *Advances in child health psychology* (pp. 167–177). University of Florida Press.

Anderson, B. J., Wolf, F. M., Burkhart, M. T., Cornell, R. G., & Bacon, G. E. (1989). Effects of peer-group intervention on metabolic control of adolescents with IDDM: Randomized outpatient study. *Diabetes Care, 12*, 179–183. https://doi.org/10.2337/diacare.12.3.179

Anderson, R. J., Freedland, K. E., Clouse, R. E., & Lustman, P. J. (2001). The prevalence of comorbid depression in adults with diabetes: A meta-analysis. *Diabetes Care, 24*, 1069–1078. https://doi.org/10.2337/diacare.24.6.1069

Atkinson, M., & Eisenbarth, G. (2001). Type 1 diabetes: New perspectives on disease pathogenesis and treatment. *The Lancet, 358*(9277), 221–229. https://doi.org/10.1016/s0140-6736(01)05415-0

Auslander, W. F. (1993). Brief family interventions to improve family communication and cooperation regarding diabetes management. *Diabetes Spectrum: A Publication of the American Diabetes Association, 6*, 330–331.

Barnard, K., Parkin, C., Young, A., & Ashraf, M. (2012). Use of an automated bolus calculator reduces fear of hypoglycemia and improves confidence in dosage accuracy in patients with type 1 diabetes mellitus treated with multiple daily insulin injections. *Journal of Diabetes Science and Technology, 6*(1), 144–149. https://doi.org/10.1177/193229681200600117

Barnard, K., Thomas, S., Royle, P., Noyes, K., & Waugh, N. (2010). Fear of hypoglycaemia in parents of young children with type 1 diabetes: A systematic review. *BMC Pediatrics, 10*, 50. https://doi.org/10.1186/1471-2431-10-50

Barnard, K. D., Lloyd, C. E., & Skinner, T. C. (2007). Systematic literature review: Quality of life associated with insulin pump use in Type 1 diabetes. *Diabetic Medicine, 24*(6), 607–617. https://doi.org/10.1111/j.1464-5491.2007.02120.x

Barnard, K. D., Wysocki, T., Allen, J. M., Elleri, D., Thabit, H., Leelarathna, L., Gulati, A., Nodale, M., Dunger, D. B., Tinati, T., & Hovorka, R. (2014). Closing the loop overnight at home setting: Psychosocial impact for adolescents with type 1 diabetes and their parents. *British Medical Journal Open Diabetes Research & Care, 2*, e000025. https://doi.org/10.1136/bmjdrc-2014-000025

Bergmans, R. S., Rapp, A., Kelly, K. M., Weiss, D., & Mezuk, B. (2021). Understanding the relationship between type 2 diabetes and depression: Lessons from genetically informative study designs. *Diabetic Medicine, 38*(2), e14399. https://doi.org/10.1111/dme.14399

Berg-Smith, S. M., Stevens, V. J., Brown, K. M., van Horn, L., Gernhofer, N., & Peters, E. (1999). A brief MI to improve dietary adherence in adolescents. *Health Education Research, 14*(3), 399–410. https://doi.org/10.1093/her/14.3.399

Bevier, W. C., Fuller, S. M., & Fuller, R. P., Rubin, R. R., Dassau, E., Doyle, F. J., Jovanovic, L., & Zisser, H. C. (2014). Artificial pancreas (AP) clinical trial participants' acceptance of future AP technology. *Diabetes Technology & Therapeutics, 16*, 590–595. https://doi.org/10.1089/dia.2013.0365

Bluestone, J. A., Herold, K., & Eisenbarth, G. (2010). Genetics, pathogenesis, and treatment in type 1 diabetes. *Nature, 464*(7293), 1293–1300. https://doi.org/10.1038/nature08933

Boltri, J. M., Davis-Smith, Y. M., Seale, J. P., Shellenberger, S., Okosun, I. S., & Cornelius, M. E. (2008). Diabetes prevention in a faith-based setting: Results of translational research. *Journal of Public Health Management and Practice, 14*(1), 29–32. https://doi.org/10.1097/01.phh.0000303410.66485.91

Breland, J. Y., Yeh, V. M., & Yu, J. (2013). Adherence to evidence-based guidelines among diabetes self-management apps. *Translational Behavioral Medicine, 3*(3), 277–286. https://doi.org/10.1007/s13142-013-0205-4

Brownson, C. A., & Heisler, M. (2009). The role of peer support in diabetes care and self-management. *The Patient, 2*(1), 5–17. https://doi.org/10.2165/01312067-200902010-00002

Cafazzo, J. A., Casselman, M., Katzman, D. K., & Palmert, M. R. (2012). Bant: An mHealth App for adolescent type I diabetes–A pilot study. *The Journal of Adolescent Health: Official Publication of the Society for Adolescent Medicine, 50*(2), S77–S78. https://doi.org/10.2196/jmir.2058

Canedo, J. R., Miller, S. T., Schlundt, D., Fadden, M. K., & Sanderson, M. (2018). Racial/ethnic disparities in diabetes quality of care: The role of healthcare access and socioeconomic status. *Journal of Racial and Ethnic Health Disparities, 5*(1), 7–14. https://doi.org/10.1007/s40615-016-0335-8

Castle, J. R., Wilson, L. M., Tyler, N. S., Espinoza, A. Z., Mosquera-Lopez, C. M., Kushner, T., Young, G. M., Pinsonault, J., Dodier, R. H., Hilts, W. W., Oganessian, S. M., Branigan, D. L., Gabo, V. B., Eom, J. H., Ramsey, K., Youssef, J. E., Cafazzo, J. A., Winters-Stone, K., & Jacobs, P. G. (2022). Assessment of a decision support system for adults with type 1 diabetes on multiple daily insulin injections. *Diabetes Technology & Therapeutics, 24*(12), 892–897. https://doi.org/10.1089/dia.2022.0252

Centers for Disease Control and Prevention. (2015). *About CDC's division of diabetes translation* [Internet]. https://www.cdc.gov/diabetes/about

Centers for Disease Control and Prevention. (2022). *National diabetes statistics report: Estimates of diabetes and its burden in the United States.* U.S. Department of Health and Human Services.

Channon, S. J., Huws-Thomas, M. V., Rollnick, S., Hood, K., Canning-John, R. L., & Rogers, C. (2007). A multicenter randomized controlled trail of motivational interviewing in teenagers with diabetes. *Diabetes Care, 30*(6), 1390–1395. https://doi.org/10.2337/dc06-2260

Chen, S. M., Creddy, D., Lin, H. S., & Wollin, J. (2012). Effects of motivational intervention on self-management, psychological, and glycemic outcomes in type 2 diabetes: A randomized controlled trial. *International Journal of Nursing Studies, 49*(6), 637–644. https://doi.org/10.1016/j.ijnurstu.2011.11.011

Cryer, P. E. (2008). The barrier of hypoglycemia in diabetes. *Diabetes, 57*(12), 3169–3176. https://doi.org/10.2337/db08-1084

Dabelea, D., Mayer-Davis, E. J., Saydah, S., Imperatore, G., Linder, B., Divers, J., Bell, R., Badaru, A., Talton, J. W., Crume, T., Liese, A. D., Merchant, A. T., Lawrence, J. M., Reynolds, K., Dolan, L., Liu, L. L., & Hamman, R. F., & SEARCH for Diabetes in Youth Study. (2014). Prevalence of type 1 and type 2 diabetes among children and adolescents from 2001 to 2009. *Journal of the American Medical Association, 311*(17), 1778–1786. https://doi.org/10.1001/jama.2014.3201

Davies, M. J., Gagliardino, J. J., Gray, L. J., Khunti, K., Mohan, V., & Hughes, R. (2013). Real-world factors affecting adherence to insulin therapy in patients with type 1 or type 2 diabetes mellitus: A systematic review. *Diabetic Medicine, 30*(5), 512–524. https://doi.org/10.1111/dme.12128

Delamater, A. M. (2006). Improving patient adherence. *Clinical Diabetes, 24*(2), 71–77. http://doi.org/10.2337/diaclin.24.2.71

Diabetes Initiative of South Carolina. (2011). *The state of diabetes initiative of South Carolina: An evaluation of the first ten year strategic plan of the diabetes initiative of South Carolina* [Internet]. http://www.scdhec.gov/Health/docs/DSC Eval Rport 3-2011.pdf

Diabetes Prevention Program. (2002). The Diabetes Prevention Program (DPP): Description of lifestyle intervention. *Diabetes Care, 25*(12), 2165–2171. https://doi.org/10.2337/diacare.25.12.2165

DiMatteo, M. R. (2004). Social support and patient adherence to medical treatment: A meta-analysis. *Health Psychology, 23*(2), 207–218. https://doi.org/10.1037/0278-6133.23.2.207

Driscoll, K. A., Raymond, J., Naranjo, D., & Patton, S. R. (2016). Fear of hypoglycemia in children and adolescents and their parents with type 1 diabetes. *Current Diabetes Reports, 16*, 77. https://doi.org/10.1007/s11892-016-0762-2

ElSayed, N. A., Aleppo, G., Aroda, V. R., Bannuru, R. R., Brown, F. M., Bruemmer, D., Collins, B. S., Hilliard, M. E., Isaacs, D., Johnson, E. L., Kahan, S., Khunti, K., Leon, J., Lyons, S. K., Perry, M. L., Prahalad, P., Pratley, R. E., Seley, J. J., Stanton, R. C., . . . Gabbay, R. A. on behalf of the American Diabetes Association. (2023). 5. Facilitating positive health behaviors and well-being to improve health outcomes: Standards of care in diabetes-2023. *Diabetes Care, 46*(Suppl. 1), S68–S96. https://doi.org/10.2337/dc23-S005

Espinosa, P. R., Garcia, L. C., Vasquez, J. J., Xiao, L., Stafford, R. S., Krenzel, L. D., Ojeda, A., & Rosas, L. G. (2022). Understanding historical trauma among urban indigenous adults at risk for diabetes. *American Indian and Alaska Native Mental Health Research, 29*(3), 43. https://doi.org/10.5820/aian.2903.2022.43

Feldman, M. A., Anderson, L. M., Shapiro, J. B., Jedraszko, A. M., Evans, M., Weil, L. E., Garza, K. P., & Weissberg-Benchell, J. (2018). Family-based interventions targeting improvements in health and family outcomes of children and adolescents with type 1 diabetes: A systematic review. *Current Diabetes Reports, 18*, 1–12. https://doi.org/10.1007/s11892-018-0981-9

Galatzer, A., Amir, S., Gil, R., Karp, M., & Laron, Z. (1982). Crisis intervention program in newly diagnosed diabetic children. *Diabetes Care, 5*, 414–419. https://doi.org/10.2337/diacare.5.4.414

Golden, S. H., Lazo, M., Carnethon, M., Bertoni, A. G., Schreiner, P. J., Diez Roux, A. V., Lee, H. B., & Lyketsos, C. (2008). Examining a bidirectional association between depressive symptoms and diabetes. *Journal of the American Medical Association, 299*(23), 2751–2759. https://doi.org/10.1001/jama.299.23.2751

Gonzalez, J. S., Kane, N. S., Binko, D. H., Shapira, A., & Hoogendoorn, C. J. (2016). Tangled up in blue: Unraveling the links between emotional distress and treatment adherence in type 2 diabetes. *Diabetes Care, 39*(12), 2182–2189. https://doi.org/10.2337/dc16-1657

Gonzalez, J. S., Peyrot, M., McCarl, L. A., Collins, E. M., Serpa, L., Mimiaga, M. J., & Safren, S. A. (2008). Depression and diabetes treatment nonadherence: A meta-analysis. *Diabetes Care, 31*(12), 2398–2403. https://doi.org/10.2337/dc08-1341

Gordon, S. (2016). *FDA approves first "artificial pancreas" for type 1 diabetes.* http://www.cbsnews.com/news/fda-approves-first-artificial-pancreas-type-1-diabetes-medtronic-minimed-670g

Harris, M. A., Antal, H., Oelbaum, R., Buckloh, L. M., White, N. H., & Wysocki, T. (2008). Good intentions gone awry: Assessing parental "miscarried helping" in diabetes. *Families, Systems, & Health, 26*(4), 393–403.

Harris, M. A., Harris, B. S., & Mertlich, D. (2005). Brief report: In-home family therapy for adolescents with poorly controlled diabetes: Failure to maintain benefits at 6-month follow-up. *Journal of Pediatric Psychology, 30*(8), 683–688. https://doi.org/10.1093/jpepsy/jsi055

Harris, M. A., Hood, K. K., & Mulvaney, S. A. (2012). Pumpers, skypers, surfers and texters: Technology to improve the management of diabetes in teenagers. *Diabetes, Obesity, & Metabolism, 14*(11), 967–972. https://doi.org/10.1111/j.1463-1326.2012.01599.x

Harris, M. A., & Mertlich, D. (2003). Piloting home-based behavioral family systems therapy for adolescents with poorly controlled diabetes. *Children's Health Care: Journal of the Association for the Care of Children's Health, 32*(1), 65–79. http://doi.org/10.1207/S15326888CHC3201_5

Hartz, J., Yingling, L., & Powell-Wiley, T. M. (2016). Use of mobile health technology in the prevention and management of diabetes mellitus. *Current Cardiology Reports, 18*(12), 130. https://doi.org/10.1007/s11886-016-0796-8

Heisler, M. (2007). Overview of peer support models to improve diabetes self-management and clinical outcomes. *Diabetes Spectrum, 20*(4), 214–221. https://doi.org/10.2337/diaspect.20.4.214

Herold, K. C., Bundy, B. N., Long, S. A., Bluestone, J. A., DiMeglio, L. A., Dufort, M. J., & Greenbaum, C. J. (2019). An anti-CD3 antibody, teplizumab, in relatives at risk for type 1 diabetes. *New England Journal of Medicine, 381*(7), 603–613. https://doi.org/10.1056/NEJMoa1902226

Hill-Briggs, F., Ephraim, P. L., Vrany, E. A., Davidson, K. W., Pekmezaris, R., Salas-Lopez, D., Alfano, C. M., & Gary-Webb, T. L. (2022). Social determinants of health, race, and diabetes population health improvement: Black/African Americans as a population exemplar. *Current Diabetes Report, 22*(3), 117–128. https://doi.org/10.1007/s11892-022-01454-3

Hill-Briggs, F., & Fitzpatrick, S. L. (2023). Overview of social determinants of health in the development of diabetes. *Diabetes Care, 46*(9), 1590–1598. https://doi.org/10.2337/dci23-0001

Hill-Briggs, F., & Gemmell, L. (2007). Problem solving in diabetes self-management and control: A systematic review of the literature. *The Diabetes Educator, 33*(6), 1032–1050. https://doi.org/10.1177/0145721707308412

Hirsch, I. B., Abelseth, J., & Bode, B. W., Fischer, J. S., Kaufman, F. R., Mastrototaro, J., Parkin, C. G., Wolpert, H. A., & Buckingham, B. (2008). Sensor-augmented insulin pump therapy: Results of the first randomized treat-to-target study. *Diabetes Technology & Therapeutics, 10*(5), 377–383. https://doi.org/10.1089/dia.2008.0068

Hood, K. K., Peterson, C. M., Rohan, J. M., & Drotar, D. (2009). Association between adherence and glycemic control in pediatric type 1 diabetes: A meta-analysis. *Pediatrics, 124*(6), e1171–e1179. https://doi.org/10.1542/peds.2009-0207

Hood, K. K., Rohan, J. M., Peterson, C. M., & Drotar, D. (2010). Interventions with adherence-promoting components in pediatric type 1 diabetes: Meta-analysis of their impact on glycemic control. *Diabetes Care, 33*(7), 1658–1664. https://doi.org/10.2337/dc09-2268

Imperatore, G., Boyle, J. P., Thompson, T. J., Case, D., Dabelea, D., Hamman, R. F., Lawrence, J. M., Liese, A. D., Liu, L. L., Mayer-Davis, E. J., Rodriguez, B. L., Standiford, D., & Search for Diabetes in Youth Study Group. (2012). Projections of type 1 and type 2 diabetes burden in the U.S. population aged <20 years through 2050: Dynamic modeling of incidence, mortality, and population growth. *Diabetes Care, 35*(12), 2515–2520. https://doi.org/10.2337/dc12-0669

Ingerski, L. M., Laffel, L., Drotar, D., Repaske, D., & Hood, K. K. (2010). Correlates of glycemic control and quality of life outcomes in adolescents with type 1 diabetes. *Pediatric Diabetes, 11*(8), 563–571. https://doi.org/10.1111/j.1399-5448.2010.00645.x

Iturralde, E., Tanenbaum, M. L., Hanes, S. J., Suttiratana, S. C., Ambrosino, J. M., Ly, T. T., Maahs, D. M., Naranjo, D., Walders-Abramson, N., Weinzimer, S. A., Buckingham, B. A., & Hood, K. K. (2017). Expectations and attitudes of individuals with type 1 diabetes after using a hybrid closed loop system. *The Diabetes Educator, 43,* 223–232. https://doi.org/10.1177/0145721717697244

Johnson, C. (2022). Conquering the health disparities of structural racism. *Journal of Public Health Management and Practice, 28*(Suppl. 1), S15–S17. https://doi.org/10.1097/PHH.0000000000001431

Johnson, S. B. (1992). Methodological issues in diabetes research: Measuring adherence. *Diabetes Care, 15,* 1658–1667. https://doi.org/10.2337/diacare.15.11.1658

King, P. S., Berg, C. A., Butner, J., Butler, J. M., & Wiebe, D. J. (2014). Longitudinal trajectories of parental involvement in Type 1 diabetes and adolescents' adherence. *Health Psychology, 33*(5), 424–432. https://doi.org/10.1037/a0032804

Kirkman, M. S., Rowan-Martin, M. T., Levin, R., Fonseca, V. A., Schmittdiel, J. A., Herman, W. H., & Aubert, R. E. (2015). Determinants of adherence to diabetes medications: Findings from a large pharmacy claims database. *Diabetes Care, 38*(4), 604–609. https://doi.org/10.2337/dc14-2098

Kostic, A. D., Gevers, D., Siljander, H., Vatanen, T., Hyötyläinen, T., Hämäläinen, A. M., Peet, A., Tillmann, V., Pöhö, P., Mattila, I., Lähdesmäki, H., Franzosa, E. A., Vaarala, O., de Goffau, M., Harmsen, H., Ilonen, J., Virtanen, S. M., Clish, C. B., Orešič, M., . . . Knip, M. on behalf of the DIABIMMUNE Study Group, & Xavier, R. J. (2015). The dynamics of the human infant gut microbiome in development and in progression toward type 1 diabetes. *Cell Host & Microbe, 17*(2), 260–273. https://doi.org/10.1016/j.chom.2015.01.001

Kutz, S. M. (1990). Adherence to diabetes regimens: Empirical status and clinical applications. *The Diabetes Educator, 16,* 50–56. https://doi.org/10.1177/014572179001600112

Laffel, L. M., Vangsness, L., Connell, A., Goebel-Fabbri, A., Butler, D., & Anderson, B. J. (2003). Impact of ambulatory, family-focused teamwork intervention on glycemic control in youth with type 1 diabetes. *The Journal of Pediatrics, 142,* 409–416. https://doi.org/10.1067/mpd.2003.138

Lal, R. A., Ekhlaspour, L., Hood, K., & Buckingham, B. (2019). Realizing a closed-loop (artificial pancreas) system for the treatment of type 1 diabetes. *Endocrine Reviews, 40*(6), 1521–1546. https://doi.org/10.1210/er.2018-00174

LeBrón, A. M. W., Spencer, M., Kieffer, E., Sinco, B., & Palmisano, G. (2019). Racial/ethnic discrimination and diabetes-related outcomes among latinos with type 2 diabetes. *Journal of Immigrant and Minority Health, 21*(1), 105–114. https://doi.org/10.1007/s10903-018-0710-0

Lewis, K. H., Moore, J. B., & Ard, J. D. (2023). Game changers: Do new medications make lifestyle-based treatment of obesity obsolete? *Obesity, 32*(2), 237–239. https://doi.org/10.1002/oby.23962

Liang, X., Wang, Q., Yang, X., Cao, J., Chen, J., Mo, X., Huang, J., Wang, L., & Gu, D. (2011). Effect of mobile phone intervention for diabetes on glycaemic control: A meta-analysis. *Diabetic medicine: A Journal of the British Diabetic Association, 28*(4), 455–463. https://doi.org/10.1111/j.1464-5491.2010.03180.x

Liese, A. D., D'Agostino, R. B., Jr., Hamman, R. F., Kilgo, P. D., Lawrence, J. M., Liu, L. L., Loots, B., Linder, B., Marcovina, S., Rodriguez, B., Standiford, D., & Williams, D. E. (2006). The burden of diabetes mellitus among US youth: Prevalence estimates from the SEARCH for diabetes in youth study. *Pediatrics, 118*(4), 1510–1518. https://doi.org/10.1542/peds.2006-0690

Ly, T. T., & Buckingham, B. A. (2015). Technology and type 1 diabetes: Closed-loop therapies. *Current Pediatrics Reports, 3,* 170–176. https://doi.org/10.1177/1359105317718615

Martens, T., Beck, R. W., Bailey, R., Ruedy, K. J., Calhoun, P., Peters, A. L., Pop-Busui, R., Philis-Tsimikas, A., Bao, S., Umpierrez, G., Davis, G., Kruger, D., Bhargava, A., Young, L., McGill, J. B., Aleppo, G., Nguyen, Q. T., Orozco, I., Biggs, W., . . . MOBILE Study Group. (2021). Effect of continuous glucose monitoring on glycemic control in patients with type 2 diabetes treated with basal insulin: A randomized clinical trial. *JAMA, 325*(22), 2262–2272. https://doi.org/10.1001/jama.2021.7444

Mayberry, L. S., Egede, L. E., Wagner, J. A., & Osborn, C. Y. (2015). Stress, depression and medication nonadherence in diabetes: Test of the exacerbating and buffering effects of family support. *Journal of Behavioral Medicine, 38*(2), 363–371. https://doi.org/10.1007/s10865-014-9611-4

Mcgrady, M. E., Laffel, L., Drotar, D., Repaske, D., & Hood, K. K. (2009). Depressive symptoms and glycemic control in adolescents with type 1 diabetes: Mediational role of blood glucose monitoring. *Diabetes Care, 32*(5), 804–806. https://doi.org/10.2337/dc08-2111

McKnight, J. A., Wild, S. H., Lamb, M. J., Cooper, M. N., Jones, T. W., Davis, E. A., Hofer, S., Fritsch, M., Schober, E., Svensson, J., Almdal, T., Young, R., Warner, J. T., Delemer, B., Souchon, P. F., Holl, R. W., Karges, W., Kieninger, D. M., Tigas, S., . . . Miller, K. M. (2015). Glycaemic control of Type 1 diabetes in clinical practice early in the 21st century: An international comparison. *Diabetic Medicine, 32*(8), 1036–1050. https://doi.org/10.1111/dme.12676

McNabb, W. L. (1997). Adherence in diabetes: Can we define it and can we measure it? *Diabetes Care, 20*, 215–218. https://doi.org/10.2337/diacare.20.2.215

Menke, A., Casagrande, S., Geiss, L., & Cowie, C. C. (2015). Prevalence of and trends in diabetes among adults in the United States, 1988–2012. *Journal of the American Medical Association, 314*(10), 1021–1029. https://doi.org/10.1001/jama.2015.10029

Michigan Diabetes Research and Training Center. (2017). *About us* [Internet]. http://diabetesresearch.med.umich.edu

Moreland, E. C., Tovar, A., Zuehlke, J. B., Butler, D. A., Milaszewski, K., & Laffel, L. M. (2004). The impact of physiological, therapeutic, and psychosocial variables on glycemic control in youth with type 1 diabetes mellitus. *Journal of Pediatric Endocrinology & Metabolism, 17*(11), 1533–1544. https://doi.org/10.1515/jpem.2004.17.11.1533

Mujahid, M. S., Maddali, S. R., Gao, X., Oo, K. H., Benjamin, L. A., & Lewis, T. T. (2023). The impact of neighborhoods on diabetes risk and outcomes: Centering health equity. *Diabetes Care, 46*(9), 1609–1618. https://doi.org/10.2337/dci23-0003

Mulvaney, S. A., Rothman, R. L., Osborn, C. Y., Lybarger, C., Dietrich, M. S., & Wallston, K. A. (2011). Self-management problem solving for adolescents with type 1 diabetes: Intervention processes associated with an Internet program. *Patient Education and Counseling, 85*, 140–142. https://doi.org/10.1016/j.pec.2010.09.018

Mulvaney, S. A., Rothman, R. L., Wallston, K. A., Lybarger, C., & Dietrich, M. S. (2010). An internet-based program to improve self-management in adolescents with type 1 diabetes. *Diabetes Care, 33*(3), 602–604. https://doi.org/10.2337/dc09-1881

Peyrot, M., Rubin, R. R., Lauritzen, T., Skovlund, S. E., Snoek, F. J., Landgraf, R., Matthews, D. R., Landgraf, R., Kleinebreil, L., & on behalf of the International DAWN Advisory Panel. (2005). Resistance to insulin therapy among patients and providers. *Diabetes Care, 28*(11), 2673–2679. https://doi.org/10.2337/diacare.28.11.2673

Peyrot, M., Rubin, R. R., Lauritzen, T., Snoek, F. J., Matthews, D. R., & Skovlund, S. E. (2005). Psychosocial problems and barriers to improved diabetes management: Results of the cross-national diabetes attitudes, wishes, and needs (DAWN) study. *Diabetic Medicine, 22*, 1379–1385. https://doi.org/10.1111/j.1464-5491.2005.01644.x

Phillip, M., Battelino, T., Rodriguez, H., Danne, T., Kaufman, F., European Society for Paediatric Endocrinology, Lawson Wilkins Pediatric Endocrine Society, International Society for Pediatric and Adolescent Diabetes, American Diabetes Association, & European Association for the Study of Diabetes. (2007). Use of insulin pump therapy in the pediatric age-group: Consensus statement from the European Society for Paediatric endocrinology, the Lawson Wilkins pediatric endocrine society, and the international society for pediatric and adolescent diabetes, endorsed by the American diabetes association and the European association for the study of diabetes. *Diabetes Care, 30*(6), 1653–1662. https://doi.org/10.2337/dc07-9922

Pierce, G. R., Sarason, B. R., Sarason, I. G., Joseph, H. J., & Henderson, C. A. (1996). Conceptualizing and assessing social support in the context of the family. In G. R. Pierce, B. R. Sarason, & I. G. Sarason (Eds.), *Handbook of social support and the family* (pp. 3–23). Plenum Press.

Polonsky, W. H., Anderson, B. J., Lohrer, P. A., Welch, G., Jacobson, A. M., Aponte, J. E., & Schwartz, C. E. (1995). Assessment of diabetes-related distress. *Diabetes Care, 18*(6), 754–760. https://doi.org/10.2337/diacare.18.6.754

Polonsky, W. H. (2007). Psychological insulin resistance: The patient perspective. *The Diabetes Educator, 33*(7), 241S–244S.

Polonsky, W. H., Fisher, L., Guzman, S., Villa-Caballero, L., & Edelman, S. V. (2005). Psychological insulin resistance in patients with type 2 diabetes: The scope of the problem. *Diabetes Care. 28*(10), 2543–2545. https://doi.org/10.2337/diacare.28.10.2543

Polonsky, W. H., Layne, J. E., Parkin, C. G., Kusiak, C. M., Barleen, N. A., Miller, D. P., Zisser, H., & Dixon, R. F. (2020). Impact of participation in a virtual diabetes clinic on diabetes-related distress in individuals with type 2 diabetes. *Clinical Diabetes, 38*(4), 357–362. https://doi.org/10.2337/cd19-0105

Polonsky, W. H., Soriano, E. C., & Fortmann, A. L. (2022). The role of retrospective data review in the personal use of real-time continuous glucose monitoring: Perceived impact on quality of life and health outcomes. *Diabetes Technology & Therapeutics, 24*(7), 492–501. https://doi.org/10.1089/dia.2021.0526

Psihogios, A. M., Fellmeth, H., Schwartz, L. A., & Barakat, L. P. (2019). Family functioning and medical adherence across children and adolescents with chronic health conditions: A meta-analysis. *Journal of Pediatric Psychology, 44*(1), 84–97. https://doi.org/10.1093/jpepsy/jsy044

Quinn, C. C., Shardell, M. D., Terrin, M. L., Barr, E. A., Ballew, S. H., & Gruber-Baldini, A. L. (2011). Cluster-randomized trial of a mobile phone personalized behavioral intervention for blood glucose control. *Diabetes Care, 34*(9), 1934–1942. https://doi.org/10.2337/dc11-0366

Rizzo, A. S., Lange, B., Suma, E. A., & Bolas, M. (2011). Virtual reality and interactive digital game technology: New tools to address obesity and diabetes. *Journal of Diabetes Science and Technology, 5*(2), 256–264. https://doi.org/10.1177/193229681100500209

Rollnick, S., Mason, P., & Butler, C. (1999). *Health behavior change: A guide for practitioners*. Churchill Livingstone.

Rothenberg, R., Zetelski, M., Sivitz, J., Klein, G., Chartoff, A., Pearson, J., Post, J., Cohen, A., Aisenberg, J., & Ghanny, S. (2015). Use of smartphone, a cellular glucometer, and social media app in the management of type 1 DM in the adolescent population: The future of diabetes care. *Hormone Research in Pediatrics, 84*, 374–375.

Russell, S. J., Hillard, M. A., Balliro, C., Magyar, K. L., Selagamsetty, R., Sinha, M., Grennan, K., Mondesir, D., Ekhlaspour, L., Zheng, H., Damiano, E. R., & El-Khatib, F. H. (2016). Day and night glycaemic control with a bionic pancreas versus conventional insulin pump therapy in preadolescent children with type 1 diabetes: A randomised crossover trial. *The Lancet. Diabetes & Endocrinology, 4*, 233–243. https://doi.org/10.1016/s2213-8587(15)00489-1

Stuckey, H., Fisher, L., Polonsky, W. H., Hessler, D., Snoek, F. J., Tang, T. S., Hermanns, N., Mundet-Tuduri, X., da Silva, M. E. R., Sturt, J., Okazaki, K., Cao, D., Hadjiyianni, I., Ivanova, J. I., Desai, U., & Perez-Nieves, M. (2019). Key factors for overcoming psychological insulin resistance: An examination of patient perspectives through content analysis. *BMJ Open Diabetes Research and Care, 7*(1), e000723. https://doi.org/10.1136/bmjdrc-2019-000723

Tanenbaum, M. L., Hanes, S. J., Miller, K. M., Naranjo, D., Bensen, R., & Hood, K. K. (2016). Diabetes device use in adults with type 1 diabetes: Barriers to uptake and potential intervention targets. *Diabetes Care, 40*(2), 181–187. https://doi.org/10.2337/dc16-1536

Tannenbaum, M. B., Hepler, J., Zimmerman, R. S., Saul, L., Jacobs, S., Wilson, K., & Albarracín, D. (2015). Appealing to fear: A meta-analysis of fear appeal effectiveness and theories. *Psychological Bulletin, 141*(6), 1178–1204. https://doi.org/10.1037/a0039729

UK Hypoglycaemia Study Group. (2007). Risk of hypoglycaemia in types 1 and 2 diabetes: Effects of treatment modalities and their duration. *Diabetologia, 50*(6), 1140–1147. https://doi.org/10.1007/s00125-007-0599-y

Vaala, S. E., Hood, K. K., Laffel, L., Kumah-Crystal, Y. A., Lybarger, C. K., & Mulvaney, S. A. (2015). Use of commonly available technologies for diabetes information and self-management among adolescents with type 1 diabetes and their parents: A web-based survey study. *Interactive Journal of Medical Research, 4*(4), 1140–1147. http://doi.org/10.2196/ijmr.4504

Wagner, D. V., Stoeckel, M., Tudor, M. E., & Harris, M. A. (2015). Treating the most vulnerable and costly in diabetes. *Current Diabetes Reports, 15*(6), 1–7. https://doi.org/10.1007/s11892-015-0606-5

Wild, D., von Maltzahn, R., Brohan, E., Christensen, T., Clauson, P., & Gonder-Frederick, L. (2007). A critical review of the literature on fear of hypoglycemia in diabetes: Implications for diabetes management and patient education. *Patient Education and Counseling, 68*(1), 10–15. https://doi.org/10.1016/j.pec.2007.05.003

World Health Organization. (2012). *World health statistics 2012*. https://www.who.int/docs/default-source/gho-documents/world-health-statistic-reports/world-health-statistics-2012.pdf

Wysocki, T. (1993). Associations among teen-parent relationships, metabolic control, and adjustment to diabetes in adolescents. *Journal of Pediatric Psychology, 18*, 441–452. https://doi.org/10.1093/jpepsy/18.4.441

Wysocki, T., Harris, M. A., Buckloh, L. M., Mertlich, D., Lochrie, A. S., Mauras, N., & White, N. H. (2007). Randomized trial of behavioral family systems therapy for diabetes: Maintenance of effects on adolescents' diabetes outcomes. *Diabetes Care, 30*(3), 555–560. https://doi.org/10.2337/dc06-1613

Wysocki, T., Harris, M. A., Buckloh, L. M., Mertlich, D., Lochrie, A. S., Mauras, N., & White, N. H. (2008). Randomized controlled trial of behavioral family systems therapy for diabetes: Maintenance and generalization of effects on parent-adolescent communication. *Behavior Therapy, 39*, 33–46. https://doi.org/10.1016/j.beth.2007.04.001

Wysocki, T., Harris, M. A., Buckloh, L. M., Mertlich, D., Lochrie, A. S., Taylor, A., Sadler, M., Mauras, N., & White, N. H. (2006). Effects of behavioral family systems therapy for diabetes on adolescents' family relationships, treatment adherence, and metabolic control. *Journal of Pediatric Psychology, 31*, 928–938. https://doi.org/10.1093/jpepsy/jsj098

Wysocki, T., Harris, M. A., Greco, P., Bubb, J., Danda, C. E., Harvey, L. M., McDonell, K., & White, N. H. (2000). Randomized, controlled trial of behavior therapy for families of adolescents with insulin-dependent diabetes mellitus. *Journal of Pediatric Psychology, 25*, 23–33. https://doi.org/10.1093/jpepsy/25.1.23

Young, H. M., Miyamoto, S., Dharmar, M., & Tang-Feldman, Y. (2020). Nurse coaching and mobile health compared with usual care to improve diabetes self-efficacy for persons with type 2 diabetes: Randomized controlled trial. *JMIR mHealth and uHealth, 8*(3), e16665. https://doi.org/10.2196/16665

Young-Hyman, D., de Groot, M., Hill-Briggs, F., Gonzalez, J. S., Hood, K., & Peyrot, M. (2016). Psychosocial care for people with diabetes: A position statement of the American Diabetes Association. *Diabetes Care, 39*(12), 2126–2140. https://doi.org/10.2337/dc16-2053

CHAPTER 16

OBESITY

LONEKE T. BLACKMAN CARR AND VERONICA R. JOHNSON

LEARNING OBJECTIVES

- Discuss the global prevalence of obesity and identify at least three associated comorbidities.
- Describe disparities in the prevalence of obesity.
- Describe the three components of the standard behavioral approach to weight loss.
- Identify at least three behavioral strategies that are commonly used in the behavioral approach to weight loss.
- Describe equity frameworks in obesity research.
- Understand the role of pharmacotherapy and metabolic and bariatric surgery in the management of overweight and obesity.

EPIDEMIOLOGY AND SIGNIFICANCE OF OBESITY

Prevalence, Comorbidities, and Significance

Overweight and obesity are defined as a body mass index (BMI) between 25.0 to 29.9 kg/m^2 and 30.0 kg/m^2 or more, respectively (Table 16.1; Centers for Disease Control and Prevention [CDC], 2022). Globally, in 2016, 11% of men and 15% of women over the age of 18 years were living with obesity (World Health Organization, 2021). In the United States, data from 2017 to 2018 showed that 30.7% of adults aged 20 years and older were overweight (Fryar et al., 2020). Obesity is present among 41.9% of men and women in the United States (Stierman et al., 2021). Disparities in obesity prevalence exist among individuals from minoritized racial and ethnic backgrounds; non-Hispanic Black adults with obesity experience the highest prevalence rate (49.9%), compared with Hispanic (45.6%), non-Hispanic White (41.4%), and non-Hispanic Asian adults (16.1% Stierman et al., 2021). Beyond disparities evident solely by race and ethnicity, disparities among people with obesity are also seen when demographic characteristics intersect. When both race/ethnicity and sex are considered, among males, obesity prevalence was highest among Hispanic (45.2%), compared with non-Hispanic White (43.1%), non-Hispanic Black (40.4%), and Asian (17.6%) adults (Stierman et al., 2021). Among females, obesity prevalence is most pronounced among non-Hispanic Black (57.9%) compared with Hispanic (45.7%), non-Hispanic White (39.6%), and Asian (14.5%) adults (Stierman et al., 2021). Obesity is a well-established risk factor for a myriad of chronic conditions, including type 2 diabetes, hypertension, cardiovascular disease, certain cancers, sleep disorders, and arthritis (Wadden et al., 2007). The disproportionately high prevalence of obesity among some marginalized groups may further exacerbate preexisting disparities in the prevalence of these chronic conditions.

Among children, obesity is defined as a BMI at or above the sex-specific 95th percentile on the U.S. CDC BMI-for-age growth charts. For children and adolescents between the ages of

TABLE 16.1 Classification of Overweight and Obesity		
	OBESITY CLASS	**BODY MASS INDEX (KG/M²)**
Underweight		<18.5
Normal		18.5–24.9
Overweight		25.0–29.9
Obesity	1	30.0–34.9
	2	35.0–39.9
Severe obesity	3	≥40

Source: From National Heart Lung and Blood Institute Obesity Education Initiative Expert Panel on the Identification Evaluation and Treatment of Overweight and Obesity. (1998). Clinical guidelines on the identification, evaluation, and treatment of overweight and obesity in adults: The evidence report. *Obesity Research, 6*(Suppl. 2), 51S–209S.

2 and 19 years, the prevalence rates are estimated at 19.7% (Stierman et al., 2021), while another 16.6% are overweight (Fryar et al., 2018). Disparities by race or ethnicity are also present within rates of pediatric obesity; compared with non-Hispanic White children and adolescents, the obesity prevalence is higher among non-Hispanic Black children and adolescents and Hispanic children and adolescents (Stierman et al., 2021).

BEHAVIORS INCLUDED IN MANAGING OVERWEIGHT AND OBESITY

Weight management is characterized by lifestyle modification, an approach that includes reduced energy intake, increased energy expenditure, and cognitive behavioral treatment, referred to as standard behavioral treatment (SBT; Digenio et al., 2009). It is indicated for individuals with obesity or with overweight in the presence of at least two risk factors for cardiovascular disease (e.g., diabetes, hypertension; NHLBI, 1998).

Dietary Modification

A key component of dietary therapy is a reduction in total caloric intake by 500 kcal/d that results in a 1 lb per week weight loss (1 lb is the equivalent of 3,500 kcal). Dietary education includes the energy value of macronutrients (e.g., fat contains 9 calories per gram compared with protein and carbohydrates, which contain 4 calories per gram), how to read food labels, the types of fat, methods to reduce fat and increase fiber and complex carbohydrate intake, portion control, and how to prepare foods to reduce caloric intake. Addressing both fat and caloric restriction is important. The calorie goal is based on the individual's baseline body weight and other factors such as sex, with for example a typical low-calorie diet containing 1,200 kilocalories for women and 1,500 kilocalories for men (National Heart Lung and Blood Institute, n.d.). Typically, the fat allowance is 20% to 30% of the total daily calories (Wing, 2004).

One approach to management of energy intake is the use of meal replacements, for example, SlimFast (Unilever, London, UK, and Rotterdam, The Netherlands). Meal replacements, in contrast to a food-based diet, can be helpful in facilitating behavior changes for several reasons. First, with relatively few options to choose from, they embody the concept of "stimulus narrowing," through which a person is likely to consume less overall than if they were faced with many different foods to choose from. Second, by simplifying the process of meal preparation (no cooking or cleanup required), meal replacements can make it easier to create and stick to a dietary plan that may require individuals to prepare and consume meals or snacks up to five times per day. Consuming meal replacements has been associated with improved weight loss and weight maintenance (Keogh & Clifton, 2012). For example, Look AHEAD Trial participants were instructed to replace two meals per day with a liquid shake and one snack with a bar for the first 6 months, and then replace one meal and one snack per day in the second half of the first year (Wadden et al., 2006). One year later, the number of meal replacements consumed was significantly associated with weight loss. However, meal replacements may not work similarly

318 III • PRIORITIZED BEHAVIORS FOR SECONDARY PREVENTION

among all racial and ethnic groups; in the Look AHEAD Trial, the use of meal replacements by Black women was associated with less robust weight loss and weight gain (West et al., 2019). Lowe et al. (2014) investigated the consumption of meal replacements in a predominately Black population recruited from the primary care setting; at 12 months, the participants had lost an average of 6.1 kg across groups, but by 24 months significant weight regain had occurred. Uptake of this and other eating behaviors may vary across racial/ethnic and sex groups.

Physical Activity

Incorporating physical activity in treatment for weight loss and maintenance is essential for successful outcomes. Recent recommendations for healthy adults from the American College of Sports Medicine (ACSM) are organized into four categories of exercise: cardiorespiratory, resistance, flexibility, and neuromotor (Garber et al., 2011). For additional information on physical activity for promoting health, please see Chapter 8, "Physical Activity." In contrast to the amount of physical activity needed for health and fitness, higher amounts of physical activity are needed to lose weight and prevent weight regain after weight loss. For a weight loss of approximately 2 to 3 kg over 4 to 6 months, moderate-intensity physical activity for at least 150 minutes per week is recommended; 225 to 420 minutes of moderate-intensity activity per week results in a 5- to 7.5-kg weight loss, over the same time period (Donnelly et al., 2009). Physical activity alone results in a 3% loss of body weight (Donnelly et al., 2009); therefore, energy restriction is necessary for additional weight loss (Curioni & Lourenco, 2005). Physical activity is also associated with cardiovascular health benefit; among adult men and women, aerobic activity reduces systolic and diastolic blood pressure. While the evidence does not support resistance exercise training as an effective tool for weight loss, it may help preserve lean muscle mass and promote percent fat loss through increases in energy expenditure (Donnelly et al., 2009). Approximately 250 to 300 minutes per week of moderate-intensity daily activity may be necessary to maintain weight loss among persons who were formerly obese (Haskell et al., 2007). Activity may be accumulated in multiple 10-minute periods throughout the day and continue to be beneficial for weight loss (Jakicic et al., 1999).

Literature suggests that race may need to be considered in the prescription of physical activity made in behavioral weight loss trials (Davis et al., 2015; Delany et al., 2014). Davis et al. (2015) observed a significantly higher amount of objective physical activity and weight loss among White compared with Black participants in an 18-month behavioral weight loss study. Importantly, physical activity was lower between these race groups at baseline, which reflects national disparities in physical activity engagement, and may indicate that factors external to the weight loss intervention may impede adoption of the behavior. For example, perceived racial composition of neighborhoods may influence physical activity engagement. According to Ray (2017), physical activity was decreased among Black men in neighborhoods perceived to be mostly White, while Black women's activity decreased in neighborhoods perceived to be mostly Black and urban (Ray, 2017). These findings reflect larger societal realities as the author states Black men's activity engagement can be disrupted due to their awareness that their presence is criminalized (Ray, 2017), which may incite unwarranted policing. A lack of perceived safety during activity likely underlies the result of less physical activity in Black women in mostly Black areas. For Black and White women and White men, activity increased as perception of a neighborhood being mostly White increased, likely reflecting the resources, including safety, necessary to support participation in activity. (Ray, 2017) The context in which physical activity is expected to occur can affect behavioral engagement and vary by race/ethnicity, sex, and other characteristics.

BEHAVIORAL STRATEGIES FOR MANAGING OBESITY

The core behavior change strategies of SBT for weight loss are based on the social cognitive theory and include goal setting, self-monitoring, cognitive restructuring, self-efficacy enhancement, and social support with feedback and guidance provided by behavioral counselors to assist with the development of problem-solving skills (Bray & Bouchard, 2014). A list of the behavioral strategies that are typically used in weight loss treatment are detailed in Table 16.2.

TABLE 16.2 Strategies Used in the Standard Behavioral Treatment Interventions for Weight Loss[a]

STRATEGY	DESCRIPTION	EXAMPLE OF STRATEGY IN PRACTICE
Goal setting	Individuals are instructed to set daily and weekly goals for calorie and fat consumption, exercise time, and behavior change.	Mr. Yang, who is participating in a weight loss program, notes that he is often hungry about an hour before lunch, and this can lead to overindulging at that meal. The nutritionist works with him to set a goal to eat a protein-rich breakfast every day and to set an alarm on his cell phone at 7 a.m. to remind him. Once he is more regularly getting protein with breakfast, his lunchtime hunger is much more manageable.
Self-monitoring	Systematically observing and recording one's behavior for the purpose of increasing one's awareness of current behaviors and the settings in which they occur. It provides opportunity to make corrective action if done in a timely manner; it also provides counselor material to provide feedback on progress.	Inspired by a New Year's resolution, Jessica downloads a diet-tracking app on her phone. She starts to record what she has for dinner each night using the app, both in terms of what foods and drinks are consumed and also how much of each item. The app then translates this into caloric consumption and breaks down the meal according to macronutrient content (how much fat, protein, and carbohydrates were consumed). This process allows her to realize that a lot of calories and carbohydrates are coming from drinking two 12-ounce sodas with dinner each night, so she makes the change to plain water.
Self-evaluation	Individuals compare their behavior with a desired standard. A perceived discrepancy between one's current performance and the desired standard/goal can prompt one into action. Satisfaction will occur if there is a close match between the performance criteria and feedback information.	A group class on weight management strategies encourages patients to compare and contrast their experiences. Mr. Jones notes that others in the class who have successfully lost weight are also reporting consistently tracking their meals, a task his dietitian recommended, but which he has not previously been motivated to do. Based on this discrepancy, he decides to start tracking all of his meals and finds that he starts to lose more weight as a result of ensuing changes in his dietary choices.
Self-reinforcement	This occurs as the evaluation process is completed, comes from seeing personal change occur. As individuals observe their behavior change, they develop a strengthened sense of efficacy for maintaining those behaviors. Thus, self-efficacy influences maintenance and self-regulation.	At first, Mrs. Smith found it hard and unpleasant to go to the gym and lift weights. She did not really know how to use the equipment, and always felt sore for a day or 2 after the workout. However, after a few weeks of sticking with the program her trainer gave her, she noticed 1 day that she was able to get on the ground and play with her 4-year-old granddaughter very easily—something she had not previously been able to do. She reflected that all of that time in the gym must be paying off, and decided to add an extra workout day each week.

(continued)

TABLE 16.2 Strategies Used in the Standard Behavioral Treatment Interventions for Weight Loss[a] (*continued*)		
STRATEGY	**DESCRIPTION**	**EXAMPLE OF STRATEGY IN PRACTICE**
Feedback	Specific, daily goals are set and one's performance in achieving these goals is evaluated; reinforcement on performance is also received. Individuals use the information recorded in their diaries as a source of feedback on their progress in changing their behavior. The interventionists monitor the recorded behavior and provide feedback and guidance.	Dr. Gupta sets a daily energy intake goal of 1200 kcal for Mrs. Young. At their next clinic visit, she reviews Mrs. Young's tracked data in a paper log that she kept of her meals and snacks. Dr. Gupta remarks that Mrs. Young did a great job with monitoring her intake, and that on most days she was very close to the recommended target of energy intake. Mrs. Young feels validated and appreciates that the doctor took the time to review the work she had done and give her feedback. It motivates her to keep going.
Stimulus control	This refers to behavioral strategies designed to help participants alter their environment, minimize cues that might trigger undesirable behaviors related to physical activity or eating, and add cues to increase activity. Individuals rearrange their environment for this purpose (e.g., remove counterproductive items from sight).	Carrie keeps a bowl of chocolate candies on her kitchen counter, right near the sink. She hates doing dishes and notices that she often rewards herself by eating a few candies when she is done. Her nutritionist suggests moving the bowl out of sight, so she puts it in a cabinet in her pantry. To make the chore more bearable, even without chocolate, she starts listening to podcasts while she does dishes.
Problem-solving	Individuals learn skills to deal with situations that interfere with achieving their goals. Problem-solving consists of five steps: identifying and defining the problem, brainstorming solutions, evaluating the pros and cons of potential solution, implementing the solution plan, and evaluating its success.	Sam and Josh are roommates. Sam is trying to lose weight but Josh, who does the cooking, tends to make very rich, high-calorie meals. They sit down together and identify this as a problem, brainstorm different solutions, and decide to try splitting the work. Sam will pick recipes and go shopping, and Josh will do the cooking. A week later, they are both enjoying the healthier meals and Josh even notes that he has less heartburn at night.
Social assertion	The skill of being assertive in social situations that threaten desirable eating and physical activity behaviors is essential to behavior change in weight loss. Individuals learn three communication styles (aggressive, passive, and assertive) and how to use assertive skills in situations that may threaten their ability to meet their eating and physical activity goals.	Regina visits her grandmother every afternoon. Her grandmother is not supportive of Regina's weight loss efforts, and tells her she looks beautiful just as she is. She even bakes fresh cookies daily and makes Regina feel guilty if she declines eating them. Regina's therapist helps her with talking points, and the next time her grandmother criticizes her weight loss efforts Regina speaks up for herself and explains that her weight loss is not about how she looks, rather she is trying to improve her health and that her grandmothers comments have been hurtful to her. Her grandmother understands, apologizes for her behavior, and agrees that they can start meeting in the park to take a walk in the afternoons instead.

STRATEGY	DESCRIPTION	EXAMPLE OF STRATEGY IN PRACTICE
Cognitive strategies	Individuals are taught how to recognize patterns of negative thought that can interfere with behavior change and weight control, such as perfectionism, all or none thinking, and self-doubt; to use cognitive techniques to counter these negative thoughts; and to use positive self-statements.	Every time Maria looked at herself in her full-length mirror as she left for work, her eyes would immediately go to her hips and thighs. Then came the intrusive thoughts about how she was never going to look the way she wanted in a pair of jeans, and no guy was going to ask out a girl who looked like this. After talking with her therapist, Maria switched to a square mirror that only showed her reflection from the waist up. Next to it, she placed a post-it note, reminding her to look in the mirror and give herself at least one compliment each day before leaving the house.
Relapse prevention	Marlatt and Gordon's relapse prevention model is used to teach participants to recognize situations that place them at risk for lapses from their dietary behavior change program (Marlatt & Gordon, 1985). They learn how to use behavioral and cognitive strategies for handling these situations in the future.	Shonti recently lost 25 lb by making major lifestyle changes. She is preparing for a family vacation, and traditionally this has meant lots of eating and drinking alcohol—things she knows are going to lead to weight regain. To try to help her navigate the situation, she schedules a visit with her nutritionist to get tips for how to navigate the vacation and have more control over what she eats and drinks. Instead of gaining the usual 10 lb on vacation, she is able to only gain 2 lb using these tools.
Portion control	Learning to recognize and control portion size is crucial to reducing food consumption.	A group class in a weight management clinic does an activity in which patients view portions of food (e.g., shredded cheese, cooked pasta, stir-fried food) and estimate the amount. They are then told the actual amount and how this compares to the recommended serving size. Afterwards, they are able to practice serving correct portions of different foods.

[a]The strategies are based on several models of motivation and behavior change.

SELF-REGULATION AND SELF-MONITORING

Programs that target behavior change such as weight loss are based on strategies that promote the individual's ability to self-regulate behavior. Kanfer's Theory of Self-Regulation, a part of the social cognitive theory, provides the theoretical basis for self-monitoring (Kanfer, 1991; Kanfer & Goldstein, 1991). Kanfer suggests that changing habits requires self-regulatory skills. He has described self-regulation as a process that includes three distinct components: self-monitoring, self-evaluation, and self-reinforcement. The behavioral strategy of self-monitoring is central to this process and includes deliberate attention to some aspect of an individual's behavior and recording details of that behavior.

Self-monitoring is the centerpiece of weight loss treatment. Burke et al. (2011) conducted a systematic review of the literature on self-monitoring in weight loss treatment programs and found consistent support for a significant association between participant self-monitoring and weight loss. Traditionally, self-monitoring includes recording one's food intake (calories and fat grams) and physical activity. More recently, self-monitoring weight has been added as an approach to increase one's awareness of weight and its relation to energy intake and expenditure, also as an aid to prevent weight regain (VanWormer et al., 2009; Wing et al., 2006). A recent systematic review indicated self-weighing is significantly associated with weight loss in behavioral weight management treatments, and it will not cause negative psychological outcomes (Zheng et al., 2015a). Furthermore, the association between self-weighing and weight change is partially mediated by adherence to diet and physical activity goals (Zheng et al., 2015b).

While SBT has been the cornerstone of weight loss interventions, "third wave" acceptance-based behavioral treatment has emerged as a means to address challenges in self-regulation and adherence to dietary and physical activity behaviors (Forman & Butryn, 2015). Acceptance-based behavioral treatment is theorized to improve self-regulation and behavior change in the midst of internal and external stimuli (Forman & Butryn, 2015). The said stimuli may cause distress, but the acceptance-based approach teaches behavioral commitment according to clear values and individual ability to override the drive to overconsume in the moment (Forman & Butryn, 2015). Three main components characterize the acceptance-based approach (Table 16.3).

Acceptance-based behavioral treatment has shown promise for obesity treatment among adults in clinical trials. A comparison of the standard versus the acceptance-based behavioral treatment among 190 adults produced significantly greater weight loss over 12 months (9.8% vs. 13.3%, respectively; Forman et al., 2016). Participants who received the acceptance-based

TABLE 16.3 Main Components of Acceptance-Based Behavioral Treatment for Obesity	
COMPONENT	DESCRIPTION
Values clarity/ commitment enhancement	Identification of goals based on participants' chosen life values guided by a structured process to connect values with diet and physical activity goals. Commitment to goals when they are challenging to practice (unpleasant) is supported by awareness skills.
Distress tolerance	Development of tolerance for unpleasant states related to eating (e.g., craving) and physical activity (e.g., discomfort) as it supports a valued goal. Willingness to accept momentary aversive states and engage in the behavior is taught.
Awareness training	Increase awareness of perceptions, thoughts, and affective experiences that influence eating and physical activity behaviors through skill development to interrupt influences that may lead to overconsumption, insufficient physical activity, and sedentary behavior. Participants learn to make conscious diet and physical activity decisions that may also address the environment.

treatment were also more likely to achieve 10% weight loss compared with those who received SBT at 12 months and beyond (Forman et al., 2016, 2019). The acceptance-based approach also shows promise among individuals who, when engaged in weight loss interventions, have only lost small to modest amounts of weight. Statistically similar weight loss was produced among Black and White participants in a trial comparing SBT with environmental and acceptance-based treatment (9.4% vs. 11.5%, respectively). Reaching at least 5% weight loss was more likely among Black participants who received the acceptance-based versus standard-only treatment (Butryn et al., 2017). Importantly, for Black participants, attendance was significantly greater among those in the acceptance versus standard study arm (Butryn et al., 2017), and greater attendance is associated with greater weight loss (Wadden et al., 2009). The trend toward higher satisfaction with the acceptance-based compared with standard treatment in Black participants observed by investigators reinforces that perhaps the acceptance-based approach holds relevance to how target behaviors are adopted (Butryn et al., 2017). The large weight losses that exceed what is typically produced among Black participants and the smaller disparity in overall weight losses between Black and White participants in Butryn et al.'s study indicate that approaches other than the SBT may hold greater relevance and produce better results among historically underrepresented groups living with a high burden of obesity.

Healthcare Provider-Directed and Patient-Centered Interventions

Assessment, diagnosis, and treatment of obesity during clinical encounters in the healthcare practitioner setting are suboptimal. In a study of 9,827 patients, only 20% of the obese patients had that diagnosis documented in their chart (Bardia et al., 2007). Even though there have been some interventions to promote health providers' adherence to current obesity clinical practice guidelines, the documentation of diagnosis and treatment plan for obesity did not significantly increase (Barnes et al., 2015). Barriers to appropriate identification and treatment of obesity have been recognized on multiple levels—provider, patient, and healthcare system. Provider barriers include negative attitude toward obesity, and lack of time and insurance reimbursement, along with lack of administrative support, training, comfort, and useful tools for delivering weight loss treatment (Findholt et al., 2013; Rao, 2010; Sebiany, 2013; Tham & Young, 2008). Patient barriers may include embarrassment, fear, patient–physician interaction, or lack of motivation, while system barriers consist of limited resources and high costs (Fujioka & Bakhru, 2010; Westerveld & Yang, 2016).

The U.S. Preventive Services Task Force recommends that practitioners offer or refer patients with a BMI of 30 kg/m² or higher to intensive, multicomponent behavioral interventions to promote weight loss and to improve glucose control and other physiological risk factors for cardiovascular diseases (Moyer, 2012); intensive counseling is defined as a minimum of two visits per month for the first 3 months (U.S. Preventive Services Task Force, 2003). Practice-based interventions that have met this intensity level resulted in significant weight losses (e.g., in a nurse practitioner-led weight loss program), patients lost a mean of 6.6 lb ($p < .05$) and 10.77 lb ($p < .05$) after 4 and 12 intensive behavioral therapy visits (Thabault et al., 2016).

Reimbursement by the Centers for Medicare & Medicaid Services (CMS) provides incentive for obesity treatment by providers. CMS will reimburse primary care providers for obesity screening and intensive behavioral therapy in settings such as physicians' offices. Medicare recipients with a BMI greater than or equal to 30 kg/m² are eligible to receive one weekly face-to-face counseling visit for 1 month and biweekly for 5 additional months. If the patient has achieved a weight loss of greater than or equal to 3 kg after the first 6 months, they may then receive monthly face-to-face counseling for an additional 6 months. However, this may prevent individuals from receiving counseling after the initial 6 months as 3-kg weight loss is an uncommon outcome among some racial/ethnic and sex groups as described earlier. CMS reimbursement for this therapy is confined to primary care settings, and it must be provided by primary care physicians or primary care practitioners (PCPs), defined as nurse practitioners, clinical nurse specialists, or physician assistants (CMS, 2011). Wadden et al. (2014) conducted a systematic review to examine the effect of behavioral counseling for patients who were overweight or obese in primary care settings. Among the reviewed studies, none reported that PCPs were following the CMS guidelines (14 sessions in 6 months). Although the policy and guidelines are supportive of obesity management in primary care, there remains a need for improvement of the application of these guidelines.

WEIGHT STIGMA AND OBESITY CONTROL

Weight stigma is defined as a social devaluation of individuals because of their body weight (Pearl, 2018). Socially, weight stigmatization can lead to negative stereotypes of laziness and a lack of self-discipline (Pearl, 2018). Weight-based discrimination can also result and lead to denial of employment and negative experiences in healthcare (Pearl, 2018). With regard to weight-related behaviors, weight stigma has been linked to unhealthy eating behaviors such as binge and emotional eating (Vartanian & Porter, 2016) and reduced physical activity (Puhl et al., 2020). In an obesity context, this stigmatization can have a negative impact at two important points, the development of obesity and obesity treatment. Weight stigma can be cyclical (**Figure 16.1**), where stigmatization acts as a psychological stressor that can increase dietary consumption and yield physiological stress response through increased cortisol levels known to promote weight gain (Tomiyama, 2014). This cycle can impair weight loss efforts among individuals who experience weight stigmatization (Tomiyama, 2014). Thus, it is important to examine the presence and impact of weight stigma and its internalization among individuals engaged in obesity treatment whether behavioral, pharmacological, or surgical (Puhl et al., 2020). During weight loss interventions, including skill development to cope with weight stigma and related stress is also recommended (Puhl et al., 2020). The influence of other identities with the experience of weight stigmatization and its internalization has received some attention. Himmelstein et al. (2017) examined survey responses on this topic and relationship to race and gender. Some important findings indicate nuances across different groups. For example, women reported more internalization than men, Black adults experienced less internalization than their White counterparts, and Hispanic women were more likely engage in disordered eating as a maladaptive coping mechanism than White women (Himmelstein et al., 2017). While more research in weight stigma, internalization and the impact in weight loss treatment is necessary, it is similarly important for an intersectional lens to be applied across these efforts to generate treatment appropriate for all.

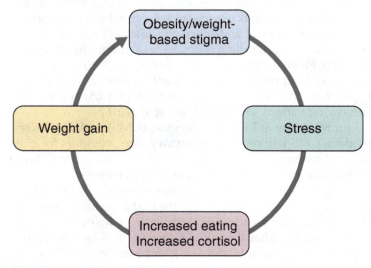

FIGURE 16.1 Cyclical obesity/weight-based stigma.

EQUITY ISSUES IN BEHAVIORAL TREATMENT FOR OBESITY

Disparities in Weight Loss Outcomes

It is well-established that the standard behavioral weight loss treatment is not as effective among certain groups, namely non-Hispanic Black and Hispanic adults (Goode et al., 2017; Wingo et al., 2014). Therefore, it is essential to understand the differential impact of current behavioral treatments by race and ethnicity. For example, while 5% to 10% weight loss is the clinical target for behavioral weight loss interventions with adults, among non-Hispanic Black women 2% to 3% weight loss is common (Goode et al., 2017). A review of interventions adapted from the Diabetes Prevention Program and conducted with Hispanic adults showed similar modest reductions in weight (McCurley et al., 2017). In the few exemplars where greater amounts of weight loss were observed, outcomes are commonly 2% to 3% lower in non-Hispanic Black versus White women (Wadden et al., 2009; West et al., 2008).

Most behavioral weight loss intervention studies are still populated by majority non-Hispanic White individuals (Haughton et al., 2018). Black adults are generally under-represented in weight control interventions (Goode et al., 2017), but when their inclusion is a target of investigators some evidence indicates appropriate levels of representation can be reached (Haughton et al., 2018). Still, adults from other marginalized racial/ethnic backgrounds remain underrepresented in weight loss trials, including Native American, Hispanic and Latino, Asian American, and Pacific Islander adults (Haughton et al., 2018). Beyond race/ethnicity, sex is a relevant demographic factor when examining who receives obesity treatment. Women continue to predominantly populate weight loss studies, which leaves a gap regarding effectiveness and needs of men during behavioral intervention. As such, it is important to consider these and other demographic characteristics that may inter-sect and deepen understanding of who may not be represented in obesity treatment or for whom the standard behavioral approach does not produce optimal weight loss.

Throughout the literature, weight loss outcomes often group participants from racial/ethnic backgrounds into a general "other" group (Haughton et al., 2018). Similarly, data are often not reported considering the intersections of identity (e.g., race/ethnicity and sex) that may be important to understand equity issues that arise at such points (Blackman Carr et al., 2022). Diminishing the disparity in obesity-related outcomes continues to be challenging due to the limited presence of racial/ethnic minorities within the sample (Goode et al., 2017). Future research must target individuals who have been underrepresented in the weight loss literature and those who represent communities that have been marginalized. Further, standards of practice may need to be set to facilitate consistent reporting of weight loss trial results by, but not limited to, race/ethnicity and sex. As weight loss interventions do not commonly produce robust results that reach clinical goals in individuals from marginalized groups, it is necessary to reexamine the components of standard behavioral practice and design more effective solutions for groups experiencing disparities in obesity and behavioral treatment.

An important component of developing effective weight loss interventions that are sensitive to varying cultural groups is identifying relevant cultural practices/beliefs that are associated with weight-related and/or dietary outcomes (e.g., cultural relationship with food) and then using this knowledge to guide intervention development (Lindberg et al., 2013). Among Hispanic individuals, culturally salient recommendations include moving beyond adapting the intervention into Spanish, constructing interventions with materials that are sensitive to literacy, and creating family-based interventions. It also is important to recognize the heterogeneity within the Hispanic population and consider the variation that may be present depending on specific ethnic heritage (e.g., Cuban, Mexican, Puerto Rican; Weinick et al., 2004). Alternatively, among Black adults, excess weight may reflect coping strategies or an increased reliance on food, in addition to the impact of neighborhood and environmental factors (Kumanyika et al., 2007; Mendez et al., 2016). Black women manage

Social Determinants of Health and Equity-Minded Frameworks

The production of more equitable obesity treatment may reside in rethinking the theoretical foundations on which behavioral weight loss interventions are constructed. Health disparity frameworks and theories are valuable because they capture the overlooked influences that may impede or modify the behavior changes that can produce weight loss. The National Institute on Minority Health and Health Disparities (NIMHD) Research Framework depicts a matrix of dimensions that influence health disparities at the cross-section of domains that can impact health (e.g., biological, behavioral, sociocultural, and built environments) and levels of influence across the social environment (e.g., individual, interpersonal, societal; Alvidrez et al., 2019). According to this framework, at the cross-section of behavioral domain of influence and the societal level of influence sit policies and laws that may influence health disparities. In an obesity disparities context, for example, this may look like zoning policies that promote a high concentration of unhealthy food retail within neighborhoods with a predominantly Black and Hispanic residents.

Similar to the NIMHD framework but specific to obesity interventions and a group experiencing high prevalence of obesity (non-Hispanic Black adults) is the Expanded Obesity Research Paradigm (Kumanyika et al., 2007). This obesity specific framework communicates that effective obesity treatment to modify weight-related behaviors must be designed with consideration for the context in which behavior change is expected to occur (Kumanyika et al., 2007). Per the framework, dietary and physical activity behaviors are influenced by three intersecting domains: historical and social contexts, cultural and psychosocial processes, and physical and built environment. To understand the influence of these domains, interdisciplinary scholarship like sociology, literature, economics, and so forth is necessary to draw knowledge from (Kumanyika et al., 2007). Content pertinent to cultural values Black adults hold and external, yet impactful, factors like historical foundations of inequity inform the knowledge domains. Further, this paradigm specifies research approaches necessary for this work, particularly qualitative methodologies and community engagement (Kumanyika et al., 2007). While this paradigm is specific to addressing obesity among non-Hispanic Black adults, its relevance to achieving equity in obesity treatment is aligned with the NIMHD framework as higher ecological levels of influence on individual behaviors such as the built environment, interpersonal influences, societal factors, and other elements are similarly represented.

The frameworks discussed and others in the field all incorporate aspects of the social determinants of health that are necessary to describe here as they are regarded as the causes of health inequities (Braveman & Gottlieb, 2014). Broadly defined, the social determinants of health are the "conditions in the environments where people are born, live, learn, work, play, worship, and age that affect a wide range of health, functioning, and quality-of-life outcomes and risks" (DHHS, n.d.). Five domains describe groupings of the social determinants of health: economic stability, education access and quality, healthcare access and quality, neighborhood and built environment, and social and community context. As SDOH underlie health inequities, it may similarly undermine the effectiveness of behavioral weight loss treatment among groups historically and systematically marginalized in American society. Table 16.4 provides examples to define and illustrate each domain and the potential influence on behavioral weight loss intervention outcomes.

The social determinants of health may affect most members of a population subgroup, and nuances may exist as individuals within a group may have dissimilar experiences (Kumanyika, 2022). Determinants of health are also societal or structural in nature and embedded into how the

TABLE 16.4 Social Determinants of Health in Behavioral Weight Loss Interventions

DOMAIN	DOMAIN FOCUS
Economic stability	Poverty alleviation; stable and sufficient incomes to meet basic needs to improve and maintain health
Education access and quality	Increased access to quality education for children and teens
Healthcare access and quality	Access to high-quality and comprehensive healthcare
Neighborhood and built environment	Safe neighborhoods and environments that promote health
Social and community context	Bolster social and community support

United States functions. Structural determinants are characterized by the economic and governance systems, social policies (e.g., racism), and norms that shape the daily context in which behaviors targeted in behavioral weight loss interventions are expected to occur (Kumanyika, 2022).

Structural racism is defined as "the totality of ways, in which societies foster racial discrimination, via mutually reinforcing inequitable systems (e.g., housing, employment, earnings, benefits, credit, media, healthcare, criminal justice, etc.)" (Bailey et al., 2017). The illustration of the structural nature of the determinants of health is clearly articulated in the definition. Several racial/ethnic groups have been marginalized through such structural determinants, including Native American, Asian Americans and Pacific Islanders, Hispanic, Latino, and non-Hispanic Black communities. Forced migration and land dispossession of Native Americans from tribal lands as part of colonization reshaped food and physical activity environments (Wiedman, 2012), limiting positive health behaviors. Considering the structural nature of SDOH requires that behavioral weight control interventions address the structural factors that have marginalized groups based on race/ethnicity, poverty, and so forth. New models for obesity control describe policy-, systems-, and environment-focused approaches to pull the levers of social and structural change that may include, for example, modification of the food environment through policy changes that establish nutrition standards for government-involved food distribution and programs, or support for community programs that focus on physical activity improvement (Kumanyika, 2019b). Importantly, Figure 16.2 depicts how exposure to SDOH and its structural manifestations can have a cumulative effect across the human life course on individuals and communities that are marginalized.

While discussions on health disparities often indicate factors that explain poor health or less than robust treatment outcomes among certain populations, frameworks also bring attention to what may support improved health. In the strengths-based (or asset-based) approach, the social environment, individual skills, physical and economic resources, and cultural and historical elements that already exist in an individual's life are valued and incorporated (Foley & Schubert, 2013). Exposure to the adverse experiences among individuals and communities may also have bred resilience and ways of coping to mitigate the negative impact of SDOH many groups experience. Through a strengths-based lens, health-promoting behaviors and cultural attributes are valued and recognized as important and necessary to counter predominantly deficit-focused research that centers the problems among marginalized populations' health and is often a perspective where the contexts that influence behavior and health are absent (Kumanyika, 2022). In obesity treatment, a strengths-based approach may look like the inclusion of traditionally healthy behaviors or maintenance of faith-based practices that were generated to cope with chronic stress (Kumanyika, 2019a). Use of research methodologies to include qualitative approaches can expand knowledge of inherent strengths to balance the predominantly quantitative and deficit-focused discourse in health behaviors (Foley & Schubert, 2013).

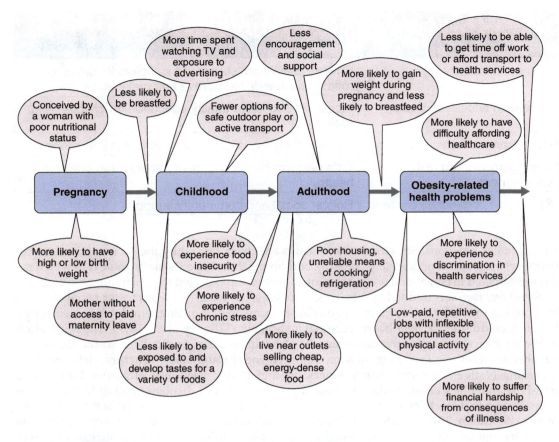

FIGURE 16.2 How inequities in obesity compound over the life course. Adverse social and economic conditions that begin before or during pregnancy or arise over time can have cumulative effects on risks of obesity, and related health problems are potential targets for policy solutions.
Source: From Kumanyika, S. K. (2022). Advancing health equity efforts to reduce obesity: Changing the course. *Annual Review of Nutrition, 42*, 453–480. https://doi.org/10.1146/annurev-nutr-092021-050805.

CASE STUDY 16.1: AUGMENTING THE DIABETES PREVENTION PROGRAM TO ACHIEVE MORE EQUITABLE OUTCOMES

Based on formative research using qualitative methodology (Tipre & Carson, 2022), a behavioral weight loss intervention was designed to address stress among Black women (Buro et al., 2022). The formative phase of research identified how Black women perceived that race- and gender-based stress impacted their weight status. The results indicated emotional eating, lack of time for exercise, and consumption of fast food as contributing factors. In the subsequent, 6-month-long randomized trial, the standard behavioral weight loss treatment approach, based on the Diabetes Prevention Program, was augmented with stress management techniques designed to address the high amount of stress experienced by Black women. The augmented arm was compared with the standard treatment alone. Stress reduction techniques are evidence-based and employ cognitive, behavioral, and coping strategies. The intervention design was created using the community-engaged approach of a community action board composed of Black women who provided personal and professional insights on stress management.

BRIEF OVERVIEW OF PHARMACOTHERAPY AND METABOLIC AND BARIATRIC SURGERY

Pharmacotherapy

Antiobesity medications (AOMs) are indicated as an adjunct to lifestyle interventions and behavior change in individuals with a BMI greater than $30 \, \text{kg/m}^2$ or a BMI greater than $27 \, \text{kg/m}^2$ with significant weight-related medical condition (e.g., type 2 diabetes, hypertension, cardiovascular disease; Apovian et al., 2015; Jensen et al., 2014). Medications should lead to at least 5% total body weight loss. However, targeting 5% to 10% total body weight loss is correlated with improvement in many metabolic, skeletal, and anatomic complications associated with excess weight; >15% total body weight loss is associated with improvement of cardiovascular outcomes (Chakhtoura et al., 2023). AOMs enhance known pathophysiological pathways primarily within the brain to regulate hunger and appetite (Apovian et al., 2015).

Prior to 2021, AOMs approved for long-term use included orlistat, phentermine-topiramate, bupropion-naltrexone, and liraglutide 3.0 mg (Apovian et al., 2015). These agents promoted no more than 10% total body weight loss on average at 52 weeks in adults with overweight and obesity (Müller et al., 2022). Despite their value in weight reduction and improvement in metabolic markers, only 1% of eligible U.S. adults were offered/prescribed these agents (Lyu et al., 2022; Washington et al., 2023). Additionally, patients are unlikely to continue beyond 12 months of use for many reasons, including decreased efficacy, unfavorable side effect profile, and cost (Kan et al., 2023).

The newest generation of AOMs are highly effective incretin-based therapies and nutrient-stimulated hormone-based (NuSH) therapies mimicking glucose-like 1 peptide (GLP-1) and glucose-dependent insulinotropic polypeptide (GIP). GLP-1 and GIP are important in glucose metabolism and promote weight loss by slowing gastric emptying and acting within various centers of the brain to increase satiety and decrease food intake (Baggio & Drucker, 2007; Hammoud & Drucker, 2023; Müller et al., 2022). Semaglutide 2.4 mg activates GLP-1 receptors to promote 15% total body weight reduction on average (Wilding et al., 2021). Tirzepatide acts on both GLP-1 and GIP receptors leading to about 22% total body weight loss on average at its highest dose of 15 mg (Jastreboff et al., 2022). Recent studies demonstrate continued use of semaglutide and tirzepatide is necessary for weight loss maintenance as patients regain weight once medications are stopped (Aronne et al., 2024).

Given the high efficacy of NuSH-based therapies, intensive lifestyle interventions have minimal impact on total weight loss (Wadden et al., 2021, 2023). Nevertheless, lifestyle interventions remain the foundation of weight management to optimize patients' body composition, cardiometabolic health, and quality of life. Lifestyle modifications and behavior change will also be important in patients who do not desire to be on medication long term due to concerns regarding safety and high cost. In the future, more pharmacotherapy options will be approved to effectively treat overweight and obesity, including cagrilintide/semaglutide (amylin/GLP-1 receptor agonist) and retatrutide (GLP-1/GIP/glucagon receptor agonist).

CASE STUDY 16.2: BARIATRIC SURGERY

Nicole is a 55-year-old female with class 3 obesity. She notes a strong genetic predisposition to excess weight and has a similar body habitus as her mother and maternal grandmother. In the past, she has tried multiple specific diet plans (i.e., Keto, Atkins, meal replacement program), increased her physical activity, and participated in several commercial diet programs (i.e., Weight Watchers, Jenny Craig) to promote weight loss. Nicole has lost up to 40 lb in the past but always manages to regain weight over time. Since menopause, Nicole has gained 25 lb and has recently been diagnosed with type 2 diabetes. She is open to use antiobesity medications as she has optimized her diet and physical activity with minimal success.

(continued)

CASE STUDY 16.2: BARIATRIC SURGERY (*continued*)

Nicole is prescribed semaglutide at her initial visit to concurrently treat her type 2 diabetes and class 3 obesity. The dose is slowly increased monthly to the highest dose of 2.4 mg weekly. At her 6-month follow-up, Nicole reports significant improvement in hunger and appetite. She notes her type 2 diabetes is better controlled (per her continuous glucose monitor), but her total weight loss is only 10 lb (approximately 5% total body weight; BMI 50 kg/m²).

Nicole is seen in clinic for follow up at 9 months and 12 months from her initial visit. She has only lost a total of 20 lb (approximately 10% total body weight; BMI 47 kg/m²). Due to her less-than-average response to semaglutide, Nicole is transitioned to tirzepatide. The dose is slowly titrated up to the maximum dose of 15 mg weekly. After 24 months from her initial visit, she has lost a total of 50 lb (approximately 20% total body weight; BMI 40 kg/m²). Nicole is pleased with the results and management of her diabetes. However, she was recently diagnosed with fatty liver disease and fear progression to nonalcoholic steatohepatitis (NASH) as her mother passed away from complications associated with NASH. While Nicole was not interested in metabolic and bariatric surgery initially, she is aware that this is the most effective tool to not only promote further weight loss but decrease her risk of having NASH.

Nicole elects to proceed with a sleeve gastrectomy (SG). She stops tirzepatide 1 week prior to surgery and continues to hold tirzepatide in the postoperative period. At 18 months post-SG, Nicole has a BMI of 27 kg/m². Her type 2 diabetes remains controlled without medication. Nicole continues a balanced low-calorie diet and has increased her physical activity to 200 minutes weekly. She continues to maintain her weight following surgery and follows up annually.

Metabolic and Bariatric Surgery

Compared with nonsurgical interventions, metabolic and bariatric surgery (MBS) is the most effective tool to promote substantial, long-term weight loss leading to improvement in metabolic disease (including type 2 diabetes), reduction in obesity-related cancer, and increased life expectancy (Eisenberg et al., 2022; Hsu & Farrell, 2024). According to the American Society for Metabolic and Bariatric Surgery (ASMBS), MBS can be offered in patients with a BMI ≥35 kg/m² (regardless of the presence of weight-related condition) or in patients with a BMI of 30 to 34.9 kg/m² (Eisenberg et al., 2022). The BMI threshold for MBS is reduced to 27.5 kg/m² in the Asian population (Eisenberg et al., 2022). Despite the lower threshold for MBS consideration, patients are more likely to obtain insurance approval based on prior guidelines established in 1991.

The last 10 years marks an increased demand for MBS. Nevertheless, only 0.5% of patients who meet the indications for surgery proceed with this intervention (Hsu & Farrell, 2024). Sleeve gastrectomy (SG) is the most common procedure in the United States, comprising more than 60% of all procedures, followed by the Roux-en-Y gastric bypass (RYGB; Hsu & Farrell, 2024). SG is the preferred surgery due to its favorable safety profile.

Once a patient considers MBS, an extensive preoperative workup is critical to ensure the patient is an appropriate candidate. The workup includes a comprehensive assessment of the patient's medical history, including screening for preexisting medical conditions, prior surgeries, current alcohol and substance use, review of laboratory tests, and screening for preexisting medical issues. A thorough psychological profile is critical to assess for mental health, emotional well-being, disordered eating, body image concerns, and understanding of the surgery and associated implications (Hsu & Farrell, 2024).

The expected total body weight loss following MBS is between 20% and 30% on average (Hsu & Farrell, 2024). Patients typically achieved this weight within 12 to 18 months post operatively. After this period, weight regain can affect up to 50% of patients (Athanasiadis et al., 2021). There are many factors contributing to weight gain, including anatomic (e.g., enlarged stomach volume), dietary (e.g., more consumption of calorie-dense foods), and psychiatric (e.g., anxiety; Athanasiadis et al., 2021). Weight regain is managed under the care of a multidisciplinary team including a dietitian, behavioral health professional, obesity medicine specialist, and bariatric surgeon. While lifestyle interventions and behavior change can assist with weight regain, use of AOMs and surgical interventions are additional treatment options to consider when appropriate.

RELAPSE PREVENTION/MAINTENANCE OF CHANGE

Long-term maintenance of weight loss has remained a formidable challenge; approximately one-third of weight lost among individuals treated with lifestyle modification is regained within 1 year (Wadden et al., 2004) and the rest within 3 to 5 years (Dulloo & Schutz, 2015; Evans et al., 2015). The behaviors required for weight loss may differ from those needed in weight loss maintenance because the goal of maintenance is to undo small weight gains before the gains become large; the goal for weight loss is generally to lose sizeable amounts of weight after a prolonged period of weight gain. Weight loss treatment is temporary and often accompanied by positive comments from others, but weight loss maintenance is long term, and ongoing reinforcement usually lapses.

A great deal of what is known about successful weight loss maintenance is a result of the National Weight Control Registry, a large registry of persons who have successfully lost 13.6 kg (30 lb) and maintained that loss for a minimum of 1 year (Klem et al., 1997). Thomas et al. reported that more than 87% of the participants in the registry were able to maintain at least a 10% weight loss 10 years after the intentional weight loss (Thomas et al., 2014). Much descriptive information has been reported on behavioral strategies used by these weight loss maintainers—increasing physical activity (approximately 1 hr/d of walking), consuming a diet moderate in calories (approximately 1800 kcal/d) and low in fat (<30% kcal from fat), regularly self-monitoring weight and food intake, limiting the variety of foods eaten, eating breakfast and eating more frequently, restricting time spent watching television, and having a consistent dietary intake across the week (Bachman et al., 2011; Ogden et al., 2012; Raynor et al., 2005, 2006). Other descriptive studies have corroborated these findings and added information related to eating low-fat, protein-rich foods and rewarding oneself for adhering to the eating and activity plan (Sciamanna et al., 2011). In contrast, internal disinhibition, decreases in physical activity, increases in energy intake from fat, and absence of monitoring one's weight have been reported as predictors of weight regain (Lillis et al., 2016; Thomas et al., 2014).

Evidence has shown that weight regain can be prevented by certain weight maintenance strategies (Dombrowski et al., 2014), but at this time interventions specifically targeting weight loss maintenance are still in infancy and the underlying mechanisms and the most effective techniques for supporting weight loss maintenance remain unclear (Sniehotta et al., 2014). Several constructs that facilitate weight loss may also be crucial in achieving weight maintenance; increasing an individual's self-efficacy, motivation, self-monitoring, and enhancing coping skills have shown to be significantly associated with better weight maintenance (Annesi & Tennant, 2012; West et al., 2011; Wing et al., 2006). Studies that focus on diet and physical activity also reported a positive result. For example, Keränen et al. reported that dietary counseling reduced emotional eating, uncontrolled eating, and binge eating symptoms during the 18-month maintenance period (Keränen et al., 2009). A three-group STOP Regain randomized controlled trial (RCT) reported significantly less weight gain in the face-to-face group compared with the control group and the internet group participants (Wing et al., 2007). The face-to-face participants rated weighing oneself, establishing a weight loss goal, tracking calories, and maintaining a log or graph of eating and exercise as more highly important than control. The three-group Treatment for Obesity in Underserved Rural Communities RCT found after 12 months that the telephone counseling and face-to-face groups gained significantly less weight than the control group. Telephone counseling and in-person counseling were equally effective, but telephone counseling was provided at half the cost (Perri et al., 2008). Nearly, 42% were able to maintain a 5% weight loss at 3.5-year follow-up (Milsom et al., 2011).

Physical activity has been emphasized as a critical element of successful weight loss maintenance. The *energy gap*, which develops after weight loss, is a contributing factor to the need for physical activity (Hill et al., 2005). It is approximated at 8 kcal/d for each pound of body weight lost and develops because of a decrease in one's total energy expenditure due to a drop in resting metabolic rate, which occurs because less energy is needed to move a smaller body size. In the current obesogenic environment with food consumed in large portions, filling this energy gap might be more easily achieved by increasing energy expenditure through physical activity (Hill et al., 2005). While the optimal amount of physical activity for weight loss maintenance has not been identified, the most recent ACSM guidelines reinforce that weight maintenance (≤3% weight gain) likely requires approximately 60 minutes of daily, moderate-intensity physical activity (e.g., brisk walking for 4 miles; Donnelly et al., 2009).

Because weight loss often peaks at 6 months after behavioral treatment begins (Jeffery et al., 2000), a plan for weight maintenance should be established at this time. Based on a joint report from the American College of Cardiology/American Heart Association/Task Force on Practice Guidelines and The Obesity Society, strategies for weight loss maintenance should include face-to-face or telephone-delivered programs that provide regular contact (monthly or more frequently) with a trained healthcare provider to help participants engage in high levels of physical activity (i.e., 200–300 min/wk), regular self-weighing (i.e., weekly or more frequently), and consume a low-calorie diet (needed to maintain lower body weight; Jensen et al., 2014).

FUTURE DIRECTIONS

Health Equity-Centered Interventions

A focus on health equity to address obesity is a necessary step to address the public health burden of obesity in effective ways across diverse populations. When health equity is the goal, intervention approaches expand to construct the most appropriate solutions to address factors that drive obesity, stymie treatment outcomes, and generate disparities. Per Kumanyika (2022), this includes prioritization of health equity issues (**Figure 16.3**). Adoption of a

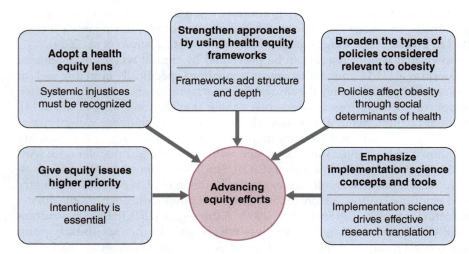

FIGURE 16.3 Five recommendations for advancing equity in obesity efforts. These actions emphasize the need for greater priority and understanding of systemic health equity issues and the varied polices that influence obesity risk and management. Implementation science offers approaches to identify effective and sustainable solutions.

Source: From Kumanyika, S. K. (2022). Advancing health equity efforts to reduce obesity: Changing the course. *Annual Review of Nutrition, 42*, 453–480. https://doi.org/10.1146/annurev-nutr-092021-050805.

lens to recognize systemic inequities and the social determinants of health that also engages communities as stakeholders in the work to address obesity is recommended. Further, use of health equity frameworks brings the context of social determinants of health to the forefront and becomes useful in identifying what and why intervention components are useful. Considering that a great swath of policies are relevant to obesity (e.g., housing, income support), potential levels to address obesity through policy change becomes important. To realize equitable intervention outcomes on a large scale, translation of rigorously designed studies to real-world settings is necessary through implementation science.

Policy-Level Interventions

From a public health perspective, policy-level interventions are needed to address obesity; these include policies that direct interventions to both dietary intake and physical activity at a societal level. One effective tactic could be for government to regulate foods that are nonnutritious, while urging (and perhaps incentivizing) companies to produce and sell more healthful foods, then making available to consumers product information that facilitates their selecting healthier foods (Farley, 2012; Vandevijvere & Swinburn, 2014). Aspects of the built environment that limit physical activity and healthy food access on a population level (e.g., neighborhood design, activity facilities, and grocery store density) must also be addressed in order to tackle obesity at the societal level (McCormack & Shiell, 2011; Mendez et al., 2016).

CONCLUSION

Obesity continues to be a public health threat. Affecting adults and children with alarming proportion, obesity requires groundbreaking and interdisciplinary strategies including innovative behavioral interventions, use of effective AOMs, and MBS to improve obesity incidence and prevalence. Moving forward, it is important for investigators to consider modernizing behavioral interventions to respond to the determinants of health, and leverage technology, policy, and community engagement to impact the vast numbers of marginalized groups that are disproportionately impacted by the obesity epidemic. Centering research and practice on the goal of health equity may produce the evidence to make significant public health progress for all.

SUMMARY KEY POINTS

- Obesity is a significant public health challenge where disparities in its prevalence exist across multiple identifiers, including, but not limited to, race, ethnicity, and sex. Thus, specific demographic groups experience greater obesity burden, which requires targeted focus to understand and address.

- Standard behavioral weight loss interventions are an efficacious treatment but are commonly less effective for certain demographic groups. Alternative behavioral approaches (e.g., acceptance-based) may be important pathways to produce highly effective and equitable obesity treatment.

- The social determinants of health should be addressed through behavioral interventions as they can influence obesity prevalence and the effectiveness of behavioral treatment.

- AOMs are increasing in efficacy to promote significant weight reduction and improvement in weight-related conditions, including type 2 diabetes, cardiovascular disease, and chronic kidney disease.

- MBS remains the most effective tool to treat obesity and should be considered at lower BMI thresholds.

DISCUSSION QUESTIONS

1. As mentioned, obesity is a well-established risk factor for chronic conditions such as type 2 diabetes, hypertension, cardiovascular disease, certain cancers, sleep disorders, and arthritis. Consider a scenario where a patient with class 2 obesity visits a healthcare provider for a non–weight-related health concern (e.g., conjunctivitis). Is it appropriate for the provider to address the patient's obesity in this visit? Or could that be a stressor for the patient, making them less likely to seek treatment when it is needed? What actions by the provider are in the patient's best interest?

2. Looking through a strengths-based lens, what health-promoting behaviors and/or cultural attributes can you identify in your own culture or community?

3. Consider neighborhoods where you have lived throughout your life. How would the attributes of these neighborhoods contribute to or protect against obesity in their residents?

4. Given the increased efficacy of AOMs, are lifestyle interventions and behavioral modifications still important? How can patients be encouraged to adopt lifestyle changes when these medications are so effective?

5. Physical activity is a critical element of weight loss maintenance. What barriers may there be to an exercise novice starting at a gym? What can be done to lift these barriers and make it more likely for them to exercise regularly?

A robust set of instructor resources designed to supplement this text is located at http://connect.springerpub.com/content/book/978-0-8261-4265-8. Qualifying instructors may request access by emailing textbook@springerpub.com.

REFERENCES

Alvidrez, J., Castille, D., Laude-Sharp, M., Rosario, A., & Tabor, D. (2019). The national institute on minority health and health disparities research framework. *American Journal of Public Health, 109*(S1), S16–S20. https://doi.org/10.2105/AJPH.2018.304883

Annesi, J. J., & Tennant, G. A. (2012-2013). Exercise program-induced mood improvement and improved eating in severely obese adults. *Int Q Community Health Educ, 33*(4), 391–402. https://doi.org/10.2190/IQ.33.4.f

Apovian, C. M., Aronne, L. J., Bessesen, D. H., McDonnell, M. E., Murad, M. H., Pagotto, U., Ryan, D. H., & Still, C. D. (2015). Pharmacological management of obesity: An endocrine Society clinical practice guideline. *The Journal of Clinical Endocrinology & Metabolism, 100*(2), 342–362. https://doi.org/10.1210/jc.2014-3415

Aronne, L. J., Sattar, N., Horn, D. B., Bays, H. E., Wharton, S., Lin, W.-Y., Ahmad, N. N., Zhang, S., Liao, R., Bunck, M. C., Jouravskaya, I., Murphy, M. A., & SURMOUNT-4 Investigators. (2024). Continued treatment with tirzepatide for maintenance of weight reduction in adults with obesity: The SURMOUNT-4 randomized clinical trial. *JAMA, 331*(1), 38–48. https://doi.org/10.1001/jama.2023.24945

Athanasiadis, D. I., Martin, A., Kapsampelis, P., Monfared, S., & Stefanidis, D. (2021). Factors associated with weight regain post-bariatric surgery: A systematic review. *Surgical Endoscopy, 35*(8), 4069–4084. https://doi.org/10.1007/s00464-021-08329-w

Bachman, J. L, Phelan, S., Wing, R. R., & Raynor, H. A. (2011). Eating frequency is higher in weight loss maintainers and normal-weight individuals than in overweight individuals. *Journal of the Academy of Nutrition and Dietetics, 111*(11), 1730–1734. https://doi.org/10.1016/j.jada.2011.08.006

Baggio, L. L., & Drucker, D. J. (2007). Biology of incretins: GLP-1 and GIP. *Gastroenterology, 132*(6), 2131–2157. https://doi.org/10.1053/j.gastro.2007.03.054

Bailey, Z. D., Krieger, N., Agenor, M., Graves, J., Linos, N., & Bassett, M. T. (2017). Structural racism and health inequities in the USA: Evidence and interventions. *Lancet. 389*(10077), 1453–1463.

Bardia, A., Holtan, S. G., Slezak, J. M., & Thompson, W. G. (2007). Diagnosis of obesity by primary care physicians and impact on obesity management. *Mayo Clinic Proceedings, 82*(8), 927–932. https://doi.org/10.4065/82.8.927

Barnes, E. R., Theeke, L. A., & Mallow, J. (2015). Impact of the Provider and Healthcare team Adherence to Treatment Guidelines (PHAT-G) intervention on adherence to national obesity clinical practice guidelines in a primary care centre. *Journal of Evaluation in Clinical Practice, 21*(2), 300–306. https://doi.org/10.1111/jep.12308

Blackman Carr, L. T., Bell, C., Alick, C., & Bentley-Edwards, K. L. (2022). Responding to health disparities in behavioral weight loss interventions and COVID-19 in black adults: Recommendations for health equity. *Journal of Racial and Ethnic Health Disparities, 9*(3), 739–747. https://doi.org/10.1007/s40615-022-01269-8

Braveman, P., & Gottlieb, L. (2014). The social determinants of health: It's time to consider the causes of the causes. *Public Health Reports, 129*(1_suppl2), 19–31. https://doi.org/10.1177/00333549141291s206

Bray, G., & Bouchard, C. (2014). *Handbook of obesity-volume 2: Clinical applications* (Vol. 2). CRC Press.

Buro, A. W., Baskin, M., Miller, D., Ward, T., West, D. S., Gore, L. R., Gwede, C. K., Epel, E., & Carson, T. L. (2022). Rationale and study protocol for a randomized controlled trial to determine the effectiveness of a culturally relevant, stress management enhanced behavioral weight loss intervention on weight loss outcomes of black women. *BMC Public Health, 22*(1), 193. https://doi.org/10.1186/s12889-022-12519-z

Burke, L. E., Wang, J., & Sevick, M. A. (2011). Self-monitoring in weight loss: A systematic review of the literature. *Journal of The American Dietetic Association, 111*(1), 92–102. https://doi.org/10.1016/j.jada.2010.10.008

Butryn, M. L., Forman, E. M., Lowe, M. R., Gorin, A. A., Zhang, F., & Schaumberg, K. (2017). Efficacy of environmental and acceptance-based enhancements to behavioral weight loss treatment: The ENACT trial. *Obesity, 25*(5), 866–872. https://doi.org/10.1002/oby.21813

Centers for Disease Control and Prevention. (2022). Defining adult overweight & obesity. https://www.cdc.gov/obesity/basics/adult-defining.html

Centers for Medicare and Medicaid Services. (2011). *Decision memo for intensive behavioral therapy for obesity*. https://www.cms.gov/medicare-coverage-database/view/ncacal-decision-memo.aspx?proposed=N&NCAId=253

Chakhtoura, M., Haber, R., Ghezzawi, M., Rhayem, C., Tcheroyan, R., & Mantzoros, C. S. (2023). Pharmacotherapy of obesity: An update on the available medications and drugs under investigation. *EClinicalMedicine, 58*, 101882. https://doi.org/10.1016/j.eclinm.2023.101882

Curioni, C. C., & Lourenco, P. M. (2005). Long-term weight loss after diet and exercise: A systematic review. *International Journal of Obesity, 29*, 1168–1174. https://doi.org/10.1038/sj.ijo.0803015

Davis, K. K., Tate, D. F., Lang, W., Neiberg, R. H., Polzien, K., Rickman, A. D., Erickson, K., & Jakicic, J. M. (2015). Racial differences in weight loss among adults in a behavioral weight loss intervention: Role of diet and physical activity. *Journal of Physical Activity and Health, 12*(12), 1558–1566. https://doi.org/10.1123/jpah.2014-0243

Delany, J. P., Jakicic, J. M., Lowery, J. B., Hames, K. C., Kelley, D. E., & Goodpaster, B. H. (2014). African American women exhibit similar adherence to intervention but lose less weight due to lower energy requirements. *International Journal of Obesity, 38*(9), 1147–1152. https://doi.org/10.1038/ijo.2013.240

Digenio, A. G., Mancuso, J. P., Gerber, R. A., & Dvorak, R. V. (2009). Comparison of methods for delivering a lifestyle modification program for obese patients: A randomized trial. *Annals of Internal Medicine, 150*(4), 255–262. https://doi.org/10.7326/0003-4819-150-4-200902170-00006

Dombrowski, S. U., Knittle, K., Avenell, A., Araújo-Soares, V., & Sniehotta, F. F. (2014). Long term maintenance of weight loss with non-surgical interventions in obese adults: Systematic review and meta-analyses of randomised controlled trials. *BMJ. 348*, g2646. https://doi.org/10.1136/bmj.g2646

Donnelly, J. E., Blair, S. N., Jakicic, J. M., Manore, M. M., Rankin, J. W., & Smith, B. K. (2009). American College of Sports Medicine Position Stand. Appropriate physical activity intervention strategies for weight loss and prevention of weight regain for adults. *Medicine and Science in Sports and Exercise, 41*(2), 459–471. https://doi.org/10.1249/MSS.0b013e3181949333

Dulloo, A. G., & Schutz, Y. (2015). Adaptive thermogenesis in resistance to obesity therapies: Issues in quantifying thrifty energy expenditure phenotypes in humans. *Current Obesity Reports, 4*(2), 230–240. https://doi.org/10.1007/s13679-015-0156-9

Eisenberg, D., Shikora, S. A., Aarts, E., Aminian, A., Angrisani, L., Cohen, R. V., De Luca, M., Faria, S. L., Goodpaster, K. P. S., Haddad, A., Himpens, J. M., Kow, L., Kurian, M., Loi, K., Mahawar, K.,

Nimeri, A., O'Kane, M., Papasavas, P. K., Ponce, J., . . . Kothari, S. N. (2022). 2022 American Society for Metabolic and Bariatric Surgery (ASMBS) and International Federation for the Surgery of Obesity and Metabolic Disorders (IFSO): Indications for metabolic and bariatric surgery. *Surgery for Obesity and Related Diseases, 18*(12), 1345–1356. https://doi.org/10.1016/j.soard.2022.08.013

Evans, E. H., Araujo-Soares, V., Adamson, A., Batterham, A. M., Brown, H., Campbell, M., Dombrowski, S. U., Guest, A., Jackson, D., Kwasnicka, D., Ladha, K., McColl, E., Olivier, P., Rothman, A. J., Sainsbury, K., Steel, A. J., Steen, I. N., Vale, L., White, M., Wright P., & Sniehotta, F. F. (2015). The NULevel trial of a scalable, technology-assisted weight loss maintenance intervention for obese adults after clinically significant weight loss: Study protocol for a randomised controlled trial. *Trials, 16*, 421. https://doi.org/10.1186/s13063-015-0931-7

Farley, T. A. (2012). The role of government in preventing excess calorie consumption: The example of New York city. *Journal of the American Medical Association, 308*(11), 1093–1094. https://doi.org/10.1001/2012.jama.11623

Findholt, N. E., Davis, M. M., & Michael, Y. L. (2013). Perceived barriers, resources, and training needs of rural primary care providers relevant to the management of childhood obesity. *The Journal of Rural Health, 29*(Suppl. 1), s17–s24. https://doi.org/10.1111/jrh.12006

Foley, W., & Schubert, L. (2013). Applying strengths-based approaches to nutrition research and interventions in Australian Indigenous communities. *Journal of Critical Dietetics, 1*(3), 11. https://doi.org/10.32920/cd.v1i3.600

Forman, E. M., & Butryn, M. L. (2015). A new look at the science of weight control: How acceptance and commitment strategies can address the challenge of self-regulation. *Appetite, 84*, 171–180. https://doi.org/10.1016/j.appet.2014.10.004

Forman, E. M., Butryn, M. L., Manasse, S. M., Crosby, R. D., Goldstein, S. P., Wyckoff, E. P., & Thomas, J. G. (2016). Acceptance-based versus standard behavioral treatment for obesity: Results from the mind your health randomized controlled trial. *Obesity, 24*(10), 2050–2056. https://doi.org/10.1002/oby.21601

Forman, E. M., Manasse, S. M., Butryn, M. L., Crosby, R. D., Dallal, D. H., & Crochiere, R. J. (2019). Long-term follow-up of the mind your health project: Acceptance-based versus standard behavioral treatment for obesity. *Obesity, 27*(4), 565–571. https://doi.org/10.1002/oby.22412

Fryar, C. D., Carroll, M. D., & Afful, J. (2020). Prevalence of overweight, obesity, and severe obesity among adults aged 20 and over: United States, 1960–1962 through 2017–2018. NCHS Health E-Stats. https://www.cdc.gov/nchs/data/hestat/obesity-adult-17-18/obesity-adult.htm#Citation

Fryar, C. D., Carroll, M. D., & Ogden, C. L. (2018). Prevalence of overweight, obesity, and severe obesity among children and adolescents aged 2–19 years: United States, 1963–1965 through 2015–2016. NCHS Health E-Stats.

Fujioka, K., & Bakhru, N. (2010). Office-based management of obesity. *Mount Sinai Journal of Medicine, 77*, 466–471. https://doi.org/10.1002/msj.20201

Garber, C. E., Blissmer, B., Deschenes, M. R., Franklin, B. A., Lamonte, M. J., Lee, I. M., Nieman, D. C., Swain, D. P., & American College of Sports Medicine. (2011). Quantity and quality of exercise for developing and maintaining cardiorespiratory, musculoskeletal, and neuromotor fitness in apparently healthy adults: Guidance for prescribing exercise. *Medicine and Science in Sports and Exercise, 43*(7), 1334–1359. https://doi.org/10.1249/MSS.0b013e318213fefb

Goode, R. W., Styn, M. A., Mendez, D. D., & Gary-Webb, T. L. (2017). African Americans in standard behavioral treatment for obesity, 2001–2015: What have we learned? *Western Journal of Nursing Research, 39*(8), 1045–1069. https://doi.org/10.1177/0193945917692115

Hammoud, R., & Drucker, D. J. (2023). Beyond the pancreas: Contrasting cardiometabolic actions of GIP and GLP1. *Nature Reviews: Endocrinology, 19*(4), 201–216. https://doi.org/10.1038/s41574-022-00783-3

Harrington, E. F., Crowther, J. H., & Shipherd, J. C. (2010). Trauma, binge eating, and the "strong Black woman". *Journal of Consulting and Clinical Psychology, 78*(4), 469–479. https://doi.org/10.1037/a0019174

Haskell, W. L., Lee, I. M., Pate, R. R., Powell, K. E., Blair, S. N., Franklin, B. A., . . . American Heart Association. (2007). Physical activity and public health: Updated recommendation for adults from the American College of Sports Medicine and the American Heart Association. *Circulation, 116*(9), 1081–1093. https://doi.org/10.1161/CIRCULATION.107.185649

Haughton, C. F., Silfee, V. J., Wang, M. L., Lopez-Cepero, A. C., Estabrook, D. P., Frisard, C., Rosal, M. C., Pagoto, S. L., & Lemon, S. C. (2018). Racial/ethnic representation in lifestyle weight loss intervention studies in the United States: A systematic review. *Preventive Medicine Reports, 9*, 131–137. https://doi.org/10.1016/j.pmedr.2018.01.012

Hill, J. O., Thompson, H., & Wyatt, H. (2005). Weight maintenance: What's missing? *Journal of the American Dietetic Association, 105*(5 Suppl. 1), 63–66. https://doi.org/10.1016/j.jada.2005.02.016

Himmelstein, M. S., Puhl, R. M., & Quinn, D. M. (2017). Intersectionality: An understudied framework for addressing weight stigma. *American Journal of Preventive Medicine, 53*(4), 421–431. https://doi.org/10.1016/j.amepre.2017.04.003

Hsu, J. L., & Farrell, T. M. (2024). Updates in bariatric surgery. *The American Surgeon™, 90*(5), 925–933. https://doi.org/10.1177/00031348231220576

Jakicic, J. M., Winters, C., Lang, W., & Wing, R. R. (1999). Effects of intermittent exercise and use of home exercise equipment on adherence, weight loss, and fitness in overweight women: A randomized trial. *Journal of the American Medical Association, 282*(16), 1554–1560. https://doi.org/10.1001/jama.282.16.1554

Jastreboff, A. M., Aronne, L. J., Ahmad, N. N., Wharton, S., Connery, L., Alves, B., Kiyosue, A., Zhang, S., Liu, B., Bunck, M. C., & Stefanski, A. (2022). Tirzepatide once weekly for the treatment of obesity. *The New England journal of medicine, 387*(3), 205–216. https://doi.org/10.1056/NEJMoa2206038

Jeffery, R. W., Drewnowski, A., Epstein, L. H., Stunkard, A. J., Wilson, G. T., Wing, R. R., & Hill, D. R. (2000). Long-term maintenance of weight loss: Current status. *Health Psychology, 19*(1S), 5–16. https://doi.org/10.1037/0278-6133.19.suppl1.5

Jensen, M. D., Ryan, D. H., Apovian, C. M., Ard, J. D., Comuzzie, A. G., Donato, K. A., Hu, F. B., Hubbard, V. S., Jakicic, J. M., & Kushner, R. F. (2014). 2013 AHA/ACC/TOS guideline for the management of overweight and obesity in adults: A report of the American College of Cardiology /American Heart Association Task Force on Practice Guidelines and The Obesity Society. *Journal of the American College of Cardiology, 63*(25 Part B), 2985–3023. https://doi.org/10.1016/j.jacc.2013.11.004

Kan, H., Bae, J. P., Dunn, J. P., Buysman, E. K., Gronroos, N. N., Swindle, J. P., Bengtson, L. G. S., & Ahmad, N. (2023). Real-world primary nonadherence to antiobesity medications. *Journal of Managed Care & Specialty Pharmacy, 29*(10), 1099–1108. https://doi.org/10.18553/jmcp.2023.23083

Kanfer, F. H. (1991). *Self-management methods* (4th ed.). Pergamon Press.

Kanfer, F. H., & Goldstein, A. P. (1991). *Helping people change: A textbook of methods* (4th ed.)., NY: Pergamon Press.

Keränen, A. M., Savolainen, M. J., Reponen, A. H., Kujari, M. L, Lindeman, S. M., Bloigu, R. S., & Laitinen, J. H. (2009). The effect of eating behavior on weight loss and maintenance during a lifestyle intervention. *Preventive Medicine, 49*(1), 32–38. https://doi.org/10.1016/j.ypmed.2009.04.011

Keogh, J. B., & Clifton, P. M. (2012). Meal replacements for weight loss in type 2 diabetes in a community setting. *Journal of Nutrition and Metabolism, 2012*, 918571. https://doi.org/10.1155/2012/918571

Klem, M., Wing, R., McGuire, M., Seagle, H., & Hill, J. (1997). A descriptive study of individuals successful at long-term maintenance of substantial weight loss. *American Journal of Clinical Nutrition, 66*(2), 239–246. https://doi.org/10.1093/ajcn/66.2.239

Kumanyika, S. (2019a). Overcoming inequities in obesity: What don't we know that we need to know? *Health Education & Behavior, 46*(5), 721–727. https://doi.org/10.1177/1090198119867319

Kumanyika, S., Whitt-Glover, M. C., Gary, T. L., Prewitt, T. E., Odoms-Young, A. M., Banks-Wallace, J., Beech, B. M., Hughes-Halbert, C., Karanja, N., Lancaster, K. J., & Samuel-Hodge, C. D. (2007). Expanding the obesity research paradigm to reach African American communities. *Preventing Chronic Disease, 4*(4), A112.

Kumanyika, S. K. (2019b). A framework for increasing equity impact in obesity prevention. *American Journal of Public Health, 109*(10), 1350–1357. https://doi.org/10.2105/AJPH.2019.305221

Kumanyika, S. K. (2022). Advancing health equity efforts to reduce obesity: Changing the course. *Annual Review of Nutrition, 42*, 453–480. https://doi.org/10.1146/annurev-nutr-092021-050805

Lillis, J., Thomas, J. G., Niemeier, H., & Wing, R. R. (2016). Internal disinhibition predicts 5-year weight regain in the National Weight Control Registry (NWCR). *Obesity Science & Practice, 2*(1), 83–87. https://doi.org/10.1002/osp4.22

Lindberg, N. M., Stevens, V. J., & Halperin, R. O. (2013). Weight-loss interventions for Hispanic populations: The role of culture. *Journal of Obesity, 2013*, 542736. https://doi.org/10.1155/2013/542736

Lowe, M. R., Butryn, M. L., Thomas, J. G., & Coletta, M. (2014). Meal replacements, reduced energy density eating, and weight loss maintenance in primary care patients: A randomized controlled trial. *Obesity (Silver Spring), 22*(1), 94–100. https://doi.org/10.1002/oby.20582

Lyu, B., Chang, A. R., Inker, L. A., Selvin, E., Grams, M. E., & Shin, J. I. (2022). Socioeconomic status and use of obesogenic and anti-obesity medications in the United States: A population-based study. *Lancet Regional Health Americas, 11*, 100249. https://doi.org/10.1016/j.lana.2022.100249

Marlatt, G. A., & Gordon, J. R. (1985). Relapse Prevention: Maintenance Strategies in the Treatment of Addictive Behaviors. New York: Guilford Press.

McCormack, G. R., & Shiell, A. (2011). In search of causality: A systematic review of the relationship between the built environment and physical activity among adults. *International Journal of Behavioral Nutrition and Physical Activity, 8*, 125. https://doi.org/10.1186/1479-5868-8-125

McCurley, J. L., Gutierrez, A. P., & Gallo, L. C. (2017). Diabetes prevention in U.S. Hispanic adults: A systematic review of culturally tailored interventions. *American Journal of Preventive Medicine, 52*(4), 519–529. https://doi.org/10.1016/j.amepre.2016.10.028

Mendez, D. D., Gary-Webb, T. L., Goode, R., Zheng, Y., Imes, C. C., Fabio, A., Duell, J., & Burke, L. E. (2016). Neighborhood factors and six-month weight change among overweight individuals in a weight loss intervention. *Preventive Medicine Reports, 4*, 569–573. https://doi.org/10.1016/j.pmedr.2016.10.004

Milsom, V. A., Ross Middleton, K. M., & Perri, M. G. (2011). Successful long-term weight loss maintenance in a rural population. *Clinical Interventions in Aging, 6*, 303–309. https://doi.org/10.2147/CIA.S25389

Moyer, V. A. (2012). Screening for and management of obesity in adults: U.S. Preventive Services Task Force recommendation statement. *Annals of Internal Medicine, 157*, 373–378. https://doi.org/10.7326/0003-4819-157-5-201209040-00475

Müller, T. D., Blüher, M., Tschöp, M. H., & DiMarchi, R. D. (2022). Anti-obesity drug discovery: Advances and challenges. *Nature Reviews Drug Discovery, 21*(3), 201–223. https://doi.org/10.1038/s41573-021-00337-8

NHLBI. (1998). *Clinical guidelines on the identification, evaluation, and treatment of overweight and obesity in adults: The evidence report.* National Institutes of Health, National Heart, Lung, and Blood Institute.

Ogden, L. G., Stroebele, N., Wyatt, H. R., Catenacci, V. A., Peters, J. C., Stuht, J., Wing, R. R., & Hill, J. O. (2012). Cluster analysis of the national weight control registry to identify distinct subgroups maintaining successful weight loss. *Obesity (Silver Spring), 20*(10), 2039–2047. https://doi.org/10.1038/oby.2012.79

Pearl, R. L. (2018). Weight bias and stigma: Public health implications and structural solutions. *Social Issues and Policy Review, 12*(1), 146–182. https://doi.org/10.1111/sipr.12043

Perri, M. G., Limacher, M. C., Durning, P. E., Janicke, D. M., Lutes, L. D., Bobroff, L. B., Dale, M. S., Daniels, M. J., Radcliff, T. A., & Martin, A. D. (2008). Extended-care programs for weight management in rural communities: The treatment of obesity in underserved rural settings (TOURS) randomized trial. *Arch Intern Med. 168*(21), 2347–2354. https://doi.org/10.1001/archinte.168.21.2347

Puhl, R. M., Himmelstein, M. S., & Pearl, R. L. (2020). Weight stigma as a psychosocial contributor to obesity. *American Psychologist, 75*(2), 274–289. https://doi.org/10.1037/amp0000538

Rao, G. (2010). Office-based strategies for the management of obesity. *American Family Physician, 81*(12), 1449–1456.

Ray, R. (2017). Black people don't exercise in my neighborhood: Perceived racial composition and leisure-time physical activity among middle class blacks and whites. *Social Science Research, 66*, 42–57. https://doi.org/10.1016/j.ssresearch.2017.03.008

Raynor, H. A., Jeffery, R. W., Phelan, S., Hill, J. O., & Wing, R. R. (2005). Amount of food group variety consumed in the diet and long-term weight loss maintenance. *Obesity Research, 13*(5), 883–890. https://doi.org/10.1038/oby.2005.102

Raynor, D. A, Phelan, S., Hill, J. O, & Wing, R. R. (2006). Television viewing and long-term weight maintenance: Results from the National Weight Control Registry. *Obesity (Silver Spring). 14*(10), 1816–1824. https://doi.org/10.1038/oby.2006.209

Sciamanna, C. N., Kiernan, M., Rolls, B. J., Boan, J., Stuckey, H., Kephart, D., Miller, C. K., Jensen, G., Hartmann, T. J, Loken, E., Hwang, K. O., Williams, R. J., Clark, M. A., Schubart, J. R., Nezu, A. M., Lehman, E., & Dellasega, C. (2011). Practices associated with weight loss versus weight-loss maintenance results of a national survey. *American Journal of Preventive Medicine, 41*(2), 159–166. https://doi.org/10.1016/j.amepre.2011.04.009

Sebiany, A. M. (2013). Primary care physicians' knowledge and perceived barriers in the management of overweight and obesity. *Journal of Family & Community Medicine, 20*(3), 147–152. https://doi.org/10.4103/2230–8229.121972

Sniehotta, F. F., Simpson, S. A., & Greaves, C. J. (2014). Weight loss maintenance: An agenda for health psychology. *British Psychological Society, 19*(3), 459–464. https://doi.org/10.1111/bjhp.12107

Stierman, B., Afful, J., Carroll, M. D., Chen, T. C., Davy, O., Fink, S., et al. (2021). National Health and Nutrition Examination Survey 2017–March 2020 prepandemic data files—Development of files and prevalence estimates for selected health outcomes. National Health Statistics Reports; no 158. Hyattsville, MD: National Center for Health Statistics. https://dx.doi.org/10.15620/cdc:106273

Thabault, P. J., Burke, P. J., & Ades, P. A. (2016). Intensive behavioral treatment weight loss program in an adult primary care practice. *Journal of the American Association of Nurse Practitioners, 28*(5), 249–257. https://doi.org/10.1002/2327–6924.12319

Tham, M., & Young, D. (2008). The role of the general practitioner in weight management in primary care—A cross sectional study in general practice. *BMC Family Practice, 9*(1), 66. https://doi.org/10.1186/1471-2296-9-66

Thomas, J. G., Bond, D. S., Phelan, S., Hill, J. O., & Wing, R. R. (2014). Weight-loss maintenance for 10 years in the National Weight Control Registry. *American Journal of Preventive Medicine, 46*(1), 17–23. https://doi.org/10.1016/j.amepre.2013.08.019

Tipre, M., & Carson, T. L. A qualitative assessment of gender- and race-related stress among black women. (2022). *Womens Health Rep (New Rochelle). 3*(1), 222–227. https://doi.org/10.1089/whr.2021.0041

Tomiyama, A. J. (2014). Weight stigma is stressful. A review of evidence for the cyclic obesity/weight-based stigma model. *Appetite, 82*, 8–15. https://doi.org/10.1016/j.appet.2014.06.108

U.S. Department of Health and Human Services. (n.d.). Social determinants of health. https://health.gov/healthypeople/priority-areas/social-determinants-health

U.S. Preventive Services Task Force. (2003). Screening for obesity in adults: Recommendations and rationale. *Annals of Internal Medicine, 139*, 930–932. https://doi.org/10.7326/0003-4819-139-11-200312020-00012

Vandevijvere, S., & Swinburn, B. (2014). Creating healthy food environments through global benchmarking of government nutrition policies and food industry practices. *Archives of Public Health, 72*(1), 7. https://doi.org/10.1186/2049-3258-72-7

VanWormer, J. J., Martinez, A. M., Martinson, B. C, Crain, A. L., Benson, G. A., Cosentino, D. L., & Pronk, N. P. (2009). Self-weighing promotes weight loss for obese adults. *American Journal of Preventive Medicine, 36*(1), 70–73. https://doi.org/10.1016/j.amepre.2008.09.022

Vartanian, L. R., & Porter, A. M. (2016). Weight stigma and eating behavior: A review of the literature. *Appetite, 102*, 3–14. https://doi.org/10.1016/j.appet.2016.01.034

Wadden, T. A., Bailey, T. S., Billings, L. K., Davies, M., Frias, J. P., Koroleva, A., Lingvay, I., O'Neil, P. M., Rubino, D. M., Skovgaard, D., Wallenstein, S. O. R., & Garvey, W. T. (2021). Effect of subcutaneous semaglutide vs placebo as an adjunct to intensive behavioral therapy on body weight in adults with overweight or obesity: The STEP 3 randomized clinical trial. *JAMA, 325*(14), 1403–1413. https://doi.org/10.1001/jama.2021.1831

Wadden, T. A., Butryn, M. L., & Wilson, C. (2007). Lifestyle modification for the management of obesity. *Gastroenterology, 132*(6), 2226–2238. https://doi.org/10.1053/j.gastro.2007.03.051

Wadden, T. A., Chao, A. M., Machineni, S., Kushner, R., Ard, J., Srivastava, G., Halpern, B., Zhang, S., Chen, J., Bunck, M. C., Ahmad, N. N., & Forrester, T. (2023). Tirzepatide after intensive lifestyle intervention in adults with overweight or obesity: The SURMOUNT-3 phase 3 trial. *Nature Medicine, 29*(11), 2909–2918. https://doi.org/10.1038/s41591-023-02597-w

Wadden, T. A., West, D. S., Delahanty, L., Jakicic, J., Rejeski, J., Williamson, D., Berkowitz, R. I., Kelley, D. E., Tomchee, C., Hill, J. O., & Kumanyika, S. (2006). The Look AHEAD study: A description of the lifestyle intervention and the evidence supporting it. *Obesity, 14*(5), 737–752. https://doi.org/10.1038/oby.2006.84

Wadden, T. A., West, D. S., Neiberg, R. H., Wing, R. R., Ryan, D. H., Johnson, K. C., Foreyt, J. P., Hill, J. O., Trence, D. L., & Vitolins, M. Z. (2009). One-year weight losses in the Look AHEAD study: Factors associated with success. *Obesity, 17*(4), 713–722. https://doi.org/10.1038/oby.2008.637

Wadden, T.A., Butryn, M. L., & Byrne, K. J. (2004). Efficacy of lifestyle modification for long-term weight control. *Obesity Research, 12 Suppl*, 151S–162S. https://doi.org/10.1038/oby.2004.282

Washington, T. B., Johnson, V. R., Kendrick, K., Ibrahim, A. A., Tu, L., Sun, K., & Stanford, F. C. (2023). Disparities in access and quality of obesity care. *Gastroenterology Clinics of North America, 52*(2), 429–441. https://doi.org/10.1016/j.gtc.2023.02.003

Weinick, R. M., Jacobs, E. A., Stone, L. C., Ortega, A. N., & Burstin, H. (2004). Hispanic healthcare disparities: Challenging the myth of a monolithic Hispanic population. *Medical Care, 42*(4), 313–320. https://doi.org/10.1097/01.mlr.0000118705.27241.7c

West, D. S., Gorin, A. A., Subak, L. L., Foster, G., Bragg, C., Hecht, J., Schembri, M., & Wing, R. R. (2011). Program to Reduce Incontinence by Diet and Exercise (PRIDE) Research Group. A motivation-focused weight loss maintenance program is an effective alternative to a skill-based approach. *Int J Obes (Lond). 35*(2), 259–269. https://doi.org/10.1038/ijo.2010.138

West, D. S., Dutton, G., Delahanty, L. M., Hazuda, H. P., Rickman, A. D., Knowler, W. C., Vitolins, M. Z., Neiberg, R. H., Peters, A., Gee, M., & Cassidy Begay, M. (2019). Weight loss experiences of African American, Hispanic, and non-Hispanic white men and women with type 2 diabetes: The Look AHEAD trial. *Obesity (Silver Spring), 27*(8), 1275–1284. https://doi.org/10.1002/oby.22522

West, D. S., Prewitt, T. E., Bursac, Z., & Felix, H. C. (2008). Weight loss of black, white, and Hispanic men and women in the Diabetes Prevention Program. *Obesity, 16*(6), 1413–1420. https://doi.org/10.1038/oby.2008.224

Westerveld, D., & Yang, D. (2016). Through thick and thin: Identifying barriers to bariatric surgery, weight loss maintenance, and tailoring obesity treatment for the future. *Surgery Research and Practice, 2016*, 8616581. https://doi.org/10.1155/2016/8616581

Wiedman, D. (2012). Native American embodiment of the chronicities of modernity: Reservation food, diabetes, and the metabolic syndrome among the Kiowa, Comanche, and Apache. *Medical Anthropology Quarterly, 26*(4), 595–612. https://doi.org/10.1111/maq.12009

Wilding, J. P. H., Batterham, R. L., Calanna, S., Davies, M., Van Gaal, L. F., Lingvay, I., McGowan, B. M., Rosenstock, J., Tran, M. T. D., Wadden, T. A., Wharton, S., Yokote, K., Zeuthen, N., & Kushner, R. F. (2021). Once-weekly semaglutide in adults with overweight or obesity. *The New England journal of medicine, 384*(11), 989–1002. https://doi.org/10.1056/NEJMoa2032183

Wing, R. R., Tate, D. F., Gorin, A. A, Raynor, H. A., Fava, J. L., & Machan, J. (2007). STOP regain: are there negative effects of daily weighing? *Journal of Consulting and Clinical Psychology, 75*(4), 652–656; https://doi.org/10.1037/0022-006X.75.4.652. *Erratum in: Journal of Consulting and Clinical Psychology, 75*(5), 715.

Wing, R. R. (2004). Behavioral approaches to the treatment of obesity. *Handbook of Obesity: Clinical Applications, 2,* 147–167.

Wing, R. R., Tate, D. F., Gorin, A. A., Raynor, H. A., & Fava, J. L. (2006). A self-regulation program for maintenance of weight loss. *The New England Journal of Medicine, 355*(15), 1563–1571. https://doi.org/10.1056/NEJMoa061883

Wingo, B., Carson, T., & Ard, J. (2014). Differences in weight loss and health outcomes among African Americans and whites in multicentre trials. *Obesity Reviews, 15,* 46–61. https://doi.org/10.1111/obr.12212

World Health Organization. (2021). *Obesity and overweight.* https://www.who.int/news-room/fact-sheets/detail/obesity-and-overweight

Zheng, Y., Klem, M. L., Sereika, S. M., Danford, C. A., Ewing, L. J., & Burke, L. E. (2015a). Self-weighing in weight management: A systematic literature review. *Obesity (Silver Spring), 23*(2), 256–265. https://doi.org/10.1002/oby.20946

Zheng, Y., Sereika, S. M., Ewing, L. J., Danford, C. A., Terry, M. A., & Burke, L. E. (2015b). Association between self-weighing and percent weight change: Mediation effects of adherence to energy intake and expenditure goals. *Journal of the Academy of Nutrition and Dietetics, 116*(4), 660–666. https://doi.org/10.1016/j.jand.2015.10.014

CHAPTER 17

MENTAL AND BEHAVIORAL HEALTH

KATHERINE SANCHEZ AND MARISOL VARGAS VILUGRON

LEARNING OBJECTIVES

- Define mental and behavioral health (BH).
- Identify social determinants of mental health.
- Explain the limits of theoretical models of disease and disorders.
- Use behavioral activation (BA) and motivational interviewing (MI) strategies for change.

WHAT IS MENTAL HEALTH?

The World Health Organization (WHO) has defined *mental health* as "a state of well-being in which the individual realizes his or her own abilities, can cope with the normal stresses of life, can work productively and fruitfully, and is able to make a contribution to his or her community." (WHO, 2014, p. 1). Mental health and substance use disorders (SUD), collectively referred to as behavioral health (BH) disorders, are a leading cause of disease burden in the United States, surpassing both cardiovascular disease and cancer (Kamal et al., 2017). As of 2019, nearly 1 in 5 adults in the United States had a diagnosed mental health condition, and 1 in 12 people over the age of 12 had a diagnosed SUD (see Chapter 9, "Tobacco, Alcohol, and Other Drugs," for more information on SUD). Individuals with BH conditions experience higher morbidity, poorer health outcomes, and a 20-year lower life expectancy than the general population (Saxena, 2018). The term *mental health* is broad and encompasses criteria-driven diagnosable mental disorders and other mental disabilities associated with impairment in functioning and risk of self-harm or harm to others. People with mental health conditions live with significant distress, and the family burden can be high, although this is not always the case.

CLINICAL PRESENTATION OF BEHAVIORAL HEALTH DISORDERS

Depression

WHO has declared depression to be the leading cause of medical disability, health burden, and increased medical cost in the United States and the world (WHO, 2021). In the United States, one in six are afflicted in their lifetime, and a chronic or relapsing course is common (Kessler, 2012; Kessler et al., 2009). Ethnic minorities have significantly lower odds of receiving adequate antidepressant treatment and guideline-concordant care (Waitzfelder et al., 2018) and experience a disproportionate burden of disability (Dwight-Johnson & Lagomasino, 2007).

Anxiety

Patients with anxiety disorders, particularly panic attacks, often present to their physicians with multiple physical complaints or irritability and may complain of a variety of symptoms that mimic heart attack and respiratory distress (Haas et al., 2005; Roy-Byrne et al., 2001). Complicating the diagnosis is the fact that as many as 75% of patients with a mental health disorder have as a chief complaint a predominantly somatic symptom. Anxiety and panic disorders are associated with numerous bodily symptoms, including hyperventilation, chest pain, dizziness, racing heart, and abdominal discomfort (Sayar et al., 2003). Patients with anxiety tend to have excessive worry around their disease, misinterpret ordinary sensations, and "catastrophize" health events. They may reject the diagnosis of a mental health disorder and insist the physician pursue the somatic complaints for an accurate diagnosis (Haas et al., 2005; Jackson & Kroenke, 2001). Additionally, the result is higher healthcare costs and worse health outcomes from overprescribing of medication to deal with symptoms (Kravitz & Ford, 2008).

Substance Use Disorders

As described in detail in Chapter 9, "Tobacco, Alcohol, and Other Drugs," SUDs for tobacco, alcohol, illicit drugs, and nonmedical use of prescription drugs contribute to substantial public health and economic problems, and racial and ethnic minoritized populations bear the greatest disease burden (Adhikari et al., 2009; Degenhardt & Hall, 2012; Degenhardt et al., 2014; Gryczynski et al., 2016). Deaths due to drug overdose have topped a million for the first time since the Centers for Disease Control and Prevention (CDC) began collecting data more than two decades ago, with increased rates for all race and Latinx-origin groups and with the largest percentage increases seen in non-Latinx Black populations (Hedegaard et al., 2021).

MENTAL HEALTH AND CHRONIC CONDITIONS

Chronic medical conditions affect nearly half of the people in the United States, and two-thirds of encounters with health practitioners are for the management of chronic conditions (Hoffman et al., 1996; Vogeli et al., 2007). It is widely understood in primary care medicine that effective treatment of chronic illness is complicated and requires significant investment on the part of the patient and their families. *Comorbidity* is defined as the presence of multiple health conditions at the same time, with one condition identified as the primary condition (Starfield, 2006). The other conditions are generally considered to be unrelated to the primary condition.

The prevalence of comorbidity increases significantly with age and represents the rule rather than the exception in primary care (Barnett et al., 2012). The simultaneous presence of multiple health problems is associated with a lower quality of life (Fortin et al., 2007), and mental health burden increases with increasing severity of chronic diseases (Fortin et al., 2006). People with multiple comorbidities have more rapid declines in their health and an increased likelihood of disability (Quiñones et al., 2016).

Adults with chronic medical disorders have high rates of depression and anxiety, which often impair self-care and compliance with treatment of their disease (Unutzer et al., 2006). Major depression increases the burden of chronic illness by increasing perception of symptoms, causing additional impairment in functioning, and increasing medical cost through overutilization of the healthcare system (Unutzer et al., 2006). Diagnosis of depression in patients with chronic illness can be challenging as it can be difficult to recognize, diagnose, and treat because of the overlay of symptoms from the physical condition. Somatic symptoms of depression include bodily pain, fatigue, weakness, and other vegetative symptoms, and are the most common presentation of depression in the medical setting (Penninx et al., 2013). Some chronic illnesses can cause people to have decreased appetite, sleep disruptions, and poor physical functioning, thereby masking the symptoms of depression (Kravitz & Ford, 2008). Many patients with comorbid depression and chronic disease may sabotage their own treatment by "focusing on the physical" and delaying treatment of mental health concerns for weeks or months. Such delays in addressing the underlying depression can not only make remission difficult, but can make treatment of the physical condition challenging (Kravitz & Ford, 2008).

Conversely, depression also appears to increase the risk of developing a chronic condition. There is now a substantial body of evidence showing that, compared with those without depression, adults with a depressive disorder or symptoms have a greater risk of developing coronary artery disease (CAD), and that patients with depression and CAD are far more likely to have a future adverse cardiovascular event, such as a heart attack or cardiac death (Gan et al., 2014). These findings hold even when controlling for smoking, lack of exercise, and other poor health behaviors that might be caused by depression. In summary, there exists a complicated and corresponding relationship between depression and chronic disease. Depression affects the prevalence and severity of chronic medical conditions and vice versa.

SOCIAL FACTORS' IMPACT ON MENTAL HEALTH

Poverty and poor health are strongly related to the presence of mental disorders (McGuire & Miranda, 2008). Data from a number of studies suggest that people from ethnic minority groups and underserved populations are particularly unlikely to receive specialty mental healthcare treatment (Jackson-Triche et al., 2000). Latinx populations and other ethnic minorities experience a disproportionate burden of disability associated with mental disorders due to these disparities in mental healthcare (Dwight-Johnson & Lagomasino, 2007). Unmet needs for mental healthcare are particularly prevalent among older adults, individuals from ethnic minority groups, and uninsured or low-income populations (Unutzer et al., 2006). The increase in worldwide disability has been attributed to social and environmental factors such as changes in family structure, substance abuse, and growing socioeconomic inequalities (Cross-National Collaborative Group, 1992; WHO, 2014).

The social determinants of health include societal conditions and psychosocial factors such as opportunities for employment, adequate income, hopefulness, and racism (Smedley, 2012). U.S. adults living in poverty are more than five times as likely to report being in fair or poor health compared with adults with incomes at least four times the federal poverty level (Heron et al., 2009). Social determinants are thought to impact health indirectly through mechanisms that may include stress associated with low socioeconomic status, experiences of disempowerment and violence, hopelessness, helplessness, and income insecurity, while they impact health more directly through reduced access to health services for physical and mental health problems (Allen et al., 2014; Lorant et al., 2003; Table 17.1).

Efforts to address the double and coexisting burden of economic disadvantage and depression are critical yet tricky to determine. An understanding of the social and environmental factors that contribute to the risk of developing mental health disorders is important for illustrating the potential for behavior change opportunities and identification of target groups and social contexts (Figure 17.1). Specifically, understanding how patient characteristics such as socioeconomic status, race, ethnicity, health beliefs and attitudes, and access to medical care influence the underutilization of services is critical (Bazargan et al., 2005; Gelberg et al., 2000; Wu et al., 2009).

TABLE 17.1 Environmental and Social Risk Factors for Mental Health Disorders

FACTOR	EXAMPLES
Environmental	Environmental factors include unsafe or unhealthy housing, proximity to highways and factories, and exposure to toxic agents and other hazards, such as overcrowding.
Educational	Education level and health literacy skills are critical to understanding basic health education communications and messaging.
Neighborhood determinants	Access to affordable healthy food or safe environments in which to exercise; stores and restaurants selling unhealthy food may outnumber markets with fresh produce or restaurants with nutritious food; residential segregation limits social cohesion, stifles economic growth, and perpetuates cycles of poverty.
Racial and ethnic determinants	Racial and ethnic minority populations are more likely to live in conditions that put their health at risk and less likely to receive specialty mental healthcare treatment.
Adverse childhood experiences	Early life stress and related adverse experiences cause enduring brain dysfunction and are a significant risk factor for the development and prevalence of a wide range of health problems throughout a person's life span, including substance misuse/abuse, depression, and obesity.

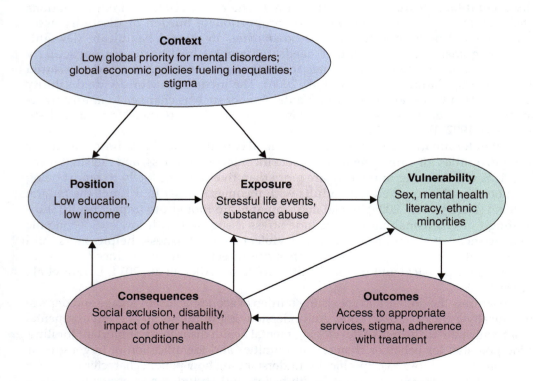

FIGURE 17.1 WHO cycle of social determinants and mental disorders.
Source: From Patel, V., Lund, C., Hatheril, S., Plagerson, S., Corrigall, J., Funk, M., & Fisher, A. (2010). Mental disorders: Equity and social determinants. In E. Blas, & A. S. Kurup (Eds.), *Equity, social determinants and public health programmes* (pp. 115–134). World Health Organization.

DIAGNOSIS OF MENTAL HEALTH DISORDERS

The most comprehensive guide for categorizing, diagnosing, and treating mental health disorders is the *Diagnostic and Statistical Manual of Mental Disorders* (*DSM-5*; American Psychiatric Association, 2013). In *DSM-5*, mood disorders are categorized based on the presentation and severity of major depressive, manic, and hypomanic episodes. *DSM-5* provides an exhaustive explanation of each type of mood disorder currently recognized by the American Psychological Association. Clinical presentations of mental health disorders commonly found in primary care are often associated with the patient's background, socioeconomic status, health, and availability of resources. The most used diagnosis in primary care is major depressive disorder (MDD), followed closely by anxiety.

The Patient Health Questionnaire-9 (PHQ-9; Kroenke & Spitzer, 2002) is a nine-question assessment that can be used to diagnose MDD and identify the severity of symptoms. It can be found online at www.apa.org/depression-guideline/patient-health-questionnaire. pdf. Scores can range between 0 and 27 and indicate mild, moderate, moderately severe, or severe depression. The PHQ-9 is often administered in conjunction with the Generalized Anxiety Disorder-7 (GAD-7; Spitzer et al., 2006), the Alcohol Use Disorders Identification Test (AUDIT; Reinert & Allen, 2002), and the Drug Abuse Screening Test (DAST; Skinner, 1982) questionnaires, which diagnose generalized anxiety order, alcohol use, and drug use, respectively. Clinicians benefit from administering all four assessments during a BH intake appointment because it provides a clear picture of the patient's BH needs, possible comorbidities, and other factors that might be contributing to their diagnosis.

Clinicians can add the Columbia-Suicide Severity Rating Scale (CSSR-S; Posner et al., 2011) as a follow-up questionnaire to assess suicide risk. The CSSR-S helps clinicians identify the patient's suicide risk and take appropriate actions such as creating a safety plan, contacting relatives/friends, and/or hospitalizing the patient. If the risk is high, it is always best to consult with a colleague or supervisor before hospitalizing the patient (especially if it is involuntary) to avoid unnecessary distress and discomfort to the patient, as well as to protect the therapeutic alliance.

Other types of depression commonly found in primary care settings include dysthymia, reactive depression, and substance/medication-induced depressive disorder. Bipolar depression or bipolar disorder is characterized by cycling mood changes, from extreme highs to extreme lows, and is most easily recognizable when presenting as mania, or in a manic cycle. A final category worth mentioning is depressive disorders that are more complex, less common, and often associated with another mental health diagnosis (e.g., posttraumatic stress disorder, bipolar disorder, schizophrenia).

TREATMENT OF MENTAL HEALTH DISORDERS

Health Belief Model

The basic tenets of the health belief model (HBM) suggest that health behaviors are shaped by perceptions of disease susceptibility, severity, barriers to health practices, benefits to treatment, self-efficacy, and cues to action. The likelihood of action is influenced by the perceived benefits to taking action weighed against the barriers associated with it. Perceived susceptibility and seriousness are in part determined by knowledge and cognitive ability and are the impetus for taking action (Rosenstock, 1974). Medication adherence varies by disease, patient characteristics, and income. Numerous other nonfinancial barriers to medication adherence have been suggested, such as disease-related knowledge, health literacy, and concerns about polypharmacy (Willis, 2018). For people struggling with mental health disorders, medication adherence behaviors may be strongly mediated by inability to recognize symptoms of serious disease, and maintain a real conviction that medications are not effective, or decide to manage their symptoms on their own. Some people with mental illness become overwhelmed with

accessing treatment, and with managing appointments, transportation, and finances (www
.nami.org). These variables affect the perceptions of seriousness, susceptibility, and benefits,
and contribute to the likelihood of taking preventive BH action (Rosenstock, 1974). All of the
factors of the HBM are thought to operate in a risk–benefit conflict that is different for each
individual, can change across time, and is influenced considerably by life circumstances.

BRINGING ABOUT BEHAVIOR CHANGE

According to the HBM, an individual's perceptions of susceptibility and seriousness are
what may lead to action. However, there are still other modifying factors, or *cues to action*,
thought to trigger preventive health behavior, such as mass public health media campaigns
(e.g., vaccines), reminder text from the dentist, or the illness of a loved one. The strength
of the cues necessary to initiate action is contingent upon the perceived seriousness of and
susceptibility to a disease. In their comprehensive review of research on the predictors of
medication compliance among patients with mood disorders, Cohen et al. (2000) examined
the utility of the HBM across numerous studies over a 15-year period (1985–2000). Adherence
with prescribed medication for depression and bipolar disorder is a prevalent obstacle to
effective treatment. A recent, comprehensive meta-analysis found the most common interventions aimed at changing medication-related behaviors included pharmacist counseling,
tailored text messages, providing information about health consequences, problem-solving,
and social support (Sheils et al., 2024). Although their findings suggested that the four factors
of the HBM were helpful to some extent in predicting adherence with treatment regimens,
a broader model that incorporates the HBM dimensions as well as physician-related factors
such as continuity of care and the quality of the doctor–patient alliance is essential to improve
both adherence and treatment outcomes (Cohen et al., 2000).

Cognitive Behavioral Theory

Cognitive behavioral theory's (CBT) primary focus is on altering a patient's behavior and
ways of thinking in ways that will lead to positive change in their relationships, work, and life
satisfaction. CBT theorists believe there is a strong and interconnected relationship between
an individual's way of thinking and subsequent behavior. They posit that a person's behavior
can affect their mood; similarly, one's mood and state of mind may influence the way an individual behaves. Because of this interconnectedness, it is important for clinicians to focus not
only on one of these areas. By working with patients to simultaneously change their behavior
and ways of thinking, clinicians are able to bring about positive changes in their patients.

CHALLENGING IRRATIONAL THINKING

Clinicians should validate patients' feelings while simultaneously challenging irrational or
maladaptive ways of thinking, often referred to as thinking traps. Thinking traps are thoughts
that patients believe to be true despite lacking evidence that this is the case. Some of the
most common thinking traps include all-or-nothing thinking, catastrophizing, minimizing,
jumping to conclusions, overgeneralizing, fortune-telling, "should" statements, and filtering
(Table 17.2). In CBT, a clinician's role is to help patients challenge thinking traps and find
more accurate and adaptive ways of interpreting their circumstances.

Bringing About Behavior Change. Similarly, in CBT, clinicians have a variety of strategies
for helping patients achieve behavior change. A common strategy is behavioral activation
(BA), or the use of pleasurable activities to improve a patient's mood (Figure 17.2). Clinicians
also focus on teaching patients to set aside time in their day for self-care. Patients often prioritize responsibilities and disregard self-care activities. Clinicians must not only motivate
patients to practice self-care, but also potentially help them brainstorm some self-care activity ideas. Bringing about behavior change also involves practicing healthy coping strategies,
exercising, and improving a patient's diet. Tobacco, alcohol, drugs, and/or sex can become

TABLE 17.2 Common Thinking Traps and Their Definitions

THINKING TRAPS	DEFINITION
All or nothing	"Making a mistake makes me a bad person."
Catastrophizing	"If I lose my job, I will lose everything I have and will never be happy."
Minimizing	"I've been taking drugs my whole life and I am completely healthy."
Mind reading	"I don't go out because people make fun of my weight behind my back."
Fortune-telling	"If I start a new relationship, I will be hurt again."
Overgeneralizing	"All men are abusive and domineering."
"Should" statements	"I should find someone to marry, or I will never be happy."
Filtering	"My life is over because I was diagnosed with diabetes and hypertension."

unhealthy coping strategies that prevent positive behavior change. Healthy, more adaptive coping strategies include but are not limited to daily exercise, a nutritious diet, arts and crafts, reading, mindfulness, relaxation exercises, time with family, time with friends, church attendance, and so forth. A patient may not be able to come up with solutions on their own due to their emotional state. Therefore, clinicians must educate patients about the importance of self-care and healthy coping strategies, motivate them to put them into practice, and help identify the ones that will best fit their needs, interests, and schedule.

Behavioral Activation

Individuals with depression commonly report lack of motivation, energy, and interest to do their daily activities. This inactivity often leads to feelings of guilt and ineffectiveness, causing the person with depression to feel stuck in a never-ending cycle of depression, fatigue, unproductivity, and guilt. BA is focused on exposure to pleasurable/accomplishment-building activities and how cognitions are related to task completion or avoidance (Figure 17.3). Teaching patients that motivation can come after beginning a task and following a plan, rather than one's mood, in completing tasks is a core cognitive component of BA.

BA is a simple and effective, evidence-based therapeutic intervention that helps patients to feel better. BA assists patients in breaking the depression cycle as they seek to engage in activities that have the potential to produce positive feelings of pleasure, sense of purpose, and achievement. Those activities can be simple, like making the bed, or more complex, like volunteering once a week. It is helpful to assist patients in selecting a combination of pleasant and productive activities, or activities that can be both pleasant and productive at the same time.

The BA approach assumes a strong relationship between avoidant behaviors and depression. Specific, behaviorally focused activation strategies include self-monitoring, structuring and scheduling daily activities, rating the degree of pleasure and accomplishment experienced during engagement in specific daily activities, exploring alternative behaviors related to achieving goals, and using role-playing to address specific behavioral deficits.

Change takes time. People who are depressed tend to focus on the negative, obsessing about the negative aspects of their life and the changes that need to be made. They might focus on end goals, which can seem unattainable and cause them to become paralyzed with doubt. Successful change demands specificity and we can guide people to behavior change that is manageable and within reach. The greatest challenge is getting patients to think small and commit to an activity that is a stepping stone to a larger goal. Patients should also not pile on

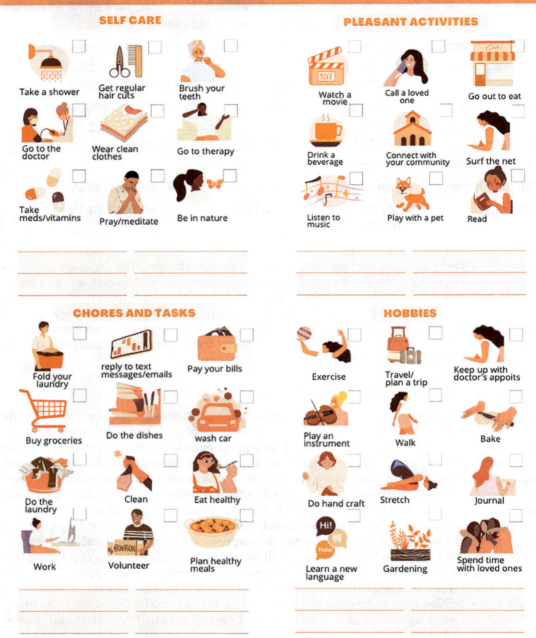

FIGURE 17.2 Pleasant, important, and productive activities. This infographic could be printed and given to a patient to put on their refrigerator and use as a checklist to see how many of these activities they can complete in a week and to reflect on when they do them/how it makes them feel.
Source: Courtesy of Marisol V. Vilugron.

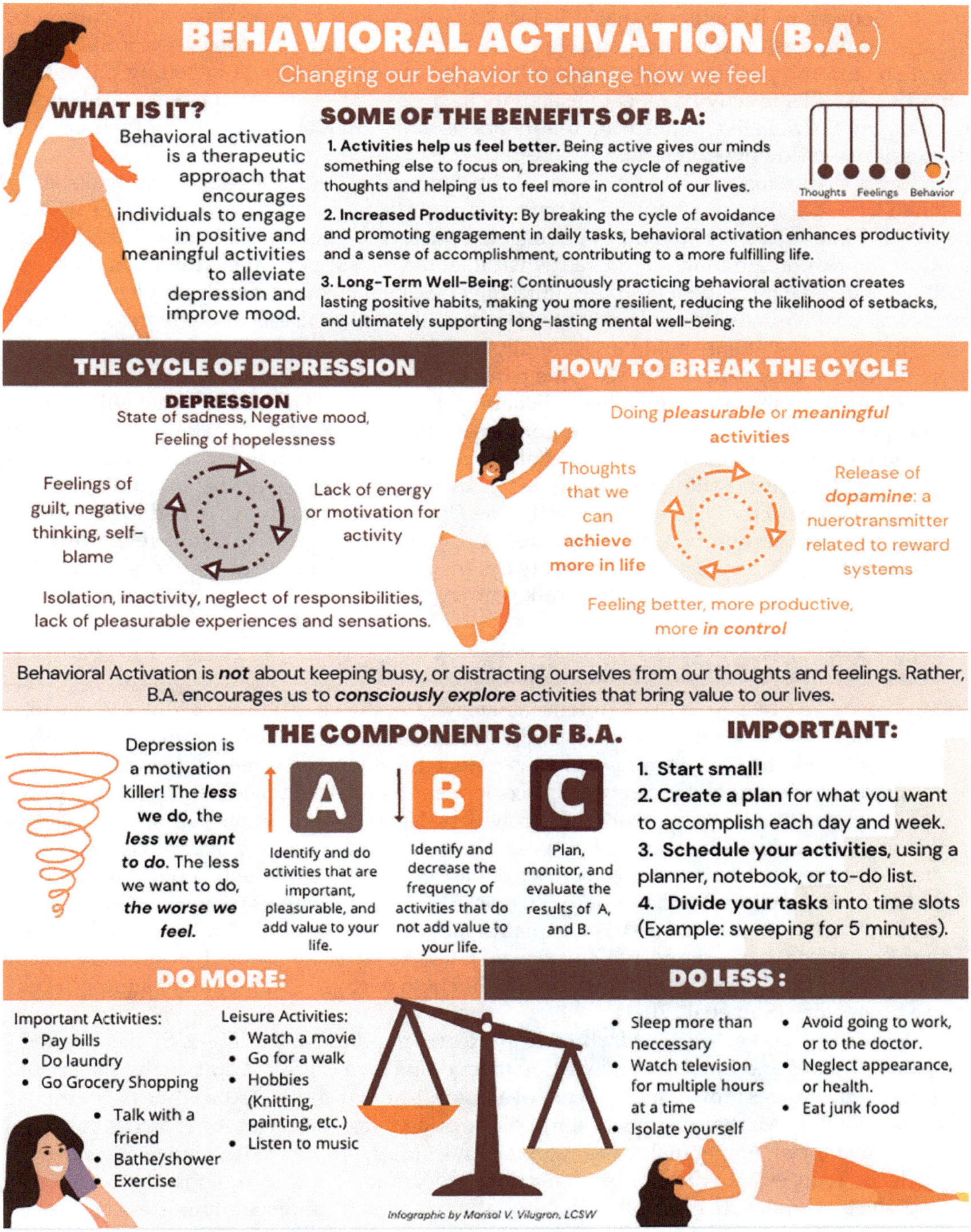

FIGURE 17.3 Behavioral activation.
Source: Courtesy of Marisol V. Vilugron.

too much change at once, pick several behaviors to change, or overhaul every aspect of their routines at once. Encourage patients to repeat the small change despite a lack of initial reward and persist in changing the negative patterns of apathy and isolation. Also, remind patients to start small and then slowly increase their activity levels until they return to their normal levels of functioning. *The key to changing how people feel is helping them change what they do.*

The pioneers of BA suggest that it is like fostering an attitude of "fake it 'til you make it" toward depression self-care—engage in an activity, in spite of a total lack of interest in doing so, and the positive feelings will follow. The greatest challenge is getting patients to commit to a realistic activity, repeat the activity in spite of a lack of initial reward, and persist in changing the negative patterns of apathy and isolation that are maintaining their cycle of depression and downward spiral.

Before a discussion can be had about *what* behavioral activities a patient can realistically begin to schedule, the patient must *create an environment that supports healthy behavior*. As with all healthy behaviors that we advise our patients to initiate, the chances of alleviating their symptoms of depression are much improved when they have a supportive environment. One key strategy is to have the patient (and the clinician, if possible) talk with family and friends about increasing positive activities and asking them to help the patient *not* focus on depressive symptoms. Instead, the patient should enlist family and friends in developing topics of discussion around positive experiences. Allowing the patient to stay in the downward, negative spiral of their depressive symptoms can have an alienating effect and lead to further social withdrawal.

The patient should have proactive conversations, even consider making a formalized agreement or *behavior contract,* with each family member and friend with whom they spend a lot of time. The contract should address specific behaviors targeted for change, and a replacement behavior or activity. For example, "I, Jane Doe, will avoid staying in bed for the entire weekend. If I do stay in bed, then my husband, John Doe, agrees to avoid rewarding the behavior by bringing me treats to cheer me up. Instead, I will get up and go for a walk, and, if I do, my husband agrees to go for a walk with me."

CASE STUDY 17.1: BEHAVIORAL ACTIVATION

Mr. Brown is a 64-year-old Black American man who receives a diagnosis of MDD during his recent medical evaluation. During the intake session, Mr. Brown shares a sense of accomplishment and pride derived from his career as a skilled welder with a reputable local welding company. However, following a workplace accident 8 months ago, he was advised to pursue early retirement. Consequently, Mr. Brown has experienced a decline in mood, increased lethargy, and a diminished sense of purpose. His recent PHQ-9 score of 18 indicates a moderately severe level of depression. Mr. Brown denies any history or current thoughts of suicide.

Mr. Brown's clinical social worker suggests BA as the treatment intervention to treat his depression. The social worker explains the rationale behind BA, emphasizing the connection between actions and emotional states. Research suggests that when patients understand the BA rationale, they are more likely to engage with treatment and perform the homework (Sun et al., 2011).

The social worker assists Mr. Brown in identifying and scheduling activities aligned with his values and interests, and writing them down on a tracker. Additionally, the social worker encourages him to rate his sense of accomplishment and pleasure while performing those activities. Mr. Brown opts to start volunteering twice a week at the local community center mentoring young males and working on welding projects in his garage. Simultaneously, he reduces activities contributing to his depression, such as prolonged screen time and sleeping more than usual. Following a few weeks of implementing these changes, Mr. Brown reports a notable improvement in his overall well-being, reporting no symptoms of depression (PHQ-9 = 4) and expressing a renewed sense of purpose and fulfillment.

Motivational Interviewing

Motivational interviewing (MI) is an evidence-based approach to behavior change (**Figure 17.4**). The most current version of MI is described in detail in Miller and Rollnick's (2013) *Motivational Interviewing: Helping People Change*. MI is a guiding style of communication that sits between following (good listening) and directing (giving information and advice). MI is

17 • MENTAL AND BEHAVIORAL HEALTH   351

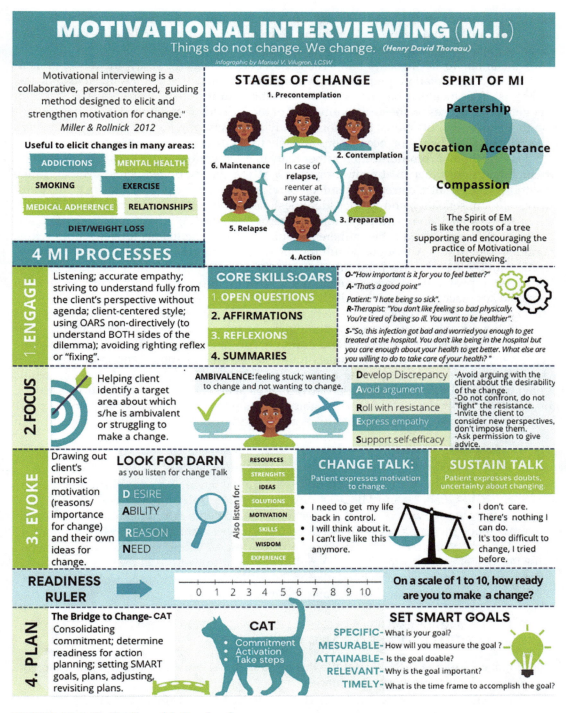

FIGURE 17.4 Motivational interviewing.
Source: Courtesy of Marisol V. Vilugron.

designed to empower people to change by drawing out their own meaning, importance, and capacity for change. MI is based on a respectful and curious way of being with people that facilitates the natural process of change and honors patient autonomy. MI requires the clinician to engage with the patient as an equal partner and refrain from unsolicited advice, confronting, instructing, directing, or warning. MI is a patient-centered, yet directive, method for enhancing intrinsic motivation to change by exploring and resolving ambivalence. A counselor using an MI style expresses empathy, develops discrepancy, reduces resistance, and supports patient self-esteem (Miller & Rollnick, 1991).

MI is similar to DiClemente and Prochaska's *stages of change model*, including precontemplation, contemplation, preparation, action, and maintenance. An unofficial sixth stage, relapse, is often included because slips are inevitable in the change process. The stages of change model focuses on the decision-making of the individual and operates on the assumption that people do not change behaviors quickly and decisively. Rather, change in behavior, especially habitual behavior, occurs continuously through a cyclical process.

MI is a method of communication rather than an intervention, sometimes used on its own or combined with other treatment approaches. MI has been applied across a broad range of settings (e.g., health, corrections, human services, education), populations (e.g., age, ethnicity, religion, sexuality, and gender identities), languages, treatment format (e.g., individual, group, telemedicine), and presenting concerns (e.g., health, fitness, nutrition, risky sex, treatment adherence, medication adherence, substance use, mental health, illegal behaviors, gambling, parenting). Although the full framework is a complex skill set that requires time, practice, and self-awareness from the clinician, the principles of MI have intuitive or common-sense appeal and its core elements can be readily applied in practice as the clinician learns the approach. It is often described as simple, but not easy.

MI compares well to other evidence-based approaches in formal research studies and is compatible with the values of many disciplines. In substance use treatment, MI increases treatment engagement and retention and improves substance abuse treatment outcomes. One meta-analysis of 72 empirical MI studies found across studies robust and enduring effects when MI is added at the beginning of treatment (Hettema et al., 2005). MI has observable behaviors and skills that allow clinicians to receive clear and objective feedback from a trainer, consultant, or supervisor. MI triggers reliable aggregate change across a range of target problems, settings, and providers, yet the effects are highly variable by site, study, and counselor.

CASE STUDY 17.2: MOTIVATIONAL INTERVIEWING

Mrs. Leticia Martinez, a 52-year-old married Latinx woman, whose preferred language is Spanish, has diabetes and MDD. During her recent consultation with her primary care physician, it was observed that Mrs. Martinez's hemoglobin A1c, a laboratory marker of average blood glucose levels, had increased from 7.4 to 9.2, and her PHQ-9 had risen from 8 to 15. Mrs. Martinez disclosed that she discontinued taking prescribed medications for her diabetes (metformin 500 mg) and depression (fluoxetine 20 mg) approximately 3 months ago. In response to her situation, Mrs. Martinez was advised to engage with a bilingual clinical social worker available at the clinic.

FOUR MI PROCESSES AND STAGES OF CHANGE REGARDING MEDICATION COMPLIANCE FOR DIABETES AND DEPRESSION

1. **Engage: Use the OARS core skills throughout an MI conversation: O**pen questions, **A**ffirmations, **R**eflections, **S**ummaries.

   The social worker was warm and friendly, helping Mrs. Martinez to feel at ease talking with a new provider. The social worker asked Leticia open-ended questions in a nonjudgmental way about her current emotional and physical well-being and her reasons for discontinuing prescribed medicines. Mrs. Martinez shared that she was "not sure" about taking medication as prescribed due to the fear of becoming dependent on her diabetes and depression medications, and expressed a preference for managing her chronic conditions through natural remedies (*precontemplation stage*).

(continued)

17 • MENTAL AND BEHAVIORAL HEALTH 353

CASE STUDY 17.2: MOTIVATIONAL INTERVIEWING (*continued*)

2. **Focus: Listen for change and sustain talk. D**evelop discrepancy; **A**void argument; Express empathy; **S**upport self-efficacy.

   The social worker suggested an exercise to identify the pros and cons of using natural remedies versus prescribed medicines. Then they reviewed the test results from the current medical visit together, and the social worker asked the patient to describe in her own words what they mean. Following this activity, Mrs. Martinez acknowledged that, despite her initial inclination toward natural remedies, it was clear that the natural remedies were not effective and that the disadvantages out-weighed the advantages in managing her diabetes and depression. Recognizing the detrimental impact of discontinuing her medications, she agreed that resuming the proposed pharmacological treatment was a prudent decision (***contemplation stage***).

3. **Evoke: Listen for DARN. D**esire, **A**bility, **R**eason, **N**eed.

   The social worker further inquired about Mrs. Martinez's motivations for effectively managing her diabetes and depression. Mrs. Martinez shared that her recent role as a grandmother heightened the importance of maintaining energy, motivation, and good health. Additionally, she emphasized the value of socializing with friends at church when not experiencing depressive episodes.

4. **Plan: Bridge to change, CAT. C**ommitment, **A**ctivation, **T**ake steps.

   To assess Mrs. Martinez's readiness to resume prescribed medications, the social worker asked her to rate her readiness/confidence on a scale from 0 to 10. Mrs. Martinez indicated an 8, and with the social worker's assistance a plan for the next steps in the action was devised (***preparation stage***).

5. **Set B-SMART goals**: **B**arriers, **S**mart, **M**easurable, **A**ttainable, **R**elevant, **T**imely.

   Mrs. Martinez's Goals and Action Plan:
   Barriers: Mrs. Martinez denied any barriers.
   Specific: Lower A1c and PHQ-9 by complying with pharmacological treatment.
   Measurable: Take metformin 500 mg and fluoxetine 20 mg once a day as prescribed.
   Attainable: Goals can be achieved in Mrs. Martinez's assessment.
   Relevant: Improve overall physical and emotional well-being.
   Time-bound: Take medicines daily at 9 a.m. after breakfast. Screen for depression using PHQ-9 in 1 month and assess A1c in 3 months with bloodwork.

CONCLUSION

As they are a leading cause of disease burden in the United States, addressing BH disorders must be a priority of any healthcare provider. In order to best address these disorders, providers must take into account social and environmental factors that can exacerbate conditions and create barriers to treatment. The most effective approach to BH incorporates dimensions of the HBM as well as physician-related factors such as continuity of care and the quality of the doctor–patient alliance.

SUMMARY KEY POINTS

- Mental health and SUD, collectively referred to as BH disorders, are a leading cause of disease burden in the United States, surpassing both cardiovascular disease and cancer.

- Depression is the leading cause of medical disability, health burden, and increased medical cost.

(*continued*)

SUMMARY KEY POINTS (continued)

- Mental health disorders such as anxiety and depression are associated with numerous bodily symptoms. This, along with the comorbidity of these disorders with chronic conditions, compounds suffering for patients and can be challenging as it can be difficult to recognize, diagnose, and treat.
- Social determinants affect a patient's mental health. It is critical to understand how patient characteristics such as socioeconomic status, race, ethnicity, health beliefs and attitudes, and access to medical care influence the underutilization of services.
- Treatment of mental health disorders can take a variety of forms, such as utilizing the health belief model, CBT, behavioral activation, and MI.

DISCUSSION QUESTIONS

1. What concerns about mental health do you have and do you hear about from friends, family members, and colleagues?
2. How would you imagine approaches to increase uptake in treatment vary by racial or ethnic background, or other sociodemographic markers?
3. Of the mechanisms to improve uptake in treatment listed in this chapter, which ones would seem to work best with people in your life and community?
4. What messages did you receive about mental health growing up? How do you feel about these messages at this point in your life?
5. Review the thinking traps in Table 17.2. Are any traps familiar to you, or do you hear them often when talking with friends or loved ones? How would these thought traps impact attitudes toward health and wellness?

A robust set of instructor resources designed to supplement this text is located at http://connect.springerpub.com/content/book/978-0-8261-4265-8. Qualifying instructors may request access by emailing textbook@springerpub.com.

REFERENCES

Adhikari, B., Kahende, J., Malarcher, A., Pechacek, T., & Tong, V. (2009, February). Smoking-attributable mortality, years of potential life lost, and productivity losses-United States, 2000–2004 (Reprinted from *MMWR*, vol. 57, pg 1226–1228, 2008) [Reprint]. *JAMA-Journal of the American Medical Association, 301*(6), 593–594.

Allen, J., Balfour, R., Bell, R., & Marmot, M. (2014). Social determinants of mental health. *International Review of Psychiatry, 26*(4), 392–407.

American Psychiatric Association. (2013). *Diagnostic and statistical manual of mental disorders* (5th ed.). Author.

Barnett, K., Mercer, S. W., Norbury, M., Watt, G., Wyke, S., & Guthrie, B. (2012, July 7). Epidemiology of multimorbidity and implications for health care, research, and medical education: A cross-sectional study. *The Lancet, 380*(9836), 37–43. https://doi.org/10.1016/S0140-6736(12)60240-2

Bazargan, M., Bazargan-Hejazi, S., & Baker, R. S. (2005, May). Treatment of self-reported depression among Hispanics and African Americans. *Journal of Health Care for the Poor and Underserved, 16*(2), 328–344.

Cohen, N. L., Parikh, S. V., & Kennedy, S. H. (2000, September). Medication compliance in mood disorders: Relevance of the Health Belief Model and other determinants. *Primary Care Psychiatry, 6*(3), 101–110.

Cross-National Collaborative Group. (1992). The changing rate of major depression. Cross-national comparisons. *JAMA, 268*(21), 3098–3105.

Degenhardt, L., Charlson, F., Mathers, B., Hall, W. D., Flaxman, A. D., Johns, N., & Vos, T. (2014, August). The global epidemiology and burden of opioid dependence: Results from the global burden of disease 2010 study. *Addiction, 109*(8), 1320–1333. https://doi.org/10.1111/add.12551

Degenhardt, L., & Hall, W. (2012, January). Extent of illicit drug use and dependence, and their contribution to the global burden of disease. *Lancet, 379*(9810), 55–70.

Dwight-Johnson, M., & Lagomasino, I. T. (2007). Addressing depression treatment preferences of ethnic minority patients. *General Hospital Psychiatry, 29*(3), 179–181.

Fortin, M., Bravo, G., Hudon, C., Lapointe, L., Dubois, M. F., & Almirall, J. (2006, September-October). Psychological distress and multimorbidity in primary care. *Annals of Family Medicine, 4*(5), 417–422. https://doi.org/10.1370/afm.528

Fortin, M., Dubois, M. F., Hudon, C., Soubhi, H., & Almirall, J. (2007, August). Multimorbidity and quality of life: A closer look. *Health and Quality of Life Outcomes, 5*, 8. https://doi.org/10.1186/1477-7525-5-52

Gan, Y., Gong, Y., Tong, X., Sun, H., Cong, Y., Dong, X., Wang, Y., Xu, X., Yin, X., Deng, J., Li, L., Cao, S., & Lu, Z. (2014, December 24). Depression and the risk of coronary heart disease: A meta-analysis of prospective cohort studies. *BMC Psychiatry, 14*(1), 371. https://doi.org/10.1186/s12888-014-0371-z

Gelberg, L., Andersen, R. M., & Leake, B. D. (2000, February). The behavioral model for vulnerable populations: Application to medical care use and outcomes for homeless people. *Health Services Research, 34*(6), 1273–1302.

Gryczynski, J., Schwartz, R. P., O'Grady, K. E., Restivo, L., Mitchell, S. G., & Jaffe, J. H. (2016, January). Understanding patterns of high-cost health care use across different substance user groups. *Health Affairs, 35*(1), 12–19. https://doi.org/10.1377/hlthaff.2015.0618

Haas, L. J., Leiser, J. P., Magill, M. K., & Sanyer, O. N. (2005, November). Management of the difficult patient. *American Family Physician, 72*(10), 2063–2068.

Hedegaard, H., Miniño, A., Spencer, M., & Warner, M. (2021). *Drug overdose deaths in the United States, 1999–2020.* NCHS Data Brief, no 428. National Center for Health Statistics. https://doi.org/10.15620/cdc:112340

Heron, M., Hoyert, D. L., Murphy, S. L., Xu, J. Q., Kochanek, K. D., & Tejada-Vera, B. (2009). *Deaths: final data for 2006* (National Vital Statistics Report), *57*(14), 1–134.

Hettema, J., Steele, J., & Miller, W. R. (2005). Motivational interviewing. *Annual Review of Clinical Psychology, 1*, 91–111. https://doi.org/10.1146/annurev.clinpsy.1.102803.143833

Hoffman, C., Rice, D., & Sung, H. Y. (1996, November). Persons with chronic conditions–Their prevalence and costs. *JAMA-Journal of the American Medical Association, 276*(18), 1473–1479.

Jackson, J. L., & Kroenke, K. (2001, May). The effect of unmet expectations among adults presenting with physical symptoms. *Annals of Internal Medicine, 134*(9), 889–897.

Jackson-Triche, M. E., Greer Sullivan, J., Wells, K. B., Rogers, W., Camp, P., & Mazel, R. (2000, May 1). Depression and health-related quality of life in ethnic minorities seeking care in general medical settings. *Journal of Affective Disorders, 58*(2), 89–97. https://doi.org/10.1016/S0165-0327(99)00069-5

Kamal, R., Cox, C., Rousseau, D., & for the Kaiser Family Foundation. (2017). Costs and outcomes of mental health and substance use disorders in the US. *JAMA, 318*(5), 415–415. https://doi.org/10.1001/jama.2017.8558

Kessler, R. C. (2012). The costs of depression. *The Psychiatric Clinics of North America, 35*(1), 1–14. https://doi.org/10.1016/j.psc.2011.11.005

Kessler, R. C., Aguilar-Gaxiola, S., Alonso, J., Chatterji, S., Lee, S., Ormel, J., Ustun, T. B., & Wang, P. S. (2009, January-March). The global burden of mental disorders: An update from the WHO World Mental Health (WMH) surveys. *Epidemiologia E Psichiatria Sociale-An International Journal for Epidemiology and Psychiatric Sciences, 18*(1), 23–33.

Kravitz, R. L., & Ford, D. E. (2008, November). Introduction: Chronic medical conditions and depression–The view from primary care. *American Journal of Medicine, 121*(11), 1–7. https://doi.org/10.1016/j.amjmed.2008.09.007

Kroenke, K., & Spitzer, R. L. (2002, September). The PHQ-9: A new depression diagnostic and severity measure. *Psychiatric Annals, 32*(9), 509–515.

Lorant, V., Deliege, D., Eaton, W., Robert, A., Philippot, P., & Ansseau, M. (2003). Socioeconomic inequalities in depression: A meta-analysis. *American Journal of Epidemiology, 157*(2), 98–112.

McGuire, T., & Miranda, J. (2008). New evidence regarding racial and ethnic disparities in mental health: Policy implications. *Health Affairs, 27*(2), 393–403.

Miller, W. R., & Rollnick, S. (1991). *Motivational interviewing: Preparing people to change addictive behavior.* New York: Guilford Press.

Miller, W. R., & Rollnick, S. (2013). *Motivational interviewing: Helping people change* (3rd ed.). New York: Guilford Press.

Patel, V., Lund, C., Hatheril, S., Plagerson, S., Corrigall, J., Funk, M., & Fisher, A. (2010). Mental disorders: Equity and social determinants. In E. Blas, & A. S. Kurup (Eds.), *Equity, social determinants and public health programmes* (pp. 115–134). World Health Organization.

Penninx, B. W. J. H., Milaneschi, Y., Lamers, F., & Vogelzangs, N. (2013, May 15). Understanding the somatic consequences of depression: Biological mechanisms and the role of depression symptom profile. *BMC Medicine, 11*(1), 129. https://doi.org/10.1186/1741-7015-11-129

Posner, K., Brown, G. K., Stanley, B., Brent, D. A., Yershova, K. V., Oquendo, M. A., Currier, G. W., Melvin, G. A., Greenhill, L., Shen, S., & Mann, J. J. (2011). The Columbia-Suicide Severity Rating

Scale: Initial validity and internal consistency findings from three multisite studies with adolescents and adults. *The American Journal of Psychiatry, 168*(12), 1266–1277. https://doi.org/10.1176/appi.ajp.2011.10111704

Quiñones, A. R., Markwardt, S., & Botoseneanu, A. (2016, June). Multimorbidity combinations and disability in older adults. *The Journals of Gerontology. Series A, Biological Sciences and Medical Sciences, 71*(6), 823–830. https://doi.org/10.1093/gerona/glw035

Reinert, D. F., & Allen, J. (2002). The Alcohol Use Disorders Identification Test (AUDIT): A review of recent research. *Alcoholism: Clinical and Experimental Research, 26*(2), 272–279.

Rosenstock, I. M. (1974). Historical origins of the health belief model. *Health Education Monographs, 2,* 328–335.

Roy-Byrne, P. P., Katon, W., Cowley, D. S., & Russo, J. (2001, September). A randomized effectiveness trial of collaborative care for patients with panic disorder in primary care. *Archives of General Psychiatry, 58*(9), 869–876.

Saxena, S. (2018). Excess mortality among people with mental disorders: A public health priority. *The Lancet Public Health, 3*(6), e264–e265. https://doi.org/10.1016/S2468-2667(18)30099-9

Sayar, K., Kirmayer, L. J., & Taillefer, S. S. (2003, March-April). Predictors of somatic symptoms in depressive disorder. *General Hospital Psychiatry, 25*(2), 108–114. https://doi.org/10.1016/s0163-8343(02)00277-3

Sheils, E., Tillett, W., James, D., Brown, S., Dack, C., Family, H., & Chapman, S. C. E. (2024). Changing medication-related beliefs: A systematic review and meta-analysis of randomized controlled trials. *Health Psychology, 43*(3), 155–170. https://doi.org/10.1037/hea0001316

Skinner, H. (1982). The drug abuse screening test. *Addictive Behaviors, 7*(4), 363–371.

Smedley, B. D. (2012). The lived experience of race and its health consequences. *American Journal of Public Health, 102*(5), 933–935. https://doi.org/10.2105/ajph.2011.300643

Spitzer, R. L., Kroenke, K., Williams, J. B. W., & Lowe, B. (2006, May). A brief measure for assessing generalized anxiety disorder–The GAD-7. *Archives of Internal Medicine, 166*(10), 1092–1097. https://doi.org/10.1001/archinte.166.10.1092

Starfield, B. (2006, March-April). Threads and yarns: Weaving the tapestry of comorbidity. *Annals of Family Medicine, 4*(2), 101–103. https://doi.org/10.1370/afm.524

Sun, G. C., Hsu, M. C., Moyle, W., Lin, M. F., Creedy, D., & Venturato, L. (2011, January). Mediating roles of adherence attitude and patient education on antidepressant use in patients with depression. *Perspect Psychiatr Care, 47*(1), 13–22. https://doi.org/10.1111/j.1744-6163.2010.00257.x

Unutzer, J., Schoenbaum, M., Druss, B. G., & Katon, W. J. (2006, January). Transforming mental health care at the interface with general medicine: Report for the President's commission. *Psychiatric Services, 57*(1), 37–47.

Vogeli, C., Shields, A. E., Lee, T. A., Gibson, T. B., Marder, W. D., Weiss, K. B., & Blumenthal, D. (2007, December). Multiple chronic conditions: Prevalence, health consequences, and implications for quality, care management, and costs. *Journal of General Internal Medicine, 22,* 391–395. https://doi.org/10.1007/s11606-007-0322-1

Waitzfelder, B., Stewart, C., Coleman, K. J., Rossom, R., Ahmedani, B. K., Beck, A., Zeber, J. E., Daida, Y. G., Trinacty, C., Hubley, S., & Simon, G. E. (2018). Treatment Initiation for new episodes of depression in primary care settings. *Journal of General Internal Medicine, 33*(8), 1283–1291.

Willis, E. (2018). Applying the health belief model to medication adherence: The role of online health communities and peer reviews. *Journal of Health Communication, 23*(8), 743–750. https://doi.org/10.1080/10810730.2018.1523260

World Health Organization. (2014). *Mental health: A state of well-being.* . https://www.who.int/features/factfiles/mental_health/en/

World Health Organization. (2021). *Depression.* https://www.who.int/news-room/fact-sheets/detail/depression

Wu, C. H., Erickson, S. R., & Kennedy, J. (2009, February). Patient characteristics associated with the use of antidepressants among people diagnosed with DSM-IV mood disorders: Results from the National Comorbidity Survey Replication. *Current Medical Research and Opinion, 25*(2), 471–482. https://doi.org/10.1185/03007990802646642

PART IV: INTERVENING IN SETTINGS AND
SYSTEMS TO MODIFY HEALTH BEHAVIORS

CHAPTER 18

SCHOOL INTERVENTIONS TO SUPPORT HEALTH BEHAVIOR CHANGE

REBEKKA M. LEE, ANDRIA B. EISMAN, AND STEVEN L. GORTMAKER

LEARNING OBJECTIVES

- Explain the benefits of situating health behavior change interventions in schools.
- Name two challenges to implementing school-based health behavior change interventions.
- Identify strategies for overcoming these barriers to implementing school-based health behaviors change interventions.
- Describe and give examples of six types of school-based health behavior change interventions.
- Describe two ways that equity can be incorporated in school-based health behavior change efforts.

WHY FOCUS ON SCHOOLS?

Promoting health behavior change within the school setting is an excellent approach to impacting population health. Because people spend most of their youth in the classroom, schools are a natural choice as settings to situate interventions that establish healthy habits early in life to prevent disease across the life course. Elementary, middle, and high schools, as well as early childcare programs and colleges and universities, have the potential for tremendous reach. This is particularly the case in the United States, where public education has been mandated since the early 1900s, but the right to healthcare is still up for debate. Schools can promote healthy behaviors and deliver services to a broad population in a way that other settings cannot. Children spend roughly 1,260 hours (180 days, 7 hours per day) at school each year, while they will likely only spend about a half hour with a primary care provider during a yearly physical exam. Although doctors and other healthcare providers play a vital role in promoting health behaviors, schools can be critical supports to reinforce health messages via educational programming, provide more constant individualized services, and model healthy environments that can shift norms throughout a child's formative years of life.

Promoting health within schools could help address health disparities and promote equity (**Figure 18.1**). While the impact of schools holds much promise, public health professionals should keep in mind that the resources and quality of schools, particularly in the United States, vary greatly. With about half of public K through 12 school funding coming from local

358   IV • INTERVENING IN SETTINGS AND SYSTEMS TO MODIFY HEALTH BEHAVIORS

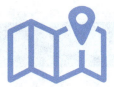

Plan implementation of evidence-based interventions to ensure children of color from schools in low income and rural areas are reached—*How can state demographic data be used to ensure equitable delivery?*

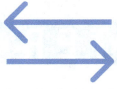

Identify mismatches between where and with whom the intervention evidence was established and each unique school context—*Are there differences in student language, race, ethnicity, social class, or staff cultural competency?*

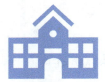

Consider how institutional racism within the school interacts with intervention implementation—*Are principals having intentional discussions about racism?*

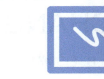

Adapt intervention materials to meet the preferences of children from different backgrounds—*How can changes be made to features of the intervention to support engagement?*

FIGURE 18.1 Approaches and questions for promoting equity in school-based interventions.
Sources: From Allen, M., Wilhelm, A., Ortega, L. E., Pergament, S., Bates, N., Cunningham, B. (2021, May 20). Applying a race(ism)-conscious adaptation of the CFIR framework to understand implementation of a school-based equity-oriented intervention. *Ethnicity & Disease, 31*(Suppl. 1), 375–388; Castro, F. G., Barrera, M., & Holleran Steiker, L. K. (2010). Issues and challenges in the design of culturally adapted evidence-based interventions. *Annual Review of Clinical Psychology, 6*, 213–239.

sources (National Center for Education Statistics, 2017) and limited U.S. funding for early care and education (Child Care State Systems Specialist Network, 2014). Therefore, initiatives within schools must be carefully planned and implemented in order to serve populations that are most in need. Equity can be promoted by focusing on purposeful implementation of evidence-based interventions in rural, low-income communities and among children of color living in cities. Furthermore, educational settings have the potential to impact health equity in emerging adulthood through similar focused implementation given the vast gaps in resources between public community colleges and vocational schools as compared with private 4-year college and universities. In addition to considering *where* evidence-based interventions are implemented to promote equity, attention should be given to *how* these interventions are implemented. For instance, interventions may need to undergo adaptations to best align with the communities where they are delivered.

INTERVENTIONS TO CHANGE HEALTH BEHAVIORS

Education as Health Intervention

Before detailing the multitude of interventions shown to be effective in schools, it is important to highlight that educational attainment, in its own right, has been a long-standing, established predictor of better health and should be acknowledged as an important strategy to promote healthy behaviors (Cohen & Syme, 2013; Pincus et al., 1987). Recognizing the profound influence of education on health and poverty, the United Nations named inclusive and equitable quality education as part of its 2030 Agenda for Sustainable Development, and the Health Promoting Schools Framework from the World Health Organization (WHO) outlines a three-pronged holistic approach emphasizing the school environment, health education, and family/community engagement (Langford et al., 2015).

Guidelines for Health Behavior Change in Schools

Leading health organizations around the world have set forth comprehensive approaches for how health should be promoted in schools, which thoughtfully take into account contextual factors and social determinants (Government of India Ministry of Health & Family Welfare, 2017; Lewallen et al., 2015; Schools for Health in Europe, n.d.). For example, in the United States, the Centers for Disease Control and Prevention (CDC) has joined forces with the Association for Supervision and Curriculum Development to create the Whole School, Whole Community, Whole Child model (**Figure 18.2**; CDC, 2023). It names 10 components for promoting health in the school setting: health education, physical education and physical activity, health services, nutrition environment and services, counseling and psychological services, social and emotional climate, physical environment, employee wellness, family engagement, and community involvement (CDC, 2023). In addition to laying out this model, the CDC supports schools with guidance documents based on the latest science and works to monitor health in schools via tools such as the Youth Risk Behavior Survey, the School Health

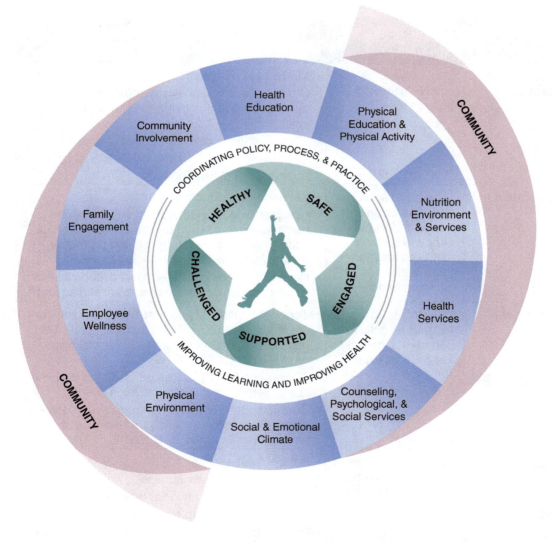

FIGURE 18.2 Whole School, Whole Community, Whole Child (WSCC) model.
Source: From Centers for Disease Control and Prevention. (2023). *Whole School, whole community, whole child (WSCC).* https://www.cdc.gov/healthyschools/wscc/index.htm.

360 IV • INTERVENING IN SETTINGS AND SYSTEMS TO MODIFY HEALTH BEHAVIORS

Profiles, the School Health Policies and Practices Study, and the Physical Education Curriculum Analysis Tool.

Types of School-Based Health Behavior Change Interventions

Promoting healthy behaviors in schools can take many forms. As a means of organizing these different approaches, we have developed a typology of school-based health behavior change interventions (Table 18.1) that displays six category types, as well as a working definition and bulleted examples for each type. This typology and the summary of evidence-based interventions present health behavior strategies from those focused most on the individual at the top to those that take the broadest population approach at the bottom. It is important to understand the impact of these levels for behavior change when taking up health initiatives in schools (Stokols, 1996). For example, interventions that rely on nurses or specialized professionals like therapists may be time-consuming and costly to deliver. They might only be available to a small part of the school population; however, the benefits to individuals most in need will likely be quite high. Conversely, policy interventions at the national, state, and

TABLE 18.1 Typology of School-Based Health Behavior Change Interventions

TYPE	DEFINITION	EXAMPLES
Patient-centered	Delivery of individualized clinical services	• Medication administration • Chronic disease management behaviors (e.g., checking blood glucose and administering insulin) • Mental health assessments and counseling • Contraceptive and pregnancy care • Substance use treatment
Education	Health lessons and messages designed to build knowledge and skills to lay the foundation for lifelong health	• Sexual health education • Comprehensive health education addressing core health areas (e.g., drug use prevention, physical activity) and cross-cutting risk and protective factors (e.g., the Michigan Model for Health). • Healthy messaging directed toward students, staff, and parents on posters, newsletters, and so forth.
Behavioral	Strategies to improve social and emotional health and development	• School-wide social and emotional learning curricula focused on skill development, self-awareness and self-management, and social awareness (Tier 1; CASEL, 2022) • Social skills training based on identified deficits (e.g., interpersonal communication; Tier 2) • Cognitive behavioral therapy on college campuses (in-person or digital) for depression or anxiety (Tier 3; Lattie et al., 2019)
System	School practices or environments that are intended to promote health	• School food service • Clean drinking water access • Ventilation and filtration for healthy air quality • Rules limiting smartphones in schools • Healthy options in vending machines on school grounds

(continued)

TABLE 18.1 Typology of School-Based Health Behavior Change Interventions (*continued*)

TYPE	DEFINITION	EXAMPLES
Policy	Regulations implemented at the national, state, district, or school level intended to promote health in schools	• District wellness policies • State law mandating vaccination • CACFP policy for snacks and meals served in early childcare
Multicomponent	Strategies intervene at multiple levels to affect behavior change	• Planet Health • NAP-SACC • Safer Choices

CACFP, Child and Adult Care Food Program; NAP-SACC, Nutrition and Physical Activity Self-Assessment for Child Care.

school level are usually relatively low in cost and easy to disseminate, resulting in a small impact to a broad population of students. Schools should seek to match the level of intervention they choose with the scope of the health problem they aim to address. Often, a mixture of individualized and population approaches, highlighted in the multicomponent type, is appropriate for meeting the needs of a given student body. Across each of these intervention types, it is essential that public health practitioners consider adaptations to ensure equity in implementation and subsequent outcomes.

PATIENT-CENTERED

Patient-centered interventions are those that deliver individualized clinical services to children within the school setting. According to 2014 data from the School Health Policies and Programs Study (SHPPS) assessment, 85% of U.S. elementary schools and 78% of middle and high schools have a part- or full-time nurse to deliver health services (National Center for HIV/AIDS, Viral Hepatitis, STD, and TB Prevention, & Division of Adolescent & School Health, 2014). Packaging behavior change interventions with traditional school-based health services like first aid and CPR and vision and hearing screenings can be an effective way to address child health needs. Moreover, schools are vital settings for ensuring medication administration and chronic disease management behaviors, such as checking blood glucose and administering insulin (Jackson et al., 2015).

Another example of patient-centered care in the school setting is the work of school-based speech-language pathologists, who work with children to improve communication behaviors and outcomes. These practitioners use a variety of behavioral strategies to address various needs, from building social communication and literacy skills to developing sound production and intelligibility, in students' individualized education plans (IEPs; Cirrin et al., 2010). While research on the effectiveness of these school interventions is limited, a review found that speech and language interventions delivered in the classroom may be similarly effective compared with traditional pullout approaches that work with students one on one (Cirrin et al., 2010). The skills fostered in these interventions advance the mental health of students as well as their ability to achieve academically in the classroom.

In just under 8% of U.S. high schools, the nurse's office has been transformed into a full-service, school-based health clinic (National Center for HIV/AIDS, Viral Hepatitis, STD, and TB Prevention, & Division of Adolescent & School Health, 2014). These clinics have been particularly important for serving as a "medical home" to teenagers in urban and rural areas who often do not receive primary care services, and in some cases provide improved access to care for the entire family (Knopf et al., 2016). Services provided in the majority of these clinics include physical and mental health assessments, vision and hearing screening, immunization, pregnancy testing, and contraceptive counseling. They take an integrated approach to care—focusing on both physical and mental health—and encourage behavior change by emphasizing the modifiable risk factors (e.g., smoking, drug use, inactivity, unsafe sexual activity, poor diet) that most contribute to health problems in youth (Knopf et al., 2016). Studies of school-based health clinics have found higher utilization of primary clinical care, improved educational outcomes, and increased contraceptive use among students (Knopf et al., 2016; Ran et al., 2016). Furthermore, a recent economic evaluation found that societal cost benefits and savings to healthcare payers such as Medicaid outweigh the operating costs of school-based health centers (Ran et al., 2016).

EDUCATION

Educational interventions include health lessons and messages designed to lay the foundation for lifelong health. They also often include skill-building lessons and activities to support students in changing their health behaviors. Health education in schools has been implemented across grade levels and can be delivered by classroom teachers or specialists, such as physical education teachers, school social workers or psychologists, or certified health educators. Data from 2014 indicate that 65% of schools had health education taught by physical education teachers or specialists (National Center for HIV/AIDS, Viral Hepatitis, STD, and TB Prevention, & Division of Adolescent & School Health, 2014).

School-based education interventions aimed at building knowledge and skills in classroom settings have been shown to increase such health-promoting behaviors as bicycle helmet wearing (Owen et al., 2011), physical activity (Community Preventive Services Task Force, 2021), fruit and vegetable consumption (Gortmaker et al., 1999), and decreasing television watching (Gortmaker et al., 1999). Research also demonstrates evidence for decreases in risk-taking behaviors such as smoking (Thomas & Perera, 2008), early drug use (Faggiano et al., 2008), unprotected sex for the prevention of unintended pregnancies (Oringanje et al., 2010), and UV sun exposure (Buller et al., 2006) if educational interventions include components on social influences and skill building, in addition to the delivery of information. The LifeSkills Training middle school program is an example of an educational program that has successfully addressed multiple risk behaviors among a diverse range of student populations, from tobacco and drug use (Spoth et al., 2008) to binge drinking (Botvin et al., 1995), to physically violent behavior.

BEHAVIORAL

For the purposes of this chapter, behavioral interventions refer to school-based strategies aimed at addressing children's behavioral health and social and emotional development. Research has shown a range of behavioral interventions at various levels (i.e., Tiers 1–3) to be effective in schools (Bruns et al., 2016). The objective of a tiered approach is to support proactive and comprehensive responses to students' academic, social-emotional, and behavioral needs to slow or prevent progression to more severe difficulties (Epperson, 2019). Tier 1 includes universal interventions for all students within a general education setting. Tier 1 is designed to meet the needs of most students (75%–90%; Epperson, 2019). Tier 1 interventions for social-emotional health may include mental health promotion interventions focused on social-emotional learning (SEL) for the entire student body and creating a supportive atmosphere in the school (Taylor et al., 2017). Those students not sufficiently responding to Tier 1 and experiencing continued difficulty may be stepped up to more focused interventions, referred to as Tier 2, such as school-based group therapy (e.g., cognitive behavioral therapy [CBT]) or social skills training (National Center on Response to Intervention, 2010). Tier 3 interventions are reserved for those students needing the most intensive treatment and support, generally <10%, and may include individual therapy or crisis interventions (e.g., for students experiencing a mental health crisis or severe distress; National Center on Response to Intervention, 2010).

A robust empirical foundation supports the effectiveness of an SEL intervention in short- and long-term youth outcomes (Hill et al., 2020). Tier 1 SEL interventions that include all youth can mitigate the impact of trauma and adversity, and reach large populations, without requiring that students are formally identified as "at-risk" (Chafouleas et al., 2019). More intensive Tier 2 programs for preventing or reducing aggressive behavior have proven successful among youth at elevated risk of poor outcomes (Wilson et al., 2003). Similarly, studies have shown reductions in symptoms of anxiety among participants in prevention and early intervention programs focused on these outcomes (Neil & Christensen, 2009). To date, most of these anxiety prevention programs have been conducted among high school-age youth employing CBT (Neil & Christensen, 2009). An example of such a program is the 6-week, group-based Blues Program, which has been shown to positively impact depression outcomes (Stice et al., 2008). A range of interventions that aim to improve young children's executive functioning, including cognitive flexibility, inhibition, and working memory, have proven effective (Diamond & Lee, 2011) This improved functioning lays the groundwork for improved health behaviors, from lower substance use and consumption of high-calorie foods to higher fruit and vegetable consumption and physical activity (Riggs et al., 2012). Children with attention deficit hyperactivity disorder (ADHD), those with lower working memory spans, and those from families with lower incomes have shown particularly high gains. While these behavioral interventions can be delivered by specialists individually, elementary school-age children have also shown significant improvements in executive functioning and declines in aggressive behavior (Crean & Johnson, 2013) via curricula delivery by classroom teachers (Diamond & Lee, 2011).

CASE STUDY 18.1: TIER 1 SCHOOL-BASED BEHAVIORAL INTERVENTION

The Michigan Model for Health™ (MMH) is a theory-based, skills-focused Tier 1 health education intervention grounded in social cognitive theory and the health belief model and centered in National Health Education Standards (Bandura, 1989; Rosenstock, 1974). The MMH, as a comprehensive health curriculum, represents a central component of the WSCC model (Whole School, Whole Child, Whole Community) that focuses on multifaceted approaches to enhancing well-being and academic success of children and youth (CDC, 2023). The curriculum has demonstrated efficacy in reducing substance use and improving mental health among high school-age students (O'Neill et al., 2011; Shope et al., 1996). The MMH curriculum has been adapted and updated to address new and emerging health issues including prescription opioid misuse, vaping, and trauma-sensitive approaches. It includes grade-specific curricula to ensure developmentally appropriate content for K through 12 students and is available at www.michiganmodelforhealth.org/.

SYSTEM

School practices or environments that are intended to promote health for youth fall under the system category of health behavior change interventions. Two major facets of the school systems that influence child health are the meals and snacks delivered via school food or dining services and the activity provided via physical education classes or movement breaks in the classroom. School feeding programs have been developed primarily as a strategy for addressing hunger among disadvantaged youth (Kristjansson et al., 2009). In lower income countries where inadequate dietary intake is a common health behavior challenge, school feeding interventions that provide nutritious meals during the school day have shown small positive effects on growth and cognition (Kristjansson et al., 2009). In higher income countries, as obesity and cardiovascular disease have increased, the health behavior of interest has shifted from providing students adequate caloric intake to promoting specific components of healthy eating in the school setting. Interventions designed to improve the healthfulness of foods and beverages served and available in schools have been successful. For instance, increases in water access have demonstrated great success. A group randomized controlled trial among after-school programs that serve school-provided snacks increased servings of water to children (Giles et al., 2012); a study of water fountain installation in German public schools showed positive effects on risk of overweight at follow-up (Muckelbauer et al., 2009); and installation of water jets on the cafeteria line has demonstrated evidence for effectiveness in reducing obesity rates (Kenney et al., 2015). In contrast to primary and secondary schools, the food environment in colleges and university is consistently associated with adverse poor dietary behaviors and weight gain (Bailey et al., 2020).

Physical education is another keystone of the school system that promotes healthy behaviors among students. Interventions to improve physical education have found some increases in child activity levels and fitness (McKenzie et al., 2004), as have after-school programs such as the Out-of-School Nutrition and Physical Activity (OSNAP) initiative that train staff to make health-promoting practice and policy changes (Cradock et al., 2015), and after-school sports have also been shown to contribute positively to students' physical activity in youth and adulthood (Bailey, 2006).

Other practice and environmental changes that have been effective at creating health behavior change in schools include delaying school start times to improve adolescents' sleep (Owens et al., 2010), interventions that promote physical activity via active recess with schoolyard improvements (Anthamatten et al., 2011), and walking to school with improved infrastructure around school grounds (Boarnet et al., 2005).

POLICY

Any regulations implemented at the national, state, district, or school level intended to promote children's health in schools are considered policies. At the local school and district level, research has shown that tobacco policies that are comprehensive and strictly enforced can decrease smoking behavior (Evans-Whipp et al., 2004), while school policies mandating nutrition guidelines can increase fruit and vegetable consumption, among other healthy eating behaviors (Jaime & Lock, 2009). Policies to promote healthy behavior even reach to the level of national policy. The passage of the Healthy Hunger-Free Kids Act (https://www.congress.gov/bill/111th-congress/senate-bill/3307), which strengthens the health requirements for the nutritional quality of foods and beverages served as school meals and competitive foods, is one example of such policy. This federal act of the U.S. Department of Agriculture in 2010 increased the school lunch reimbursement rate and streamlined processes to improve access of reduced price and free meals and after-school snacks to low-income students. Furthermore, updated school meal standards required access to drinking water at meals; increases in fruits, vegetables, and whole grains served; and reductions in sodium and sugar content. As noted above, there is good evidence that aspects of the Healthy Hunger-Free Kids Act are cost-effective strategies to reduce childhood obesity (Kenney et al., 2020).

The COVID-19 pandemic has highlighted the importance of policies to control the spread of infectious disease in schools. One strategy that has proven very cost-effective in the past is mandated vaccination (Walsh et al., 2016). All states have some vaccine requirements for school entry, and national programs provide financial resources for child vaccines. Consequently, vaccination rates are quite high, and inequities have narrowed over time. However, adoption of the COVID-19 vaccine has been highly politicized, and initial implementation has been poor, with some states barring vaccine requirements.

MULTICOMPONENT

Multicomponent health behavior interventions are any strategies that contain two or more of the intervention types detailed above; this could include a curriculum that is implemented in conjunction with changes to the practices and environment within a school, or a state policy that mandates implementation of clinical services for a high-risk population of students in the school setting. Planet Health is a successful example of a multicomponent schools-based interventions designed to improve child physical activity and nutrition behaviors for the prevention of child obesity (Franckle et al., 2017; Gortmaker et al., 1999). In Planet Health, educational and skill-building lessons promoting healthy changes in nutrition and physical activity behaviors were accompanied by changes to the physical education lessons and practices delivered in the school. The results showed that these two strategies reduced television viewing and increased fruit and vegetable consumption among middle school students; the prevalence of obesity among girls decreased (Franckle et al., 2017; Gortmaker et al., 1999), as did disordered weight control behaviors (Austin et al., 2005). Similar multicomponent obesity prevention efforts have been successful at creating behavior change in after-school settings as well. The OSNAP initiative, which utilized a combination of learning collaborative trainings with program staff to change practices at their programs to provide healthier snacks and opportunities for more physical activity, along with an evidence-based education curriculum (https://www.hsph.harvard.edu /prc/projects/food-fun/), yielded increases in daily vigorous physical activity and improvements in diet among elementary school-age children (Cradock et al., 2015; Lee et al., 2018). Safer Choices is an excellent demonstration of a multicomponent intervention designed to address students' sexual health risk behaviors (Coyle et al., 1999). The results indicate that this intervention that uses five components—school health promotion councils at the school organization level, curriculum and staff development, peer leadership, parent education, and activities to connect students to services within their community—increased condom and contraceptive usage (Coyle et al., 1999; Kirby et al., 2004). Additionally, SunSafe is a community-based program that brought schools together with recreation departments, coaches, and primary care clinicians to successfully improve sun-protective behaviors (Olson et al., 2007). Finally, a multicomponent asthma intervention that provided individual education to students, support for linking parents and students to physicians and nurses, and a school action committee has proven effective at improving young children's self-management behaviors (Bartholomew et al., 2006).

CHALLENGES IN WORKING WITH SCHOOLS

The first, and probably most evident, challenge for those hoping to promote healthy behaviors within schools is the fact that school's primary mission is learning. All patient-centered health initiatives, health education, behavioral health interventions, system and environmental change efforts, and health policies should be designed to align with current school practices and mission to be most effective and sustainable over time. Interventions that explicitly aim to promote academic objectives, such as building skills in reading, writing, and math, while working to meet health goals will likely achieve the most support from teachers and school administrators (Gortmaker et al., 1999).

It is also important that school-based interventions are designed to be easily adaptable across a range of school norms and cultures. This flexibility allows for local relevance that is also essential for buy-in from teachers, parents, students, and administrators. For example, nutrition interventions should allow for adaptation based on differences in the types of whole grains and produce that have the best cultural fit with the diets of the school population. Emphasizing the healthy choices available in people's regular diet, such as serving corn tortillas over refined grain options in a school that predominately serves youth who are Latinx, may have more acceptability than introducing unfamiliar whole grains such as quinoa or bulgur to a school menu. Intervention implementation should also take into account the infrastructure of school buildings to ensure success. For instance, the aging water fixtures may influence the feasibility of implementing drinking water interventions in schools (Kenney, Daly et al., 2019).

Traditionally, there has been a limited focus on the cost of different strategies in school settings, and a limited research base for the cost-effectiveness of strategies (Levin, 2001). Promoting health in public schools where budgets are tight and resources must be allocated carefully is particularly challenging, and cost-effectiveness analysis can be seen as an important tool for making health promotion appealing to education leaders, teachers, policy makers, and taxpayers. Interventions that have a broad reach and make use of existing personnel and infrastructure can be particularly cost-effective and may even be cost-saving in the long run

(Vos et al., 2010). One example of this type of cost-effective strategy is the middle school nutrition and physical activity curriculum Planet Health, which weaves grade and subject-specific lessons into existing class time, is led by classroom teachers, and requires minimal materials to implement (Gortmaker et al., 1999; Wang et al., 2003). Providing drinking water in school lunch settings has also been found to be a very cost-effective strategy (Kenney, Cradock et al., 2019). A number of school-based physical activity interventions have likewise been identified as exhibiting good cost-effectiveness outcomes (Cradock et al., 2017).

With instability of resources, schools often depend on grant funding that can lead to continuous adoption of new interventions and limit the opportunity for sustainment of effective interventions. Intentional deimplementation is also an important consideration when interventions are found to be ineffective or potentially harmful (McKay et al., 2018; Poole, Lee et al., 2023). For instance, schools have attempted to charge nurses with tackling the prevention of obesity—measuring body mass index that becomes part of a "report card" with tailored information and advice for behavior change delivered to all parents with the weight status of their children, with limited success and potential for initiating harmful disordered eating behaviors (Poole, Gortmaker et al., 2023). While cost is a major challenge for creating change in educational settings, thoughtful planning and prioritization, along with data on cost-effectiveness, population impact, and impact on disparities, can help ensure the right interventions are implemented for optimal impact on the health of all students.

FUTURE DIRECTIONS

Although this overview demonstrates that there are numerous effective strategies for promoting healthy behaviors in schools, there is still much room to advance the field and make the most out of the school setting. As researchers are developing new school-based health interventions, they should apply community-engaged research principles to involve students, teachers, parents, administrators, and other school personnel as partners in all stages of the research process (Israel et al., 1998). They use their real-world experience to help researchers determine if they are asking the right questions, designing and testing suitable interventions, and interpreting results appropriately. School-based health interventions developed using community-engaged principles are likely to address equity considerations, meet the needs of teachers, and fit better into the daily practices of schools. Furthermore, health behavior change strategies designed with early feedback from partners have promise in making a sustained impact on child health over time.

Because health is not the first priority in schools, funds, resources, and staff time must first go toward academic subjects. Finding additional cost-effective strategies across health outcomes for supporting behavior change is an important area for future research that can potentially promote long term buy-in among school administrators and policy makers. Cost-effectiveness analyses identify some best value-for-money strategies; this includes studies of specific programs like Planet Health (Wang et al., 2003), the Project Toward No Tobacco Use (Wang et al., 2001), and the Safer Choices sexual health intervention (Wang et al., 2000). In addition, comparative effectiveness studies have recently documented how some interventions, like policy changes including water jets on school lunch, can be very cost-effective strategies (Kenney, Cradock et al., 2019).

The science of dissemination and implementation is an emerging field of research that needs further application in the study of school-based health initiatives. This is particularly important given the striking finding that less than 3% of U.S. schools report implementing evidence-based wellness interventions (Kenney et al., 2017). Studying dissemination and implementation shifts the focus from determining the efficacy of school-based interventions to investigating whether (and how) intervention can be implemented as intended by school personnel and maintained over time (Lee et al., 2023). Researchers looking specifically at school-based interventions have determined that factors related to the intervention design, such as its cost and time, the quality and amount of training required, and how well the

18 • SCHOOL INTERVENTIONS TO SUPPORT HEALTH BEHAVIOR CHANGE

intervention is standardized and incorporated into typical school practices, influence its effectiveness (Payne & Eckert, 2010). Factors beyond the intervention, such as the characteristics of the teacher or other school personnel (e.g., years of experience, motivation, education level), may also influence effectiveness in schools (Payne & Eckert, 2010). Looking beyond the classroom, researchers have also investigated how school and external community factors influence the success of health behavior interventions in schools (Payne & Eckert, 2010). The field of dissemination and implementation science is new and growing; future research is needed to understand the degree to which each of these types of factors influences health behavior change intervention success.

CASE STUDY 18.2: NATIONAL POLICY TO PROMOTE HEALTH

The Child and Adult Care Food Program (CACFP) is a national program administered by the U.S. Department of Agriculture Food and Nutrition Service. The CACFP provides reimbursements for nutritious meals and snacks served to over four million children who are enrolled in early childcare settings and after-school programs (USDA, 2023). The program addresses equity by providing higher reimbursements to settings that serve a greater number of children from households with lower incomes. The CACFP programs have healthier environments and local site policies compared with programs that do not participate (Kenney et al., 2023). Some studies have shown benefits of the program on dietary quality outcomes, such as serving and consumption of fruits, vegetables, and whole grains, as well as food insecurity (Kenney et al., 2023).

SUMMARY KEY POINTS

- Promoting health behavior change within the school setting is an excellent approach to impacting population health because the setting reaches many people and helps establish healthy behaviors early in life.

- Researchers and practitioners should attend to the issues of differential school resources and adaptation needs to ensure equity in school-based health intervention implementation.

- Promoting healthy behaviors in schools can take many forms across levels of delivery, ranging from patient-focused intervention to policy strategies.

- Many health behaviors have been successfully addressed through school-based interventions, including mental and behavioral health, nutrition and physical activity, contraceptive and pregnancy care, vaccination, and substance use.

- School-based health behavior change interventions should be designed to align with school practices and focus on learning to be most effective, acceptable, and sustainable.

DISCUSSION QUESTIONS

1. Think back to your childhood and your experience in school. What messages did you receive about health? What was your school environment's impact on your health behavior?

2. Consider the role of schools in a child's health along with the role of the parents. Can you imagine any scenarios where what the school considers to be in the best interest of the child's health is at odds with the beliefs of the parent or vice versa? What would be some examples? In these cases, what is in the best interest of the child?

(continued)

DISCUSSION QUESTIONS (continued)

3. Was there a nurse's office when you attended school? If so, what was the role of the nurse? Did you and other students feel the health center at your school was a valuable resource? If there was not a nurse at your school, how do you think that impacted your school life?

4. Consider your own community, either where you grew up, where you live now, or another place where you once lived. What are the most pressing concerns about school-age children in this community? Do you feel the school environment adequately addresses these concerns? If not, what more could be done? What obstacles would you imagine could be in the way to making programs more effective?

5. If you were to implement a school-based health behavior change intervention in a school setting from your past, what would it be and why?

 A robust set of instructor resources designed to supplement this text is located at http://connect.springerpub.com/content/book/978-0-8261-4265-8. Qualifying instructors may request access by emailing textbook@springerpub.com.

REFERENCES

Anthamatten, P., Brink, L., Lampe, S., Greenwood, E., Kingston, B., & Nigg, C. (2011). An assessment of schoolyard renovation strategies to encourage children's physical activity. *International Journal of Behavioral Nutrition and Physical Activity, 8*(1), 27. https://doi.org/10.1186/1479-5868-8-27

Austin, S. B., Field, A. E., Wiecha, J., Peterson, K. E., & Gortmaker, S. L. (2005). The impact of a school-based obesity prevention trial on disordered weight-control behaviors in early adolescent girls. *Archives Pediatrics & Adolescent Medicine, 159*(3), 225–230. https://doi.org/10.1001/archpedi.159.3.225

Bailey, C. P., Sharma, S., Economos, C. D., Hennessy, E., Simon, C., & Hatfield, D. P. (2020). College campuses' influence on student weight and related behaviours: A review of observational and intervention research. *Obesity Science Practice, 6*(6), 694–707. https://doi.org/10.1002/osp4.445

Bailey R. (2006, Oct). Physical education and sport in schools: a review of benefits and outcomes. *Journal of School Health, 76*(8), 397–401. https://doi.org/10.1111/j.1746-1561.2006.00132.x

Bandura, A. (1989). Human agency in social cognitive theory. *The American Psychologist, 44*(9), 1175–1184. https://doi.org/10.1037/0003-066x.44.9.1175

Bartholomew, L. K., Sockrider, M. M., Abramson, S. L., Swank, P. R., Czyzewski, D. I., Tortolero, S. R., Markham, C. M., Fernandez, M. E., Shegog, R., & Tyrrell, S. (2006). Partners in school asthma management: Evaluation of a self-management program for children with asthma. *Journal of School Health, 76*(6), 283–290. https://doi.org/10.1111/j.1746-1561.2006.00113.x

Boarnet, M. G., Anderson, C. L., Day, K., McMillan, T., & Alfonzo, M. (2005). Evaluation of the California Safe Routes to School legislation–Urban form changes and children's active transportation to school. *American Journal of Preventive Medicine, 28*(2), 134–140. https://doi.org/10.1016/j.amepre.2004.10.026

Botvin, G. J., Baker, E., Dusenbury, L., Botvin, E. M., & Diaz, T. (1995). Long-term follow-up results of a randomized drug abuse prevention trial in a white middle-class population. *JAMA, 273*(14), 1106–1112.

Bruns, E. J., Duong, M. T., Lyon, A. R., Pullmann, M. D., Cook, C. R., Cheney, D., & McCauley, E. (2016). Fostering SMART partnerships to develop an effective continuum of behavioral health services and supports in schools. *The American Journal of Orthopsychiatry, 86*(2), 156–170. https://doi.org/10.1037/ort0000083

Buller, D. B., Taylor, A. M., Buller, M. K., Powers, P. J., Maloy, J. A., & Beach, B. H. (2006). Evaluation of the sunny days, healthy ways sun safety curriculum for children in kindergarten through fifth grade. *Pediatric Dermatology, 23*(4), 321–329. https://doi.org/10.1111/j.1525-1470.2006.00270.x

CASEL. (2022). *Program guide CASEL: Collaborative for academic social and emotional learning*. Program Guide. https://pg.casel.org/

Centers for Disease Control and Prevention. (2023). *Whole School, whole community, whole child (WSCC)*. https://www.cdc.gov/healthyschools/wscc/index.htm

Chafouleas, S., Koriakin, T., Roundfield, K., & Overstreet, S. (2019). Addressing childhood trauma in school settings: A framework for evidence-based practice. *School Mental Health, 11*(1), 40–53. https://doi.org/10.1007/s12310-018-9256-5

Child Care State Systems Specialist Network. (2014). *Federal and state funding for child care and early learning.* https://childcareta.acf.hhs.gov/sites/default/files/federal_and_state_funding_for_child_care_and_early_learning_edited.pdf

Cirrin, F. M., Schooling, T. L., Nelson, N. W., Diehl, S. F., Flynn, P. F., Staskowski, M., Torrey, T, Z., & Adamczyk, D. F. (2010). Evidence-based systematic review: Effects of different service delivery models on communication outcomes for elementary school-age children. *Language Speech and Hearing Services in Schools, 41*(3), 233–264. https://doi.org/10.1044/0161-1461(2009/08-0128)

Cohen, A. K., & Syme, S. L. (2013). Education: A missed opportunity for public health intervention. *American Journal of Public Health, 103*(6), 997–1001. https://doi.org/10.2105/ajph.2012.300993

Community Preventive Services Task Force. (2021). *Physical activity: Classroom-based physical activity break interventions.* https://www.thecommunityguide.org/findings/physical-activity-classroom-based-physical-activity-break-interventions

Coyle, K., Basen-Engquist, K., Kirby, D., Parcel, G., Banspach, S., Harrist, R., Baumler, M., & Weil, M. (1999). Short-term impact of safer choices: A multicomponent, school-based HIV, other STD, and pregnancy prevention program. *Journal of School Health, 69*(5), 181–188. https://doi.org/10.1111/j.1746-1561.1999.tb06383.x

Cradock, A. L., Barrett, J. L., Giles, C. M., Lee, R. M., Kenney, E. L., deBlois, M. E., Thayer, J. C., & Gortmaker, S. L. (2015). Promoting physical activity with the out of school nutrition and physical activity (OSNAP) initiative: A cluster-randomized controlled trial. *JAMA Pediatrics, 170*(2), 1–9. https://doi.org/10.1001/jamapediatrics.2015.3406

Cradock, A. L., Barrett, J. L., Kenney, E. L., Giles, C. M., Ward, Z. J., Long, M. W., Resch, S. C., Pipito, A. A., Wei, E. R., & Gortmaker, S. L. (2017). Using cost-effectiveness analysis to prioritize policy and programmatic approaches to physical activity promotion and obesity prevention in childhood. *Preventive Medicine, 95*, S17–S27. https://doi.org/10.1016/j.ypmed.2016.10.017

Crean, H. F., & Johnson, D. B. (2013). Promoting Alternative Thinking Strategies (PATHS) and elementary school aged children's aggression: Results from a cluster randomized trial. *American Journal of Community Psychology, 52*(1–2), 56–72. https://doi.org/10.1007/s10464-013-9576-4

Diamond, A., & Lee, K. (2011). Interventions shown to aid executive function development in children 4 to 12 years old. *Science, 333*(6045), 959–964. https://doi.org/10.1126/science.1204529

Epperson, A. (2019). *What is MTSS? PBIS rewards.* https://www.pbisrewards.com/blog/what-is-mtss/

Evans-Whipp, T., Beyers, J. M., Lloyd, S., Lafazia, A. N., Toumbourou, J. W., Arthur, M. W., & Catalano, R. F. (2004). A review of school drug policies and their impact on youth substance use. *Health Promotion. International, 19*(2), 227–234. https:doi.org/10.1093/heapro/dah210

Faggiano, F., Vigna-Taglianti, F. D., Versino, E., Zambon, A., Borraccino, A., & Lemma, P. (2008, May). School-based prevention for illicit drugs use: A systematic review. *Preventive Medicine, 46*(5), 385–396. https://doi.org/10.1016/j.ypmed.2007.11.012

Franckle, R. L., Falbe, J., Gortmaker, S., Barrett, J. L., Giles, C., Ganter, C., Blaine, R. E., Buszkiewicz, J., Taveras, E. M., Kwass, J. A., & Land, T. (2017). Student obesity prevalence and behavioral outcomes for the Massachusetts childhood obesity research demonstration project. *Obesity, 25*(7), 1175–1182. https://doi.org/10.1002/oby.21867

Giles, C. M., Kenney, E. L., Gortmaker, S. L., Lee, R. M., Thayer, J. C., Mont-Ferguson, H., & Cradock, A. L. (2012). Increasing water availability during afterschool snack evidence, strategies, and partnerships from a group randomized trial. *American Journal of Preventive Medicine, 43*(3), S136–S142. https://doi.org/10.1016/j.amepre.2012.05.013

Gortmaker, S. L., Peterson, K., Wiecha, J., Sobol, A. M., Dixit, S., Fox, M. K., & Laird, N. (1999). Reducing obesity via a school-based interdisciplinary intervention among youth: Planet Health. *Archives of Pediatrics & Adolescent Medicine, 153*(4), 409–418. https://doi.org/10.1001/archpedi.153.4.409

Government of India Ministry of Health & Family Welfare. (2017, March 3). *School health programme.* http://www.mohfw.nic.in/index1.php?lang=1&level=2&sublinkid=667&lid=658

Hill, K. G., Bailey, J. A., Steeger, C. M., Hawkins, J. D., Catalano, R. F., Kosterman, R., Epstein, M., & Abbott, R. D. (2020). Outcomes of childhood preventive intervention across 2 generations: A nonrandomized controlled trial. *JAMA Pediatrics, 174*(8), 764–771. https://doi.org/10.1001/jamapediatrics.2020.1310

Israel, B. A., Schulz, A. J., Parker, E. A., & Becker, A. B. (1998). Review of community-based research: Assessing partnership approaches to improve public health. *Annual Review Public Health, 19*, 173–202. https://doi.org/10.1146/annurev.publhealth.19.1.173

Jackson, C. C., Albanese-O'Neill, A., Butler, K. L., Chiang, J. L., Deeb, L. C., Hathaway, K., Kraus, E., Weissberg-Benchell, J., Yatvin, A. L., & Siminerio, L. M. (2015). Diabetes care in the school setting: A position statement of the American diabetes association. *Diabetes Care, 38*(10), 1958–1963. https://doi.org/10.2337/dc15-1418

370 IV • INTERVENING IN SETTINGS AND SYSTEMS TO MODIFY HEALTH BEHAVIORS

Jaime, P. C., & Lock, K. (2009). Do school based food and nutrition policies improve diet and reduce obesity? *Preventive Medicine, 48*(1), 45–53. https://doi.org/10.1016/j.ypmed.2008.10.018

Kenney, E. L., Barrett, J. L., Bleich, S. N., Ward, Z. J., Cradock, A. L., & Gortmaker, S. L. (2020). Impact of the healthy, hunger-free kids act on obesity trends. *Health Affairs (Millwood), 39*(7), 1122–1129. https://doi.org/10.1377/hlthaff.2020.00133. Erratum in: Health Aff (Millwood). (2020) Sep; 39(9): 1650.

Kenney, E. L., Cradock, A. L., Long, M. W., Barrett, J. L., Giles, C. M., Ward, Z. J., & Gortmaker, S. L. (2019). Cost-effectiveness of water promotion strategies in schools for preventing childhood obesity and increasing water intake. *Obesity (Silver Spring), 27*(12), 2037–2045. https://doi.org/10.1002/oby.22615

Kenney, E. L., Daly, J. G., Lee, R. M., Mozaffarian, R. S., Walsh, K., Carter, J., & Gortmaker, S. L. (2019). Providing students with adequate school drinking water access in an era of aging infrastructure: A mixed methods investigation. *International Journal of Environmental Resarch and Public Health, 17*(1), 62. https://doi.org/10.3390/ijerph17010062

Kenney, E. L., Gortmaker, S. L., Carter, J. E., Howe, M. C., Reiner, J. F., & Cradock, A. L. (2015). Grab a cup, fill it up! An intervention to promote the convenience of drinking water and increase student water consumption during school lunch. *American Journal of Public Health, 105*(9), 1777–1783. https://doi.org/10.2105/AJPH.2015.302645

Kenney, E. L., Tucker, K. T., Plummer, R. S., Mita, C., & Andreyeva, T. (2023). The child and adult care food program and young children's health: A systematic review. *Nutriton Reviews, 81*(11), 1402–1413. https://doi.org/10.1093/nutrit/nuad016

Kenney, E. L., Wintner, S., Lee, R. M., & Austin, S. B. (2017). Obesity prevention interventions in US public schools: Are schools using programs that promote weight stigma? *Preventing Chronic Disease, 14*, E142. https://doi.org/10.5888/pcd14.160605

Kirby, D. B., Baumler, E., Coyle, K. K., Basen-Engquist, K., Parcel, G. S., Harrist, R., & Banspach, S. W. (2004). The "Safer choices" intervention: Its impact on the sexual behaviors of different subgroups of high school students. *Journal of Adolescent Health, 35*(6), 442–452. https://doi.org/10.1016/j.jadohealth.2004.02.006

Knopf, J. A., Finnie, R. K., Peng, Y., Hahn, R. A., Truman, B. I., Vernon-Smiley, M., Johnson, V. C., Johnson, R. L., Fielding, J. E., Muntaner, C., Hunt, P. C., Phyllis Jones, C., Fullilove, M. T., & Community Preventive Services Task Force. (2016). School-based health centers to advance health equity: A community guide systematic review. *American Journal of Preventive Medicine, 51*(1), 114–126. https://doi.org/10.1016/j.amepre.2016.01.009

Kristjansson, B., P. M., MacDonald, B., Krasevec, J., Janzen, L., Greenhalgh, T., Wells, G. A., MacGowan, J., Farmer, A. P., Shea, B., Mayhew, A., Tugwell, P., & Welch, V. (2009). School feeding for improving the physical and psychosocial health of disadvantaged students. *The Cochrane Library*, (1), CD004676. https://doi.org/10.1002/14651858.CD004676.pub2

Langford, R., Bonell, C., Jones, H., Pouliou, T., Murphy, S., Waters, E., Komro, K., Gibbs, L., Magnus, D., & Campbell, R. (2015). The World Health Organization's Health Promoting Schools framework: A Cochrane systematic review and meta-analysis. *BMC Public Health, 15*(1), 130. https://doi.org/10.1186/s12889-015-1360-y

Lattie, E. G., Adkins, E. C., Winquist, N., Stiles-Shields, C., Wafford, Q. E., & Graham, A. K. (2019). Digital mental health interventions for depression, anxiety, and enhancement of psychological well-being among college students: Systematic review. *Journal of Medical Internet Research, 21*(7), e12869. https://doi.org/10.2196/12869

Lee, R. M., Eisman A. B., & Gortmaker, S. L. (2023). Health dissemination and implementation within Schools. In R. C. Brownson, G. A. Colditz, & E. K. Proctor (Eds.), *Dissemination and implementation research in health: Translating science to practice* (3rd ed.). Oxford University Press.

Lee, R. M., Giles, C. M., Cradock, A. L., Emmons, K. M., Okechukwu, C., Kenney, E. L., Thayer, J., & Gortmaker, S. L. (2018). Impact of the Out-of-School Nutrition and Physical Activity (OSNAP) group randomized controlled trial on children's food, beverage, and calorie consumption among snacks served. *Journal of the Academy of Nutrition and Dietetics, 118*(8), 1425–1437. https://doi.org/10.1016/j.jand.2018.04.011

Levin, H. M., & McEwan, P. J. (2001). *Cost-effectiveness analysis: Methods and applications*. Vol. 4. Sage.

Lewallen, T. C., Hunt, H., Potts-Datema, W., Zaza, S., & Giles, W. (2015). The whole school, whole community, whole child model: A new approach for improving educational attainment and healthy development for students. *Journal of School Health, 85*(11), 729–739. https://doi.org/10.1111/josh.12310

McKay, V. R., Morshed, A. B., Brownson, R. C., Proctor, E. K., & Prusaczyk, B. (2018). Letting go: Conceptualizing intervention de-implementation in public health and social service settings. *American Journal of Community Psychology, 62*(1–2), 189–202. https://doi.org/10.1002/ajcp.12258

McKenzie, T. L., Sallis, J. F., Prochaska, J. J., Conway, T. L., Marshall, S. J., & Rosengard, P. (2004). Evaluation of a two-year middle-school physical education intervention: M-SPAN. *Medicine and Science in Sports and Exercise, 36*(8), 1382–1388. https://doi.org/10.1249/01.mss.0000135792.20358.4d

Muckelbauer, R., Libuda, L., Clausen, K., Toschke, A. M., Reinehr, T., & Kersting, M. (2009). Promotion and provision of drinking water in schools for overweight prevention: Randomized, controlled cluster trial. *Pediatrics, 123*(4), e661–e667. https:doi.org/10.1542/peds.2008-2186

National Center for Education Statistics. (2017). *Public school revenue sources.* https://nces.ed.gov/programs/coe/indicator_cma.asp

National Center for HIV/AIDS, Viral Hepatitis, STD, and TB Prevention, & Division of Adolescent & School Health. (2014). *Results from the school health policies and practices study.* https://www.cdc.gov/healthyyouth/data/shpps/results.htm

National Center on Response to Intervention. (2010). *Essential components of RTI–A closer look at response to intervention.* U.S. Department of Education, Office of Special Education Programs.

Neil, A. L., & Christensen, H. (2009). Efficacy and effectiveness of school-based prevention and early intervention programs for anxiety. *Clinical Psychology Review, 29*(3), 208–215. https://doi.org/10.1016/j.cpr.2009.01.002

Olson, A. L., Gaffney, C., Starr, P., Gibson, J. J., Cole, B. F., & Dietrich, A. J. (2007). SunSafe in the middle school years: A community-wide intervention to change early-adolescent sun protection. *Pediatrics, 119*(1), e247–e256. https://doi.org/10.1542/peds.2006-1579

O'Neill, J., Clark, J., & Jones, J. (2011). Promoting mental health and preventing substance abuse and violence in elementary students: A randomized control study of the Michigan Model for Health. *The Journal for School Health, 81*(6), 320–330. https://doi.org/10.1111/j.1746-1561.2011.00597.x

Oringanje, C., Meremikwu, M. M., Eko, H., Esu, E., Meremikwu, A., & Ehir, I. J. E. (2010). Interventions for preventing unintended pregnancies among adolescents. *The Cochrane Library,* (2), CD005215. https://doi.org/10.1002/14651858.cd005215.pub3

Owen, R., Kendrick, D., Mulvaney, C., Coleman, T., & Royal, S. (2011). Non-legislative interventions for the promotion of cycle helmet wearing by children. *Cochrane Database of Systematic Reviews,* (11), CD003985. https://doi.org/10.1002/14651858.cd003985.pub3

Owens, J. A., Belon, K., & Moss, P. (2010). Impact of delaying school start time on adolescent sleep, mood, and behavior. *Archives of Pediatrics & Adolescent Medicine, 164*(7), 608–614. https://doi.org/10.1001/archpediatrics.2010.96

Payne, A. A., & Eckert, R. (2010). The relative importance of provider, program, school, and community predictors of the implementation quality of school-based prevention programs. *Prevention Science, 11*(2), 126–141. https://doi.org/10.1007/s11121-009-0157-6

Pincus, T., Callahan, L. F., & Burkhauser, R. V. (1987). Most chronic diseases are reported more frequently by individuals with fewer than 12 years of formal education in the age 18–64 United-States population. *Journal of Chronic Diseases, 40*(9), 865–874. https:doi.org/10.1016/0021-9681(87)90186-x

Poole, M. K., Gortmaker, S. L., Barrett, J. L., McCulloch, S. M., Rimm, E. B., Emmons, K. M., Ward, Z. J., & Kenney, E. L. (2023). The societal costs and health impacts on obesity of BMI report cards in US schools. *Obesity (Silver Spring), 31*(8), 2110–2118. https:doi.org/10.1002/oby.23788

Poole, M. K., Lee, R. M., Kinderknecht, K. L., & Kenney, E. L. (2023). De-implementing public health policies: A qualitative study of the process of implementing and then removing body mass index (BMI) report cards in Massachusetts public schools. *Implementation Science Communications, 4*(1), 63. https://doi.org/10.1186/s43058-023-00443-1

Ran, T., Chattopadhyay, S. K., Hahn, R. A., & Community Preventive Serv Task, F. (2016). Economic evaluation of school-based health centers a community guide systematic review. *American Journal of Preventive Medicine, 51*(1), 129–138. https://doi.org/10.1016/j.amepre.2016.01.017

Riggs, N. R., Spruijt-zetz, D., Chou, C. P., & Pentz, M. A. (2012). Relationships between executive cognitive function and lifetime substance use and obesity-related behaviors in fourth grade youth. *Child Neuropsychology, 18*(1), 1–11. https://doi.org/10.1080/09297049.2011.555759

Rosenstock, I. M. (1974). Historical origins of the health belief model. *Health Education Monographs, 2*(4), 328–335. https://doi.org/10.1177/109019817400200403

Schools for Health in Europe. (n.d.). Improving the health of children and young people in the European region and central Asia. https://www.schoolsforhealth.org/

Shope, J., Copeland, L., Maharg, R., & Dielman, T. (1996). Effectiveness of a high school alcohol misuse prevention program. *Alcoholism Clinical and Experimental Research, 20*(5), 791–798. https://doi.org/10.1111/j.1530-0277.1996.tb05253.x

Spoth, R. L., Randall, G. K., Trudeau, L., Shin, C., & Redmond, C. (2008). Substance use outcomes 5½ years past baseline for partnership-based, family-school preventive interventions. *Drug and Alcohol Dependence, 96*(1–2), 57–68. https://doi.org/10.1016/j.drugalcdep.2008.01.023

Stice, E., Rohde, P., Seeley, J. R., & Gau, J. M. (2008). Brief cognitive-behavioral depression prevention program for high-risk adolescents outperforms two alternative interventions: A randomized efficacy trial. *Journal of Consulting and Clinical Psychology, 76*(4), 595–606. https://doi.org/10.1037/a0012645

Stokols, D. (1996). Translating social ecological theory into guidelines for community health promotion. *American Journal of Health Promotion, 10*(4), 282–298. https://doi.org/10.4278/0890-1171-10.4.282

Taylor, R. D., Oberle, E., Durlak, J. A., & Weissberg, R. P. (2017). Promoting positive youth development through school-based social and emotional learning interventions: A meta-analysis of follow-up effects. *Child Development, 88*(4), 1156–1171. https://doi.org/10.1111/cdev.12864

Thomas, R., & Perera, R. (2008). School-based programmes for preventing smoking. *The Cochrane Library,*(4), CD001293. https://doi.org/10.1002/14651858.CD001293.pub3

USDA. (2023). Child and adult care food program. https://www.fns.usda.gov/cacfp

Vos, T., Carter, R., Barendregt, J., Mihalopoulos, C., Veerman, J., Magnus, A., Wallance, A., & for the ACE–Prevention team (2010). *Assessing Cost-Effectiveness in Prevention (ACE–Prevention): Final report.* https://public-health.uq.edu.au/files/571/ACE-Prevention_final_report.pdf

Walsh, B., Doherty, E., & O'Neill, C. (2016). Since the start of the vaccines for children program, uptake has increased, and most disparities have decreased. *Health Affairs (Millwood), 35*(2), 356–364. https://doi.org/10.1377/hlthaff.2015.1019

Wang, L. Y., Crossett, L. S., Lowry, R., Sussman, S., & Dent, C. W. (2001). Cost-effectiveness of a school-based tobacco-use prevention program. *Archives Pediatrics & Adolescent Medicine, 155*(9), 1043–1050. https://doi.org/10.1001/archpedi.155.9.1043

Wang, L. Y., Davis, M., Robin, L., Collins, J., Coyle, K., & Baumler, E. (2000). Economic evaluation of Safer Choices: A school-based human immunodeficiency virus, other sexually transmitted diseases, and pregnancy prevention program. *Archives Pediatrics & Adolescent Medicine, 154*(10), 1017–1024. https://doi.org/10.1001/archpedi.154.10.1017

Wang, L. Y., Yang, Q., Lowry R., & Wechsler, H. (2023). Economic analysis of a school-based obesity prevention program. *Obesity Research, 11*(11), 1313–1324. https://doi.org/10.1038/oby.2003.178

Wilson, S. J., Lipsey, M. W., & Derzon, J. H. (2003). The effects of school-based intervention programs on aggressive behavior: A meta-analysis. *Journal of Consulting and Clinical Psychology, 71*(1), 136–149.

CHAPTER 19

CHRONIC DISEASE PREVENTION IN THE WORKSITE

ELIZABETH ABLAH, MARY T. IMBODEN, AND ANNA L. ZENDELL

LEARNING OBJECTIVES

- Improve policies, programs, services, and organizational performance.
- Identify factors that affect the health of a worksite.
- Explain how systems, policies, and programs at a worksite are associated with behaviors associated with chronic disease.
- Describe strategies that engage individuals and teams to achieve worksite health goals.

TERMINOLOGY

In this chapter, we predominantly use the term *worksite* to refer to an organization or business where work occurs. This is in contrast to "workplace," which might suggest a facility on a specific property. We are cognizant of the significant growth in remote and hybrid work and therefore use "worksite" to reflect the organizations (whether industry, schools, hospitals, or local government) that employ the workforce.

THE WORKING POPULATION IN THE UNITED STATES

Adults in the U.S. workforce are ethnically and racially diverse. In 2020, the workforce consisted of workers who were White (77%), Latinx (18%), Black (13%), and Asian American (6%; Bureau of Labor Statistics [BLS], 2021a). The U.S. workforce is also diverse in age, with a higher percentage of older adults than in previous decades. Between 2000 and 2020, the percentage of employed workers older than 60 doubled among men and women (National Academies of Sciences, Engineering, and Medicine [NASEM], 2022). This is a result of the aging U.S. population, as well as changes in labor force participation at all ages, higher participation rates among those of older ages, and lower rates among those of younger ages.

Nearly 61% of those 16 years or older are in the civilian workforce, and many employed individuals spend a significant amount of their time at work. In recent decades, the workforce has shifted to include a larger proportion of sedentary occupations. Duffy et al. (2021) note that physically demanding occupations now constitute fewer than 20% of all jobs. Additionally, the location in which the employed population works has shifted in recent years. The onset of the COVID-19 pandemic precipitated a dramatic change in global business operations and employment strategies. One of the most notable changes for many employers was the rapid shift to a remote work environment. In the United States alone, the number of people working remotely has nearly tripled since 2019 (United States Census Bureau [USCB],

2022). At the close of 2022, an estimated 25% of all professional jobs in the United States were remote, and it is projected that the number of remote opportunities will continue to increase (BLS, 2021b; The Ladders, 2021). In 2022, 53% of U.S. workers were hybrid workers.

As a result of these changes, employers are reimagining their health and well-being initiatives. This is more important than ever as the stay-at-home orders and distress brought on by the pandemic led to harmful health behaviors, including poor nutrition and overeating, excessive sedentary behavior and lack of physical activity, increased consumption of alcohol and use of tobacco, as well as an increase in screen time, causing impaired sleep (Lange & Nakamura, 2020).

LEADING CAUSES OF MORBIDITY AND MORTALITY IN THE UNITED STATES

Chronic diseases such as heart disease, diabetes, and cancer have been the leading causes of death and disability in the United States for decades (Kava et al., 2022; National Center for Chronic Disease Prevention and Health Promotion [NCCDPHP], n.d.-b). These chronic conditions are also major contributors to the cost of health insurance premiums and employee medical claims; this is significant for employers since employer-based health insurance covers more than 54% of the U.S. population and employers typically pay into health insurance premiums (USCB, 2022). The aging workforce has contributed substantially to higher healthcare costs because many chronic conditions are more prevalent among older individuals. However, chronic disease is increasingly common among younger Americans, with more younger adults in the workforce living with cardiovascular conditions, obesity, and other chronic conditions than in prior generations (NCCDPHP, n.d.-b; Watson et al., 2022). Many chronic diseases are preventable through behavior modification of key chronic disease risks, including tobacco use, physical inactivity, poor nutrition, and stress (Moy et al., 2017).

WORKSITE AS A PRIORITY INTERVENTION SETTING FOR HEALTH

Given that many working adults spend most of their waking hours at work, worksite and occupational factors such as long hours, shift work, insufficient sleep, and high-demand, low-control work environments have a strong influence on employees' behaviors and health. The worksite offers an important opportunity to promote health behaviors among working adults, a substantial proportion of the U.S. adult population (Wong et al., 2019).

As a setting for implementing strategies to improve health behaviors, worksites offer several opportunities. Workplaces typically have organizational structures, internal communication mechanisms, shared physical spaces for work, or places where food and beverages are offered. All these can be used to support health. Common features to facilitate employee health include health insurance and other employee benefits, occupational health and safety departments, human resource departments with an employee health mission, interior and exterior physical plant attributes, and cafeterias and vending services, among others. Worksites have access to concentrated, sometimes large, and relatively stable populations of people who often share geographic proximity, as well as sociodemographic characteristics (Goetzel & Ozminkowski, 2008).

The worksite is also recognized as a priority setting for health promotion beyond employers. The U.S. Department of Health and Human Services (USDHHS) and the Office of Disease Prevention and Health Promotion established the Healthy People 2030 objectives to improve the health and well-being of the United States over the decade (USDHHS, n.d.) and track goals related to worksite wellness. These include strengthening the workforce by promoting health and well-being; increasing the proportion of worksites that offer employee health promotion, physical activity, and nutrition programs; and increasing the proportion of worksites with policies to ban indoor smoking. Several initiatives, such as the Centers for Disease Control and Prevention's (CDC) Workplace Health Promotion, the Community Guide to Preventive Services, and the U.S. National Physical Activity Plan also include worksite wellness recommendations (CDC, 2019; Community Preventive Services Task Force [CPSTF], 2023; Physical Activity Alliance [PAA], 2016).

RISK FACTORS FOR CHRONIC ILLNESS AT WORKSITES

Worksite and occupational factors can influence employees' behaviors and risk for developing or worsening chronic conditions. Worksites often constitute obesogenic environments. Many jobs worldwide are sedentary, often requiring high amounts of sitting or standing without adequate movement. Shifting trends over the decades have led to more workers driving or riding to and from work, with less active commuting like walking or biking. The large amount of time spent working indicates that a substantial number of calories are typically consumed while working, making dietary intake in the workplace critical to energy balance.

Since the COVID-19 pandemic, there has been a rise in remote and hybrid worksites, and the sedentary nature of work has increased even more. Since worksites pay for many expenses related to healthcare for approximately 55% of non-older adults (Congressional Research Services [CRS], 2023) and bear the impacts of chronic disease-related workforce costs and absences (Roemer et al., 2022), it is essential that worksites have opportunities and resources to implement best practices that will improve their employees' health and decrease healthcare costs.

The risk of chronic disease is inversely associated with income and education level, and populations of color experience the highest rates of chronic disease diagnoses and health disparities (National Institute of Allergy and Infectious Disease [NIAD], n.d.). Accordingly, by implementing practices that improve the healthfulness of worksites, employees' health can be improved, and healthcare costs can be reduced.

FOUR BEHAVIORS AND PREVENTION AT WORKSITES

It is well-established that three modifiable behaviors (i.e., not using tobacco, engaging in physical activity, and consuming nutritious foods) can prevent common and costly chronic diseases such as heart disease, diabetes, some cancers, and lung disease (Roemer et al., 2022). Additionally, it has been argued that a fourth behavior, the prevention and management of stress, must be addressed to promote health at work. For 70% of employed Americans, work serves as a significant source of stress (American Psychological Association [APA], 2020). Factors at work associated with stress include high work demands and low decision or perceived control over responsibilities, which is further exacerbated when employees experience low support from their supervisors (Bjornstadt, 2014). Other factors can include long hours, heavy workload, organizational changes, tight deadlines, job role changes, job insecurity, and a lack of promotional opportunity. Work that is boring or unrewarding, being under skilled for the job, being micromanaged, experiencing poor working conditions, or a lack of resources can all lead to vocational stress. Extreme situations such as discrimination, harassment, poor relationships with colleagues or leadership, or crisis incidents also lead to extreme stress.

Focus on promoting modifiable health behaviors by using comprehensive intervention strategies allows employers to create environments for their employees, where the default behavior they practice is healthy as a function of working in that space (Ablah et al., 2020). When employers create environments that support employees in practicing healthy behaviors, all employees benefit. Employees benefit regardless of whether or not they have a chronic disease, whether or not they are motivated to practice these behaviors, and whether or not they practice these behaviors elsewhere (Kahn-Marshall & Gallant, 2012). Everyone benefits from refraining from tobacco use, being physically active, and consuming healthy foods and beverages. Therefore, it is to the worksite's advantage, for the health of employees and the economic health of the worksite, to contribute to the development and maintenance of environments that prompt employees to practice these behaviors (Goetzel et al., 2019; Henke et al., 2019).

Moreover, prevention strategies are less expensive than treatment. Prevention strategies are perceived as positive, as they engage employees through messages of health rather than disease. Primary prevention strategies are preferred, as they reduce or eliminate the problem. Regarding stress, for instance, a manager may identify that an employee's skills and abilities differ considerably from their responsibilities. The manager can redesign the employee's work to improve fit and decrease stress. Secondary prevention strategies provide at-risk employees with tools to shield them from stress, such as stress management training. Tertiary prevention, which may be necessary if health and productivity have been impacted from prolonged exposure to stress, might include the provision and promotion of employee assistance programs (EAPs), especially for the associated mental and behavioral health benefits.

THE NEED FOR EQUITY

Even as the COVID-19 pandemic exposed stark disparities in our healthcare system, worksite inequities were more fully exposed, especially regarding socioeconomic status. According to the BLS (2022), more than six million people were considered working poor, making an income that falls below the official federal poverty level. Many employees earning low wages live a food- and housing-insecure existence. They may work overtime or juggle multiple jobs to support themselves and their families. In-person and hybrid employees may spend their breaks running errands, making phone calls, and other nonwork tasks, potentially limiting their ability to partake in work-based wellness initiatives. Part-time workers may lack health insurance, which forms the backbone of most health interventions in this country. To successfully establish and sustain a worksite wellness intervention, these concerns must be addressed. If not, employees who could derive the most benefit from the wellness programs may not be able to participate in a meaningful way.

For worksites that want to make a difference in the wellness of their workers, investing in boosting income, advancement opportunities, and health insurance with affordable premiums is an important precursor to successful worksite wellness programming. Leaders must ask their employees what they need and want to feel their best. For worksites that are struggling financially, this may need to be a process of incremental change from the top down.

CONSIDERATIONS FOR PLANNING AND IMPLEMENTING WELLNESS INTERVENTIONS

To establish effective and sustainable worksite wellness intervention programs that include engaging employees and management, several factors must be considered and planned prior to implementation. First and foremost, the work needs to be led by a wellness committee that is representative of employees at the worksite. Effective wellness committees must be diverse, representing different departments and management levels; different shifts, levels of interest in health, and work location; and employee race, ethnicity, age, and gender (Ablah et al., 2020; Duffy et al., 2021). The wellness committee is instrumental in planning and leading health initiatives.

Engagement and buy-in of upper management is essential. Midlevel and senior executives can provide support through words and action. Upper management is vital in the creation of the worksite's culture (Ablah et al., 2020; HERO Health, 2016) as they control funding and resource allocation that may be necessary to move the initiative forward. The wellness committee must be empowered by upper management to implement the committee's work plan as part of worksite operations.

It is best practice for worksites to identify at least one person whose position description includes wellness initiatives at the worksite. However, implementing and maintaining health and well-being initiatives in the workplace is a shared responsibility. Those in authority need to demonstrate support and commitment to the importance of the initiative. All employees can be a part of ongoing review and evaluation of initiatives to ensure that resources remain relevant and effective.

Moreover, other stakeholders, such as middle management and frontline workers, must be engaged. Stakeholder mapping can be a useful tool for wellness committees to identify potential stakeholders (O'Malley & Cebula, 2015). This process allows committees to identify their various stakeholders' personal or professional interests with respect to the topic (e.g., tobacco), the degree to which they are needed to ensure success of the initiative (from 1, not that important, to 10, which signifies they must be on board), and the details about who will engage these stakeholders and how they will be engaged. One common stakeholder group identified by worksites is employees who are not supportive of change or health initiatives. As negative comments are often "heard" louder than positive comments, worksite wellness committees often need to attend to feedback from the stakeholders garnering 8s, 9s, and 10s (whose engagement is required for the success of the initiative) and decide collectively when to adjust. Unless a negative comment originates from a stakeholder in authority (an 8, 9, or 10), it is advised that wellness committees identify the people with negative comments as "5s" or less, instead dedicating their efforts to ensuring support from those identified as extremely important stakeholders.

Finally, it is an issue of equity that employers offer opportunities that are accessible and appropriate for all employees. For example, it is important to avoid overincentivizing or penalizing participation in wellness programs, as not all employees have access to resources needed to engage in wellness programs. Some may have complicated feelings about their health or bodies, hidden health conditions, barriers to affordable and high-quality healthcare, or other obstacles. For example, an after-work yoga class may be unfeasible for a single parent or employee dependent on public transportation. Infusing health initiatives into working hours allows for greater employee participation.

INTERVENTION STRATEGIES TO DEVELOP HEALTHY WORKSITES

Worksite wellness initiatives can address a range of health behaviors (e.g., tobacco, physical activity, food and beverage, stress) or health outcomes (e.g., hypertension control, diabetes management, mental health). Worksite health and well-being initiatives consist of employer-coordinated initiatives, including multiple strategies (information, programs, benefits, policies, and environmental supports) designed to facilitate healthy behaviors and improve health or well-being of all employees (CDC, 2019). Strategies employers offer within these initiatives range from the provision of informational materials (e.g., posters), programs (i.e., short-lived opportunities, usually designed for individuals to opt-in), benefit design strategies (e.g., paid time off), written policy to codify the desired behaviors (e.g., worksite tobacco ban), and environmental changes (e.g., sit-to-stand desks). Worksite wellness initiatives are offered with the intention of improving employee health and decreasing the financial burden that employers incur due to poor employee health, absenteeism, presenteeism, and poor productivity.

To fully address the complexity of each health behavior, it is to the worksite's advantage to implement a comprehensive set of strategies (multiple interventions using information, program, benefit design, policy, and environment) to achieve the significant change needed to promote health. Comprehensive worksite initiatives focus on *organizational* health promotion, as opposed to individual health promotion strategies. In organizational health promotion, the focus is on modifying the worksite. Intentionally developed and implemented policies, systems, and environmental changes (PSEs) can promote and improve health among employees as a group. Worksites often implement organizational policies to protect the safety of employees and the employer. Many research-informed organizational policies, such as a ban on employees having or using tobacco at the worksite, can improve the health of the worksite as well as the health of employees (who may or may not have the internal motivation to adopt a behavior change). In this sense, worksites can "level the playing field," ensuring equal opportunities for all employees to practice healthy behaviors and work in better environments, as a function of being employed through the worksite.

As a result, it is best for a worksite wellness committee to focus on one health behavior (e.g., tobacco use) at a time, developing a suite of interventions to address the specific health behavior comprehensively and holistically, until all strategies have been implemented (Ablah et al., 2020). In other words, to make impactful change, worksites need to address one health behavior at a time, comprehensively, and maintain those strategies when preparing to address the next health behavior. Once a behavior has been implemented and is in sustainment mode, another health behavior can be chosen.

Such approaches are consistent with social-ecological models (described in detail in Chapter 21, "The Roles of the Built Environment in Supporting Health Behavior Change"). Social-ecological models provide a useful framework for understanding how the worksite can affect the health and well-being of employees as a population, and in turn how worksite wellness interventions can be designed (Sallis & Owen, 2015; **Figure 19.1**). The idea of implementing a comprehensive set of strategies (e.g., programs, policies, environmental changes) is consistent with the social-ecological model, where effectiveness and sustainability are more likely when multiple strategies are all addressing the same topic. This demonstrates to the employee that the employer is serious about the specific health behavior, as the employer is dedicating time and resources to promote significant organizational culture change.

The social-ecological model can also serve as a useful framework for worksite wellness committees and those in authority at the worksite to recognize that, regardless of whether the worksite is being intentional about the environments they have created for employees, they are very much affecting their employees' health and well-being. When wellness committees make changes to their worksite's culture or environment, they are simply being intentional about the health behaviors they want to affect.

It can be important for worksites to consider participation strategies used to promote their health and well-being initiatives. Specifically, initiatives addressing behavior changes (e.g., physical activity, nutrition, smoking cessation) may benefit from multiple strategies tailored toward employees as well as the neighborhoods and communities where employees reside.

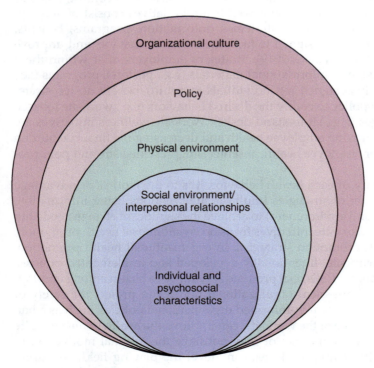

FIGURE 19.1 Social-ecological model for worksite wellness initiatives.

Worksites can consider social strategies that encourage participation such as peer support; affinity groups connecting people with common interests or characteristics; group goal setting or activities; competitions/challenges; supporting a cause; and/or allowing family members, friends, or community members to participate.

Finally, communication is key! It is important to align the communication method and format with the population the worksite wants to serve. Further, the use of specific and tailored content can increase participation (HERO Health, 2016). This may include intending to provide information to employees with specific roles in the worksite or for subgroups based on demographics or health status.

Research-Informed Worksite Interventions

Implementing comprehensive strategies can create a culture of health within worksites through efforts that influence the physical and social environment to promote health and well-being, and involve leaders, managers, peers, and employees (Kent et al., 2016).

TOBACCO

For example, a comprehensive approach to addressing tobacco at a worksite might include adopting a policy prohibiting tobacco products on-site with clear guidance as to what is and is not allowed, reducing or eliminating employee out-of-pocket costs for tobacco cessation counseling and medication, making counseling and medication easily accessible, posting signs that state that tobacco use is prohibited, distributing information and campaigns, and ensuring that the worksite remains tobacco-free (Table 19.1). Wellness initiatives that are composed of multiple components and using multiple strategies can achieve greater impact.

A tobacco cessation case study illustrates how a tobacco comprehensive intervention can be implemented. In 2019, Gove County Medical Center, in rural Quinter, Kansas, employed almost 200 individuals. They wanted to reduce tobacco use among their employees, patients, and visitors. The wellness committee developed a comprehensive plan, including information, program, benefit design, policy, and environmental strategies. The cornerstone of the comprehensive plan was the development and implementation of policy.

Information strategies included informing employees about available services and resources for tobacco cessation, coverage for counseling and medication through the medical center, the worksite's tobacco-free policy, consequences of policy noncompliance, policy enforcement, and how to report violations. The medical center used posters, graphics, and email campaigns, including Tips From Former Smoker, SmokefreeTXT, and managing cravings.

Program strategies included promoting tobacco cessation counseling, medication, and the state quitline, KanQuit. The worksite also encouraged tobacco users to combine multiple cessation aids (e.g., medications, in-person counseling, phone support) to support their quit attempts.

Benefit design strategies included worksite promotion of their EAP tobacco cessation counseling, and the elimination of out-of-pocket costs for Food and Drug Administration (FDA)-approved prescription cessation medications and over-the-counter nicotine replacement products.

The tobacco-free policy developed by the medical center was effective January 1, 2020. It prohibited all forms of tobacco (e.g., cigarettes, chew, e-cigarettes, cigars) for all indoor and outdoor worksite property, including parking lots, company vehicles, personal vehicles on worksite property, sidewalks, roads, and property adjoined to the medical center's owned or operated property. Moreover, as this is a healthcare facility, employees who smelled of smoke were asked to change clothes.

Finally, the medical center removed tobacco receptacles and designated tobacco use areas. The worksite posted signs stating that smoking is prohibited by state law. It displayed the international "no smoking" symbol and information about its tobacco-free policy.

TABLE 19.1 Comprehensive Intervention Strategies to Address Tobacco at a Worksite

STRATEGY	EXAMPLE
Information	
Share services and resources available for tobacco cessation	Post a flier about tobacco cessation programs, counseling, and/or medications in in the break room and/or restrooms.
Widely promote the worksite's tobacco-free policy	Add policy language in company-wide new hire training documents, policies, and procedures, such as the worksite's tobacco policy, the consequences of noncompliance, how the policy is enforced, and who violations are reported to.
Promote tobacco-free campaigns	Share tips from a former smoker.
Promote tobacco cessation at home	Use telephone counseling and text message reminders/check-ins.
Program	
Access to counseling	Provide individual, group, or telephone counseling; provide employees with an adequate number of sessions free of charge.
Access to seven FDA-approved medications	Provide access to nicotine replacement therapies (patch, gum, lozenge, nasal spray, inhaler) and nonnicotine medications (bupropion, varenicline).
Quitline	This works best when the individual is ready to quit tobacco.
Benefit design	
Make treatment available	Reduce or eliminate employee out-of-pocket costs for tobacco cessation counseling and medication.
Policy	
Worksite does not permit the use of tobacco products on-site	Provide a tobacco-free environment for all employees and visitors. Add clear statement to the organization's policies: "No use of any tobacco product or electronic device that delivers nicotine or other substance to the person using the product/device is permitted within the facilities or on the property of [employer] at any time. This policy covers the smoking of any tobacco product, the use of oral tobacco products, the use of e-cigarettes ('vaping')."
Environment	
Signage	Post signs that state that tobacco use is prohibited; display the international "no smoking" symbol.
Convert designated tobacco areas to nontobacco uses	Convert a smoking gazebo to a bike shelter or garden.

FDA, Food and Drug Administration.

The medical center has implemented a system to document the tobacco use status of all hospitalized patients and offers tobacco dependence treatment to all hospitalized patients who use tobacco. The hospital formulary includes FDA-approved tobacco dependence medications, and it ensures compliance with The Joint Commission regulations mandating that all sections of the hospital be smoke-free and that patients receive cessation treatments. Staff are trained that first-line medications may be used to reduce nicotine withdrawal symptoms, even if a patient is not intending to quit.

During the initiative, some members of the wellness committee reported that some managers felt uncomfortable confronting visitors about the new policy. WorkWell KS made employees little cards indicating that the facility was tobacco-free, that their cooperation was appreciated, and providing quitline information. The medical center held a press release to inform the community of the changes. The wellness committee reported very little pushback once the policy was in place.

Cigarette use among employees decreased from 19% at baseline to 8% at follow-up, and e-cigarettes and chewing tobacco also decreased. Greater proportions of employees reported trying to quit cigarettes (19% compared with 13% at baseline) and chew (5% compared with 4% at baseline). The medical center was aware of at least four employees who had requested nicotine replacement therapy provided through a WorkWell KS initiative. At follow-up, more employees (83%) reported 0 days being exposed to secondhand smoke at work (from the prior 7 days) than at baseline (76%).

PHYSICAL ACTIVITY

Regular physical activity reduces one's risk of chronic diseases, including heart disease, cancer, and diabetes; improves one's mental health by decreasing symptoms of anxiety, depression, and stress; and enhances one's immune response (Ross et al., 2016; Sharma et al., 2006). Physical activity guidelines recommend that adults participate weekly in at least 150 minutes of moderate-intensity aerobic physical activity and spend at least 2 days a week doing a muscle-strengthening activity to achieve substantial health benefits (USDHHS, 2018). However, in 2023, 28% of Americans are meeting physical activity guidelines (Abildso et al., 2023).

During the COVID-19 pandemic, physical activity levels declined due to community-level mitigation strategies, such as stay-at-home orders and business closures, which restricted access to places for adults to be active. One study suggested that working from home was associated with an additional 2 hours of sitting time compared with employees working entirely in-person (9.2 vs. 7.3 hours of sitting time, respectively; Streeter et al., 2021). Another study suggested that average daily step counts declined at the onset of the pandemic from 10,000 to 4,600 steps per day (Giuntella et al., 2021).

Research has reported that the primary barrier to physical activity participation is time and pointed to the employer's role in combating physical inactivity by offering opportunities for employees to be active during the workday. Table 19.2 provides strategies that employers can implement to promote physical activity and/or discourage sedentary behavior.

TABLE 19.2 Comprehensive Intervention Strategies to Address Physical Inactivity and/or Sedentary Behavior at a Worksite	
STRATEGY	**EXAMPLE**
Information	
Educating employees about the benefits of safe physical activity	Offer training on how to walk safely, including posture, footwear, and identification of safe indoor/outdoor spaces to walk.

(continued)

382 IV • INTERVENING IN SETTINGS AND SYSTEMS TO MODIFY HEALTH BEHAVIORS

TABLE 19.2 Comprehensive Intervention Strategies to Address Physical Inactivity and/or Sedentary Behavior at a Worksite (*continued*)

STRATEGY	EXAMPLE
Providing information about accessibility for people with mobility or other limitations	Place accessibility signs for safe places for people with mobility challenges to be active. Ensure all wellness programs contain information about ways people with mobility challenges or differing abilities can participate. Partner with health professionals to ensure information accuracy.
Giving remote employees information on how to be physically active at their work location or in their community	Provide a list of stretches that can be performed at one's desk, and information on the benefits of breaking sitting time up with standing time; information is inclusive in terms of visual, auditory, physical, and other mobility abilities.
Program	
Fitness challenges	Use physical activity trackers to incorporate physical activity challenges that all can participate in. If doing a step challenge, consider allowing employees to convert other activities into steps for those who may not be ambulatory.
Group exercise classes on-site	Offer instructor-led yoga class when employees are available to take a break (e.g., lunch hour). Instructor offers and models adaptation and alternative movements based on ability levels.
Stretch/physical activity breaks	Incorporate stretch breaks before or after team meetings. Provide modifications to stretches to increase accessibility. Offer software on work computers to prompt breaks and physical activity. Incorporate language into your policies and procedures to support these opportunities for employees.
Benefit design	
Discounted gym memberships or stipend for exercise equipment	Provide funds for each employee that can be used toward a gym membership, virtual exercise classes, or exercise equipment.
Discounts for active commuting options	Provide employee discounts on active apparel and free bike valet, and allow space for safe bicycle/equipment storage.
Policy	
Paid time to exercise	Allow employees to be physically active while on the clock and provide spaces on-site for physical activity, including accessible options. Allow 90 minutes for lunch if the employee is engaging in physical activity during their break.
Flextime for physical activity	Allow employees to "flex" or shift their work schedules within a certain time frame to allow time to be physically active, while maintaining their expected number of work hours.
Walking meetings	Allow employees to have walking meetings as part of their workday, especially during brainstorming or creativity sessions.
Environment	
Creating a built environment that supports physical activity in the workplace	Provide on-site gyms, walking trails, indoor walking options, and standing desks; modify workspaces to support stretching and movement during the workday; ensure accessible areas.

Workplace wellness physical activity and sedentary behavior interventions often inadvertently leave out or marginalize employees with physical limitations, including those with mobility issues. Table 19.2 includes strategies to support people with disabilities in participating in physical activity and sedentary behavior prevention programs. There are unique concerns for people with physical limitations in engaging in physical activity interventions. People who use wheelchairs may be more prone to problems with bone density and therefore are at a high risk for injury if participating in some activities. Hybrid employees with significant visual impairments or brain injuries may have difficulty navigating internal and external environments due to unfamiliarity, unexpected or distressing stimuli, and other factors. As the Inclusive Worksite Wellness Guide authors assert, individuals living with a disability can maintain and promote their health and must have the access to do so in their communities, including their worksites (National Center on Health, Physical Activity, and Disability [NCHPAD], 2019).

NUTRITION

Regular consumption of healthy foods and beverages is associated with reduced risk of chronic diseases such as heart disease, type 2 diabetes, and some cancers. MyPlate is based on the Dietary Guidelines for Americans (DGA) 2020–2025 and offers guidance on the approximate amounts and types of foods that are needed by American adults (DGA, n.d.). Compared with its predecessor, the Food Pyramid, MyPlate provides recommended portions. A significant change from the Food Pyramid is that MyPlate recommends that fruits and vegetables make up half of all the foods an adult consumes every day. Although recommendations vary by gender and age, it is recommended that adults consume 1 ½ to 2 ½ cups of whole fruits and 2 ½ to 4 cups of varied vegetables daily. Whole grains and lean proteins make up the remaining half of the recommended foods. Regarding daily beverage consumption, the U.S. NASEM (2005) report determined that approximately 15.5 cups (125 ounces) and 11.5 cups (91 ounces) of fluids for men and women, respectively, is adequate.

To address equity and to lower healthcare costs, it is to a worksite's advantage to improve the food and beverage environment at the worksite. Table 19.3 provides strategies that employers can implement to improve the food and beverage environment at a worksite.

TABLE 19.3 Comprehensive Intervention Strategies to Address Foods and Beverages at a Worksite	
STRATEGY	**EXAMPLE**
Information	
Share benefits on the adoption of a Mediterranean diet.	Offer a Mediterranean diet "lunch and learn" with a local dietitian.
Offer more fruits and vegetables at worksite; share strategies to eat more fruits and vegetables.	In canteens, catering, and cafeterias, provide recipes that incorporate vegetables to common dishes, such as adding squash to meatloaf recipe.
Post nutritional information.	Provide nutrition fact panel for dishes served at worksite, especially if it is not offering a 100% healthy food and beverage environment.
Campaign to increase consumption of healthy foods/beverage consumption.	Implement 5 A Day program: a simple and practical message to increase fruit and vegetable consumption.

(continued)

TABLE 19.3 Comprehensive Intervention Strategies to Address Foods and Beverages at a Worksite (*continued*)

STRATEGY	EXAMPLE
Program	
Host a farmer's market.	Invite local producers and farmers to worksites regularly and during special events when hybrid/remote employees are at the worksite.
Invest in community-supported agriculture for worksite.	Worksite pays for x number of shares of producer/farmer's goods, and the worksite receives the equivalent produce.
Benefit design	
Reward employees with benefits.	Employees receive a premium reduction or contribution to health savings account if they complete 12 weeks of 5 A Day program.
provide free/low-cost nutrition consult.	Provide tailored feedback on diet and clinical values from a dietitian.
Policy	
Adopt standards that define "healthy" foods and beverages.	Standards include fruits, vegetables, whole grains, and lean proteins, and exclude foods with high sodium, saturated fats, trans fats, added sugar, and refined grains.
Adopt a policy that governs the offering of foods and beverages at the worksite.	Only coffee, unsweetened tea, and water are provided by the employer. Foods and beverages purchased by the employer must meet the worksite's food and beverage standards.
Environment	
Make it available!	Make fruits, vegetables, and/or cool drinking water available in the break room in sufficient quantities, on a consistent basis, at prices that are either affordable or free, and promote them!
Decrease availability of unhealthy foods and beverages.	Sugar-sweetened beverages (diet and otherwise) are not purchased or made available for employees.

CASE STUDY 19.1: ARKANSAS CITY POLICE DEPARTMENT

In early 2020, the Arkansas City Police Department (ACPD) in rural Kansas employed approximately 30 individuals. The police department's wellness committee established a vision of having healthy, productive, and safe employees. Their short-term goal was, "As a result of working at the ACPD, employees will consume healthy foods and beverages."

The wellness committee developed a comprehensive plan, including information, program, benefit design, policy, and environmental strategies. First, the committee assessed employee food and beverage consumption to determine the baseline level of healthful food and beverage consumption, and if their initiative was effective at a 1-year follow-up assessment. Their baseline assessment revealed that 78% of the employees did not meet dietary recommendations for fruit and vegetable consumption.

(continued)

19 • CHRONIC DISEASE PREVENTION IN THE WORKSITE   385

CASE STUDY 19.1: ARKANSAS CITY POLICE DEPARTMENT (*continued*)

Next, the wellness committee launched a campaign, "Taking care of YOU so you can take care of THEM." The goal was to increase the number of accessible healthy foods and beverages. Posters promoting healthy foods and beverages were placed across the worksite.

Several initiatives were offered. A new program, "Arrest Unhealthy Snacks," encouraged healthy snack and beverage consumption between meals by offering fruits, vegetables, and healthy beverages in the workplace as a substitute for unhealthy snacks. In addition, employees were offered up to two free dietetic consultations per year. Communication of these offerings occurred through email and meetings.

ACPD adopted several policies related to food and beverage. To define healthy foods and beverages at the worksite, ACPD adopted nutrition guidelines. Further, ACPD enacted a policy stating that healthy foods and beverages (that comply with their guidelines) would be available at internal meetings and events. Failure to comply with the policy could result in disciplinary action. Preference was given to caterers that pledged to prepare healthy foods for the community. A second policy was a No Dumping Policy, where employees were asked to ensure that the foods and beverages they bring to share with fellow employees met policy guidelines. Both policies were posted on the employee intranet and in the employee break room and were effective July 1, 2020.

As for the environment, ACPD increased access to water and other healthy beverages. Second, ACPD provided a greater proportion (85%) of snacks that met their nutritional guidelines in their vending machine. Third, the break room was stocked with fresh fruits and vegetables multiple times each week. These changes became effective on August 15, 2020.

From baseline to 1-year follow-up, the mean self-reported daily intake of fruits and vegetables increased from 3 to 4 cups per day. At baseline, 22% of respondents reported meeting dietary guidelines for intake of fruits and vegetables. At follow-up, 50% of respondents reported meeting dietary guidelines.

STRESS AND MENTAL HEALTH

Mental health consists of our emotional, psychological, and social well-being—all of which influence peoples' daily thoughts, feelings, and actions, both at home and in the workplace. Mental health conditions are among the most common health conditions, with an estimated one in five American adults (one in eight globally) experiencing mental illness in a given year, with many more going undiagnosed (National Institute of Mental Health [NIMH], 2023; World Health Organization [WHO], 2022).

The COVID-19 pandemic has negatively affected many people's mental health, increasing the prevalence of anxiety and major depressive disorders by 25% (WHO, 2022). Individuals with untreated mental illness are at risk for absenteeism and presenteeism, as well as for worse outcomes from common medical conditions such as diabetes, respiratory diseases, and musculoskeletal disorders, resulting in increased medical costs (CDC, 2018).

The Health Enhancement Research Organization Health and Well-Being Best Practices Scorecard, in collaboration with Mercer (HERO Scorecard, HERO, 2016), is a tool designed to help organizations learn about best practices for promoting workplace health and well-being. The HERO Scorecard can provide worksites discovery opportunities to improve and measure progress over time with a mental health and well-being best-practice score. Organizations can take the HERO Scorecard and receive a mental health and well-being best-practice score to learn about best practices for promoting workforce mental health and well-being. Further, the HERO Scorecard provides organizations with social determinants of health score and a diversity, equity, and inclusion score—two areas known to contribute significantly to an employee's mental health and well-being.

With the growing need for mental health support, it is important for employers to implement strategies and solutions that meet their employees' needs and create a culture that supports mental health and well-being in the workplace. **Table 19.4** provides strategies that employers can implement to improve the stress and well-being environment at a worksite.

TABLE 19.4 Comprehensive Intervention Strategies to Address Stress and Well-Being at a Worksite

STRATEGY	EXAMPLE
Information	
Posters and signs	Work Free Zone sign; posters describing the benefits of taking care of your mental health and well-being
Program	
Promoting relaxation	Meditation class, yoga, relaxation, or restorative breaks
Enhancing professionalism skills	Problem-solving, time management, and conflict resolution training, especially for managers
Improving emotional intelligence	Assertiveness, interpersonal skills training
Stress management	Nature-based stress management class
Addressing burnout	Promoting a healthy work–life balance, setting realistic expectations, recognizing great work
Benefit design	
Employee assistance program	24-hour, 365 days/year, direct access to professional counseling
Connecting benefit with important program accomplishment	Rewarding employees for participating in a financial planning class by contributing funds into their flexible spending account; reduced premium for employee attendance in a mindfulness class
Ensuring access to mental healthcare	Mental health screening, access to mental health provider/treatment, access to cognitive behavioral therapy
Family-friendly benefits	Offering childcare on-site; infants up to 6 months may be brought to work
Employee-friendly benefits	Separating sick from vacation leave, meaningful and regular recognition of employees, internal promotions, financial rewards
Policy	
Booster break	Allowing employees to take 10- to 15-minute "rest" or "booster" breaks
Flex-time	Employees working the same number of hours, with agreed-upon start and finish times; might include a required period (e.g., 10 a.m. to 2 p.m.) with bandwidths (e.g., 6 a.m. to 10 p.m.) to ensure an adequate number of hours are worked
Adequate staffing	Useful for worksites that require minimum staffing levels; ensures worksite has a sufficient number of staff in proportion to the required work

(continued)

TABLE 19.4 Comprehensive Intervention Strategies to Address Stress and Well-Being at a Worksite (*continued*)	
STRATEGY	**EXAMPLE**
Stable shift	Worksite not rotating employees to different shifts; third shift remains third shift unless a permanent change is made
Overtime	Banning mandatory overtime for nonexempt employees—mandatory overtime in healthcare settings is associated with errors, poor patient care, and legal liabilities; offering voluntary overtime for time and a half pay when working beyond a set threshold
Time and accommodations to access care	Time accommodations to ensure access to mental healthcare, including stress management classes
Human resources	Policies to prevent and address sexual harassment and bullying; worksite ensures enforcement
Environment	
Offering a designated nonworkspace	"Zen" comfort or relaxation room
Creating a healthy environment	Offering personal, private spaces with access to natural light and nature inside (e.g., plants)

Many worksites focus their health and well-being initiatives on employee mental health and well-being, including reducing levels of depression, anxiety, stress, and burnout. HERO has developed a guide that provides case study examples highlighting organizations that have adopted many recommended worksite mental health and well-being practices and discusses their implementation strategies (HERO Health, 2020). Additionally, HERO offers an infographic of six workplace mental health and well-being best practices (**Figure 19.2**).

LESSONS LEARNED

Three lessons learned can help employers and wellness committees develop and implement a successful intervention. First, shared responsibility and accountability are critical in worksite wellness initiatives. All the burden of figuring out how to engage in initiatives must not fall on the employees; the worksite must actively provide environments that are conducive to engaging in healthy behaviors (Ablah et al., 2019).

Second, when developing a worksite wellness plan, it is imperative to create feasible goals and objectives so that effectiveness can be evaluated. This promotes an initiative that can have a strong benefit for employees and promotes transparency for those participating.

Finally, it is essential to focus on modifiable behaviors that can lead to chronic disease—tobacco, physical inactivity, poor nutrition, and stress. Many employers and wellness committees immediately consider a focus on weight, and an important lesson emerging in the literature is the fallibility of relying on weight loss to promote health. Particularly troubling is the reliance on body mass index (BMI) as a diagnostic measure for body fat or health. BMI cannot distinguish between lean and fat mass and cannot provide an indication of body fat distribution. In addition, other metrics may be better predictors of chronic diseases. Concerns have also been raised about inconsistencies in measuring body fat, especially between men and women, and across racial and ethnic groups. Rather, direct metrics associated with modifiable behaviors that lead to overall better health need to be the focus of worksite health and well-being data collection, as these are more appropriate for worksites to assess. Further, worksites can promote these factors to influence true health change.

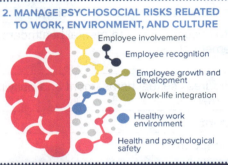
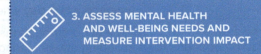

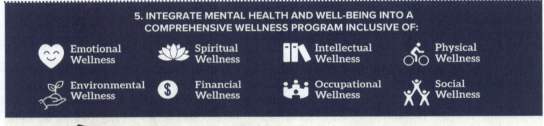

FIGURE 19.2 Six workplace mental health and well-being best practices.
Source: Adapted from Health Enhancement Research Organization. (2020). *Employee mental health and well-being: Emerging best practices and case study examples.* https://hero-health.org/wp-content/uploads/2020/09/HERO_MHWB_BestPractices_CaseExamples_091520.pdf.

Moreover, it is essential to avoid high stakes contests, like the Biggest Loser, where there is a lack of medical best practices to undergird the wellness initiative. As Ablah et al. (2019) note, these types of programs can induce rapid weight cycling, which can cause significant physical harm, as well as potential emotional harm. Employers and wellness committees would benefit from a focus on physical activity or other modifiable behaviors associated with chronic disease and leave weight-associated interventions to physicians when prescribed.

SUMMARY KEY POINTS

- Modifiable behaviors (tobacco, consumption of unhealthy foods and beverages, physical inactivity, and stress) significantly contribute to the leading chronic diseases in the United States.
- Modifiable behaviors associated with chronic disease can be targeted to improve the health of employees. These might include tobacco cessation, consumption of healthy foods and beverages, physical activity, and stress prevention and management.

(continued)

SUMMARY KEY POINTS (*continued*)

- Worksites serve an important role in the health of employees, regardless of whether the influence is positive or negative. A leadership-supported worksite wellness committee allows a worksite to demonstrate its commitment to improving employees' health.
- There are many research-informed strategies that can assist worksites in improving the health of the worksite and its employees. Implementation of these strategies is recommended, rather than developing strategies that are untested or may harm employees.
- Chronic disease prevention at the worksite is achievable. It is ideal to implement primary prevention strategies, addressing one topic (e.g., tobacco cessation) at a time. Once the topic has been fully addressed using multiple strategies (e.g., information, program, benefit design, policy, environment) and the initiative is being maintained, the worksite wellness committee may then move on to another topic.

DISCUSSION QUESTIONS

1. Select one of the chronic diseases profiled in this chapter. How do worksites contribute to its development? Take one factor you have chosen and propose an initiative that will help the worksite address this factor.
2. Consider an organization where you currently work or have worked in the past. What would the ideal worksite wellness committee look like? What roles would be represented? How would you engage employees who may be reluctant to engage in health initiatives?
3. Is it more beneficial for worksites to focus on making changes to one behavior at a time or to offer a menu of behavior change choices for their employees? How would you choose which behavior(s) to focus on? What information would you gather to help with your decision?
4. What barriers hinder employers from making worksite-level changes that are associated with a health behavior (e.g., tobacco, sedentary behavior)? How might you use worksite policy to alleviate one or more of these barriers?
5. To what extent is it the employer's responsibility to provide a healthy worksite for employees? How can employers embrace equity as they make significant contributions to the health infrastructure they offer employees?

A robust set of instructor resources designed to supplement this text is located at http://connect.springerpub.com/content/book/978-0-8261-4265-8. Qualifying instructors may request access by emailing textbook@springerpub.com.

REFERENCES

Abildso, C. G., Daily, S. M., Meyer, M. R. U., Perry, C. K., & Eyler, A. (2023). Prevalence of meeting aerobic, muscle-strengthening, and combined physical activity guidelines during leisure time among adults, by rural-urban classification and region–United States, 2020. *American Journal of Transplantation, 23*(3), 443–446. https://doi.org/10.1016/j.ajt.2023.01.021

Ablah, E., Wilcox, E., & Honn, A. (2019). The cons of traditional worksite wellness interventions and a proposed model. *Public Health Reports, 134*(4), 319–323. https://doi.org/10.1177/0033354919845683

Ablah, E., Wilcox, E. A., Umansky, E., Honn, A., O'Malley, E., & Usher, J. (2020). A model for developing comprehensive initiatives to improve the health of the worksite: The WorkWell KS strategic framework. *Workplace Health & Safety, 68*(6), 293–299. https://doi.org/10.1177/2165079919894364

American Psychological Association. (2020). *Stress in America 2020: A national mental health crisis.* https://www.apa.org/news/press/releases/stress/2020/report-october

Bjornstadt, S. (2014). *Nature contact during working hours: Benefits related to stress reduction, health and sick leave* [Master's thesis]. Norwegian University of Life Sciences.

Bureau of Labor Statistics. (2021a). *Labor force characteristics by race and ethnicity, 2020.* https://www.bls.gov/opub/reports/race-and-ethnicity/2020/home.htm

Bureau of Labor Statistics. (2021b). *2020 results of the business response survey.* Business Response Survey. https://www.bls.gov/brs/2020-results.htm

Bureau of Labor Statistics. (2022). *Civilian labor force participation by age, sex, race, and ethnicity.* https://www.bls.gov/emp/tables/civilian-labor-force-participation-rate.htm

Centers for Disease Control and Prevention. (2018). *Mental health in the workplace.* Mental health disorders and stress affect working-age Americans. https://www.cdc.gov/workplacehealthpromotion/tools-resources/workplace-health/mental-health/

Centers for Disease Control and Prevention. (2019). *Workplace health model.* https://www.cdc.gov/workplacehealthpromotion/model/index.html

Community Preventive Services Task Force. (2023). *Worksite health.* The Community Guide to Preventive Services. https://www.thecommunityguide.org/topics/worksite-health.html#cc-widget-14b8

Congressional Research Services. (2023, February 6). *U.S. health care coverage and spending.* https://crsreports.congress.gov/product/pdf/IF/IF10830.

Dietary Guidelines for Americans. (n.d.). *Dietary guidelines for Americans, 2020–2025.* Retrieved from https://www.dietaryguidelines.gov/resources/2020-2025-dietary-guidelines-online-materials

Duffy, E. Y., Hiremath, P. G., Martinez-Amezcua, P., Safeer, R., Schrack, J. A., Blaha, M. J., Michos, E. D., Blumenthal, R. S., Martin, S. S., & Cainzos-Achirica, M. (2021). Opportunities to improve cardiovascular health in the new American workplace. *American Journal of Preventive Cardiology, 5,* 100136. https://doi.org/10.1016/j.ajpc.2020.100136

Giuntella, O., Hyde, K., Saccardo, S., & Sadoff, S. (2021). Lifestyle and mental health disruptions during COVID-19. *Proceedings of the National Academy of Sciences of the United States of America, 118*(9), e2016632118. https://doi.org/10.1073/pnas.2016632118

Goetzel, R. Z., Fabius, R., Roemer, E. C., Kent, K. B., Berko, J., Head, M. A., & Henke, R. M. (2019). The stock performance of American companies investing in a culture of health. *American Journal of Health Promotion, 33*(3), 439–447. https://doi.org/10.1177/0890117118824818

Goetzel, R. Z., & Ozminkowski, R. J. (2008). The health and cost benefits of work site health-promotion programs. *Annual Review of Public Health, 29,* 303–323. https://doi.org/10.1146/annurev.publhealth.29.020907.090930

Henke, R. M., Head, M. A., Kent, K. B., Goetzel, R. Z., Roemer, E. C., & McCleary, K. (2019). Improvements in an organization's culture of health reduces workers' health risk profile and health care utilization. *Journal of Occupational and Environmental Medicine, 61*(2), 96–101. https://doi.org/10.1097/jom.0000000000001479

HERO Health. (2016). *The HERO Health and well-being best practices scorecard in collaboration with Mercer.* https://hero-health.org/wp-content/uploads/2016/10/HERO-Scorecard-2016-Progress-Report_digitalREV.pdf

HERO Health. (2020). *Employee mental health and well-being: Emerging best practices and case study examples.* https://hero-health.org/wp-content/uploads/2020/09/HERO_MHWB_BestPractices_CaseExamples_091520.pdf

HERO Scorecard. HERO. (2016). Retrieved January 15, 2024, from https://url.us.m.mimecastprotect.com/s/SyzEC1wnBPUMNQEWAsLdIIJ?domain=hero-health.org/; https://hero-health.org/hero-scorecard/

Kahn-Marshall, J. L., & Gallant, M. P. (2012). Making health behaviors the easy choice for employees: A review of the literature on environmental and policy changes in worksite health promotion. *Health Education & Behavior, 39*(6), 752–776. https://doi.org/10.1177/1090198111434153

Kava, C. M., Strait, M., Brown, M. C., Hammerback, K., Harris, J. R., Alongi, J., & Hannon, P. A. (2022). Partnerships to expand worksite wellness programs - A qualitative analysis of state and local health department perspectives. Inquiry: *The Journal of Health Care Organization, Provision, and Financing, 59.* https://doi.org/10.1177/00469580221092822

Kent, K., Goetzel, R. Z., Roemer, E. C., Prasad, A., & Freundlich, N. (2016). Promoting healthy workplaces by building cultures of health and applying strategic communications. *Journal of Occupational and Environmental Medicine, 58*(2), 114–122. https://doi.org/10.1097/JOM.0000000000000629

Lange, K. W., & Nakamura, Y. (2020). Lifestyle factors in the prevention of COVID-19. *Global Health Journal, 4*(4), 146–152. https://doi.org/10.1016/j.glohj.2020.11.002

Moy, E., Garcia, M. C., Bastian, B., Rossen, L. M., Ingram, D. D., Faul, M., Massetti, G. M., Thomas, C. C., Hong, Y., Yoon, P. W., & Iademarco, M. F. (2017). Leading causes of death in nonmetropolitan and metropolitan areas–United States, 1999–2014. *Morbidity and Mortality Weekly Report, 66*(1), 1–8. https://doi.org/10.15585/mmwr.ss6601a1

National Academies of Sciences, Engineering, and Medicine. (2005). *Dietary reference intakes for water, potassium, sodium, chloride, and sulfate.* https://nap.nationalacademies.org/read/10925/chapter/1

National Academies of Sciences, Engineering, and Medicine. (2022). The emerging older workforce. In T. Becker & S. T. Fiske (Eds.). *Understanding the aging workforce: Defining a research agenda.* National Academies Press.

National Center for Chronic Disease Prevention and Health Promotion. (n.d.-a). *About chronic diseases.* Centers for Disease Control and Prevention. Retrieved June 14, 2024, from https://www.cdc.gov/chronicdisease/about/index.htm

National Center for Chronic Disease Prevention and Health Promotion. (n.d.-b). *Workplace health promotion.* Retrieved June 14, 2024, from https://www.cdc.gov/chronicdisease/resources/publications/factsheets/workplace-health.htm

National Center on Health, Physical Activity, and Disability. (2019). *Inclusive worksite wellness: Strategies for including employees of all abilities in wellness initiatives.* https://www.nchpad.org/fppics/Inclusive%20Worksite%20Wellness%20Guide.pdf

National Institute of Allergy and Infectious Disease. (n.d.). *Minority health and health disparities.* Retrieved June 14, 2024, from https://www.niaid.nih.gov/research/minority-health-disparities

National Institute of Mental Health. (2023). *Mental illness.* https://www.nimh.nih.gov/health/statistics/mental-illness

O'Malley, E., & Cebula, A. (2015). *Your leadership edge: Lead any time, anywhere.* Bard Press.

Physical Activity Alliance. (2016). *National physical activity plan.* https://paamovewithus.org/wp-content/uploads/2020/07/National-PA-Plan.pdf

Roemer, E. C., Kent, K. B., Goetzel, R. Z., Krill, J., Williams, F. S., & Lang, J. E. (2022). The CDC worksite health scorecard: A tool to advance workplace health promotion programs and practices. *Preventing Chronic Disease, 19*(32), 210375. https://doi.org/10.5888/pcd19.210375

Ross, R., Blair, S. N., Arena, R., Church, T. S., Després, J. P., Franklin, B. A., Haskell, W. L., Kaminsky, L. A., Levine, B. D., Lavie, C. J., Myers, J., Niebauer, J., Sallis, R., Sawada, S. S., Sui, X., & Wisløff, U. (2016). Importance of assessing cardiorespiratory fitness in clinical practice: A case for fitness as a clinical vital sign: A scientific statement from the American Heart Association. *Circulation, 134*(24), e653–e699. https://doi.org/10.1161/cir.0000000000000461

Sallis, J. F., & Owen, N. (2015). *Ecological models of health behavior.* In K. Glanz, B. K. Rimer, & K. V. Viswanath (Eds.), *Health behavior: Theory, research, and practice.* (pp. 43–64). Jossey-Bass/Wiley.

Sharma, A., Madaan, V., & Petty, F. D. (2006). Exercise for mental health. *Primary Care Companion to the Journal of Clinical Psychiatry, 8*(2), 106. https://doi.org/10.4088/pcc.v08n0208a

Streeter, J., Roche, M., & Friedlander, A. (2021). *From bad to worse: The impact of work-from-home on sedentary behaviors and exercising.* https://longevity.stanford.edu/wp-content/uploads/2021/05/Sedentary-Brief.pdf

The Ladders. (2021). *25% of all professional jobs in North America will be remote by end of next year.* https://www.theladders.com/press/25-of-all-professional-jobs-in-north-america-will-be-remote-by-end-of-next-year

United States Census Bureau. (2022). *The number of people primarily working from home tripled between 2019 and 2021.* https://www.census.gov/newsroom/press-releases/2022/people-working-from-home.html

U.S. Department of Health and Human Services. (n.d.). *Healthy people 2030.* Office of Disease Prevention and Health Promotion. Retrieved June 14, 2024, from https://health.gov/healthypeople

U.S. Department of Health and Human Services. (2018). *Physical activity guidelines for Americans*, (2nd ed.). Author.

Watson, K. B., Carlson, S. A., Loustalot, F., Town, M., Eke, P. I., Thomas, C. W., & Greenlund, K. J. (2022). Chronic conditions among adults aged 18–24–United States, 2019. *MMWR Morbidity and Mortality Weekly Report, 17*(30), 964–970. https://doi.org/10.15585/mmwr.mm7130a3

Wong, K., Chan, A. H. S., & Ngan, S. C. (2019). The effect of long working hours and overtime on occupational health: A meta-analysis of evidence from 1998 to 2018. *International Journal of Environmental Research and Public Health, 16*(12), 2102. https://doi.org/10.3390/ijerph16122102

World Health Organization. (2022). *World mental health report: Transforming mental health for all.* https://www.who.int/publications/i/item/9789240049338

CHAPTER 20

HEALTHCARE PROVIDER AND SYSTEM INTERVENTIONS PROMOTING HEALTH BEHAVIOR CHANGE

KRISTINA H. LEWIS

LEARNING OBJECTIVES

- Identify the key benefits of targeting healthcare providers and healthcare systems to effect health behavior change.
- Identify three challenges in targeting healthcare systems for health behavior change.
- Describe an example of how system supports or practice redesign could improve health behavior change interventions in primary care settings.

INTRODUCTION

As highlighted in this book, there are effective interventions for modifying a wide range of health behaviors. To be maximally effective, strategies need to address not just the individual, but also healthcare providers and systems. Expanding beyond individual approaches results in a broader impact on the population in a shorter period of time. For example, system interventions such as incorporating clinical decision support tools in electronic health records (EHRs) are associated with increased assessment of tobacco use, counseling on tobacco cessation, and prescribing of tobacco cessation medications in ambulatory care settings (Bae et al., 2016).

The primary care setting, where the majority of healthcare occurs, is a particularly important arena for implementing health system interventions. In addition, this setting has seen significant increases in rates of behavioral health-related visits (Olfson et al., 2014). The primary care setting is also an important venue for delivering health behavior interventions that have the potential for significant population health impact. Owing to these factors, and because the majority of available evidence stems from the primary care setting, this chapter focuses primarily on interventions targeting primary care staff, providers, and healthcare systems of service delivery. However, although these settings are often ideal for implementing behavior change-related interventions in healthcare, they have important limitations. First, physicians and other primary care providers (PCPs) are already more burdened than their specialist colleagues with respect to EHR-based prompts and tasks and thus may be less likely open to or able to sustainably implement additional workflow changes to address patients' behavioral needs (Rotenstein et al., 2021). Additionally, reliance solely on PCPs to deliver most

---

The author acknowledges the contributions of Anne C. Dobmeyer, PhD, ABPP; Jeffrey L. Goodie, PhD, ABPP; and Christopher L. Hunter, PhD, ABPP, to this chapter as it appeared in earlier editions.

interventions in the healthcare space may exacerbate existing inequities in behavior-related outcomes because patients from minoritized or lower income backgrounds are less likely to have PCPs compared with non-Latinx White patients or those from middle or higher income backgrounds (Hawks et al., 2020; Levine et al., 2020). These caveats are important to bear in mind while considering the evidence base summarized in this chapter.

CHALLENGES IN HEALTHCARE SYSTEMS

Despite the ubiquitous need for evidence-based health behavior interventions in primary care settings, multiple barriers have interfered with the widespread adoption of these approaches. Although recent changes may decrease these barriers, they have historically affected how medical providers are trained, providers' attitudes and beliefs about health behavior change, and the healthcare system itself.

Medical Education

The opening of the Johns Hopkins Medical School in 1893 and the publication of the "Flexner Report" in 1910 guided the redesign of the American medical education system between the 1870s and 1920s (Cuff & Vanselow, 2004; Ludmerer, 1999). Until recently, however, this fundamental training model remained largely unchanged, with the first 2 years of medical education focused on preclinical basic science and the last 2 years on clinical studies and disease management. This curriculum design left little room for formal instruction on counseling patients to improve unhealthy behaviors with a goal of primary or secondary prevention (Moser & Stagnaro-Green, 2009). After evaluating medical education, the Institute of Medicine (IOM; Cuff & Vanselow, 2004) concluded that medical schools inadequately teach methods for targeting problem health behaviors (e.g., tobacco use, diet, and inactivity). Limited exposure to health behavior change skills during medical school decreased the likelihood that future physicians would value and apply these skills. Medical education is now adapting for the 21st century.

Beliefs and Attitudes

Research suggests that health behavior change is often not discussed by providers during patient encounters (Barnes & Schoenborn, 2012). In part, this is because providers may view such discussions as futile. Using tobacco cessation counseling as an example, many physicians believe that patients are not motivated to quit, that patients usually fail to quit, that there is not enough appointment time to target quitting, and that there are other priorities besides tobacco cessation during the appointment (Association of American Medical Colleges [AAMC], 2007; Vogt et al., 2005). Additionally, most physicians report low confidence in their ability to motivate patients to stop smoking (AAMC, 2007). Additional studies indicate that, compared with addressing tobacco use, physicians believe that their patients would find discussions about diet, weight, and physical activity more embarrassing and difficult and would be unlikely to follow their advice (Dolor et al., 2010; Steeves et al., 2015). These beliefs are suggestive of underlying antiobesity bias or weight stigma, which is known to be common among medical providers, and suggest even more significant barriers to targeting weight-related health behaviors compared with something like tobacco use (Puhl & Suh, 2015; Puhl et al., 2016).

Lack of Systems to Support Primary Care Provider Intervention

It is essential that there are systems to support quick assessments, decision-making, and referrals in primary care. Often, algorithms derived from clinical guidelines and evidence-based reviews serve to inform decision-making. Pairing these algorithms with EHRs and other integrated systems can help quickly identify patients who may benefit from more intensive treatment and facilitate referrals to specialty care. The absence of these algorithms and systems to support health behavior change serves as another barrier to promoting behavior change.

Inadequate Intensive Treatment Options

The referral process to and options for intensive behavior change treatment are often limited and difficult to access (Rowan et al., 2013; Walker et al., 2015). For PCPs, this means that even if they identify the need to target health-related behaviors and determine that a patient needs specialty or more intensive care, there are significant barriers and limited options, such as shortage of providers, lack of availability, or restrictions on benefits (Rowan et al., 2013; Walker et al., 2015). It becomes easier for healthcare providers to focus on the aspects of care for which they have treatment options available and that they believe they can affect.

Reimbursement and Financial Barriers

Healthcare organizations that have not valued or viewed chronic care management as important are unlikely to reimburse and reward efforts to reduce chronic disease through health behavior change (Bodenheimer et al., 2002). Relative to other treatment-oriented interventions (e.g., prescriptions or procedures), preventive interventions have lower reimbursement rates (Levine et al., 2019). The example of tobacco cessation supports is illustrative of this tension. Despite the enormous health impacts that tobacco cessation can have, most physicians describe the limited coverage for tobacco cessation and limited reimbursement for physicians' time as significant barriers to targeting tobacco use (AAMC, 2007). In environments where financial reimbursement must be considered, there is less incentive to prioritize behavior change counseling. Providing reimbursement for health behavior change (e.g., tobacco cessation) has been shown to have an impact on the likelihood that the health behavior will be targeted in some situations (e.g., Ramsay et al., 2016). However, even with changes in healthcare laws, coverage for counseling remains variable (Jamal et al., 2015; McAfee et al., 2015). For example, as of 2017, the Centers for Disease Control and Prevention (CDC) reports that Medicaid plans in 33 states cover individual counseling and only 10 states cover group counseling for tobacco cessation for all populations. In contrast, there was much more consistent Medicaid coverage for prescription medications used to support tobacco cessation, with all 50 states providing coverage for bupropion and 46 of 50 covering nicotine replacement therapy patches (DiGiulio et al., 2018).

Lack of Access to Physician Extenders, Behavioral Health, and Other Provider Types

Although it is essential for PCPs to discuss and initiate conversations about behavior change, they are not working at their peak scope of practice if they bear complete responsibility for the assessment, initiation, and maintenance of behavior change counseling. Team-based care integrates other primary care staff, such as nurses, advanced practice professionals, behavior specialists, registered dietitians, and medical technicians, who could assist with behavior change counseling across the population served in the clinic (Mitchell et al., 2012). Even systemic efforts to integrate behavioral health specialty assets into primary care do not necessarily improve the PCP's ability to implement health behavior change (Hunter & Goodie, 2010).

Placing behavioral health providers and other team members who are better equipped to provide behavior change counseling near the PCP's point of care may ease the referral process and increase communication between the PCP and the behavioral health provider. However, as long as separate standards of care are maintained and each provider is separately responsible for the care provided, there is limited opportunity for medical providers to learn how they could change their practice using health behavior change methods (Williams et al., 2006). In order to generate evidence to support integrated care models, many health systems are now pursuing pilot programs of these models and have begun to publish on observed outcomes (Kim et al., 2023).

The many individual and systemic barriers to health behavior change interventions are long-standing and have stifled the integration of behavior change counseling into routine healthcare (Arora et al., 2016). A broad range of changes are needed to affect the practice of physicians and the healthcare systems in which they provide care.

TRAINING FOR THE 21ST CENTURY

Medical education and healthcare systems are undergoing radical changes presenting opportunities for improving how health behavior change is taught. Many medical schools are undertaking curriculum reform and reconsidering the Flexner model of education. A Carnegie Foundation study and subsequent recommendations made by Cook et al. (2010), which have been called "Flexner II," were important in guiding the process of curriculum reform. The authors use the four goals of medical education introduced by Flexner (standardization, integration, habits of inquiry and improvement, and professional formation) to identify challenges and make recommendations for improvement. To achieve the goal of integration, the authors specifically encourage the integration of basic, clinical, and social sciences, as well as interprofessional education and teamwork. To promote habits of inquiry and improvement, the authors encourage participation in initiatives focusing on population health and quality improvement. These recommendations, along with the awareness of the impact of health behaviors on morbidity and mortality (Mokdad et al., 2004), provided the rationale and opportunities to integrate health behavior change training into medical education.

Much work was also based on a 2004 report by the National Academy of Medicine (NAM; previously known as the IOM). The NAM developed five recommendations for improving the integration of behavioral and social science training (**Box 20.1**; Cuff & Vanselow, 2004). The NAM report identified important behavioral and social science curriculum content organized across five domains: biological, psychological, social, behavioral, and economic. In the psychological and behavioral domains, the NAM encouraged using the transtheoretical model of change to address maladaptive behavior patterns of patients, including health risk behaviors.

BOX 20.1 NATIONAL ACADEMY OF MEDICINE'S RECOMMENDATIONS FOR INTEGRATING BEHAVIORAL AND SOCIAL SCIENCE INTO MEDICAL SCHOOL CURRICULA

Recommendations
- Develop and maintain a database on behavioral and social science curricular content, teaching techniques, and assessment methodologies in U.S. medical schools.
- Provide an integrated 4-year curriculum in the behavioral and social sciences. Medical students should demonstrate competency in the following domains:
  - Mind–body interactions in health and disease
  - Patient behavior
  - Physician role and behavior
  - Physician–patient interactions
  - Social and cultural issues in healthcare
  - Health policy and economics
- Establish a career development award strategy to produce leaders in the behavioral and social sciences in medical schools.
- Establish curriculum development demonstration project awards that fund demonstration projects in behavioral and social science curriculum development at U.S. medical schools.
- Increase behavioral and social science content on the U.S. Medical Licensing Examination.

Source: From Cuff, P. A., & Vanselow, N. A. (Eds.). (2004). *Improving medical education: Enhancing the behavioral and social science content of medical school curricula*. National Academies Press.

The AAMC published a 2011 report on the behavioral and social science foundations for future physicians, which states: "A complete medical education must include, alongside physical and biological science, the perspectives and findings that flow from the behavioral and social sciences" (AAMC, 2011, p. 5). The report adopted the recommendations of the 2004 NAM report (Cuff & Vanselow, 2004), along with additions from the Royal College of Physicians and Surgeons of Canada, to create a framework on how to teach and apply behavioral and social sciences across clinical, educational, and curriculum applications (Frank, 2005).

Knowledge of behavioral sciences also impacts who is selected for medical training. Starting in 2015, the Medical College Admission Test (MCAT), the prerequisite standardized exam used to guide decisions about medical school acceptance, included a section on the psychological, social, and biological foundations of behavior, requiring applicants to medical school to have a basic understanding of the social and behavioral sciences (Kaplan et al., 2012). Scores on this new section have been found to correlate with academic performance on preclerkship courses and subscores on the U.S. Medical Licensing Examination Step 1 exam related to behavioral sciences concepts (AAMC, 2016).

The increased emphasis on behavioral and social sciences is also growing in graduate medical education. Although family medicine has required residents to be exposed to the behavioral sciences, the Accreditation Council for Graduate Medical Education (ACGME) has proposed that family medicine residencies have faculty dedicated to the integration of behavioral health; that residents are able to diagnose, manage, and coordinate the care for common behavioral issues in patients of all ages; and that behavioral health is integrated into the residents' total educational experience (ACGME, 2017). The ACGME requires exposure to behavioral science for other primary care specialties (e.g., internal medicine and pediatrics); however, the requirements are not nearly as specific as those proposed for family medicine. In the context of all these recommendations for changes, there is a growing body of evidence that teaching health behavior change to medical students can change their knowledge, attitudes, and skills related to health behavior change counseling (Martino et al., 2007; Moser & Stagnaro-Green, 2009; Spollen et al., 2010).

Medical School/Internship/Residency

A systematic review of efforts to teach health behavior change interventions during medical school and residency demonstrated that these efforts can be successful (Hauer et al., 2012). Effective interventions were based on existing frameworks such as the National Cancer Institute's five As (Ask, Advise, Assess, Assist, and Arrange) and/or motivational interviewing within a stages of change framework (e.g., Katz et al., 2008; Prochaska et al., 2008). These educators used active learning strategies, structured practice with feedback to learners, and/or opportunities to practice after receiving feedback. Many of these efforts emphasize training brief, effective behavior change interventions that could be used in primary care settings. Medical schools are experimenting with distributed learning and "flipping the classroom." Some researchers are examining how to couple classroom learning experiences with distributed learning methods that use a range of technologies and media (e.g., electronic text, pictures, files, video, and discussion boards) to allow students to engage with course content from anywhere, anytime, and at their own pace (Bouwmeester et al., 2016; Ramnanan & Pound, 2017). Distributed learning methods may use the electronically based, bidirectional communication methods of distance learning, but distributed learning is a broader educational model that includes teaching methods that can be incorporated into traditional face-to-face classroom experiences (Fleming & Hiple, 2004). When researchers have used flipped classroom techniques, they have found that medical students engage with the material, increase their knowledge, and value the approach (Bouwmeester et al., 2016; Ramnanan & Pound, 2017). Additionally, there is an increased focus on interprofessional training throughout medical schools (West et al., 2016). Although much of the interprofessional training occurs between students in medicine, nursing, and pharmacy, this focus opens opportunities for medical and behavioral health providers to train and learn from each other.

Exposure to Effective Integrated Collaborative Care Models During Training

As we highlight throughout the chapter, integrating behavioral health providers into primary care settings provides an important opportunity for not only delivering behavior change counseling, but also teaching other providers and team members how to implement behavior change counseling. Current ACGME program requirements for graduate medical education in family medicine require that there are behavioral specialists on faculty, familiar with evidence-based health behavior change assessments and interventions, who are specifically designated to teach modern behavioral and psychiatric principles to residents.

Increased Exposure to Resources to Support Health Behavior Change Interventions

Although there are interprofessional organizations (e.g., American Psychosomatic Society, Collaborative Family Healthcare Association, Society of Behavioral Medicine) and journals (e.g., *Families, Systems and Health*; *Psychosomatic Medicine*; *Translational Behavioral Medicine*) where the science regarding health behavior change is presented and discussed, most PCPs are not exposed to these conferences and articles. It is therefore important for health behavior change experts to present at and write for the venues where PCPs *do* attend or subscribe, and to translate the science into clinically relevant and meaningful concepts. For example, behavior change counseling experts should collaborate with medical colleagues to prepare appropriate manuscripts for journals that are commonly read by practicing physicians in order to translate the health behavior change science for the broader medical community. Taking the science to the PCPs and other medical providers, rather than expecting them to seek out that science and those resources, may help shape current PCP behavior. Additionally, the U.S. Preventive Services Task Force is finding that behavioral health counseling is valuable in improving overall health (e.g., LeFevre, 2014a, 2014b). Such findings will likely reinforce the perceived importance of offering these interventions throughout the healthcare system.

CHANGING THE HEALTHCARE SYSTEM

Improving the education of physicians about health behavior interventions is an important start, but unless the healthcare system is re-envisioned to support the promotion of health behavior change, it will be difficult for providers to act on what they have learned and for the system to sustain these changes. Primary care organizations have endorsed joint principles for integrating behavioral healthcare into a model called the patient-centered medical home (PCMH; Table 20.1; Baird et al., 2014). According to the Agency for Healthcare Research and Quality (AHRQ), the PCMH encompassed five key characteristics: (a) providing team-based comprehensive care; (b) providing care that is patient-centered and consistent with "each patient's unique needs, culture, values and preferences"; (c) providing care that is coordinated with other groups, such as any specialists or community-based providers; (d) delivering services in a physically, time-oriented, and economically accessible way; and (e) providing high-quality and evidence-based care (AHRQ, 2022). The themes of this chapter (e.g., finances, systems interventions, integration of behavioral health providers) touch on these principles. Additionally, the passage of the Medicare Access and CHIP Reauthorization Act of 2015 (MACRA), which pushed the U.S. healthcare system from a "fee-for-service" toward a "fee-for-performance" system, and the 21st Century Cures Act, which strengthened mental health parity requirements and allowed Medicaid payments for same-day mental primary care and mental health services, represents positive developments for supporting behavioral health interventions in and out of primary care settings.

TABLE 20.1 Joint Principles: Integrating Behavioral Healthcare Into the Medical Home

PRINCIPLES	BRIEF DESCRIPTION WITH FOCUS ON BEHAVIOR HEALTH INTEGRATION	HEALTH EQUITY CONSIDERATIONS
Personal physician	Every patient has a personal physician.	Not all patients have equal access to PCPs. Those living in rural areas, patients from lower income neighborhoods, and patients from minoritized groups are all less likely to have a PCP (Levine 2020). Efforts to increase the proportion of patients with a personal physician must also address these existing inequities in order to avoid further exacerbating health disparities.
Physician-directed medical practice	The physician and team of healthcare professionals integrate the physical, mental, emotional, and social aspects of the patient's healthcare needs.	Clinics caring for underserved communities may have fewer physicians, as well as reduced access to other types of healthcare professionals, including behavioral health providers. Thus, the ability to operationalize these principles may be much more challenging in resource-constrained settings.
Whole person orientation	Given the prevalence of behavioral health disorders, the role of psychosocial factors in health, and the personal care plans requiring health behavior change, behavioral healthcare is fully incorporated into the medical home.	
Coordinated or integrated care	Healthcare, including behavioral healthcare, must be coordinated and integrated via shared registries, shared medical records (especially shared problem and medication lists), shared decision-making, shared revenue streams, and shared responsibility for the patient's care plan.	Clinics caring for underserved communities may have more rudimentary electronic health records that do not harmonize or share data easily with those from large academic centers, and revenue streams may be harder to predict because many patients may be unable to afford to pay the full price of their medical bills. This may limit the ability of these clinics to adapt to truly integrated or coordinated care models using modern data systems.
Quality and safety	Partnerships with the physician, the patient, and the patient's family must include behavioral health clinicians. Electronic health records must incorporate behavioral health notes and outcomes, and providers must attend to behavioral healthcare issues.	

(continued)

TABLE 20.1 Joint Principles: Integrating Behavioral Healthcare Into the Medical Home (*continued*)

PRINCIPLES	BRIEF DESCRIPTION WITH FOCUS ON BEHAVIOR HEALTH INTEGRATION	HEALTH EQUITY CONSIDERATIONS
Enhanced access	Physical integration of behavioral health professionals is an attractive strategy for improving care, and sites with these providers should consider having open access to these providers.	Clinics caring for underserved populations may have less physical space and/or capital funds for expansion to allow for physical integration of behavioral health providers within the office. This could make it more difficult for these clinics to address the enhanced physical access to behavioral health providers that the principle outlines.
Payment	Appropriate recognition of the value of behavioral healthcare and payment is directed toward this care and toward collaboration between primary care providers and behavioral health clinicians.	Payment models in clinics serving lower income populations may differ and often allow patients to pay only as much as they feel they are able to based on a sliding scale. These clinics may also have a large proportion of Medicaid-insured patients, which will lead to lower average reimbursement for the same service compared with what would be paid by a commercial insurance plan. Thus, payment of behavioral health professionals in such settings will be lower compared with clinics serving a predominantly commercially insured or well-off population. This could act as a disincentive to behavioral health professionals considering whether to practice in such settings.

PCP, primary care provider.

Source: From Baird, M., Blount, A., Brungardt, S., Dickinson, P., Dietrich, A., Epperly, T., Green, L., Henley, D., Kessler, R., Korsen, N., Miller, B., Pugno, P., Roberts, R., Schirmer, J., Seymour, D., Degruy, F., McDaniel, S., & Working Party Group on Integrated Behavioral Healthcare. (2014). Joint principles: Integrating behavioral health care into the patient-centered medical home. *Annals of Family Medicine, 12*(2), 183–185. https://doi.org/10.1370/afm.1633.

Chronic Care Model

In an effort to broaden the focus of healthcare from acute to more chronic problems, the chronic care model was developed to guide quality improvement efforts (Bodenheimer et al., 2002; Wagner et al., 2001). The model recommends that a patient with a chronic medical condition has a primary care team organizing and coordinating their care. The team reviews data and collaborates with the patient, sets goals and promotes self-management, applies behavioral interventions intended to maximize health, and ensures continuous follow-up. In the chronic care model, the health system is assumed to be part of a community. The chronic care model has six primary elements (Table 20.2), many of which overlap with the principles of the PCMH. Improving these six elements fundamentally assists providers in their ability to target health behaviors contributing to disease. Importantly, however, these principles may be easier to operationalize and sustain in clinics or health systems serving a higher income population, which has important implications for health equity. In order for the chronic care model and PCMHs to truly improve health equity, additional resources, research, and careful community engagement will be needed from current and future members of the behavioral and healthcare workforce.

Evidence suggests that care redesigned around the chronic care model results in improved patient care and health outcomes (Baptista et al., 2016; Coleman et al., 2009), and it is recommended for the management of behavioral health conditions (McLellan et al., 2013). The chronic care model promotes changing the focus from the "tyranny of the urgent" to a broader and life-course perspective on healthcare.

System Supports and Practice-Level Redesigns

There is a growing body of research suggesting that system support/practice-level redesign for the delivery of health behavior change interventions by PCPs can be effective. Key evidence-based components of systems supports or practice redesign to successfully promote health behavior change in clinical practice include the following:

- Careful review of staff roles, workflows, and office systems, and creation of clinic–community connections to allow for referral to outside supporting resources
- Training of all clinical staff on "The 5 As" (Assess, Advise, Agree, Assist and Arrange) approach to address health-related behaviors
- Creating effective interventions that leverage electronic data platforms to screen for unhealthy behaviors, including using reminders, prompts, and other processes to integrate such screening into daily clinical practice

TABLE 20.2 Components of the Chronic Care Model	
CHRONIC CARE MODEL COMPONENT	**DESCRIPTION**
Health systems	Create a culture and practice of promoting safe and high-quality care.
Community resources and policies	Mobilize community programming, counseling, and support groups to meet patient needs.
Self-management support	Empower and prepare patients to manage their health.
Delivery system design	Ensure delivery of effective and efficient clinical care and self-management support.
Decision support	Promote evidence-based clinical care consistent with patient preferences.
Clinical information system	Organize patient and population data to facilitate efficient and effective care.

Source: Adapted from Bodenheimer, T., Wagner, E. H., & Grumbach, K. (2002). Improving primary care for patients with chronic illness. *Journal of the American Medical Association, 288*(14), 1775–1779. https://doi.org/10.1001/jama.288.14.1775 and www.improvingchroniccare.org.

- Employing a team approach to deliver health behavior change interventions; front-office staff, medical assistants and nurses may screen patients for health behavior problems and deliver counseling interventions prior to or after the patient appointment, while physicians, who have limited time, serve more to reinforce the health behavior change message

With the increased use of EHRs, clinical decision support systems (CDSS) are likely to play a growing role in effective PCP and team member behavior change interventions. CDSS are:

designed to aid directly in clinical decision making, in which characteristics of individual patients are used to generate patient specific interventions, assessments, recommendations, or other forms of guidance that are then presented to a decision-making recipient or recipients that can include clinicians, patients, and others involved in care delivery (HealthIT.gov, 2017, p. 1).

Roshanov et al. (2013) previously assessed the effectiveness of 166 randomized controlled trials (RCTs) using CDSS in six systematic reviews assessing its effectiveness in prescribing and management of drugs, monitoring and dosing of narrow therapeutic index drugs, primary prevention and screening, chronic disease management, and acute care. CDSS improved process of care in 52% to 64% of studies across all six reviews, with 15% to 31% showing positive health impact on patient outcomes. Roshanov and colleagues also ran analyses on 150 of the RCTs meeting sufficient criteria to examine CDSS characteristics' impact on outcomes. They found the following factors had statistically significant associations with outcomes:

- Systems that provided advice for patients
- Systems that required a reason for a provider to override advice
- Advice presented in electronic charting or order entry systems

We recommend clinics review CDSS development guidance (HealthIT.gov, 2017) prior to initiating a CDSS initiative to ensure they have an effective CDSS build plan to produce desired results.

CASE STUDY 20.1: IMPLEMENTING AN ELECTRONIC HEALTH RECORD-BASED SUGARY DRINK SCREENER IN PEDIATRIC PRACTICES

BACKGROUND

Sugary drink consumption in childhood increases the risk of obesity and numerous other health conditions. As a result, clinical guidelines for pediatricians recommend that providers ask and counsel on sugary drink intake. Historically, this practice has been implemented in ways that are difficult to track over time, may differ between providers, and may not result in counseling or interventions to address identified overconsumption.

CHANGING PRACTICE AROUND SUGARY DRINK SCREENING

In 2017, a large academic health system in Southeastern United States developed and implemented an EHR-based screening tool to promote more regular and standardized collection of sugary drink consumption information in pediatrics and to facilitate behavior change counseling and intervention when needed. The developers of the tool first worked with clinical stakeholders to identify the optimal timing in clinic workflows for inclusion of the screener, and determined that medical assistants, not physicians, were optimally positioned to administer screening. The EHR-based tool was set up to fire automatically and use simple point-and-click, multiple-choice responses rather than requiring free-text entry. All clinical

(continued)

CASE STUDY 20.1: IMPLEMENTING AN ELECTRONIC HEALTH RECORD-BASED SUGARY DRINK SCREENER IN PEDIATRIC PRACTICES (*continued*)

staff were trained on the techniques for screening and brief counseling points to share with parents and patients. Because staff and clinicians endorsed very little free time to add more counseling to their workflows, automated, technology-enabled educational resources were developed to pair with EHR-based screening, including an educational video and information sent to parents automatically after the pediatrician visit.

DID IT WORK? INITIAL RESULTS

In the initial year of screening at participating practices, over 20,000 children were screened using the EHR-based tool, representing 91% of all patients seen during this time. Consistent with national estimates, the screening tool identified higher reported intake than is recommended, with 41% of respondents indicating they regularly consumed more than one sugary beverage per day, and disparities in consumption such that intake was higher among children from racial or ethnic minority backgrounds. In a telephone survey among 200 randomly selected screened families, the parents indicated a high level of support and comfort with the screening process and desire for additional resources to help their families make a change in this behavior. Among those who received information from their pediatrician's office about sugary drink intake, over half indicated that this had prompted them to reduce their child's sugary drink consumption (Lewis et al., 2018).

INTEGRATED COLLABORATIVE BEHAVIORAL HEALTHCARE

Integrating behavioral health providers into healthcare settings, particularly primary care, offers opportunities for PCPs to expose patients to evidence-based behavioral health interventions. Although various approaches to integrated collaborative care have been described in the literature, only a small number of approaches constitute models of care with clearly delineated operational and clinical processes. The collaborative care model (CoCM) and the primary care behavioral health (PCBH) model represent two prominent models of integrated collaborative care commonly implemented in primary care settings. Each model has different principal goals, which shape their methods and influence how much of the practice population is exposed to evidence-based interventions. In some cases, these two models are both introduced to produce a blended model of CoCM and PCBH models to maximize the strengths and minimize the weaknesses of each model (Hunter et al., 2014; Kearney et al., 2014).

Collaborative Care Model

In CoCM (Unutzer & Park, 2012), clinics implement specific pathways for enhancing identification and evidence-based treatment of discrete clinical problems, such as depression or anxiety. PCPs refer identified patients to a care manager (e.g., registered nurse or provider with a master's degree in a behavioral health field), who assists the patient in adhering to the PCP's recommended behavioral health treatment plan (often psychotropic medication) through a series of planned, protocol-driven telephone contacts at scheduled intervals (Figure 20.1). During these contacts, the care manager assesses clinical progress using a standardized measure to determine whether symptoms are improving. Information regarding patient progress is provided to the PCP, who can then make determinations regarding modifying the treatment plan, if needed. The care manager also monitors and reinforces the patient's adherence to the treatment plan. For example, if the PCP prescribed a medication, the care manager might assess whether the patient has filled the prescription and begun taking the medication. The care manager might also ask about any barriers to following the plan (e.g., side effects, cost) and work with the patient on problem-solving.

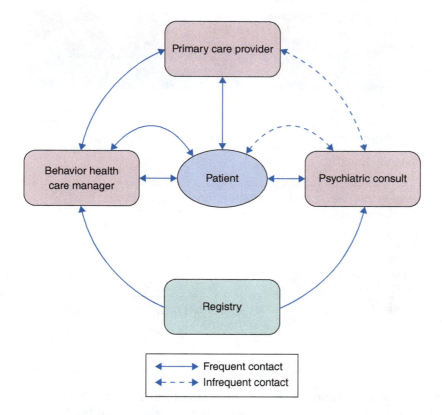

FIGURE 20.1 Collaborative care model.

Some CoCM approaches incorporate additional behavioral health resources to enhance behavioral health treatment in primary care. For example, a consulting psychiatrist (external to primary care) may routinely staff cases with the care manager and provide consultative treatment recommendations (e.g., change in medication, recommended referrals) to the PCP (Oxman et al., 2002). In other settings, the presence of an integrated primary care behavioral health consultant (BHC) in addition to a care manager provides the opportunity for a "blended" model, in which the care manager assists with tracking progress and reinforcing the behavior change plan for patients seen by the PCP and/or a BHC for a variety of concerns (Hunter et al., 2014).

A robust evidence base provides support for CoCM, particularly in the treatment of depression. A 2012 Cochrane report of CoCM for depression and anxiety reviewed 79 RCTs and concluded that CoCM led to reduced symptoms of anxiety and depression compared with usual primary care treatment. Positive results were also found on a number of secondary outcomes, including medication use, mental health quality of life, and patient satisfaction with care (Archer et al., 2012). Thus, CoCM enhances the likelihood that primary care patients are exposed to evidence-based treatments and experience clinical improvement in targeted symptoms. However, this model has limited reach into the broader primary care population and limited health impact beyond the one or two areas of clinical focus, as only those patients diagnosed with the discrete, targeted clinical problem receive enhanced care.

Primary Care Behavioral Health Model

The PCBH model is a fundamentally different model of targeting health behaviors (Robinson & Reiter, 2016; Strosahl, 1998). In the PCBH model, BHCs are integrated into the primary care clinic as team members and follow the standards of care within that clinic. These standards of care are different from those in specialty care (Table 20.3). Patients are referred to the BHC

TABLE 20.3 Comparison of Behavioral Health Standards of Care in Specialty Mental Health and Primary Care Settings

CHARACTERISTIC	SPECIALTY MENTAL HEALTHCARE	PRIMARY CARE BEHAVIORAL HEALTH
Appointment time	50–120 minutes	15–30 minutes
Initiation of care	Self-referral or formal referral from clinic	Patient presents directly to appointment or makes appointment in same clinic
Responsibility of care	Behavioral health provider	PCP
Assessments	Extensive interviews and psychological testing	Targeted functional analyses, brief assessment measures
Interventions	6–12 weeks	1–4 contacts
Documentation	Comprehensive, multipage reports, separate record keeping	Brief, integrated part of the medical record
Follow-up	1–2 week follow-ups	Not at all, next day, 1 week, 1 month, 3–6 months

PCP, primary care provider.

and are typically seen one to four times in 15- to 30-minute appointment slots. The focus is on targeted, evidence-based interventions for problem behaviors. Patients can book future appointments to see the BHC or may be taken directly from the medical provider to the BHC on the same day for a "warm handoff." When managing a chronic medical problem (e.g., chronic pain and obesity), patients may be seen periodically over time (e.g., one appointment per month) by the BHC alone or in conjunction with the PCP or other team members to target complex health behaviors. These adaptations allow the BHC to seamlessly operate within the context of the primary care clinic and interact with a broad swath of the population.

Embedding and integrating BHCs into the primary care environment is a healthcare system intervention for changing how health behavior change counseling occurs. Like their PCP counterparts, the embedded BHC can conduct assessments, interventions, and/or consultation for anyone served by the clinic. The PCBH model has the potential to be applied to a broad range of health behavior and behavioral health concerns (Hunter, Goodie et al., 2017; Robinson & Reiter, 2016), and has been shown to be effective in improving outcomes for patients presenting with heterogeneous problems (Bryan et al., 2012), anxiety and depression (e.g., Angantyr et al., 2015), insomnia (Goodie et al., 2009), and posttraumatic stress disorder (PTSD; Cigrang et al., 2015). However, this model of care needs far more research and rigorous testing to determine its overall efficacy and effectiveness (Hunter, Funderburk et al., 2017).

The PCBH model has the potential to improve the skills of the PCPs in implementing health behavior change interventions with patients. The BHCs directly interact with PCPs around specific patient needs and provide focused BHC interventions, as well as consultative recommendations on what the PCP might target and how they might deliver focused interventions in their follow-up appointments. BHC recommendations are evidence-based/informed and can be delivered by the PCP in 1 to 3 minutes. When PCPs see the skills used by the BHC and the positive outcomes on patient behavior, the PCP's comfort level and willingness to develop their own skills for implementing health behavior change interventions may improve. PCPs see more directly how health behavior change counseling can work, even in the fast-paced environment of primary care. As discussed earlier, if PCPs rely heavily on consultations with colleagues to guide their own clinical interventions, working side by side with a behavioral expert allows for easy access to a collegial voice for health behavior interventions. When BHCs are integrated into primary care settings, patients and PCPs report high levels of satisfaction with the delivery of behavioral health services, and PCPs report improved recognition and treatment of behavioral health concerns (e.g., Angantyr et al., 2015; Funderburk et al., 2012). Despite these potential benefits, the widespread implementation of the PCBH model has been limited by many of the same barriers discussed for the healthcare system.

CASE STUDY 20.2: THE TEAM UP PROGRAM

BACKGROUND ON TEAM UP

Children living in poverty are at increased risk of mental health disorders but are less likely to be diagnosed or to have access to appropriate care for these conditions compared with children from households not in poverty. In many urban communities in the United States, children living in poverty obtain their medical care from clinics designated as "Federally-Qualified Health Centers" (FQHCs). An FQHC is a not-for-profit clinic that serves medically underserved populations and agrees to provide primary care services to patients regardless of their ability to pay for the services, often using a sliding scale fee schedule (Healthcare.gov, n.d.).

In 2016, a program was initiated in three FQHCs in Massachusetts to better integrate mental health services into pediatric primary care. The "Transforming and Expanding Access to Mental Health in Urban Practices (TEAM UP)" model was based on four pillars or categories of activities: *(a) transform care:* modifying care delivery to allow for improved support for families as they parent in early childhood, improving rates of screening children for social, developmental, and behavioral issues, improving access to health system resources that address these needs, and helping connect families to community-based resources and early childhood intervention specialists as well; *(b) strengthen foundations:* by shifting culture and engaging clinical leaders and champions as well as engaging community members, readying the environment by optimizing EHRs and other clinical workflow components to better support this type of work, and augmenting the staff team to support team-based care; *(c) create a learning community:* by training team members on new skills, and tracking and reacting to data metrics that show how/whether changes are having an impact; and *(d) leading system-level change:* by growing the community of practices using this model, supporting advancements in data monitoring capabilities to measure impact, and investing in additional workforce growth as well as career development and advancement opportunities for existing team members; and lastly, by engaging in advocacy at the local and state level to continue to expand the model to other systems.

DID IT WORK? INITIAL RESULTS

In 2023, using the data metrics that were built as part of the TEAM UP program (TEAM UP for Children, n.d.), an evaluation of the project's impact was published. Kim et al. reported on over 20,000 children who received care at a participating health center or nonparticipating control center between 2014 and 2017. Their results were striking and emphasize the importance of systematic and thoughtful integration of these services into primary care: Receipt of care in a TEAM UP clinic was associated with higher rates of diagnosis of mental health conditions, greater use of mental health treatment services, and less use of psychotropic medications in children (Kim et al., 2023).

PERSON-CENTERED PROVIDER AND SYSTEM INTERVENTIONS

It is well-known that patients' level of readiness for behavior change constitutes an important variable in treatment success. Interventions tailored to match the patients' level of readiness have been widely promoted in effective health behavior change efforts. A similar focus can be taken when the healthcare provider or system is the target of behavior change interventions.

Like the patients they serve, medical students, PCPs, staff, and healthcare systems fall along a continuum of readiness to embrace the use of health behavior change interventions. Some will not have substantial awareness of the need to change their approach to practice, while others may be aware of the need to alter their approach but believe they do not have the resources, time, or skills to do so. Still others may be highly motivated and ready to actively implement health behavior change strategies with their patients. Therefore, adopting a person- or system-centered, supportive approach to behavior change may be just as important when working with medical providers, staff, and systems as it is when assisting individual patients in changing health behaviors.

An initial step in moving toward a person- or system-centered approach to promoting adoption of health behavior change strategies involves assessing readiness for change. This assessment can be accomplished through informal or formal means. Informal discussions regarding proposals for changing a PCP's (or clinic's) approach to trying out a different approach toward health behavior change promotion may yield fruitful and rich information. Hallway or break room discussions about a topic, such as implementing a reminder system within the EHR to prompt providers to ask tobacco users if they would consider a quit attempt within the next month, are likely to engender some debate and yield good information regarding readiness to approach such an endeavor. Additionally, a formal assessment of PCPs or clinic staff and leadership can be conducted to determine levels of readiness to change specific aspects of provider or system behavior. Robinson and Reiter (2016) provided a questionnaire to assess PCPs' perceived barriers to altering their referral and consultation behaviors with integrated BHCs in their clinics. The results assist in understanding sources of low utilization of BHCs and can be used to develop a tailored intervention plan to increase desired PCP behavior. In one example, the results of the assessment might reveal the following three barriers to PCP use of BHCs: (a) unsure how to refer, (b) discomfort in discussing a referral to the BHC with patients, and (c) belief that behavioral health consultation is unlikely to benefit patients. A plan to increase PCPs' use of the BHC, therefore, might need to include educational components, as well as skill- and efficacy-building elements.

Thus, provider and system interventions can be tailored to match levels of readiness to change practices related to promoting health behavior change in patients. This involves meeting PCPs at their level of readiness and working with them to gradually build their skills and confidence to increase their readiness to take even small steps toward change. A PCP may not be ready, for example, to work with patients with depression on increasing their social or enjoyable activities, but might be able to learn and implement a brief intervention to increase adherence to taking prescribed antidepressants. On a broader system level, a primary care clinic might not be ready to implement a full clinical pathway for managing obesity in primary care, but might be ready to start a patient registry of obese patients and implement a clinical reminder to cue PCPs to develop small, feasible behavior change plans with patients (e.g., related to eating or physical activity) and to refer patients for more intensive treatment when necessary.

Addressing One Component Is Not Enough

For system changes to be maximally effective in leading to positive health behavior change, there is a need for multicomponent interventions. A "cradle to grave" approach, with multiple factors or contingencies in place, would allow distinct interventions to complement and potentially augment each other.

At a foundational level, there is a need to expose medical students early in training to behavior change principles and interventions. This exposure should expand and continue throughout their training and lifelong continuing education of PCPs. Healthcare systems need to be changed to support provider interventions for health behavior change. Financial factors need to be addressed, either with a financial incentive for integrated CoCMs, or at minimum with finance-neutral programs, to promote uptake of changing the service delivery system from separate primary care and behavioral health systems to integrated models of care. Technology should be leveraged to capitalize on innovations in EHR and other data systems capabilities (e.g., automated prompts for PCP behavior, patient registries). When integrated CoCMs are feasible, efforts need to be made to ensure they fit into primary care clinic workflow, and that the behavioral health components can be supported by multiple primary care team members. Contingencies in integrated collaborative care clinics need to support and reinforce behavior change (e.g., consequences tied to screening rate targets, etc.). When integrated CoCMs are not feasible (for financial, personnel availability, or other reasons), clinics should be encouraged to use alternative system approaches incorporating screening and treatment algorithms, technology assistance, and automated referral processes to increase the primary care team's ability to deliver effective health behavior change interventions.

CONCLUSION

Healthcare provider and system interventions are crucial for expanding the impact of health behavior change interventions. Moving forward requires innovation and effort at multiple levels, most importantly in the areas of training, healthcare policy reform, health equity, and research. Future directions for training efforts need to expand the available training for behavioral health providers seeking to work in primary care environments. Experts in health behavior change should collaborate with medical school administrators and faculty to capitalize on current curriculum reform efforts to inject the fundamentals of health behavior change into the earliest medical school classes. As students move from medical school clerkships to internships and residencies, health behavior change experts should promote teaching and evaluation of health behavior change skills, across all medical specialties.

Enacted healthcare policy reforms, particularly related to funding and reimbursement for models involving system approaches for health behavior change (e.g., integrated CoCMs such as PCBH and CoCM), may reduce some of the previously existing barriers. Even expertly trained BHCs and prepared primary care practices and providers will not result in sustainable implementation of integrated care approaches without the financial business plan to support it. To this end, research to identify effective, key components of these system approaches, with a focus on addressing the associated costs and benefits, is needed. Additionally, further studies demonstrating that provider and system approaches can effectively lead to behavior change in patients, with subsequent impact on symptoms, functioning, quality of life, and healthcare utilization patterns, are warranted. Although evidence is strong in some problem areas (e.g., care management for depression, systematic screening for tobacco), other problem areas, behaviors, and outcomes are understudied. Bolstering the evidence that provider and system interventions effectively lead to improved patient outcomes in a cost-effective manner will help drive the case for continued healthcare policy reform.

SUMMARY KEY POINTS

- Health system-based interventions, and in particular primary care-based interventions, to address health and mental health behaviors offer a way to reach a broader segment of the population and increase the impact of behavioral interventions compared with traditional individual-level outreach and interventions.

- Modern medical education paradigms increasingly feature training in health behavior change counseling, for medical students as well as higher level trainees such as residents and fellows. Such training has been integrated to address a common barrier to implementing behavioral interventions in clinical settings: lack of provider skill and knowledge about health behaviors and mental health.

(continued)

SUMMARY KEY POINTS (continued)

- The U.S. healthcare system has several structural barriers that make widespread use of behavioral health interventions difficult in clinical settings. These include reimbursement and financial systems that prioritize more treatment-oriented interventions, and a paucity of external intensive treatment programs to which patients can be referred.
- Improving referral and care coordination with behavioral providers using the CoCM and integrating dedicated behavioral health professionals into clinical settings using the PCBH model are two approaches that have shown great promise for improving patient access to mental health and intensive behavioral health treatment programs, which may improve health outcomes in other areas as well.
- Models such as the chronic care model and the PCMH provide a road map for how behavioral health could be meaningfully integrated into clinical settings; however, careful attention to existing inequities is needed for all patients to benefit from the application of these ideals.
- Building brief interventions into clinician workflows via the EHR (e.g., CDSS) is a promising way to engage clinicians in at least initiating discussions about health behaviors and ideally connecting patients with providers or programs that are better equipped to support long-term behavior changes.

DISCUSSION QUESTIONS

1. Consider your own relationship with your PCP. What process did you go through to find a PCP? What obstacles did you have to overcome to establish a PCP? Or conversely, if you do not have a PCP, reflect on what barriers are in your way to obtain one.
2. What do you believe the role of a PCP should be in mental or behavior health? Are there reasons a patient may feel more comfortable speaking about their mental health concerns with their PCP rather than seeking specialized mental healthcare?
3. Have you had any experience with distributed learning methods? If so, how did these supplements enhance or change your learning experience? If not, do you believe such methods would be useful to your education? Why or why not?
4. Review the five key characteristics of the PCMH. Select one characteristic and relate it to your place of primary care (or, if you do not currently have a PCP, a known PCP resource in your community). Rate how well the PCP represents this characteristic, examples of how it does so, and how it can improve if needed.
5. Review Case Study 20.2 on the TEAM UP program. Why do you think TEAM UP is associated with less use of psychotropic medications in this population of children?

A robust set of instructor resources designed to supplement this text is located at http://connect.springerpub.com/content/book/978-0-8261-4265-8. Qualifying instructors may request access by emailing textbook@springerpub.com.

REFERENCES

Accreditation Council for Graduate Medical Education. (2017). *ACGME program requirements for graduate medical education in family medicine.* www.acgme.org

Agency for Healthcare Research and Quality. (2022). *Defining the PCMH.* https://www.ahrq.gov/ncepcr/research/care-coordination/pcmh/define.html

Angantyr, K., Rimner, A., & Norden, T. (2015). Primary care behavioral health model: Perspectives of outcome, client satisfaction, and gender. *Social Behavior and Personality, 43*(2), 287–302.

Archer, J., Bower, P., Gilbody, S., Lovell, K., Richards, D., Gask, L., Dickens, C., & Coventry, P. (2012). Collaborative care for depression and anxiety problems. *Cochrane Database of Systematic Reviews,* (10), CD006525. https://doi.org/10.1002/14651858.CD006525.pub2

Arora, P. G., Stephan, S. H., Becker, K. D., & Wissow, L. (2016). Psychosocial interventions for use in pediatric primary care: An examination of providers' perspectives. *Families, Systems, & Health, 34*(4), 414–423. https://doi.org/10.1037/fsh0000233

Association of American Medical Colleges. (2007). *Physician behavior and practice patterns related to smoking cessation.* Author.

Association of American Medical Colleges. (2011). *Behavioral and social science foundations for future physicians.* Author. https://www.aamc.org/download/271020/data/behavioralandsocialsciencefoundationsforfuturephysicians.pdf

Association of American Medical Colleges. (2016). *Using MCAT data in 2017 medical student selection.* Author. www.aamc.org

Bae, J., Ford, E. W., & Huerta, T. R. (2016). The electronic medical record's role in support of smoking cessation activities. *Nicotine and Tobacco Research, 18*(5), 1019–1024. https://doi.org/10.1093/ntr/ntv270

Baird, M., Blount, A., Brungardt, S., Dickinson, P., Dietrich, A., Epperly, T., Green, L., Henley, D., Kessler, R., Korsen, N., Miller, B., Pugno, P., Roberts, R., Schirmer, J., Seymour, D., Degruy, F., McDaniel, S., & Working Party Group on Integrated Behavioral Healthcare. (2014). Joint principles: Integrating behavioral health care into the patient-centered medical home. *Annals of Family Medicine, 12*(2), 183–185. https://doi.org/10.1370/afm.1633

Baptista, D. R., Wiens, A., Pontarolo, R., Regis, L., Reis, W. C. T., & Correr, C. J. (2016). The chronic care model for type 2 diabetes: A systematic review. *Diabetology & Metabolic Syndrome, 8,* 7. https://doi.org/10.1186/s13098-015-0119-z

Barnes, P. M., & Schoenborn, C. A. (2012). *Trends in adults receiving a recommendation for exercise or other physical activity from a physician or other health professional* (pp. 1–8). US Department of Health and Human Services, Centers for Disease Control and Prevention, National Center for Health Statistics. https://www.cdc.gov/nchs/data/databriefs/db86.pdf

Bodenheimer, T., Wagner, E. H., & Grumbach, K. (2002). Improving primary care for patients with chronic illness. *Journal of the American Medical Association, 288*(14), 1775–1779. https://doi.org/10.1001/jama.288.14.1775

Bouwmeester, R. A., de Kleijn, R. A., ten Cate, O. T. J., van Rijen, H. V., & Westerveld, H. E. (2016). How do medical students prepare for flipped classrooms? *Medical Science Educator, 26*(1), 53–60.

Bryan, C. J., Corso, M. L., Corso, K. A., Morrow, C. E., Kanzler, K. E., & Ray-Sannerud, B. (2012). Severity of mental health impairment and trajectories of improvement in an integrated primary care clinic. *Journal of Consulting and Clinical Psychology, 80*(3), 396–403. https://doi.org/10.1037/a0027726

Cigrang, J. A., Rauch, S. A. M., Mintz, J., Brundige, A., Avila, L. L., Bryan, C. J., Goodie J. L., Peterson, A. L., & STRONG STAR Consortium. (2015). Treatment of active duty military with PTSD in primary care: A follow-up report. *Journal of Anxiety Disorders, 36,* 110–114. https://doi.org/10.1016/j.janxdis.2015.10.003

Coleman, K., Austin, B. T., Brach, C., & Wagner, E. H. (2009). Evidence on the chronic care model in the new millennium. *Health Affairs, 28*(1), 75–85. https://doi.org/10.1377/hlthaff.28.1.75

Cook, M., Irby, D. M., & O'Brien, B. C. (2010). *Educating physicians: A call for reform of medical school and residency.* Jossey-Bass.

Cuff, P. A., & Vanselow, N. A. (Eds.). (2004). *Improving medical education: Enhancing the behavioral and social science content of medical school curricula.* National Academies Press.

DiGiulio, A., Jump, Z., & Yu, A., Babb, S., Schecter, A., Williams, K. S., Yembra, D., & Armour, B. S. (2018). State medicaid coverage for tobacco cessation treatments and barriers to accessing treatments–United States, 2015–2017. *MMWR Morbidity Mortality Weekly Report, 67*(13), 390–395. https://doi.org/10.15585/mmwr.mm6713a3

Dolor, R. J., Østbye, T., Lyna, P., Coffman, C. J., Alexander, S. C., Tulsky, J. A., Brouwer, R. J., Esoimeme, I., & Pollak, K. I. (2010). What are physicians' and patients' beliefs about diet, weight, exercise, and smoking cessation counseling? *Preventive Medicine, 51*(5), 440–442. https://doi.org/10.1016/j.ypmed.2010.07.023

Fleming, S., & Hiple, D. (2004). Distance education to distributed learning: Multiple formats and technologies in language instruction. *CALICO Journal, 22,* 63–82.

Frank, J. R. (2005). *The CanMEDS 2005 physician competency framework.* The Royal College of Physicians and Surgeons of Canada. http://meds.queensu.ca/medicine/obgyn/pdf/CanMEDS2005.booklet.pdf

Funderburk, J. S., Fielder, R. L., DeMartini, K. S., & Flynn, C. A. (2012). Integrating behavioral health services into a university health centers: Patient and provider satisfaction. *Families, Systems, & Health, 30*(2), 130–140. https://doi.org/10.1037/a0028378

Goodie, J. L., Isler, W., Hunter, C. L., & Peterson, A. L. (2009). Using behavioral health consultants to treat insomnia in primary care: A clinical case series. *Journal of Clinical Psychology, 65*(3), 294–304. https://doi.org/10.1002/jclp.20548

Hauer, K. E., Carney, P. A., Chang, A., & Satterfield, J. (2012). Behavior change counseling curricula for medical trainees: A systematic review. *Academic Medicine, 87*(7), 956–968. https://doi.org/10.1097/acm.0b013e31825837be

Hawks, L., Himmelstein, D. U., Woolhandler, S., Bor, D. H., Gaffney, A., & McCormick, D. (2020). Trends in unmet need for physician and preventive services in the United States, 1998–2017. *JAMA Internal Medicine, 180*(3), 439–448. https://doi.org/10.1001/jamainternmed.2019.6538

HealthCare.gov. (n.d.). *Federally Qualified Health Center (FQHC)*. Retrieved November 7, 2023, from https://www.healthcare.gov/glossary/federally-qualified-health-center-fqhc/

HealthIT.gov. (2017). *Clinical decision support rule*. www.healthit.gov

Hunter, C. L., Funderburk, J. S., Polaha, J., Bauman, D., Goodie, J. L., & Hunter, C. M. (2017). Primary Care Behavioral Health model (PCBH) research: Current state of the science and a call to action. *Journal of Clinical Psychology in Medical Settings, 25*(2), 127–156. https://doi.org/10.1007/s10880-017-9512-0

Hunter, C. L., & Goodie, J. L. (2010). Operational and clinical components for integrated-collaborative behavioral healthcare in the patient-centered medical home. *Families, Systems, & Health, 28*(4), 308–321. https://doi.org/10.1037/a0021761

Hunter, C. L., Goodie, J. L., Dobmeyer, A. C., & Dorrance, K. A. (2014). Tipping points in the Department of Defense's experience with psychologists in primary care. *American Psychologist, 69*(4), 388–398. https://doi.org/10.1037/a0035806

Hunter, C. L., Goodie, J. L., Oordt, M. S., & Dobmeyer, A. (2017). *Integrated behavioral health in primary care; Step-by-step guidance for assessment and intervention* (2nd ed.). American Psychological Association.

Jamal, A., Homa, D. M., O'Connor, E., Babb, S. D., Caraballo, R. S., Singh, T., Hu, S. S., & King, B. A. (2015). Current cigarette smoking among adults–United States, 2005–2014. *Morbidity and Mortality Weekly Report, 64*(44), 1233–1240. https://doi.org/10.15585/mmwr.mm6444a2

Kaplan, R. M., Satterfield, J. M., & Kington, R. S. (2012). Building a better physician–The case for the new MCAT. *New England Journal of Medicine, 366*(14), 1265–1268. https://doi.org/10.1056/NEJMp1113274

Katz, D. L., Shuval, K., Comerford, B. P., Faridi, Z., & Njike, V. Y. (2008). Impact of an educational intervention on internal medicine residents' physical activity counselling: The Pressure System Model. *Journal of Evaluation in Clinical Practice, 14*(2), 294–299. https://doi.org/10.1111/j.1365-2753.2007.00853.x

Kearney, L. K., Post, E. P., Pomerantz, A. S., & Zeiss, A. M. (2014). Applying the interprofessional patient aligned care team in the Department of Veterans Affairs. *American Psychologist, 69*(4), 399–408. https://doi.org/10.1037/a0035909

Kim J., Sheldrick, R. C., Gallagher, K., Bair-Merritt, M. H., Durham, M. P., Feinberg, E., Morris, A., & Cole, M. B. (2023). Association of integrating mental health into pediatric primary care at federally qualified health centers with utilization and follow-up care. *JAMA Network Open, 6*(4), e239990. https://doi.org/10.1001/jamanetworkopen.2023.9990

LeFevre, M. L. (2014a). Behavioral counseling interventions to prevent sexually transmitted infections: US Preventive Services Task Force recommendation statement behavioral counseling interventions to prevent STIs. *Annals of Internal Medicine, 161*, 894–901.

LeFevre, M. L. (2014b). Behavioral counseling to promote a healthful diet and physical activity for cardiovascular disease prevention in adults with cardiovascular risk factors: US Preventive Services Task Force recommendation statement behavioral counseling in adults with cardiovascular risk factors. *Annals of Internal Medicine, 161*(8), 587–593. https://doi.org/10.7326/m14-1796

Levine, D. M., Linder, J. A., & Landon, B. E. (2020). Characteristics of Americans with primary care and changes over time, 2002–2015. *JAMA Internal Medicine, 180*(3), 463–466. https://doi.org/10.1001/jamainternmed.2019.6282

Levine, S., Malone, E., Lekiachvili, A., & Briss, P. (2019). Health care industry insights: Why the use of preventive services is still low. *Preventing Chronic Disease, 16*, 180625. https://doi.org/10.5888/pcd16.180625

Lewis, K. H., Skelton, J. A., Hsu, F. C., Ezouah, P., Taveras, E. M., & Block, J. P. (2018). Implementing a novel electronic health record approach to track child sugar-sweetened beverage consumption. *Preventive Medicine Reports, 11*, 169–175. https://doi.org/10.1016/j.pmedr.2018.06.007

Ludmerer, K. M. (1999). *Time to heal: American medical education from the turn of the century to the era of managed care*. Oxford University Press.

Martino, S., Haeseler, F., Belitsky, R., Pantalon, M., & Fortin, A. H. (2007). Teaching brief motivational interviewing to year three medical students. *Medical Education, 41*(2), 160–167. https://doi.org/10.1111/j.1365-2929.2006.02673.x

McAfee, T., Babb, S., McNabb, S., & Fiore, M. C. (2015). Helping smokers quit–Opportunities created by the Affordable Care Act. *New England Journal of Medicine, 372*(1), 5–7. https://doi.org/10.1056/NEJMp1411437

McLellan, A. T., Starrels, J. L., Tai, B., Gordon, A. J., Brown, R., Ghitza, U., Gourevitch, M., Stein, J., Oros, M., Horton, T., Lindblad, R., & McNeely, J. (2013). Can substance use disorders be managed using the chronic care model? Review and recommendations from a NIDA consensus group. *Public Health Reviews, 35*(2), 1–14.

Mitchell, P., Wynia, M., Golden, R., McNellis, B., Okun, S., Webb, C. E., Rohrbach, V., & Von Kohorn, I. (2012). *Core principles & values of effective team-based health care.* Institute of Medicine.

Mokdad, A. H., Marks, J. S., Stroup, D. F., & Gerberding, J. L. (2004). Actual causes of death in the United States, 2000. *Journal of the American Medical Association, 291*(10), 1238–1245. https://doi.org/10.1001/jama.291.10.1238

Moser, E. M., & Stagnaro-Green, A. (2009). Teaching behavior change concepts and skills during the third-year medicine clerkship. *Academic Medicine, 84*(7), 851–858. https://doi.org/10.1097/acm.0b013e3181a856f8

Olfson, M., Kroenke, K., Wang, S., & Blanco, C. (2014). Trends in office-based mental health care provided by psychiatrists and primary care physicians. *The Journal of Clinical Psychiatry, 75*(3), 247–253. https://doi.org/10.4088/jcp.13m08834

Oxman, T. E., Dietrich, A. J., Williams, J. W., & Kroenke, K. (2002). A three-component model for reengineering systems for the treatment of depression in primary care. *Psychosomatics, 43*(6), 441–450. https://doi.org/10.1176/appi.psy.43.6.441

Prochaska, J. J., Fromont, S. C., Leek, D., Hudmon, K. S., Louie, A. K., Jacobs, M. H., & Hall, S. M. (2008). Evaluation of an evidence-based tobacco treatment curriculum for psychiatry residency training programs. *Academic Psychiatry, 32*(6), 484–492. https://doi.org/10.1176/appi.ap.32.6.484

Puhl, R., & Suh, Y. (2015). Health consequences of weight stigma: Implications for obesity prevention and treatment. *Current Obesity Report, 4*(2), 182–190. https://doi.org/10.1007/s13679-015-0153-z

Puhl, R. M., Phelan, S. M., Nadglowski, J., & Kyle, T. K. (2016). Overcoming weight bias in the management of patients with diabetes and obesity. *Clinical diabetes: A publication of the American Diabetes Association, 34*(1), 44–50. https://doi.org/10.2337/diaclin.34.1.44

Ramnanan, C. J., & Pound, L. D. (2017). Advances in medical education and practice: Student perceptions of the flipped classroom. *Advances in Medical Education and Practice, 8*, 63–73. https://doi.org/10.2147/amep.s109037

Ramsay, P. P., Shortell, S. M., Casalino, L. P., Rodriguez, H. P., & Rittenhouse, D. R. (2016). A longitudinal study of medical practices' treatment of patients who use tobacco. *American Journal of Preventive Medicine, 50*(3), 328–335. https://doi.org/10.1016/j.amepre.2015.07.005

Robinson, P. J., & Reiter, J. T. (2016). *Behavioral consultation and primary care: A guide to integrating services* (2nd ed.). Springer Publishing.

Roshanov, P. S., Fernandes, N., Wilczynski, J. M., Hemens, B. J., You, J. J., Handler, S. M., Nieuwlaat, R., Souza, N. M., Beyene, J., Van Spall, H. G., Garg, A. X., & Haynes, R. B. (2013). Features of effective computerized clinical decision support systems: Meta-regression of 162 randomised trials. *British Medical Association, 346*, f657. https://doi.org/10.1136/bmj.f657

Rotenstein, L. S., Holmgren, A. J., Downing, N. L., & Bates, D. W. (2021). Differences in total and after-hours electronic health record time across ambulatory specialties. *JAMA Internal Medicine, 181*(6), 863–865. https://doi.org/10.1001/jamainternmed.2021.0256

Rowan, K., McAlpine, D. D., & Blewett, L. A. (2013). Access and cost barriers to mental health care, by insurance status, 1999–2010. *Health Affairs, 32*(10), 1723–1730. https://doi.org/10.1377/hlthaff.2013.0133

Spollen, J. J., Thrush, C. R., Dan-Vy, M., Woods, M. B., Tariq, S. G., & Hicks, E. (2010). A randomized controlled trial of behavior change counseling education for medical students. *Medical Teacher, 32*(4), e170–e177. https://doi.org/10.3109/01421590903514614

Steeves, J. A., Liu, B., Willis, G., Lee, R., & Smith, A. W. (2015). Physicians' personal beliefs about weight-related care and their associations with care delivery: The US National survey of energy balance related care among primary care physicians. *Obesity Research & Clinical Practice, 9*(3), 243–255. https://doi.org/10.1016/j.orcp.2014.08.002

Strosahl, K. (1998). Integrating behavioral health and primary care services: The primary mental health care model. In A. Blount (Ed.), *Integrated primary care: The future of medical and mental health collaboration* (pp. 139–166). Norton.

TEAM UP for Children. (n.d.). *TEAM UP for children transformation model.* https://teamupforchildren.org/our-work

Unutzer, J., & Park, M. (2012). Strategies to improve the management of depression in primary care. *Primary Care: Clinics in Office Practice, 39*(2), 415–431. https://doi.org/10.1016/j.pop.2012.03.010

Vogt, F., Hall, S., & Marteau, T. M. (2005). General practitioners' and family physicians' negative beliefs and attitudes towards discussing smoking cessation with patients: A systematic review. *Addiction, 100*(10), 1423–1431. https://doi.org/10.1111/j.1360-0443.2005.01221.x

Wagner, E. H., Austin, B. T., Davis, C., Hindmarsh, M., Schaefer, J., & Bonomi, A. (2001). Improving chronic illness care: Translating evidence into action. *Health Affairs, 20*(6), 64–78. https://doi.org/10.1377/hlthaff.20.6.64

Walker, E. R., Cummings, J. R., Hockenberry, J. M., & Druss, B. G. (2015). Insurance status, use of mental health services, and unmet need for mental health care in the United States. *Psychiatric Services, 66*(6), 578–584. https://doi.org/10.1176/appi.ps.201400248

West, C., Graham, L., Palmer, R. T., Miller, M. F., Thayer, E. K., Stuber, M. L., Awdishu, L., Umoren, R. A., Wamsley, M. A., Nelson, E. A., Tysinger, J. W., George, P., Carney, P. A., & Joo, P. A. (2016). Implementation of Interprofessional Education (IPE) in 16 US medical schools: Common practices, barriers, and facilitators. *Journal of Interprofessional Education & Practice, 4*, 41–49.

Williams, J., Shore, S. E., & Foy, J. M. (2006). Co-location of mental health professionals in primary care settings: Three North Carolina models. *Clinical Pediatrics, 45*(6), 537–543. https://doi.org/10.1177/0009922806290608

CHAPTER 21

THE ROLES OF THE BUILT ENVIRONMENT IN SUPPORTING HEALTH BEHAVIOR CHANGE

ANGIE L. CRADOCK

LEARNING OBJECTIVES

- Define the built environment and identify how it is measured in research and practice.
- Describe ways the built environment can impact health behaviors and health equity.
- Identify example interventions in the built environment that promote behavior change.
- Outline ways that policy and systems influence the built environment.
- Introduce additional directions for research and practice related to health behavior change and the built environment.

WHY PRIORITIZE THE BUILT ENVIRONMENT FOR HEALTH BEHAVIOR CHANGE?

The notion that the environment can influence our health is not new. Historically, urban planning and public health have had strong links through interventions implemented to address and alleviate communicable diseases (Corburn, 2004). More recently, these links have been rekindled via interdisciplinary research addressing health disparities, chronic and infectious diseases, and their associated health-related behaviors. Theoretically, features of the built environment can influence health behaviors directly via differential access or exposure to health-promoting or damaging environments, or they may enhance or inhibit the impact of health behavior change interventions. The built environment is considered a key social determinant of health and key to promoting greater health equity (https://health .gov/healthypeople). Interventions directed at physical surroundings—the environments we create and within which we live, work, play, socialize, and shop—may initiate and sustain meaningful health-related behavior change and prevent adverse exposures.

This chapter reviews research on aspects of the built environment related to health behaviors and health behavior change, including the various ways in which features of the built environment are measured in research and practice. Examples of built environment interventions and related research illustrate the contexts and mechanisms by which the built environment may shape and define health and health-related behaviors. Finally, a discussion of new directions and technologies for research and practice provides ideas for innovation in understanding the links between the built environment and health behavior and in designing and evaluating health behavior change interventions that can promote greater equity and support resilient communities.

Defining the Built Environment

The "built environment" comprises human-made structures and systems that physically define regions, communities, and neighborhoods, including the buildings, streets, green spaces, and physical systems that serve them (**Figure 21.1**). The domains, definitions, and measures of the built environment used in research vary considerably in the scientific literature, in part because of the large number of features or characteristics that researchers have studied and measured (Brownson et al., 2009). Broadly defined as separate from the natural environment (e.g., air quality and water quality) and the social environment (e.g., social support and social capital), the built environment is often characterized by domains such as access (e.g., proximity, density) and attributes of amenities (e.g., quality), including transportation systems, stores, libraries, and sidewalks. The built environment can be conceptualized and measured at specific geographic scales and is frequently defined for research and intervention at multiple nested levels (**Figure 21.2**). These levels can include community-level characteristics or neighborhood design features (e.g., regional bicycle networks and

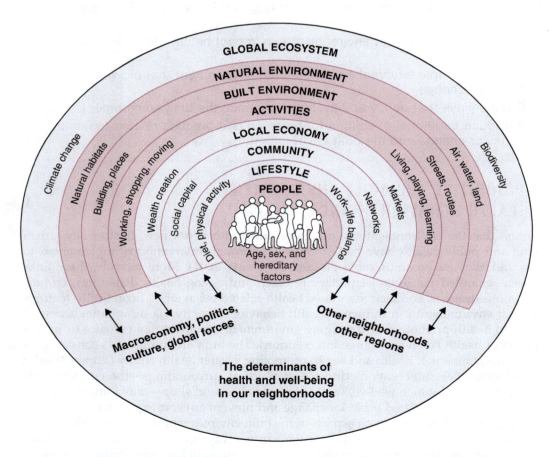

FIGURE 21.1 Determinants of health and well-being in local neighborhoods.
Source: Reprinted from Rao, M., Prasad, S., Adshead, F., & Tissera, H. (2007). The built environment and health. *The Lancet, 370*(9593), 1111–1113. https://doi.org/10.1016/s0140-6736(07)61260-4. Copyright 2007, with permission from Elsevier.

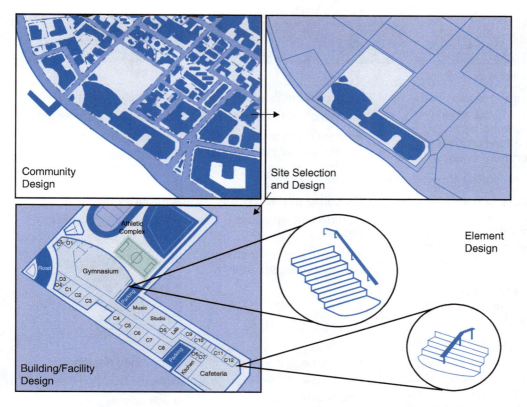

FIGURE 21.2 Examples of geographic scales of the built environment.
Source: Courtesy of Brett Otis.

community zoning), building site selection and design (e.g., the location and siting of new school buildings), street and building design (e.g., square footage for physical activity), and element design (e.g., width and lighting of stairwell or sidewalk; Zimring et al., 2005).

Measurement of the Built Environment

Various assessments can be used to measure the built environment (**Table 21.1**), and measures vary enormously from study to study. Researchers have measured the built environment via a self-reported questionnaire. This type of survey data measures the respondents' perceptions of characteristics of the built environment, such as their access to neighborhood parks or recreational facilities. One such survey measure of the built environment is the Neighborhood Environment Walkability Scale (NEWS; Cerin et al., 2006), which can be used to characterize perceptions of access via questions such as: "About how long would it take you to walk from your home to the nearest basketball court?" While self-reported assessment of the built environment may have several benefits, it can be difficult for study participants to disentangle the perception of their environment from their usual health-related behavior practices (Diez Roux, 2007). For example, independent of actual measured distance, regular walkers may report their local grocery as quite accessible via walking more often than those who are less inclined or able to walk longer distances.

Systematic social observations (SSOs) or environmental audits (Brownson et al., 2009) have increased in popularity as a tool to measure the built environment. Traditional SSOs are in-person assessments of neighborhoods or physical spaces such as stores or building features. When conducting SSOs, researchers can assess various built environment features via walking or driving, using handheld computers, or simply documenting features using

IV • INTERVENING IN SETTINGS AND SYSTEMS TO MODIFY HEALTH BEHAVIORS

TABLE 21.1 Built Environment Assessments

TYPE OF ASSESSMENT	KEY FEATURES	RELEVANT SCALE OF MEASURE
Self-reported questionnaires		
these are questionnaires that are designed to characterize personal perceptions of local built environment features.	+ Ease of administration + Individualized information – Perception may be related to behavior of interest	Community design Site selection and design Building/facility design Element design
Traditional systematic social observation		
these are in-person assessments of the neighborhood, including assessing various built environment features via walking or driving, using handheld computers, or simply with a paper and pencil.	+ Objective assessment – Can be time-/resource-intensive – Required level of training to conduct assessments	Community design Site selection and design Building/facility design Element design
Geographic information system		
Geographic information system technology, which facilitates storing, managing, analyzing, and presenting data that are linked to a location, can measure the built environment.	+ Can manage and store many types of data + Visual display – Not always available in all areas or covering all relevant elements	Community design Site selection and design Building/facility design
Web-enabled applications, wearable sensing devices		
Web-enabled applications and wearable sensing devices use cameras or other sensors that are carried or worn on the body and can be used to capture features of the built environment.	+ Collects data in real time with relevant behaviors + Captures features/elements of personal environment – Sometimes, using costly equipment – Can be limited to daytime collection	Site selection and design Building/facility design Element design
Remote sensing and webcams		
Web cameras collect images of spaces that can be used to characterize built environment characteristics.	+ Longitudinal monitoring + Timely data + Low-burden collection + Collects data in real time with relevant behaviors – Inconsistent image properties – Sometimes cannot characterize specific features/elements	Community design Site selection and design Element design

(continued)

21 • THE ROLES OF THE BUILT ENVIRONMENT IN SUPPORTING HEALTH BEHAVIOR CHANGE

TABLE 21.1 Built Environment Assessments (*continued*)		
TYPE OF ASSESSMENT	**KEY FEATURES**	**RELEVANT SCALE OF MEASURE**
Web-based geospatial data and Big Data		
Web-based data can be used to measure the built environment. Big Data integrates multiple sources of unstructured or structured linked, georeferenced data.	+ Accessibility + Can be historic or timely data + Geographic coverage − Sometimes cannot characterize specific features/elements − Requires substantial data storage, management, processing, and analysis capacity	Community design Site selection and design Building/facility design

a paper-and-pencil tool. Usually, these observations are based on an existing tool, such as the Environmental Assessment of Public Recreation Spaces (EAPRS) tool (Saelens et al., 2006). This method of assessing the built environment can be particularly time-intensive and requires well-trained data collectors to ensure reliable and valid assessments. Researchers have used methods that rely more upon technology-based methods to overcome these limitations.

Geographic information system (GIS) methods are commonly used to measure features and characteristics of the built environment (Pontin et al., 2022). GIS technology facilitates storing, managing, analyzing, and presenting data that are linked with a specific geographic location. Although complete GIS data layers are not always readily accessible for all geographic regions, researchers and practitioners can obtain or create GIS data layers and then perform various functions in a GIS package (e.g., ArcGIS) to assess and define measures such as geographic proximity or density measures (e.g., distance to grocery store and park density). Some studies have coupled GIS analysis with global positioning system (GPS) technology to track people's movements in order to link behaviors or exposures with characteristics of the built environments as study participants move through space and time. This strategy of capturing behavior within its context is also a focus of web-enabled applications using internet-enabled handheld devices like smartphones or tablets in conjunction with activity trackers or logged data to allow individuals to report on or characterize aspects of a specific location (King et al., 2015; Schootman et al., 2016).

Wearable sensing methods and remote assessment are more recently developed tools for characterizing the built environment. Wearable sensing methods, including cameras or other sensing and recording systems, can measure one's built environment. For example, the SenseCam is a small, lightweight wearable camera worn via a lanyard around the neck that captures up to 3,000 first-person, point-of-view images daily (Doherty et al., 2011). The ability to collect these measurement data in real time in conjunction with behavioral data and to capture aspects of the built environment that other methods cannot (e.g., physical obstructions such as construction work and parked cars in cycle lanes) are unique features of these tools and techniques. However, these methods currently cannot capture images in dark environments, managing the large amounts of data retrieved can be difficult (Doherty et al., 2011), and the device and its use in research can be costly. Smartphones are increasingly incorporated into study design and measures.

Remote assessment technologies are emerging tools for observing and measuring the built environment. Web cameras collect images of public (or private) spaces that are streamed to computers and maintained on computer networks (Schootman et al., 2016). One example of this technology is Google Street View, where omnidirectional cameras mounted on vehicles capture images that can be used to characterize the local environment (Koo et al., 2022). In other applications, the location of cameras is fixed, allowing for assessment of the same locations over time under various conditions. The Archive of Many Outdoor Scenes (AMOS) is a resource for the collection of long-term imagery from publicly accessible outdoor webcams (https://mvrl.cse.wustl.edu/datasets/amos/; Hipp et al., 2013). Remote sensing strategies can allow researchers to easily access images from many locations or at the same location over time. However, limitations may include incomplete coverage in all locations of interest, inconsistent image quality, and privacy concerns (Schootman et al., 2016).

Web-based geospatial technologies and Big Data are emerging tools for measuring and characterizing the built environment. For example, the web-based Walk Score tool (freely available at www.walkscore.com) is popular due to its accessibility, international scale, and use of timely data. Walk Score allows a user to enter any query location into the online interface on its website and receive the Walk Score assigned to that location, which is calculated based on the distance to various categories of "walkable" amenities (e.g., schools, stores, parks, and libraries). Walk Score can accurately characterize several aspects of the built environment (e.g., the density of retail destinations, density of recreational open space, intersection density, and residential density) across geographies and spatial scales (Duncan et al., 2011), but only provides an overall assessment of neighborhood walkability, rather than characterizing specific features that may be of interest for certain purposes.

Big Data strategies integrate aspects of many of these assessment strategies in characterizing the built environment. The term *Big Data* can refer to structured and unstructured data that are generated naturally or linked purposefully to allow for a complex and integrated characterization of the built environment (Thakuriah et al., 2017). For example, researchers can connect user-generated survey content with remote sensing data, administrative records, and other sources of measurement, such as satellite or light detection and ranging (LiDAR) data, to create composite characterizations of place. Challenges of Big Data include the vast quantities of data management and processing used to capture and characterize the environment and the unstructured nature of the information, privacy, and data quality concerns (Thakuriah et al., 2017).

Each of these built environment measurement tools has strengths and limitations in characterizing important aspects of the built environment. Existing methods may also not capture all aspects that might be relevant to specific segments of the population (e.g., people with mobility issues, older persons). The use of multiple methods of measuring the built environment may provide a fuller picture of environmental conditions. A particular method (or methods) may be used because of cost or implementation concerns or its utility in characterizing the specific features or geographic scale of the environment that is the point for understanding and intervention.

Life-Course Perspective and Context-Specific Behaviors

The impact and importance of the built environment in health behavior change interventions will differ according to the behaviors, context, and population of interest. For example, features within the built environment of the street setting, such as a sidewalk or crossing signal, may be particularly relevant to interventions promoting walking behaviors among children, older individuals, and other populations with different visual or mobility levels. In many cases, context is a key consideration. School environments are relevant contexts in the lives of children and adolescents. They may be particularly pertinent for nutrition and physical activity interventions among younger persons, while the work environment is likely central to many adult behavioral interventions. Other built environment contexts, for example,

21 • THE ROLES OF THE BUILT ENVIRONMENT IN SUPPORTING HEALTH BEHAVIOR CHANGE   419

community parks where people "play" and socialize, may be important to interventions focused on increasing participation in moderate and vigorous physical activity or restricting tobacco use in park areas. Therefore, successful research and intervention studies must use measurement strategies relevant to the specific behavior being studied and the context in which the behavior occurs and capture and assess the built environment at an appropriate geographic scale to quantify its potential impact. The following provides some examples of the associations between features of the built environment and behaviors, including physical activity, healthy eating, tobacco and alcohol use, injury prevention, and traffic safety.

PHYSICAL ACTIVITY

Built environments can promote physical activity via physical activity-promoting facilities and environments (**Figure 21.3**) while providing opportunities for socialization (de Toit et al., 2007). Physical activity behaviors and built environment characteristics that influence them have been studied extensively (Pontin et al., 2022). Physical activity, measured objectively via monitoring devices or self-report from study participants, is often segmented into various domains (e.g., transport and recreational) or activity types (e.g., walking and cycling) in studies of the built environment–physical activity links. Among adults, cycling for transportation has been associated with amenities such as dedicated cycle routes or other road structures

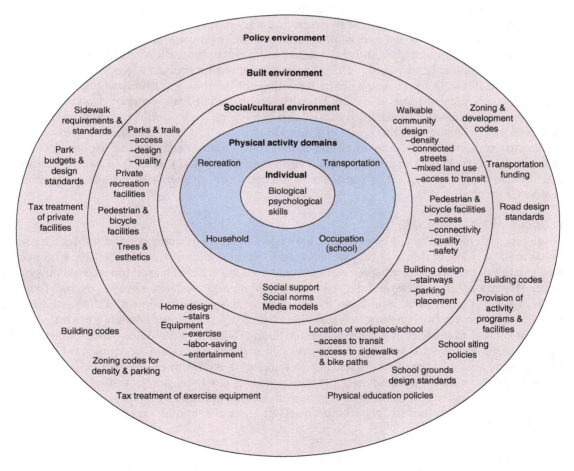

FIGURE 21.3 An ecological model of physical activity behaviors.
Source: From Sallis, J. F., Floyd, M. F., Rodriquez, D. A., & Saelens, B. E. (2012). Role of built environments in physical activity, obesity, and cardiovascular disease. *Circulation, 125*(5), 729–737. https://doi.org/10.1161/CIRCULATIONAHA.110.969022.

enhancing the separation of bicyclists from other traffic, as well as with factors such as high population density and distance. Similarly, attributes of destinations (e.g., presence and proximity) and routes (e.g., sidewalks and street connectivity) are frequent correlates of both utilitarian and recreational walking (see Pontin et al., 2022, for a recent review). Among children and adolescents, research suggests walkability, traffic speed/volume, access/proximity to recreational facilities, and the urban form characteristics of land-use mix and residential density are some important correlates of physical activity participation (Ding et al., 2011).

NUTRITION-RELATED BEHAVIORS

Local stores, supermarkets, and fast-food restaurants can influence nutrition-related behaviors via access and marketing of foods and beverages. Additionally, access to healthy foods is not uniform across all settings, including areas with high proportions of households with low-income, or racial and ethnic minoritized groups, and in rural areas (Larson, Story, & Nelson, 2009). The larger geographic-scale built environment for food access broadly shaped by policy and organizational factors (Story et al., 2008) is often characterized according to the measures of availability (e.g., number of stores with healthy items) or access (e.g., distance to supermarket and density of fast-food establishments; Lytle & Sokol, 2017).

Research that has evaluated a variety of different dietary patterns, foods, or nutrients suggests evidence for association with nutrition-related built environments. In many cases, measures of perceived availability are linked to healthy nutritional behaviors, while objective accessibility measures receive less support from the literature. Researchers suggest this may be because the distance-based accessibility measures fail to capture other relevant measures of the food environment that influence purchasing, including affordability, acceptability, and accommodation (Caspi et al., 2012). For example, within the same geographic context, perceived and objective GIS-based characterizations of the food environment are associated but are not identical (Moore et al., 2012). Additionally, small-scale element designs within retail settings can also influence nutrition-related behaviors. For example, the location of food or beverage choices within the space of a single retail environment and the ways in which choices are presented to the consumer, sometimes called "choice architecture" (Johnson et al., 2012), influence specific product selection (Thorndike et al., 2012). There is a need for more attention to the measurement of food access and food environments at various geographic scales (Caspi et al., 2012).

TOBACCO AND ALCOHOL USE

Some research has evaluated associations between the built environment and substance use behaviors, positing that access can influence use. Studies suggest that the density, number, and locational proximity of tobacco retailers are associated with increased tobacco use among youth (Henriksen et al., 2008) and decreased cessation among moderate/heavy smokers (Halonen et al., 2014). Similarly, over time, increases in local liquor store densities are associated with increases in alcohol consumption (Brenner et al., 2015), and shorter distance to an alcohol outlet is related to more heavy alcohol consumption (Halonen et al., 2013). Decision-makers are increasingly interested in policy strategies such as direct regulation, licensing, and zoning strategies as a way to promote a more health-enhancing environment by reducing both the density and the number of retailers of harmful products like tobacco (Ackerman et al., 2017). Reducing the density and number of retailers could also address the disproportionate presence of marketing for harmful tobacco products in areas of economic or social disadvantage (Lee et al., 2015).

INJURY PREVENTION AND TRAFFIC SAFETY

As programs and public health campaigns promote physically active transportation, the safety of pedestrians and bicyclists becomes an important concern. Deaths among pedestrians have increased substantially since 2009, with nearly 18 people per day having been struck and killed while walking in 2020. Disparities exist in pedestrian deaths by geographic location and by demographic characteristics, with greater numbers of traffic deaths occurring among older persons, individuals in lower socioeconomic positions, and people of color, perhaps due to differential hazard exposures (Smart Growth America, 2022). Targeted investments in infrastructure and physical improvements may prevent injury and decrease potential barriers to active transport. Proven effective environmental changes (sometimes called "countermeasures") such as speed bumps can contribute to a reduction in vehicle operating speeds. In contrast, safe crossing strategies such as the provision of marked crosswalks and wide, raised medians result in more pedestrians crossing at identified crossing locations and fewer pedestrian crashes, respectively (Albee & Bobitz, 2021).

INTERVENTIONS IN THE BUILT ENVIRONMENT: OPPORTUNITIES AND CHALLENGES

Interventions within the built environment to influence health behaviors can reach populations of individuals defined by geographic context and the potential for sustainability over time. However, several challenges are related to identifying and disseminating effective built environment interventions. These include identifying specific and effective strategies for a given context that can prioritize populations experiencing the greatest risks, the potential long-time course and cost associated with larger scale built environment interventions, and the need for development of cross-sector or cross-organizational partners to implement multisector or multisystem interventions.

Health Disparities, Inequities, and the Built Environment

Health disparities or health inequalities are differences in health outcomes (or their determinants) among populations based on categories of social, geographic, demographic, or environmental attributes. Health inequities, a subset of disparities, are modifiable, often occur among disadvantaged groups, and are unjust (Truman et al., 2011). The built environment is considered a key social determinant of health (*Healthy People 2030*). Interventions within the built environment can be used to promote social and environmental justice and reduce health inequities by eliminating the differential exposures to health-promoting or health-harming environments that are found among particular populations defined by social, demographic, or geographic attributes. For example, studies have shown that individuals from some racial or ethnic groups and communities with more individuals with low-income are exposed to features of the built environment that may contribute to obesity (e.g., fewer parks and recreational facilities, as well as fewer supermarkets; Lovasi et al., 2009).

Identifying Effective Built Environment Interventions

Research on the role of the built environment in health behavior change as communities and organizations undertake to implement and evaluate new evidence-based or evidence-informed initiatives in the built environment. As with the built environment itself, built environment interventions vary considerably regarding their scale, from smaller scale efforts in changing specific design features inside a building to larger scale efforts such as the design and construction of a network of bicycling pathways. In many cases, random assignment to intervention condition is not an option due to the nature of these changes. Frequently, research opportunities come through natural experiments, where actions to change the built environment are planned or already underway, and an evaluation can be conducted around them.

Training programs, community assessment tools, and educational settings provide opportunities for educating students, professionals, and the public regarding the roles of the built environment in influencing health behaviors and other health-related outcomes. Table 21.2 outlines examples of resources that can be used to develop and evaluate interventions in a variety of settings for multiple health-related behaviors.

Tools for transport and planning practitioners (Table 21.2) and initiatives that include training public health practitioners and community members on methods for measuring and assessing the built environment are an approach to promote and enhance health and health-related behaviors used increasingly in interventions by public health agencies and health departments (see several examples at www.cdc.gov/nccdphp/dnpao/state-local -programs/). Training programs for transportation professionals address topics including pedestrian safety, pedestrian and bicycle planning, and pedestrian and bicycle facility design (Dill & Weigand, 2010), building on interdisciplinary model curricula that have been outlined (Botchwey et al., 2009). Interdisciplinary collaborations have led to evidence-based design

TABLE 21.2 Resources for Identifying and Implementing Built Environment Interventions		
RESOURCE	**HEALTH BEHAVIOR AREA(S)**	**SOURCE AND RESOURCE TYPE**
The Community Guide: Environmental and Policy Approaches to Increase Physical Activity: Street-Scale Urban Design Land Use Policies	Physical activity	www.thecommunityguide.org/pa /environmental-policy/streetscale .html Summary and support materials related to the recommendation for urban design and land-use policies and practices that support physical activity
Healthy Eating Design Guidelines for School Architecture	Healthy eating	www.cdc.gov/pcd/issues /2013/12_0084.htm Design guidelines that cover 10 domains of the school food environment and 5 core healthy eating design principles
Physical Activity Design Guidelines for School Architecture	Physical activity	http://dx.doi.org/10.1371/journal .pone.0132597 Design guidelines that cover 10 domains of the school physical environment to promote school spaces that enable healthy physical activity
U.S. Green Building Council (Leadership in Energy and Environmental Design)	Climate resilience	https://www.usgbc.org/ Green building certification program for multiple phases of design and building types
Smart Growth Tools	Multiple	https://www.epa.gov/smartgrowth /smart-growth-tools https://smartgrowthamerica.org/ Tools and resources to help communities learn about and implement smart growth approaches

(continued)

TABLE 21.2 Resources for Identifying and Implementing Built Environment Interventions (*continued*)

RESOURCE	HEALTH BEHAVIOR AREA(S)	SOURCE AND RESOURCE TYPE
Active Design Guidelines	Multiple	https://www.nyc.gov/site/planning/plans/active-design-guidelines/active-design-guidelines.page Tools and resources to help cities learn about and implement planning approaches to create streets and buildings that support and promote the physical health and well-being of residents
Pedestrian and Bicycle Information Center	Multiple	www.pedbikeinfo.org A clearinghouse of pedestrian and bicycle information about health, safety, engineering, advocacy, education, enforcement, access, and mobility
Policy and legal frameworks to address health-related features of communities	Multiple	https://www.changelabsolutions.org/ A source for laws and policies that promote healthier built environments and health equity

guidelines for the siting, construction, and renovation of key community facilities and institutions such as schools (Brittin et al., 2015; Huang et al., 2013), buildings (City of New York, 2010), and healthcare facilities (https://www.fgiguidelines.org/) to promote healthy behaviors such as healthy eating, infection control, and fall prevention practices.

Time Courses, Cost, and Sustainability

Generally, built environmental interventions could be considered sustainable interventions in that they influence the structure and function of the physical environment in which health behaviors occur but do not require repeated introduction to be maintained. Depending on the intervention strategy and the scale at which it is implemented, the cost and the time frame for execution may be important considerations in both intervention evaluation study design and the replication or dissemination of effective built environment interventions. Increasingly, studies have sought to evaluate or report intervention implementation costs and conduct cost-effectiveness analysis studies of built environment interventions, a developing research area (McKinnon et al., 2016).

Developing Necessary Partnerships Across Sectors

Many interventional strategies necessitate the development of partnerships to ensure appropriate implementation and effectiveness. However, interventions within the built environment can require new or cross-sector partnerships, particularly for interventions using a system perspective that requires changes across multiple sectors within a system to implement (Giles-Corti et al., 2022). Such collaborations can include urban planners, parks/recreation officials, transportation engineers, and public health officials. Transport system

INTERVENTIONS TO CHANGE BEHAVIORS

Intervention within the built environment can be instrumental in helping to influence health behavior in at least three ways. First, through modification of the built environment directly, interventions may create prompts or structure the built environment to make the desired health behavior easier or even automatic, while less desirable health behaviors are made more difficult. This interventional strategy is often included as a component of multicomponent health behavior change interventions. Second, the built environment may also serve to modify interventional impact by moderating the effects of a behavioral intervention that has been introduced. Third, characteristics of the built environment may require that existing health behavior change interventions be modified (or adapted) prior to implementation to achieve fidelity of the interventional implementation and maximum intervention effectiveness (Chaix, 2009). The following sections provide examples of these types of influence across a number of sectors that impact health behavior.

Physical Spaces to Promote Health

Schools are important environments for influencing the health-related behaviors of students. Interventions within the built environments of schools have been developed to address dietary behaviors, as well as physical activity and tobacco use. Often, making "the healthy choice the easy choice" in school-based interventions has included a mix of a physical infrastructure change intervention, as well as awareness and education.

Many students consume food and beverages while on school property, making the built environment of schools a popular setting for interventions to promote healthy eating and drinking behaviors. Adequate fruit and vegetable intake is recommended to promote health and reduce chronic disease risk and may help with maintaining a healthy weight when consumed in place of more calorically dense foods (U.S. Department of Agriculture and U.S. Department of Health and Human Services, 2020). In the Los Angeles Unified School District, school building infrastructure changes, including the addition of salad bars to the cafeteria and the promotion of the salad bar as an option for a reimbursable school lunch program, were accompanied by an increase in reported fruit and vegetable consumption among students (Slusser et al., 2007). In some instances, the school environment may serve as a barrier. For example, promoting adequate water intake among students may produce health benefits, as water provides a calorie-free source of hydration. However, in some schools, drinking water access is poor due to inadequate plumbing or contaminated drinking water sources. To implement an intervention to promote tap water as a primary beverage during after-school snack periods, participants had to modify the intervention activities and provide alternate drinking water sources due to the lack of potable tap water in some schools (Giles et al., 2012).

School playgrounds are a common context for play and physical activity among students. Several studies have evaluated the physical activity changes associated with interventions that include modification to the playground environments. Among preschool-age students, physical activity-friendly equipment appropriate for younger children was added to the outdoor play area in a childcare center to promote active play. The young attendees significantly decreased the percentage of outdoor playtime spent in sedentary behavior and increased light, moderate, and vigorous physical activity over 5 days of measurement following the intervention (Hannon & Brown, 2008). Among older children, researchers found that setting up painted playground markings identifying appropriate activity-specific play areas, and installing physical structures, including goal posts and basketball hoops, fencing, and seating areas, led to increased time that students attending these schools spent in moderate and vigorous physical activity over 6 months compared with students attending schools who did not receive the environmental intervention (Ridgers et al., 2007). The newness and level of physically active play-promoting attributes of built environment interventions may also be important considerations for physical activity. Researchers found that, although playground utilization was greater, physical activity levels did not increase in a playground intervention study incorporating art, shade structures, and garden elements into playground environments (Anthamatten et al., 2011) and that over longer periods, even effective renovation intervention impacts may diminish (Ridgers et al., 2010).

CASE STUDY 21.1: PLAY ACROSS BOSTON

In one community, a research collaboration identified inequities in access to (distance to and density of) quality playgrounds and programmatic opportunities for physical activity via a community-wide survey and GIS analysis of on-site built environment assessments initiated to understand how community resources and household characteristics might combine to influence physical activity. City officials, researchers, and community partners collaborated in a participatory process in efforts that identified and then created actions reducing documented disparities in access to physical activity facilities. Monitoring included a follow-up assessment of playground quality among a subset of public parks and a survey of local bicycle and pedestrian transportation infrastructure that might influence access to these public resources. City budget data were also reviewed to estimate citywide playground renovation rates before and after the report was released. Findings indicated improvements in playground quality and an equitable park renovation schedule since the baseline assessment (Cradock et al., 2005; Hannon et al., 2006). This initiative included assessments of community- and location-specific measures of the built environment, highlighting the importance of considering both the metric and scale of assessments in research and intervention (Duncan et al., 2012). The participatory project activities point to the important roles of community input and collaboration in interventions to address inequalities (Hannon et al., 2006). In this case, the community collaborations led to more equity in access to quality recreation facilities over time (Barrett et al., 2011).

Prompting Healthy Behaviors in Other Everyday Environments

The built environment may be used to promote and prompt healthy behaviors in everyday activities and environments beyond schools as well. For example, taking the stairs is one way to be more physically active in everyday environments and has been associated with improvements in fitness over short intervention periods (Boreham et al., 2005). Examples of interventions promoting stair use in place of elevators and escalators have generally relied on point-of-decision signage, frequently demonstrating statistically significant increases in stair use with potential for longer term sustainability (Soler et al., 2010). However, research suggests building feature design characteristics can impede or promote stair use. Relevant features include the number of floors in a building (and the visibility of stairs; Bungum et al., 2007). Stairwell lighting, restrictions or key access, and the number of stairs between floors are additional factors associated with stair use (Titze et al., 2001). For example, researchers conducted an innovative natural experiment in an office setting that was designed to promote stair use. In one study group, the workers' offices clustered around the skip-stop elevator, an elevator that was designed not to stop at every floor but located adjacent to an open stairway, whereas other workers' offices accessed an elevator that stopped at each floor with nearby enclosed fire exit stairs. Researchers measured stair use with infrared monitors and card-reader activity logs and found that the skip-stop stair design was used 33 times more than the enclosed stair of the traditional elevator core (Nicoll & Zimring, 2009).

The purpose of innovative health facility design is not only to provide adequate functionality for the performance of services but also to underscore how the facility itself can help promote appropriate health behaviors, remove exposures to environmental stressors, and encourage positive distraction and emotion that may influence health outcomes directly (https://www.fgiguidelines.org/; Olmsted, 2016). Studies have looked at ways in which built environment features of healthcare settings, such as access to natural views and gardens and decreased exposure to noise through facility element design features, may help alleviate stress and promote recovery (Drahota et al., 2012; Ulrich et al., 2008). Public health and design professionals have jointly developed evidence-based guiding principles for healthcare facility design for ICUs, including outlining access to hand hygiene facilities (Thompson et al., 2012). Handwashing behaviors are a key component for infection control and public health. Both hygienic soap and alcohol solutions can be used to beneficial effect and are considered important features of adequate health facility design for infection control. Appropriate access to handwashing facilities through proper placement of accessible dispensers and density of dispensers per hospital bed results in better compliance with accepted hand hygiene protocols (Bischoff et al., 2000).

Other examples of interventions to prompt and improve health-related behaviors occur outside of buildings on the streets of cities and towns. Transportation planning professionals use several design features for streets and street crossings to prompt and encourage appropriate driving speeds and traffic safety behaviors among pedestrians to reduce potential for injury and make these environments more walkable and safer for all users (Albee & Bobitz, 2021). For example, installations of marked crosswalks identify for pedestrians and drivers the expected and appropriate locations for pedestrian road crossings and may also contribute to safer vehicle speeds (Schultz et al., 2015). Accessible pedestrian crossing countdown signals, visual signals that provide information on the amount of time remaining on signalized intersections, as well as auditory information for pedestrians with visual can prompt safe street-crossing behaviors, thereby decreasing the potential for pedestrian injury. Installation of traffic-calming measures, including speed feedback signs, speed bumps to reduce traffic speed, and designing streets with special features such as chicanes (midblock bump-outs on alternate sides of the street) are strategies used to reduce traffic speed and cut-through on residential streets (Bunn et al., 2009). These types of interventions are often employed together in areas with heightened pedestrian and vehicle conflict or in places where improved walkability is desired to promote physically active transportation modes.

Using Planning, Design, and Transportation to Influence and Modify Community Spaces: System Perspectives

Land-use planning, design, and transportation are three key systems used to promote health-related behaviors while simultaneously preventing or reducing injury or unwanted environmental exposures (Rydin et al., 2012). Integrated systems strategies that promote safe and sustainable walking, cycling, and public transport options while reducing motor vehicle dependence can promote health (Giles-Corti et al., 2022). Using system perspectives, built environment interventions can be implemented across entire communities as they are being developed or redeveloped. For example, the Smart Growth movement often involves multidisciplinary partners from planning, design, transportation, the environment, and health as well as safety sectors, among others (Geller, 2003). It is based on 10 principles (Emerine et al., 2006) that can be followed in the development and redevelopment policies and practices at the local, state, and federal levels to support communities that promote health and well-being (Geller, 2003).

In other cases, communities may work locally within a single system. Domestically and internationally, bicycling planning, policy, and infrastructure development have led to variations in bicycling across communities of various sizes (Pucher et al., 2010). Interventions within the transportation system to increase the share of road users who travel via bicycle and foster safe travel focus on provision of bikeway facilities that may include on-street bike lanes, on-street bike paths (or cycle tracks), and off-street bike paths. Minneapolis, Minnesota, and Portland, Oregon are examples of two cities that have substantially increased per capita bicycling infrastructure such as bike lanes and paths. These infrastructure improvements have come with complementary features, including bicycle parking and improved integration with transit or local bicycle sharing programs, which accompanied twofold to fivefold increases in bicycling rates among commuters (Pucher et al., 2011) and important reductions in severe accidents and fatalities (Pucher & Buehler, 2016). In Boston, the expansion of Boston's bicycle infrastructure from 0.034 miles in 2007 to over 92 miles in 2014 was associated with a threefold increase in bicycle use and significantly improved cyclist safety (Pedroso et al., 2016). Community and transportation planners have also undertaken initiatives to improve access and promote safety across entire neighborhoods. Area-specific, traffic-calming interventions appear to contribute to injury reduction and safety improvements (Bunn et al., 2009; Elvik, 2001), and improved reported physical health, increased local pedestrian activity, and decreased traffic nuisance (Morrison et al., 2004). These types of "complete streets" initiatives are becoming more commonly integrated transportation system strategies that aim to enhance safety, walkability, and mobility in communities (Gregg & Hess, 2019).

Using Local, State, and National Policy to Influence the Built Environment

Policy change can be an important component and contributor to intervention in the built environment. Relevant policy may exist within organizations or at various levels of government, including federal, state, or local authority levels, and include administrative policy enacted and implemented in counties, cities, and through other legal entities. Policy-focused interventions may begin with the identification of relevant policies followed by efforts to identify the relevant policy-making body with legal authority to change or implement specific policy. Relevant policy may be assistive policies that enable modifications to the built environment to promote certain types of health behaviors (e.g., federal policy requiring water access in meal service areas for schools participating in the National School Lunch Program), whereas other types of policies may be restrictive, thereby inhibiting changes to the built environment in order to decrease exposure to unhealthy built environments (Perdue et al., 2003).

Some local policies can determine how and where physical infrastructure is developed. Local zoning policies can influence developments in the structure of locales, including the land-use mix, connectivity of streets, the planned infrastructure for pedestrians or bicyclists, and other neighborhood aesthetics (Lopez, 2012). Recent uptake of more physical activity friendly zoning has been documented in municipal policy elements since 2014 (Webber et al., 2023). Because local zoning and building ordinances also define appropriate land uses, they may be used to restrict certain unwanted uses or types of development. For example, studies suggest links between the density of tobacco retail outlets around schools or homes and smoking prevalence (Henriksen et al., 2008) and decreased cessation among moderate/heavy smokers (Halonen et al., 2014). In some communities, zoning ordinances, conditional use permits, and direct regulation have restricted the location of tobacco retail establishments within a certain distance of schools and other community resources like parks and playgrounds (Center for Tobacco Policy & Organizing, 2011). Policy strategies such as moratorium ordinances can prevent new tobacco retailers from entering the market in a community, while establishing tobacco retailer licensing laws enables enforcement of compliance with federal, state, and local tobacco-related laws for existing businesses (Pearson, 2014).

Policy can also serve to facilitate access to existing built environment infrastructure. For example, shared-use arrangements, or creating sharing agreements that facilitate public use of community resources, such as schools or recreation facilities, are one of the strategies included in the National Physical Activity Plan (www.physicalactivityplan.org). In many cases, the sharing of these community resources is facilitated by written contracts or legal arrangements. These shared or joint-use agreements specify liability, use, maintenance, and responsibilities of the parties engaged in the facility-sharing arrangements (Public Health Law & Policy, 2010). Community-use policy strategies may be one way to alleviate the lack of available recreational facilities in some communities, particularly in areas with populations at high risk for disease or lower income communities or neighborhoods with higher proportions of residents of color, where studies have documented disparities in physical activity promoting amenities (Powell et al., 2006) and recreational open space (Duncan et al., 2013). An intervention focused on community use of an existing renovated school playground was associated with a measurable increase in the number of children who were physically active on the school grounds and in the local neighborhoods when compared with a similar-sized neighborhood and school that had not been renovated nor opened for community use (Farley et al., 2007). Model community-use agreement templates may be important facilitators in the dissemination of these policies to local communities and school districts (Eyler & Swaller, 2012); however, the prevalence of municipal shared-use policies has declined since 2014 (Webber et al., 2023).

CASE STUDY 21.2: MOVING MORE IN RURAL SETTINGS

Many rural areas are unique in their proximate access to natural amenities that facilitate recreational physical activity and resources in the built environment, such as abandoned rail beds that have transitioned to rail trails, that enable both transportation-related and recreational physical activity. An ecological approach specific to rural contexts may be needed to promote different types of physical activity behaviors (e.g., recreational, household, or occupational; Umstattd Meyer et al., 2016). Rural areas are less likely than urban locales to have several local-level physical activity-promoting policies (Webber et al., 2023) and more likely to have higher levels of deadly motor vehicle crashes (Beck et al., 2017). In response, the Federal Highway Administration (FHWA) put forward the Small Town and Rural Multimodal Networks guide (https://www.fhwa.dot.gov/environment/bicycle _pedestrian/publications/small_towns/fhwahep17024_lg.pdf) as a design resource and idea book to help meet the specific needs of rural settings to support changes in the built environments to support safe, accessible, and active travel for people of all ages and abilities. The guide provides design information for a variety of transportation facility types that are particularly relevant for small towns and rural settings. For example, it included multiple design strategies for rural areas that consider the volume and speeds of existing rural roadways, the multimodal network (i.e., the collection of interconnected pedestrian and bicycle transportation facilities that are used for mobility), and land uses (e.g., higher density in built-up areas of small rural town centers to less dense areas with limited local destinations). Keys for use in rural settings were the considerations of common challenges unique to rural built environments, such as state highways that pass through town centers and constrained terrain due to agricultural uses that could be addressed through innovations in design and planning for the rural setting. These context-sensitive planning and design strategies may be useful in tailoring and adapting intervention strategies for different rural settings to ensure their success.

Creating a Healthy Community Through Multicomponent Built Environment Interventions

Multicomponent built environment interventions include changes to the built environment in addition to other behavior change intervention components, including informational strategies and behavior modification. For example, as walking and bicycling to school can help kids be more physically active (Faulkner et al., 2009), Safe Routes to School (SRTS) programs in the United States were created as part of federal transportation policy that provided funding to support local programs in each state. These programs work to create safe and convenient opportunities for children to walk and bicycle to school via changes in the built environment (engineering) and use education, promotion, and enforcement strategies at the school and community levels (Guide to Community Preventive Services, 2019). Evaluation of the local implementation of safe routes programs suggests that interventions have varied from focusing primarily on making built environment improvements to providing information to families on navigating obstacles safely and effectively within the built environment. However, the most promising examples include multicomponent intervention strategies, and evidence reviewed suggests they are effective in increasing walking among students and reducing risks for traffic-related injury (Guide to Community Preventive Services, 2019).

Multicomponent interventions can also support healthy eating behaviors. In a collaboration in design and health promotion in Virginia, partners outlined plans for school designs that promote procurement, preparation, and storage of foods to preserve nutritional value, teaching kitchen areas for student educational activities and extracurricular use, serving zones designed to promote display of healthy foods and minimize visibility of less-healthy options, water access, and on-site food production facilities. This application of evidence and theory-based behavioral science principles is intended to facilitate the implementation of multifaceted and multicomponent education, communication, and marketing activities to prompt teachers and students toward more healthy nutrition behaviors through their daily interactions with the built environment of the school itself (Huang et al., 2013). Future iterations of interventional research will benefit from advances in tools and technology to assess and interact with the built environment and the identification of new ways to use these tools to address environmental sustainability and inequities in access to health-promoting built environments.

ADDITIONAL DIRECTIONS FOR INTERVENTIONS IN THE BUILT ENVIRONMENT

There is a greater understanding regarding the many impacts of climate change on health (Giles-Corti et al., 2022). These impacts include exposure to extreme weather events and wildfires; decreased air quality; and diseases transmitted by insects, food, and water. Mitigation efforts that aim to reduce emissions of heat-trapping gases and particles can help reduce the negative impact of climate change on human health (Melillo & Richmond, 2014). Increasingly, governments are trying ways to promote behaviors that improve physical health and slow emissions by changing the built environment. For example, in 2010, the New York City Department of Design and Construction (DDC), Department of Health and Mental Hygiene, Department of Transportation (DOT), and City Planning jointly released *Active Design Guidelines: Promoting Physical Activity and Health in Design* (City of New York, 2010). These guidelines were directed at those responsible for street, neighborhood, and building planning and construction. Strategies that encourage healthy and sustainable behaviors, such as physically active transportation options, cover each scale of the built environment, from large-scale urban land-use planning to small-scale design elements such as the specifics of stairway construction. The design guidelines apply to a variety of different project types, locations, and settings (e.g., public and private, urban and suburban) to encourage wide adoption of such healthy design practices. Four supplements have also been subsequently developed, focusing on sidewalks, community engagement, housing, and safety. Tools and guidance plans have also been developed and promoted specifically to address sustainable building design and neighborhood development through the U.S. Green Building Council. A variety of voluntary LEED (Leadership in Energy and Environmental Design), consensus-based standards, and guidance documents are available to promote sustainable construction and design practices for buildings and communities (new.usgbc.org/leed). Locally, zoning codes, such as Boston's Green Buildings Article 37, promote sustainable development of the city to minimize environmental impacts, conserve energy, and improve the local environment. These standards for development address transportation demand issues, open space, and water recharging and energy generation standards. These codes, which dictate how the built environment is constructed and developed, can promote active transportation options by incentivizing siting new development near transit to foster transit use and promoting nonvehicle alternative transportation options by creating facilities for bicycles and bicycle parking. Globally, there is a stated urgency to take action to support healthy and sustainable cities through actions in governance, policy and benchmarking, and monitoring of indicators of changes in the built environment (Giles-Corti et al., 2022).

Additionally, newer technologies, particularly remote sensing, georeferencing technology, and associated spatial analysis techniques that can incorporate multiple input sources, have altered the potential for place-specific intervention strategies focused on promoting health-related behaviors and environments that are conducive to positive health outcomes. GIS-based methods can be used to identify and characterize areas in need of environmental intervention to increase safety and reduce injury (Poulos et al., 2012; Rodgers, 2010) or to tailor individually focused behavioral interventions (e.g., identifying neighborhood facilities and dispensing walking prescriptions by healthcare providers; Duncan et al., 2011). These advances will enable focused efforts to promote a healthier built environment and reduce health inequities.

CONCLUSION

Researchers and practitioners use various methods and metrics to measure the built environment that can also be used to design and evaluate interventions within the built environment that influence health and health behavior change. Interventions to promote healthy behaviors have been implemented in contexts including school settings, worksites, and communities. The built environment may influence health behaviors directly or indirectly. New tools, technologies, and directions in research and practice may help advance built environment interventions to promote population health and equitable health outcomes.

SUMMARY KEY POINTS

- The built environment comprises human-made structures and systems that physically define regions, communities, and neighborhoods, including the buildings, streets, greenspaces, and physical systems that serve them.

- Researchers and practitioners use various methods and metrics to measure the built environment, which can be assessed at various geographic scales.

- Interventions directed at physical surroundings may initiate and sustain meaningful health-related behavior change and prevent adverse exposures.

- Characteristics of the built environment can make desirable health behaviors easier or more automatic, moderate the effects of a behavioral intervention, or necessitate existing health behavior change interventions be modified (or adapted) prior to implementation to ensure effectiveness.

- New tools, technologies, and directions in research and practice may help advance and adapt built environment interventions to promote population health and more equitable health outcomes.

DISCUSSION QUESTIONS

1. Think about the built environment features in the area around where you live or study. Name two aspects or features of the built environment in this area and describe how they might either directly or indirectly impact transportation modes, access to local destinations, or other health-related behaviors among people who live in or visit that area.

2. Consider an intervention strategy in the built environment to promote healthy behaviors in or around schools for a particular health behavior topic of your choice. Try to identify potential policy levels at more than one level that might influence the built environment (i.e., federal, state, community, school district, or school level) that you may need to consider when implementing your strategy. Describe these and how they might be related to your selected health behavior topic.

3. Consider one aspect of the built environment relevant to promoting more resilient communities that encourage physically active transportation or land uses. At what geographic scale would you want to assess this aspect? What assessment tool(s) would be most relevant and why did you select them?

4. The 2030 public health goals for the United States (*Healthy People 2030*) consider the built environment to be a social determinant of health, a factor that has an impact on people's health, well-being, and quality of life. Consider two ways that the built environment may also contribute to health disparities or inequities.

5. Consider a store that you recently visited to purchase food, beverages, or other household supplies. Were there aspects within the building design and product placement itself that influenced your purchases? Were there features of accessibility to the store in relation to your home or ease of visiting the store itself that made you select that store or location? What change in the built environment might influence others' purchases or store visits?

ACKNOWLEDGMENTS

Dustin T. Duncan contributed his expertise in the planning and development of an earlier edition of this book chapter. Additionally, Brett Otis developed the graphic design and layout for Figure 21.2. I am grateful for their valuable contributions to this chapter.

 A robust set of instructor resources designed to supplement this text is located at http://connect.springerpub.com/content/book/978-0-8261-4265-8. Qualifying instructors may request access by emailing textbook@springerpub.com.

REFERENCES

Ackerman, A., Etow, A., Bartel, S., & Ribisl, K. M. (2017). Reducing the density and number of tobacco retailers: Policy solutions and legal issues. *Nicotine & Tobacco Research, 19*(2), 133–140. https://doi.org/10.1093/ntr/ntw124

Albee, M., & Bobitz, P. (2021). *Making our roads safer. Final report FHWA-SA-21-070*. Federal Highway Administration Office of Safety. https://highways.dot.gov/safety/proven-safety-countermeasures

Anthamatten, P., Brink, L., Lampe, S., Greenwood, E., Kingston, B., & Nigg, C. (2011). An assessment of schoolyard renovation strategies to encourage children's physical activity. *International Journal of Behavioral Nutrition and Physical Activity, 8*, 27. https://doi.org/10.1186/1479-5868-8-27

Barrett, J. L., Hannon, C., Keefe, L., Gortmaker, S. L., & Cradock, A. L. (2011). Playground renovations and quality at public parks in Boston, Massachusetts, 1996–2007. *Preventing Chronic Disease, 8*(4), A72. http://www.cdc.gov/pcd/issues/2011/jul/10_0118.htm

Beck, L. F., Downs, J., Stevens, M. R., & Sauber-Schatz, E. K. (2017). Rural and urban differences in passenger-vehicle–occupant deaths and seat belt use among adults–United States, 2014. *MMWR Surveillance Summaries, 66*(17), 1–13. https://doi.org/10.15585/mmwr.ss6617a1

Bischoff, W. E., Reynolds, T. M., Sessler, C. N., Edmond, M. B., & Wenzel, R. P. (2000). Handwashing compliance by health care workers–The impact of introducing an accessible, alcohol-based hand antiseptic. *Archives of Internal Medicine, 160*(7), 1017–1021. https://doi.org/10.1001/archinte.160.7.1017

Boreham, C. A. G., Kennedy, R. A., Murphy, M. H., Tully, M., Wallace, W. F. M., & Young, I. (2005). Training effects of short bouts of stair climbing on cardiorespiratory fitness, blood lipids, and homo-cysteine in sedentary young women. *British Journal of Sports Medicine, 39*(9), 590–593. https://doi.org/10.1136/bjsm.2002.001131

Botchwey, N. D., Hobson, S. E., Dannenberg, A. L., Mumford, K. G., Contant, C. K., McMillan, T. E., Jackson, R. J., Lopez, R., & Winkle, C. (2009). A model curriculum for a course on the built environment and public health training for an interdisciplinary workforce. *American Journal of Preventive Medicine, 36*(Suppl. 2), S63–S71. https://doi.org/10.1016/j.amepre.2008.10.003

Brenner, A. B., Borrell, L. N., Barrientos-Gutierrez, T., & Diez Roux, A. V. (2015). Longitudinal associations of neighborhood socioeconomic characteristics and alcohol availability on drinking: Results from the Multi-Ethnic Study of Atherosclerosis (MESA). *Social Science & Medicine, 145*, 17–25. https://doi.org/10.1016/j.socscimed.2015.09.030

Brittin, J., Sorensen, D., Trowbridge, M., Lee, K. K., Breithecker, D., Frerichs, L., & Huang, T., (2015). Physical activity design guidelines for school architecture. *PLoS One, 10*(7), e0132597. https://doi.org/10.1371/journal.pone.0132597

Brownson, R., Hoehner, C., Day, K., Forsyth, A., & Sallis, J. (2009). Measuring the food and physical activity environments: State of the science. *American Journal of Preventive Medicine, 36*(Suppl. 4), 25.

Bungum, T., Meacham, M., & Truax, N. (2007). The effects of signage and the physical environment on stair usage. *Journal of Physical Activity & Health, 4*(3), 237–244. https://doi.org/10.1123/jpah.4.3.237

Bunn, F., Collier, T., Frost, C., Ker, K., Steinback, R., Roberts, I., & Wentz, R. (2009). Area wide traffic calming for preventing traffic related injuries. *Cochrane Database of Systematic Reviews*, (1), CD003110.

Caspi, C. E., Sorensen, G., Subramanian, S. V., & Kawachi, I. (2012). The local food environment and diet: A systematic review. *Health & Place, 18*(5), 1172–1187. https://doi.org/10.1016/j.healthplace.2012.05.00

Center for Tobacco Policy & Organizing. (2011). *Matrix of local ordinances restricting tobacco retailers within a certain distance of schools*. http://www.center4tobaccopolicy.org

Cerin, E., Saelens, B. E., Sallis, J. F., & Frank, L. D. (2006). Neighborhood environment walkability scale: Validity and development of a short form. *Medicine and Science in Sports and Exercise, 38*(9), 1682–1691. https://doi.org/10.1249/01.mss.0000227639.83607.4d

Chaix, B. (2009). Geographic life environments and coronary heart disease: A literature review, theoretical contributions, methodological updates, and a research agenda. *Annual Review of Public Health, 30*, 81–105. https://doi.org/10.1146/annurev.publhealth.031308.100158

City of New York. (2010). *The active design guidelines: Promoting physical activity through design*. www.nyc.gov/adg

Corburn, J. (2004). Confronting the challenges in reconnecting urban planning and public health. *American Journal of Public Health, 94*(4), 541–546. https://doi.org/10.2105/ajph.94.4.541

Cradock, A. L., Kawachi, I., Colditz, G. A., Hannon, C., Melly, S. J., Wiecha, J. L., & Gortmaker, S. L. (2005). Playground safety and access in Boston neighborhoods. *American Journal of Preventive Medicine, 28*(4), 357–363. https://doi.org/10.1016/j.amepre.2005.01.012

de Toit, L., Cerin, E., Leslie, E., & Owen, N. (2007). Does walking in the neighborhood enhance local sociability? *Urban Studies, 44*(9), 1677–1695. https://doi.org/10.1080/00420980701426665

Diez Roux, A. V. (2007). Neighborhoods and health: Where are we and where do we go from here? *Revue d'epidemiologie et de sante publique, 55*(1), 13–21. https://doi.org/10.1016/j.respe.2006.12.003

Dill, J., & Weigand, L. (2010). Incorporating bicycle and pedestrian topics in university transportation courses: A national scan. *Transportation Research Record, 2198*, 1–7. https://doi.org/10.3141/2198-01

Ding, D., Sallis, J. F., Kerr, J., Lee, S., & Rosenberg, D. E. (2011). Neighborhood environment and physical activity among youth: A review. *American Journal of Preventive Medicine, 41*(4), 442–455. https://doi.org/10.1016/j.amepre.2011.06.036

Doherty, A. R., Caprani, N., Conaire, C. O., Kalnikaite, V., Gurrin, C., Smeaton, A. F., & O'Connor, N. E. (2011). Passively recognising human activities through lifelogging. *Computers in Human Behavior, 27*(5), 1948–1958. https://doi.org/10.1016/j.chb.2011.05.002

Drahota, A., Ward, D., Mackenzie, H., Stores, R., Higgins, B., Gal, D., & Dean, T. P. (2012). Sensory environment on health-related outcomes of hospital patients. *Cochrane Database of Systematic Reviews,* (3), 362. https://doi.org/10.1002/14651858.CD005315.pub2

Duncan, D. T., Aldstadt, J., Whalen, J., Melly, S. J., & Gortmaker, S. L. (2011). Validation of walk score (R) for estimating neighborhood walkability: An analysis of four US metropolitan areas. *International Journal of Environmental Research and Public Health, 8*(11), 4160–4179. https://doi.org/10.3390/ijerph8114160

Duncan, D. T., Aldstadt, J., Whalen, J., White, K., Castro, M. C., & Williams, D. R. (2012). Space, race, and poverty: Spatial inequalities in walkable neighborhood amenities? *Demographic Research, 26*(17), 409–448. https://doi.org/10.4054/DemRes.2012.26.17

Duncan, D. T., Kawachi, I., White, K., & Williams, D. R. (2013). The geography of recreational open space: Influence of neighborhood racial composition and neighborhood poverty. *Journal of Urban Health, 90*(4), 618–631. https://doi.org/10.1007/s11524-012-9770-y

Elvik, R. (2001). Area-wide urban traffic calming schemes: A meta-analysis of safety effects. *Accident Analysis and Prevention, 33*(3), 327–336. https://doi.org/10.1016/s0001-4575(00)00046-4

Emerine, D., Shenot, C., Bailey, M. K., Sobel, L., & Susman, M. (2006). *This is smart growth.* www.smart growth.org

Eyler, A. A., & Swaller, E. M. (2012). An analysis of community use policies in Missouri school districts. *Journal of School Health, 82*(4), 157–179. https://doi.org/10.1111/j.1746-1561.2011.00683.x

Facility Guidelines Institute. (2014). *Guidelines for design and construction of hospitals and outpatient facilities.* American Society for Healthcare Engineering of the American Hospital Association.

Farley, T. A., Meriwether, R. A., Baker, E. T., Watkins, L. T., Johnson, C. C., & Webber, L. S. (2007). Safe play spaces to promote physical activity in inner-city children: Results from a pilot study of an environmental intervention. *American Journal of Public Health, 97*(9), 1625–1631. https://doi.org/10.2105/ajph.2006.092692

Faulkner, G. E. J., Buliung, R. N., Flora, P. K., & Fusco, C. (2009). Active school transport, physical activity levels and body weight of children and youth: A systematic review. *Preventive Medicine, 48*(1), 3–8. https://doi.org/10.1016/j.ypmed.2008.10.017

Geller, A. L. (2003). Smart growth: A prescription for livable cities. *American Journal of Public Health, 93*(9), 1410–1415. https://doi.org/10.2105/ajph.93.9.1410

Giles, C. M., Kenney, E. L., Gortmaker, S. L., Lee, R. M., Thayer, J. C., Mont-Ferguson, H., & Cradock, A. L. (2012). Increasing water availability during afterschool: Evidence, strategies and partnerships from the OSNAP Group Randomized Trial. *American Journal of Preventive Medicine, 43*(3), S136–S142. https://doi.org/10.1016/j.amepre.2012.05.013

Giles-Corti, B., Moudon, A. V., Lowe, M., Cerin, E., Boeing, G., Frumkin, H., Salvo, D., Foster, S., Kleeman, A., Bekessy, S., de Sá, T. H., Nieuwenhuijsen, M., Higgs, C., Hinckson, E., Adlakha, D., Arundel, J., Liu, S., Oyeyemi, A. L., Nitvimol, K., & Sallis, J. F. (2022). What next? Expanding our view of city planning and global health, and implementing and monitoring evidence-informed policy. *Lancet Global Health, 10*(6), e919–e926. https://doi.org/10.1016/S2214-109X(22)00066-3

Gregg, K., & Hess, P. (2019). Complete streets at the municipal level: A review of American municipal complete streets policy. *International Journal of Sustainable, 13*(6), 407–418.

Guide to Community Preventive Services. (2019). *TFFRS–physical activity: Interventions to increase active travel to school.* https://www.thecommunityguide.org/pages/tffrs-physical-activity-interventions -increase-active-travel-school.html

Halonen, J. I., Kivimäki, M., Kouvonen, A., Pentti, J., Kawachi, I., Subramanian, S. V., & Vahtera, J. (2014). Proximity to a tobacco store and smoking cessation: A cohort study. *Tobacco Control, 23*(2), 146–151. https://doi.org/10.1136/tobaccocontrol-2012-050726

Halonen, J. I., Kivimaki, M., Virtanen, M., Pentti, J., Subramanian, S. V., Kawachi, I., & Vahtera, J. (2013). Living in proximity of a bar and risky alcohol behaviors: A longitudinal study. *Addiction, 108*(2), 320–328. https://doi.org/10.1111/j.1360-0443.2012.04053

Hannon, J. C., & Brown, B. B. (2008). Increasing preschoolers' physical activity intensities: An activity-friendly preschool playground intervention. *Preventive Medicine, 46*(6), 532–536. https://doi .org/10.1016/j.ypmed.2008.01.006

Hannon, C., Cradock, A., Gortmaker, S. L., Wiecha, J., El Ayadi, A., Keefe, L., & Harris, A. (2006). *Play across Boston: A community initiative to reduce disparities in access to after-school physical activity programs for inner-city youths.* Preventing Chronic Disease. http://www.cdc.gov/pcd/issues/2006 /jul/05_0125.htm

Henriksen, L., Feighery, E. C., Schleicher, N. C., Cowling, D. W., Kline, R. S., & Fortmann, S. P. (2008). Is adolescent smoking related to the density and proximity of tobacco outlets and retail cigarette advertising near schools? *Preventive Medicine, 47*(2), 210–214. https://doi.org/10.1016/j.ypmed .2008.04.008

Hipp, J. A., Adlakha, D., Eyler, A. A., Chang, B., & Pless, R. (2013). Emerging technologies: Webcams and crowd-sourcing to identify active transportation. *American Journal of Preventive Medicine, 44*(1), 96–97. https://doi.org/10.1016/j.amepre.2012.09.051

Huang, T. T. K., Sorensen, D., Davis, S., Frerichs, L., Brittin, J., & Celentano, J. (2013). Healthy eating design guidelines for school architecture. *Preventing Chronic Disease, 10,* E27. https://doi.org/10.5888/pcd10.120084

Johnson, E. J., Shu, S. B., Dellaert, B. G., Fox, C., Goldstein, D. G., Häubl, G., Larric, R. P., Payne, W. J., Peters, E., Schkade, D., Wansink, B., & Weber, E. U. (2012). Beyond nudges: Tools of a choice architecture. *Marketing Letters, 23*(2), 487–504. https://doi.org/10.1007/s11002-012-9186-1

King, A. C., Glanz, K., & Patrick, K. (2015). Technologies to measure and modify physical activity and eating environments. *American Journal of Preventive Medicine, 48*(5), 630–638. https://doi.org/10.1016/j.amepre.2014.10.005

Koo, B. W., Guhathakurta, S., & Botchwey, N. (2022). Development and validation of automated microscale walkability audit method. *Health Place, 73,* 102733. https://doi.org/10.1016/j.healthplace.2021.102733

Lee, J. G., Henriksen, L., Rose, S. W., Moreland-Russell, S., & Ribisl, K. M. (2015). A systematic review of neighborhood disparities in point-of-sale tobacco marketing. *American Journal of Public Health, 105*(9), e8–18. https://doi.org/10.2105/AJPH.2015.302777

Lopez, R. P. (2012). *The built environment and public health* (1st ed.). Jossey-Bass.

Lovasi, G. S., Hutson, M. A., Guerra, M., & Neckerman, K. M. (2009). Built environments and obesity in disadvantaged populations. *Epidemiological Review, 31,* 7–20. https://doi.org/10.1093/epirev/mxp005

Lytle, L. A., & Sokol, R. L. (2017). Measures of the food environment: A systematic review of the field, 2007–2015. *Health Place, 44,* 18–34. https://doi.org/10.1016/j.healthplace.2016.12.007

McKinnon, R. A., Siddiqi, S. M., Chaloupka, F. J., Mancino, L., & Prasad, K. (2016). Obesity-related policy/environmental interventions: A systematic review of economic analyses. *American Journal of Preventive Medicine, 50*(4), 543–549. https://doi.org/10.1016/j.amepre.2015.10.021

Melillo, J. M., Terese, T. C., Richmond., & Yohe, W. W. (Eds.). (2014). *Highlights of climate change impacts in the United States: The third national climate assessment.* U.S. Global Change Research Program.

Moore, L. V., Roux, A. V. D., & Franco, M. (2012). Measuring availability of healthy foods: Agreement between directly measured and self-reported data. *American Journal of Epidemiology, 175*(10), 1037–1044. https://doi.org/10.1093/aje/kwr445

Morrison, D. S., Thomson, H., & Petticrew, M. (2004). Evaluation of the health effects of a neighbourhood traffic calming scheme. *Journal of Epidemiology and Community Health, 58*(10), 837–840. https://doi.org/10.1136/jech.2003.017509

Nicoll, G., & Zimring, C. (2009). Effect of innovative building design on physical activity. *Journal of Public Health Policy, 30,* S111–S123. https://doi.org/10.1057/jphp.2008.55

Olmsted, R. N. (2016). Construction and renovation of health care facilities for patient safety and infection prevention. *Infectious Disease Clinics of North America, 30*(3), 713–728. https://doi.org/10.1016/j.idc.2016.04.005

Pearson, A. (2014). *Local strategies to regulate vape shops & lounges.* Change Lab Solutions. http://changelabsolutions.org/sites/default/files/Vapor_Lounges_FINAL_20140926_1.pdf

Pedroso, F. E., Angriman, F., Bellows, A. L., & Taylor, K. (2016). Bicycle use and cyclist safety following Boston's bicycle infrastructure expansion, 2009–2012. *American Journal of Public Health, 106*(12), 2171–2177. https://doi.org/10.2105/AJPH.2016.303454

Perdue, W. C., Stone, L. A., & Gostin, L. O. (2003). The built environment and its relationship to the public's health: The legal framework. *American Journal of Public Health, 93*(9), 1390–1394. https://doi.org/10.2105/ajph.93.9.1390

Pontin, F. L., Jenneson, V. L., Morris, M. A., Clarke, G. P., & Lomax, N. M. (2022). Objectively measuring the association between the built environment and physical activity: A systematic review and reporting framework. *The International Journal of Behavioral Nutrition and Physical Activity, 19*(1), 119. https://doi.org/10.1186/s12966-022-01352-7

Poulos, R. G., Hatfield, J., Rissel, C., Grzebieta, R., & McIntosh, A. S. (2012). Exposure-based cycling crash, near miss and injury rates: The safer cycling prospective cohort study protocol. *Injury Prevention, 18*(1), e1. https://doi.org/10.1136/injuryprev-2011-040160

Powell, L. M., Slater, S., Chaloupka, F. J., & Harper, D. (2006). Availability of physical activity-related facilities and neighborhood demographic and socioeconomic characteristics: A national study. *American Journal of Public Health, 96*(9), 1676–1680. https://doi.org/10.2105/AJPH.2005.065573

Public Health Law & Policy. (2010). *Summary of legal rules governing liability for recreational use of school facilities public health law and policy.* http://changelabsolutions.org/sites/phlpnet.org/files/Liability_RecUse_JU_FINAL_2010.03.19_revised_20111213.pdf

Pucher, J., & Buehler, R. (2016). Safer cycling through improved infrastructure. *American Journal of Public Health, 106*(12), 2089–2091. https://doi.org/10.2105/AJPH.2016.303507

Pucher, J., Buehler, R., & Seinen, M. (2011). Bicycling renaissance in North America? An update and re-appraisal of cycling trends and policies. *Transportation Research Part A-Policy and Practice, 45*(6). 443–453. https://doi.org/10.1016/j.tra.2011.03.001

Pucher, J., Dill, J., & Handy, S. (2010). Infrastructure, programs, and policies to increase bicycling: An international review. *Preventive Medicine, 50,* S106–S125. https://doi.org/10.1016/j.ypmed.2009.07.028

Rao, M., Prasad, S., Adshead, F., & Tissera, H. (2007). The built environment and health. *The Lancet, 370*(9593), 1111–1113. https://doi.org/10.1016/s0140-6736(07)61260-4

Ridgers, N. D., Fairclough, S. J., & Stratton, G. (2010). Twelve-month effects of a playground intervention on children's morning and lunchtime recess physical activity levels. *Journal of Physical Activity & Health, 7*(2), 167–175. https://doi.org/10.1123/jpah.7.2.167

Ridgers, N. D., Stratton, G., Fairclough, S. J., & Twisk, J. W. R. (2007). Long-term effects of a playground markings and physical structures on children's recess physical activity levels. *Preventive Medicine, 44*(5), 393–397. https://doi.org/10.1016/j.ypmed.2007.01.009

Rodgers, S. E., Jones, S. J., Macey, S. M., & Lyons, R. A. (2010). Using geographical information systems to assess the equitable distribution of traffic-calming measures: Translational research. *Injury Prevention, 16*(1), 7–11. https://doi.org/10.1136/ip.2009.022426

Rydin, Y., Bleahu, A., Davies, M., Dávila, J. D., Friel, S., De Grandis, G., Groce, N., Hallal, P. C., Hamilton, I., Howden-Chapman, P., Lai, K. M., Lim, C. J., Martins, J., Osrin, D., Ridley, I., Scott, I., Taylor, M., Wilkinson, P., & Wilson, J. (2012). Shaping cities for health: Complexity and the planning of urban environments in the 21st century. *The Lancet, 379*(9831), 2079–2108. https://doi.org/10.1016/S0140-6736(12)60435-8

Saelens, B. E., Frank, L. D., Auffrey, C., Whitaker, R. C., Burdette, H. L., & Colabianchi, N. (2006). Measuring physical environments of parks and playgrounds: EAPRS instrument of development and inter-rater reliability. *Journal of Physical Activity and Health, 3*(1S), S190–S207. https://doi.org/10.1123/jpah.3.s1.s190

Sallis, J. F., Floyd, M. F., Rodriquez, D. A., & Saelens, B. E. (2012). Role of built environments in physical activity, obesity, and cardiovascular disease. *Circulation, 125*(5), 729–737. https://doi.org/10.1161/CIRCULATIONAHA.110.969022

Schootman, M., Nelson, E. J., Werner, K., Shacham, E., Elliott, M., Ratnapradipa, K., Lian, M., & Mcvay, A. (2016). Emerging technologies to measure neighborhood conditions in public health: Implications for interventions and next steps. *International Journal of Health Geographics, 15*(1), 20. https://doi.org/10.1186/s12942-016-0050-z

Schultz, C. L., Sayers, S. P., Wilhelm Stanis, S. A., Thombs, L. A., Thomas, I. M., & Canfield, S. M. (2015). The impact of a signalized crosswalk on traffic speed and street-crossing behaviors of residents in an underserved neighborhood. *Journal of Urban Health, 92*(5), 910–922. https://doi.org/10.1007/s11524-015-9979-7

Shinkle, D., Rall, J., Wheet, A., Rockefeller Foundation, & National Conference of State Legislatures. (2012). *On the move: State strategies for 21st century transportation solutions.* National Conference of State Legislatures.

Slusser, W. M., Cumberland, W. G., Browdy, B. L., Lange, L., & Neumann, C. (2007). A school salad bar increases frequency of fruit and vegetable consumption among children living in low-income households. *Public Health Nutrition, 10*(12), 1490–1496. https://doi.org/10.1017/s1368980007000444

Smart Growth America. (2022). *Dangerous by design, 2022.* Smart Growth America. https://smartgrowthamerica.org/wp-content/uploads/2022/07/Dangerous-By-Design-2022-v3.pdf

Soler, R. E., Leeks, K. D., Buchanan, L. R., Brownson, R. C., Heath, G. W., Hopkins, D. H., & Task Force Community Preventive Services. (2010). Point-of-decision prompts to increase stair use. A systematic review update. *American Journal of Preventive Medicine, 38*(2), S292–S300. https://doi.org/10.1016/j.amepre.2009.10.028

Story, M., Kaphingst, K. M., Robinson-O'Brien, R., & Glanz, K. (2008). Creating healthy food and eating environments: Policy and environmental approaches. *Annual Review of Public Health, 29,* 253–272. https://doi.org/10.1146/annurev.publhealth.29.020907.090926

Thakuriah, P., Tilahun, N. Y., Zellner, M. (2017). Big data and urban informatics: Innovations and challenges to urban planning and knowledge discovery. In P. Thakuriah, N. Tilahun, & M. Zellner (Eds.), *Seeing Cities Through Big Data. Springer Geography.* Springer, Cham. https://doi-org.ezp-prod1.hul.harvard.edu/10.1007/978-3-319-40902-3_2

Thompson, D. R., Hamilton, D. K., Cadenhead, C. D., Swoboda, S. M., Schwindel, S. M., Anderson, D. C., Schmitz, E. V., St Andre, A. C., Axon, D. C., Harrell, J. W., Harvey, M. A., Howard, A., Kaufman, D. C., & Petersen, J. (2012). Guidelines for intensive care unit design. *Critical Care Medicine, 40*(5), 1486–1600. https://doi.org/10.1097/CCM.0b013e3182413bb2

Thorndike, A. N., Sonnenberg, L., Riis, J., Barraclough, S., & Levy, D. E. (2012). A 2-phase labeling and choice architecture intervention to improve healthy food and beverage choices. *American Journal of Public Health, 102*(3), 527–533. https://doi.org/10.2105/ajph.2011.300391

Titze, S., Martin, B. W., Seiler, R., & Marti, B. (2001). A worksite intervention module encouraging the use of stairs: Results and evaluation. *Sozial-Und Praventivmedizin, 46*(1), 13–19. https://doi.org/10.1007/bf01318794

Truman, B. I., Smith, C. K., Roy, K., Chen, Z., Moonesinghe, R., Zhu, J., Crawford, C. G., & Zaza, S. (2011). Rationale for regular reporting on health disparities and inequalities–United States. *Morbidity and Mortality Weekly Report, 60*(1), 3–10.

Ulrich, R. S., Zimring, C., Zhu, X., DuBose, J., Seo, H.-B., Choi, Y.-S., Quan X., & Joseph, A. (2008). A review of the research literature on evidence-based healthcare design. *Herd-Health Environments Research & Design Journal, 1*(3), 61–125. https://doi.org/10.1177/193758670800100306

Umstattd Meyer, M. R., Moore, J. B., Abildso, C., Edwards, M. B., Gamble, A., & Baskin, M. L. (2016). Rural active living: A call to action. *Journal of Public Health Management and Practice, 22*(5), E11–E20. https://doi.org/10.1097/PHH.0000000000000333

U.S. Department of Agriculture and U.S. Department of Health and Human Services. (2020, December) *Dietary Guidelines for Americans, 2020–2025* (9th ed.). http://www.dietaryguidelines.gov/

Webber, B. J., Whitfield, G. P., Moore, L. V., Stowe, E., Omura, J. D., Pejavara, A., Galuska, D. A., & Fulton, J. E. (2023). Physical activity–friendly policies and community design features in the US, 2014 and 2021. *Preventing Chronic Disease, 20*, 220397. https://doi.org/10.5888/pcd20.220397

Zimring, C., Joseph, A., Nicoll, G. L., & Tsepas, S. (2005). Influences of building design and site design on physical activity–Research and intervention opportunities. *American Journal of Preventive Medicine, 28*(2), 186–193. https://doi.org/10.1016/j.amepre.2004.10.025

INDEX

AAMC. *See* Association of American Medical Colleges

ACA. *See* Affordable Care Act

acamprosate, 175

ACC. *See* American College of Cardiology

accelerometers, 103, 149

acceptance-based behavioral treatment, 322–323

access to healthcare, 33, 185
- cancer screening, 256, 262, 266
- during COVID-19 pandemic, 94
- and HIV prevention, 23, 25, 26, 223
- of women, 215, 219

accounting, 4

Accreditation Council for Graduate Medical Education (ACGME), 396, 397

ACEs. *See* adverse childhood experiences

ACGME. *See* Accreditation Council for Graduate Medical Education

ACIP. *See* Advisory Committee on Immunization Practices

ACPD. *See* Arkansas City Police Department

ACSM. *See* American College of Sports Medicine

actigraphy, 103, 106

Active Design Guidelines: Promoting Physical Activity and Health in Design (City of New York), 423, 429

active living, 140

actor-partner interdependence model (APIM), 47, 51–52

ADA. *See* American Diabetes Association

ADHD. *See* attention deficit hyperactivity disorder

adolescence/adolescents, 11. *See also* children
- adverse experiences, and CVD, 275
- behavioral family systems therapy, 50–51
- with diabetes, 43, 48, 296, 297, 302–303, 307
- eating behavior of, 121
- HPV vaccination for, 221, 222
- identity development, 87
- obesity in, 316–317
- pediatric weight management programs targeting, 88–89
- physical activity of, 145, 147, 152
- and substance use, 176, 180–181
- vaccination programs, issues facing, 197–198

adverse childhood experiences (ACEs), 275, 281, 344

adverse selection, 8

Advisory Committee on Immunization Practices (ACIP), 193

Affordable Care Act (ACA), 8, 10, 13, 256

Agency for Healthcare Research and Quality (AHRQ), 397

AHA. *See* American Heart Association

AHRQ. *See* Agency for Healthcare Research and Quality

alcohol use, 174
- and built environment, 420
- in children/adolescents, 180
- epidemiology of, 174–175
- pharmacology of alcohol, 175
- during pregnancy, 174, 181
- screening for, 174

alcohol use disorder (AUD), 166
- diagnosis of, 174
- medications for, 175
- motivational interviewing for treating, 175

Alcohol Use Disorders Identification Test–Consumption (AUDIT–C), 174

alcohol-impaired driving, 242–243

American Association of Cardiovascular and Pulmonary Rehabilitation, 282

American Association of Diabetes Educators, 307

American Cancer Society, 256, 258

American College of Cardiology (ACC), 276, 282, 332

American College of Sports Medicine (ACSM), 319, 332

American Diabetes Association (ADA), 300, 301, 306

American Heart Association (AHA), 275, 276, 280, 282, 332

American Psychological Association (APA), 86, 345

American Society for Metabolic and Bariatric Surgery (ASMBS), 330

AMOS. *See* Archive of Many Outdoor Scenes

anal cancer, 220

anthrax, 22

antidepressants, 298, 341, 406

anti-obesity medications (AOMs), 329–330

antiretroviral therapy (ART), 223–224

anti-vaccine movements, 203, 204, 205

anxiety, 83, 89, 342, 363, 385, 403

anxiety prevention programs, 363

AOMs. *See* anti-obesity medications

APA. *See* American Psychological Association

APIM. *See* actor-partner interdependence model

Appalachian Access Project, 32

Archive of Many Outdoor Scenes (AMOS), 418

438 INDEX

Arkansas City Police Department (ACPD), 384–385
ART. *See* antiretroviral therapy
Asian Americans, 2
Ask-Provide-Verify approach, 197, 199, 200
ASMBS. *See* American Society for Metabolic and Bariatric Surgery
Association for Supervision and Curriculum Development, 359
Association of American Medical Colleges (AAMC), 396
asymmetric information
    addressing with health policy, 9–10
    definition of, 8
attention deficit hyperactivity disorder (ADHD), 82–83, 89, 363
attitudes toward behavior (theory of reasoned action), 65, 66
AUD. *See* alcohol use disorder
AUDIT, 345
audit and feedback approaches, 261
AUDIT–C. *See* Alcohol Use Disorders Identification Test–Consumption
augmented reality, 151

BA. *See* behavioral activation
BAC. *See* blood alcohol content
bant (mobile app), 307
behavior change wheel, 124
behavior contract, 350
behavioral activation (BA), 346, 347, 349–350
behavioral economics, 12–13, 243–244
behavioral family systems therapy (BFST), 50–51, 305
behavioral family systems therapy for diabetes (BFST-D), 51, 303, 304
behavioral health. *See* mental health
behavioral health consultants (BHCs), 403–405, 406
behavioral observation methods, 103, 104, 106
Behavioral Risk Factor Surveillance System (BRFSS), 113, 140
benzodiazepines, 177
BFST. *See* behavioral family systems therapy
BFST-D. *See* behavioral family systems therapy for diabetes
BHCs. *See* behavioral health consultants
bicycling, 421, 426–427, 428–429
big data, 417, 418
biochemical analysis, 106, 107
bioecological theory, 83, 86
biomarkers, 106–107, 142, 259
bipolar disorder, 345
birth control movement, 215–216
Black Americans, 4. *See also* race/ethnicity
    cancer screening of, 258, 260, 264, 266
    community trust on healthcare providers, 195
    CVD in, 274, 275, 280
    diabetes in, 306

HIV/AIDs in, 223
    identity development, 87
    lung cancer in, 4, 260, 266
    and obesity management, 318, 323
    representation in behavioral weight loss intervention studies, 325
    social networks of, 147
    social support of, 147
    stress management, 328
    substance use among, 174, 176, 178, 179, 182
blood alcohol content (BAC), 242–243
blood pressure lowering agents, 276, 277
Blues Program, 363
BMI. *See* body mass index
body mass index (BMI), 12, 53, 112, 131, 276, 316, 323, 329, 330, 366, 387
brain development, impact of substance use on, 181
breast cancer screening, 257, 258, 262
BRFSS. *See* Behavioral Risk Factor Surveillance System
built environment, 333, 413–414
    defining, 414–415
    geographic scales of, 415
    injury prevention and traffic safety, 420–422
    life-course perspective and context-specific behaviors, 418–421
    measurement of, 415–418
    and nutrition, 420, 429
    objective measures of, 109, 112
    and physical activity, 148–149, 419–420
    and tobacco/alcohol use, 420
built environment interventions
    additional directions for, 429–430
    community collaborations, 425
    development of partnerships across sectors, 423–424
    effective, identification of, 421–423
    health disparities/inequities, 421, 425
    multicomponent, 428–429
    physical spaces for health promotion, 424–425
    prompting healthy behaviors in everyday environments, 425–426
    rural areas, 428
    system perspectives, 426–427
    time courses, cost, and sustainability of, 423
buprenorphine, 178–179, 185
bupropion, 173, 394
bupropion-naltrexone, 329
buspirone, 177

CACFP. *See* Child and Adult Care Food Program
CAD. *See* coronary artery disease
CAGE. *See* Cut down, Annoyed, Guilty, Eye-opener
cagrilnitide/semaglutide, 329
CALO-RE taxonomy, 151–152

CAM. *See* complementary and alternative medicine practitioners, vaccine attitudes among

Canadian Task Force on Preventive Health Care, 256

cancer screening
  and age, 258, 259–260, 263
  breast cancer, 257, 258, 262
  cervical cancer, 257, 258–259, 263
  colorectal cancer, 257, 259–260, 265
  and community partnership, 264
  direct mail campaign intervention, 262
  equity in, 264–267, 268
  evidence-based interventions, 263–264
  future, key health equity challenges for, 267
  incidence and mortality rates of cancer, 253, 254
  interventions, gaps, and future needs for, 264
  lack of diversity in clinical trials, 267
  lung cancer, 255, 257, 260, 262, 263, 266, 267
  opportunistic *vs.* organized screening, 256
  overuse of, 268
    and inequities, 266
    reducing, 262–263
  potential benefits and harms of, 254–255
  potential to reduce and widen inequities, 266
  rates of, 255–256, 268
  recommendations, 256–257
  and social determinants of health, 264, 266
  use, increasing, 261–262

cannabis use, 176
  and cannabis legalization, 176–177
  in children/adolescents, 180
  pharmacology of cannabis, 177
  during pregnancy, 181
  and stigma, 184

cannabis use disorder (CUD)
  diagnosis of, 176
  epidemiology of, 176
  treatments for, 177

cardiac rehabilitation (CR), 282–283, 285

cardiovascular disease (CVD)
  behavior change interventions for management and secondary prevention of, 277–282
  cardiac rehabilitation, 282–283, 285
  and diet, 276
  epidemiology and significance of, 274–275
  health behaviors central to management of, 276–277
  life-course approaches for prevention and management of, 275–276
  mHealth and eHealth, 279–280
  multicomponent interventions, 281–282, 284–285
  and patient adherence, 276–277, 279
  patient education and therapeutic patient education, 278–279
  promotion of cardiovascular health, 275
  provider-delivered interventions, 279
  risk factors for, 275

Cardiovascular Risk in Young Finns Study (YFS), 275

care managers, 402, 403

CareCoach, 307

CBA. *See* cost-benefit analysis

CBPR. *See* community-based participatory research

CBRC. *See* Centre for Behavioural Research in Cancer, Australia

CBT. *See* cognitive behavioral therapy

CDC. *See* U.S. Centers for Disease Control and Prevention

CDSSs. *See* clinical decision-support systems

CEFMU. *See* child, early, and forced marriages and unions

Centers for Medicare and Medicaid Services (CMS), 282, 323–324

Centre for Behavioural Research in Cancer (CBRC), Australia, 245

cervical cancer, 212, 220–221
  screening, 257, 258–259, 263
  types of, 220

cervical cytology. *See* Pap test

CGMs. *See* continuous glucose monitors

child, early, and forced marriages and unions (CEFMU), 226–227

Child and Adult Care Food Program (CACFP), 367

children, 11. *See also* adolescence/adolescents; developmental influences on behavior/health; school-based interventions; vaccines
  adverse childhood experiences, 275, 281, 344
  COVID-19 vaccines for, 95
  with diabetes, 48, 108, 295, 296, 300
  eating behavior of, 121
  EHR-based sugary drink screening, 401–402
  and gender identity development, 88
  HPV vaccination for, 221
  obesity in, 112, 316–317
  parent and family factors framework, 48–49
  physical activity of, 144, 145, 151, 152
  in poverty, 405
  self- and family-management framework, 44
  substance use in, 180–181

choice architecture, 132, 420

cholera, 22

chronic care model, 399–400

chronic diseases, 44, 50, 55, 153, 155, 374. *See also* cardiovascular disease (CVD); diabetes; worksite wellness interventions
  epidemiology of, 22
  and mental health, 342–343
  and obesity, 316
  and patient adherence, 276
  and physical activity, 142
  at worksites, risk factors for, 375

440 INDEX

chronic obstructive pulmonary disease (COPD), 171
chronic pain, 48–49
CHWs. *See* community health workers
citizen science, 149, 155
civil rights movement, 87
Clean Air Act of 1970, 8
climate change, 25, 429
clinical decision-support systems (CDSSs), 401
closed loop automated insulin delivery systems, 306–307
CM. *See* contingency management
CMS. *See* Centers for Medicare and Medicaid Services
COACH. *See* Community Outreach and Cardiovascular Health Trial
cocaine use, 179
cocaine use disorder, 179
CoCM. *See* collaborative care model
coercion in family planning programs, 216
coffee, 166
cognitive behavioral therapy (CBT), 181, 346–347, 348
cognitive development, 84
cognitive strategies for weight loss, 321
collaborative care model (CoCM), 402–403, 407
collectivism, 94–95
colonoscopy, 259
colorectal cancer screening, 257, 259–260, 265
Columbia-Suicide Severity Rating Scale (CSSR-S), 345
common fate model, 47, 52–53
The Community Guide: Environmental and Policy Approaches to Increase Physical Activity: Street-Scale Urban Design Land Use Policies, 422
Community Guide to Preventive Services, 375
community health workers (CHWs), 261–262, 281–282, 284
Community Outreach and Cardiovascular Health (COACH) Trial, 281–282
Community Preventive Services Task Force, 264
community-based family planning program, 216
community-based interventions, 282, 365
  for diabetes management, 303–305
  dietary interventions, 121
community-based participatory research (CBPR), 27–29
  for developing interventions through Engaged for Change, 29–32
  empowerment theory-based community forum, 32–34
  HOLA, 26–27
community(ies). *See also* built environment
  -based physical activity opportunities for people living with disabilities, 145
  -based prevention of substance use, 167

citizen science, 149, 155
  and eating behavior change, 132
  engagement, 28, 56, 185–186, 366, 400
  norms, 244
  social support interventions in, 150
  -wide education campaigns, 150
community-level health behavior measurement, 101, 108–109
  built environment and neighborhood characteristics, 109, 112
  objective measures, 109–110, 112
  subjective measures, 111, 112–113
community-use agreements, 428
co-morbidity, 342–343
comparative advantage, 6, 8
competitive hypothesis testing, 75
complementary and alternative medicine (CAM) practitioners, vaccine attitudes among, 195–196
complementary goods, 6–8, 15
complete streets, 427
computer vision modeling, 109
condoms, 24–25, 224
conflict resolution hypothesis of motivational interviewing, 198
contingency management (CM), 179, 181
continuous glucose monitors (CGMs), 108, 296, 297, 306
continuous subcutaneous insulin infusion (CSII), 296, 297, 306
contraception demand, 218–219. *See also* family planning and contraception
  drivers of, 218
  inhibitors of, 218–219
  interventions to address, meet, and generate, 219
  measures, 217–218
contraceptive prevalence, 217
control beliefs (theory of reasoned action), 65
Controlled Substance Act, 184
COPD. *See* chronic obstructive pulmonary disease
coping skills training (CST), 48
coronary artery disease (CAD), 343
correlational approaches to theory testing, 74
cost to outcomes ratio, 14
cost-benefit analysis (CBA), 15–16
cost-effectiveness analysis, 15–16
cost-minimization analysis, 15
cost-utility analysis (CUA), 15, 16
counseling, 397, 404. *See also* motivational interviewing (MI)
  family planning, 219
  group, 128
  for obese patients, 323–324, 331
  reimbursement for, 394
  telephone, 70, 131, 331

tobacco cessation, 379, 393
covert antecedents (relapse prevention model), 69
COVID-19 pandemic, 1, 94–95
  developmentally focused health behavior change strategies during, 89
  HIV management during, 25
  HPV vaccination during, 222
  and life expectancy, 2
  measurement of mask wearing/social distancing behaviors during, 102
  and mental health, 94, 385
  physical activity during, 381
  and policies in schools, 364
  and remote work environment, 373, 375
  social support during, 147
  vaccination incentivization campaign, 16
  vaccination mandates, 11, 12, 194–195, 364
CR. *See* cardiac rehabilitation
crack cocaine, 179, 184
crash (dummy) test standards, 239
crosswalks, 421, 426
cryotherapy, 220
CSII. *See* continuous subcutaneous insulin infusion
CSSR-S. *See* Columbia-Suicide Severity Rating Scale
CST. *See* coping skills training
CT colonography, 259
CT scan, 260
CUA. *See* cost-utility analysis
CUD. *See* cannabis use disorder
cue to action (health belief model), 62, 63, 203, 346
cultural acceptability, 90
cultural humility, 90, 91, 92–93
cultural influences on behavior/health, 82, 90
  COVID-19 pandemic, 94–95
  global health issues, 91–92
  global mental health, 94
  health equity, 91
cultural responsiveness, 91
cultural sensitivity, 91
culture
  and adaptability of school-based interventions, 365
  and behavioral weight loss interventions, 325
  cultural adaptation of motivational interviewing, 130
  definitions of, 90
  role in gender identity development, 88
Cut down, Annoyed, Guilty, Eye-opener (CAGE), 174
CVD. *See* cardiovascular disease

dangerous driving, 244
DAST, 345
DCCT. *See* Diabetes Control and Complications Trial

decision aids, 265
deep-vein thrombosis (DVT), 15–16
depression, 341, 350, 385, 403
  behavioral activation for, 347
  and chronic diseases, 342–343
  and diabetes management, 298–299
  diagnosis of, 345
  symptoms of, 342–343
descriptive norms (theory of reasoned action), 65
developmental influences on behavior/health, 82, 83
  bioecological theory, 83, 86
  developmentally focused health behavior change strategies, 88–89
  domains of development, 84–85
  identity development, 87–88
  roles of interactive media use, 86–87
developmental milestones, 83
developmental model of self- and social regulation, 47, 53–54
developmental transitions, 83, 89
device-based measures of physical activity, 103, 140, 141, 149
diabetes, 294
  epidemic of, 295–296
  public health impact of, 295
  types of, 295
Diabetes Control and Complications Trial (DCCT), 294, 297
diabetes distress, 299
Diabetes Initiative of South Carolina (DSC), 305
diabetes management
  adherence to prescribed management regimens, 297
  behavioral family systems therapy for diabetes, 303, 304
  community-based interventions, 303–305
  depression, 298–299
  differences and similarities by type, 296
  emotional barriers to, 298–300
  evidence base, 301
  family barriers to, 300–301
  family-based interventions, 302–303
  fear of hypoglycemia, 299–300
  link between adherence and health outcomes, 297
  motivational interviewing, 302
  multicomponent interventions, 301–302
  psychological insulin resistance, 299
  psychosocial care guidelines, 300
  reducing health disparities in diabetes care, 306
  role of technology, 306–307
  system-based interventions, 305
Diabetes Prevention Program (DPP), 303–305, 325, 328

442 INDEX

diabetes self-management education (DSME), 301, 305

Diagnostic and Statistical Manual of Mental Disorders, 5th edition (*DSM-5*), 165, 166, 171, 172, 174, 176, 179, 345

diaries, 107, 108, 140

diet education, 123–124, 317

diet history interviews, 107

Dietary Guidelines for Americans, 119, 121

diffusion of innovations theory, 131

digital interventions, 39, 54, 55, 56, 61, 70–71, 131, 152, 224, 279–280. *See also* mobile health (mHealth)

digital natives, 86

diphtheria-tetanus-pertussis (DTP) vaccine, 193, 194, 203

direct objective measures of individual-level health behaviors, 103–104, 106

directly observed therapy (DOT), 106

disabilities, people with
physical activity of, 145–146
unintentional injuries among, 240
worksite physical activity interventions for, 383

dissemination and implementation science, 366–367

distributed learning, 396

disulfiram, 175

dogs as sources of social support, 147

DOT. *See* directly observed therapy

doubly labeled water method, 106, 141

DPP. *See* Diabetes Prevention Program

drinking and driving, 242–243

drinking water, access to, 364, 365, 366, 385, 424

dronabinol, 177

drug user health hubs, 170

DSC. *See* Diabetes Initiative of South Carolina

DSM-5. See Diagnostic and Statistical Manual of Mental Disorders, 5th edition

DSME. *See* diabetes self-management educationDTP. *See* diphtheria-tetanus-pertussis vaccine

DVT. *See* deep-vein thrombosis

dynamic computational model of social cognitive theory, 71

EAPRS. *See* Environmental Assessment of Public Recreation Spaces tool

eating behaviors, change in, 119–120, 121, 326
assessment of eating behaviors, 101, 103, 106, 107
barriers to healthy eating, 122–123, 129
behavior change wheel, 124
behavior theories and constructs, 124–127
biology of eating, 120–121
built environment interventions, 424, 429

clinics, 132–133
communities/schools, 132
diet education, 123–124
food choice model, 126
gaps in current knowledge, 133
goal setting, 127
and habituation, 123
individual dietary behavior change, 121–122
intuitive eating, 130
motivational interviewing, 130
multicomponent interventions, 429
problem solving and decision making, 128–129
promotion of healthy eating, 123–127
self-monitoring, 127–128
social support, 128
technology and mHealth, 131–132
workplace, 132

EBCCP. *See* evidence-based cancer control programs

e-cigarettes, 174, 180, 381

ecological momentary assessment (EMA), 107, 151

ecological systems theory, 83, 215

ecological theory of development. *See* ecological systems theory

economic analysis, 13

economic costs associated with policy/program/ intervention implementation, 14

economic evaluations, 13–16

economic stability, 4

economics, 3, 4
making the best choice, 5
market failures, 8–9
markets, 6
Opportunity Atlas, 5
principles, and health policy development, 4–9
relationships between goods, 6–8
supply and demand relationships, 7

ECS. *See* endocannabinoid system

education, 4, 27
for changing speeding behavior, 241–242
community-wide education campaigns, 150
diabetes self-management education, 301
diet, 123–124, 317
educational interventions in schools, 362
as health intervention, 358
level, and mental health, 344
level, and physical activity, 145
nutrition, 122, 123
patient, 261, 264, 268, 278–279
physical, 363, 364, 365
sexual, 214

efficacy expectations (social cognitive theory), 63–64

eHealth, 70. *See also* mobile health (mHealth)
for CVD management/secondary prevention, 277, 279–280

-delivered CR programs, 283
for eating behavior change, 131–132
EHRs. *See* electronic health records
electronic health records (EHRs), 113, 392, 393, 401–402
electronic monitoring of health behaviors, 103, 104
EMA. *See* ecological momentary assessment
emerging adulthood
health equity in, 358
identity development, 87
psychological development in, 82–83
empathy, 133, 198, 302
employer-based health insurance, 374
empowerment theory-based community forum, 32–34
endocannabinoid system (ECS), 177
energy gap, 332
Engaged for Change, 29–32
Environmental Assessment of Public Recreation Spaces (EAPRS) tool, 417
environmental audits, 415
EPI. *See* Expanded Program on Immunization
epidemiology, 21–22
Epworth Sleepiness Scale (ESS), 107
eradication of disease, 193
ESS. *See* Epworth Sleepiness Scale
ethnicity. *See* race/ethnicity
EUROACTION trial, 281
evidence-based cancer control programs (EBCCP), 263–264
ex ante moral hazard, 9
ex post moral hazard, 9
exercise, 48, 52, 74, 139, 276, 282, 318. *See also* physical activity
Expanded Obesity Research Paradigm, 326
Expanded Program on Immunization (EPI), 193
externality (economics), 8–9, 10

fall prevention, 246–247
family barriers to diabetes management, 300–301
family medicine, 396
family planning and contraception
coercion in family planning programs, 216
contraception demand, 217–219
counseling, 219
engagement of men in, 219, 220
history of family planning programs, 215–216
Malawi Male Motivators Project, 220
family system, 39–40
defining, 40, 42–43
developmental model of self- and social regulation, 47, 53–54
future directions of interventions, 55–56
levels of intervention, 41, 43, 44
social ecological theory, 41, 44, 45, 48–50

typological approaches, 55
family system-illness (FSI) model, 46, 50–51
family systems theory, 40, 42–43, 44, 46
actor-partner interdependence model, 47, 50–51
common fate model, 47, 52–53
family-based interventions, 41, 43, 55, 150
for diabetes management, 302–303
for obesity management, 325
family-focused interventions, 41, 43, 48
Family/friend Activation to Motivate Self-care (FAMS), 53
family-level interventions, 41, 43
FAMS. *See* Family/friend Activation to Motivate Self-care
fatal injuries, 237, 238, 239
FDA. *See* Food and Drug Administration
Federal Highway Administration (FHWA), 428
Federally-Qualified Health Centers (FQHCs), 405
feedback (systems theory), 42–43, 53–54
feedback (weight loss strategy), 320
fentanyl, 178, 179, 180
FHWA. *See* Federal Highway Administration
finance, 4
flexible sigmoidoscopy, 259
flipped classroom, 396
Food and Drug Administration (FDA), 173, 174, 175, 177, 178, 179, 180, 381
food choice model, 126
food frequency questionnaires, 107
forced sterilization, 216
FQHCs. *See* Federally-Qualified Health Centers
FSI. *See* family system-illness model
functional support (social support), 146

gabapentin, 177
GAD-7, 345
games/gaming
applications, 71
digital, 224
interventions, 131, 151, 224
video, 64
gay, bisexual, queer, and other men who have sex with men (GBQMSM), 24, 26–27, 32, 33
GBQMSM. *See* gay, bisexual, queer, and other men who have sex with men
gender. *See also* women
-based violence, 215, 225–227
and CVD, 275
equality *vs.* equity, 215
gender identity development, 88
inequality, 214
and physical activity, 144, 147
gender role development, theory of, 88
geographic information systems (GIS), 109, 112, 148, 416, 417, 420, 425, 430

444 INDEX

geo-referencing, 430
germ theory of disease, 22
gFOBT. *See* high-sensitivity guaiac fecal occult
blood test
GirlTrek, 149
GIS. *See* geographic information systems
global health
issues, 91–92
mental health, 94
global positioning system (GPS), 70, 141, 417
globalization, 155
GlucoMe Insulin Pen Monitor cap, 106
goal setting
diabetes management, 307
eating behavior change, 127
weight loss, 319
GOMER (Get Out of My Emergency Room), 184
Google Street View, 109, 418
Gove County Medical Center, 379, 381
GPS. *See* global positioning system
guanfacine, 177
guideline directed medical therapy, 277

habituation, and eating behaviors, 123
handwashing behaviors, 426
harm reduction (substance use), 166, 182, 183, 185
current progress in, 169
historical origins of, 168
integration and specialization, 170
lessons learned, 169
services, innovation in, 170
HARTS Lab, 149
HBM. *See* health belief model
Health and Well-being Best Practices Scorecard
(HERO Scorecard), 385
health behavior measurement, 100
community/population-level, 101, 108–113
considerations, 102–103, 113–114
future directions, 113–114
individual-level, 101, 103–108
methods, 102–103
psychometric properties, 102, 108
socioecological model and intersectionality,
101
and structural stigma/discrimination, 113–114
health belief model (HBM), 23, 61–63, 70, 72–73,
125, 200, 202–203, 222, 245, 345–346, 363
Health Chat campaign, 53
health disparities, 2, 28
and built environment, 421
childhood obesity, 112
community engagement in addressing, 56
and CVD, 274, 275
definition of, 91
in diabetes care, reducing, 306
and digital healthcare, 280

frameworks, 326
and HIV/AIDS, 33, 223
HPV vaccination coverage, 221
injuries, 239–240
mental healthcare, 343
and obesity, 316–317, 325, 326
sexual and reproductive health, 215
and stigma/discrimination in policies, 113–114
substance use, 174, 177, 178, 182
and systems of oppression and privilege, 101
Health Enhancement Research Organization
(HERO)
HERO Scorecard, 385
workplace mental health and well-being best
practices, 388
health equity, 2, 28, 61, 101, 130
and built environment, 421, 425
and cancer screening, 258, 264–267, 268
and culture, 91
and digital healthcare, 280
issues, in behavioral treatment for obesity,
325–328
obesity interventions centered on, 332–333
and school-based interventions, 357–358
in SUD outcomes, public policies that promote,
183–184
Health ICT, 150
health insurance, 376
and asymmetric information, 8
and cancer screening, 255, 265, 266
employer-based, 374
and market failures, 10–11
and moral hazard, 9
penalties, 11
reimbursement, 323, 394
health literacy, 123, 344
health policies, 17
addressing asymmetric information with, 9–10
addressing externalities with, 10
for decreasing consumption of soda, 15
economic principles for developing, 4–9
economic rationale for policy intervention, 9–12
evaluation of, 13–17
for remedying market failures, 10–11
role in influencing health, 3–4
sin taxes, 11–12
and substitutes/compliments, 7–8
healthcare system, 393
beliefs and attitudes about health behavior
change, 393
chronic care model, 399–400
inadequate intensive treatment options, 394
lack of access to physician extenders,
behavioral health and other provider types,
394
lack of systems to support primary care
provider intervention, 393

medical education system, 393
  patient-centered medical home, 397, 398–399
  reimbursement and financial barriers, 323, 394
  system supports and practice-level redesigns, 400–402
  system-centered approach to behavior change, 405–407
Healthy Eating Design Guidelines for School Architecture, 422
Healthy Hunger-Free Kids Act, 364
Healthy People 2030, 2, 3–4, 374
HERO. *See* Health Enhancement Research Organization
heroin, 166, 167
HFS-P. *See* Hypoglycemia Fear Survey for Parents
highly potent synthetic opioids (HPSO), 178
high-risk human papillomavirus testing, 259
high-sensitivity guaiac fecal occult blood test (gFOBT), 259
Hip Hop HEALS (Healthy Eating And Living in Schools), 64
HIV/AIDS, 212
  epidemic, global evolution of, 222–223
  injection-related, 168
  prevention, 23, 33, 223
    multilevel strategy for, 26–27
    social and behavioral changes for improving, 224–225
    socioecological models for, 24–26
  treatment, social and behavioral changes for improving, 223–224
HOLA, 26–27
housing, 5
HPSO. *See* highly potent synthetic opioids
HPV. *See* human papillomavirus
human papillomavirus (HPV), 220–221, 259
  disparities in vaccination coverage, 221
  feminization of, 222
  interventions at different levels of socioecological model, 221–222
  vaccination, 194, 195, 220–222, 259
human–animal companionship, 147
hypoglycemia
  fear of, 299–300
  nighttime, 108
Hypoglycemia Fear Survey for Parents (HFS-P), 108

I-Change model, 73
ICPD. *See* International Conference on Population and Development
ICT. *See* information and communication technologies
identity development, 87
  gender identity, 88

racial and ethnic identity, 87
IEPs. *See* individualized education plans
IMB. *See* Information-Motivation-Behavioral skills model
immediate determinants (relapse prevention model), 68–69
impedance plethysmography (IPG), 15–16
income, 4, 5, 11, 12
  and access to primary care physicians, 393
  and CVD, 274
  and physical activity, 145
increasing vaccination model, 200
incremental cost to outcome ratio, 16
independent observations, 44
indirect objective measures of individual-level health behaviors, 104–105, 106–107
individualism, 94–95
individualized education plans (IEPs), 361
individual-level dietary behavior change, 121–122
individual-level health behavior measurement, 101
  direct objective measures, 103–104, 106
  indirect objective measures, 104–105, 106–107
  subjective measures, 105, 107–108
  youth with type 1 diabetes mellitus, 108
individual-level theories of health behavior, 60–61
  application to multiple health behaviors change, 75–76
  application to technology-enabled interventions, 70–71
  biological underpinnings/consequences and social context, 75
  comparison of, 72–73
  future directions, 74–76
  health belief model, 61–63, 72–73
  link between theory use and intervention effectiveness, 74
  relapse prevention model, 68–69, 72–73
  social cognitive theory, 63–64, 72–73, 150
  theories of within-person behavioral variability, 71
  theory of planned behavior, 65–67, 72–73
  theory testing, 74–75
  transtheoretical model, 67–68, 72–73
inferior goods, 6
information, 123–124. *See also* education
  asymmetric, 8, 9–10
  campaigns, 7, 9, 10
  ecological, 102
  informational interventions for physical activity, 150–151
  provision, 10, 13, 199
information and communication technologies (ICT), 150, 151

446 INDEX

Information-Motivation-Behavioral skills (IMB) model, 220
injuries, 236–237. *See also* unintentional injuries
Institute of Medicine (IOM), 29, 393
insulin, 296, 297, 299, 306
insulin pen, 297
insulin pumps. *See* continuous subcutaneous insulin infusion (CSII)
integrated behavioral model, 73
integrated theory of health behavior change, 73
integrated-collaborative behavioral healthcare, 402
    collaborative care model, 402–403
    primary care behavioral health model, 403–405
intensive behavioral change treatment, 394
intentional injuries, 236
interactive media use, impact on development, 86–87
interdependence (systems theory), 40, 42, 51, 52
interdependent observations, 44
intergenerational economic mobility, 4
International Conference on Population and Development (ICPD), 212, 214, 220
International Physical Activity Questionnaire (IPAQ), 140
interprofessional training, 396
intersectionality, 93, 101
intimate partner violence (IPV), 215, 225
intuitive eating, 130
IOM. *See* Institute of Medicine
IPAQ. *See* International Physical Activity Questionnaire
IPG. *See* impedance plethysmography
IPV. *See* intimate partner violence

Jacobson v. Massachusetts (1905), 194
JITAIs. *See* just-in-time adaptive interventions
The Joint Commission, 381
Joint United Nations Programme on HIV/AIDS (UNAIDS), 222–223
just-in-time adaptive interventions (JITAIs), 151

Koch, Robert, 22
Koch's postulates, 22

language development, 83
latex condoms, 224
Latinx people
    diabetes in, 306
    HIV/AIDs in, 223
    HOLA, 26–27
    radionovelas for addressing vaccine hesitancy, 221–222
    Salud Con La Familia (Health with the Family) program, 53

social networks of, 147
social support of, 147
LEEP. *See* Loop Electrosurgical Excision Procedure
legislation for behavior change, 242–243
leisure-time physical activity, 145, 147
life expectancy, 2–3, 22
life-course approaches, 154
    built environment, 418–421
    for prevention and management of CVD, 275–276
Life-Simple 7 score, 280
LifeSkills Training middle school program, 362
lifestyle, 69
    and CVD management/prevention, 276, 280, 281–282, 283, 284
    and diabetes management, 296, 297, 303
    and health belief model, 200
    and obesity management, 317, 329, 331
    and SCT, 64
    and SDOH, 2
    tracking (mHealth), 128
liraglutide, 329
Loeffler, Frederich, 22
Loeffler, Koch, 22
logs, 107, 140
Loop Electrosurgical Excision Procedure (LEEP), 220
Los Angeles Unified School District, 424
lung cancer
    deaths, 3–4, 171, 253
    screening, 255, 257, 260, 262, 263, 266, 267

MACRA. *See* Medicare Access and CHIP Reauthorization Act of 2015
Malawi Male Motivators Project, 220
mammography, 258
Managed Alcohol Programs (MAP) model, 166
MAP. *See* Managed Alcohol Programs model
marked crosswalks, 421, 426
market equilibrium, 6, 7
market failures, 8–9, 10–12
markets, 6
mask wearing during COVID-19 pandemic, 89, 95, 102
match–mismatch experiment, 67
MBS. *See* metabolic and bariatric surgery
MCAT. *See* Medical College Admission Test
MDRTC. *See* Michigan Diabetes Research and Training Center
meal replacements, 318–319
measles, 193, 195, 203–204
measles, mumps, and rubella (MMR) vaccine, 194, 204
Med-eMonitor, 106
Medicaid, 394, 397

Medical College Admission Test (MCAT), 396
medical education/training, 393, 395–396, 406
    curriculum reform, 395–396
    exposure to effective integrated-collaborative
        care models during, 397
    exposure to resources to support health
        behavior change interventions, 397
    medical school/internship/residency, 396–397
    NAM recommendations for integrating
        behavioral and social sciences into medical
        school curricula, 395
medical treatment engagement, measurement of,
    101, 106, 107, 108
Medicare Access and CHIP Reauthorization Act
    of 2015 (MACRA), 397
medication adherence, 50, 62–63, 406
    during adolescence, 83
    ART, 223–224
    and CVD management, 276–277, 282
    and diabetes management, 297
    measurement of, 107
    of people with mental health disorders, 345,
        346
Medication Event Monitoring System (MEMS),
    106
medications
    for alcohol use disorder, 175
    for cannabis use disorder, 177
    for diabetes, 296, 298
    for opioid use disorder, 178–179
    for tobacco use disorder, 173
    for weight loss, 329–330
MEMS. See Medication Event Monitoring System
men who have sex with men (MSM), 220, 223
mental health, 361
    and chronic conditions, 342–343
    clinical presentation of behavioral health
        disorders, 341–342
    cognitive behavioral therapy, 346–347, 348
    definition of, 341
    global, 94
    impact of social and environmental factors on,
        343–344
    outcomes, impact of physical activity on,
        141–142
    Transforming and Expanding Access to Mental
        Health in Urban Practices (TEAM UP)
        model, 404
    worksite wellness interventions, 385–387, 388
mental health disorders
    behavioral activation, 346, 347, 349–350
    diagnosis of, 345
    health belief model, 345–346
    motivational interviewing, 350–353
    treatment of, 345–353
mental health insurance laws/mental health
    parity laws, 10–11

Mercer, 385
meta-analyses, 61, 155
metabolic and bariatric surgery (MBS), 330–331
metformin, 298
methadone, 178, 179, 185
mHealth. See mobile health (mHealth)
mHealth+CarePartner, 49–50
MI. See motivational interviewing
miasma, 21–22
Michigan Diabetes Research and Training Center
    (MDRTC), 305
Michigan Model for Health™ (MMH), 363
Millennium Development Goals, 212
mindful eating, 130
mindfulness-based relapse prevention, 69
mindless eating, 123
mirtazapine, 177
miscarried helping, 300
MMH. See Michigan Model for Health™
MMR. See measles, mumps, and rubella vaccine
Mobile App Rating Scale, 131
mobile health (mHealth), 49–50, 55, 70, 71, 87, 151
    for CVD management/secondary prevention,
        278, 279–280
    -delivered CR programs, 283
    for diabetes management, 307
    for eating behavior change, 131–132
    for improving ART adherence, 224
    self-monitoring tools, 128
mobile methadone programs, 185
mood disorders, 345, 346
moral hazards, 9
moratorium ordinances, 427
motivational interviewing (MI), 130, 181, 396
    for alcohol use disorder, 175
    clinical interview, questions used in, 172
    for CVD management/secondary prevention,
        278–279
    for diabetes management, 302
    for mental health disorders, 350–353
    for tobacco use disorder, 171–172
    for vaccination conversations, 196, 197,
        198–200
MSM. See men who have sex with men
multicomponent interventions, 406–407
    built environment interventions, 428–429
    for CVD management/secondary prevention,
        281–282, 284–285
    for diabetes management, 301–302
    for obesity management, 323
    in schools, 364–365
multidisciplinary team-based approaches,
    281–282, 284
MULTIFIT program, 281
multi-method, multi-informant assessment
    approach, 102
multimethodological theory-testing framework, 75

448 INDEX

multiple health behaviors change
    application of individual-level health behavior
        theories to, 75–76
    interventions, for physical activity, 153–154
mutual influence (systems theory), 40, 42
MyPlate, 383

N-acetyl cysteine (NAC), 177
Na Mikimiki Project, 70
nabilone, 177
nabiximols, 177
NAC. *See* N-acetyl cysteine
naloxone (Narcan), 169, 180
naltrexone, 175, 177, 178
NAM. *See* National Academy of Medicine
Narcotic Treatment Administration (NTA), 167
National Academy of Medicine (NAM), 395
National Cancer Institute, 263, 396
National Comprehensive Cancer Network, 256
National Health and Nutrition Examination
    Survey (NHANES), 119, 140
National Health Education Standards, 363
National Health Interview Survey (NHIS), 140, 171
National Highway Traffic Safety Administration,
    243
National Household Travel Survey (NHTS), 140
National Immunization Technical Advisory
    Groups (NITAGs), 192, 193–194
National Institute on Minority Health and Health
    Disparities Research Framework, 326
National Institutes of Health (NIH), 28, 29, 172,
    245
National Lung Screening Trial, 260, 267
National Physical Activity Plan, 427
National Survey of Children's Health (NSCH), 140
National Survey on Drug Use and Health
    (NSDUH), 174–175, 176, 178
National Weight Control Registry, 331
Native Americans, 4, 327
NCDs. *See* non-communicable diseases
neighborhood characteristics. *See also* built
    environment
    and diabetes, 306
    and eating behavior, 123
    and economic opportunities, 5
    measurement of, 109, 112
    and mental health, 344
    and physical activity, 148–149, 318
Neighborhood Environment Walkability Survey
    (NEWS), 415
NEMS. *See* Nutrition Environment Measurement
    Survey
NEWS. *See* Neighborhood Environment
    Walkability Survey
NHANES. *See* National Health and Nutrition
    Examination Survey
NHIS. *See* National Health Interview Survey

NHTS. *See* National Household Travel Survey
NICH. *See* Novel Interventions in Children's
    Healthcare
nicotine, 171
nicotine replacement therapy (NRT), 173, 394
nighttime hypoglycemia, 108
NIH. *See* National Institutes of Health
NITAGs. *See* National Immunization Technical
    Advisory Groups
non-binary people, 32, 92, 215
non-communicable diseases (NCDs), 22. *See also*
    chronic diseases
nonfatal injuries, 237, 238
nonsummativity (systems theory), 42, 52–53
North Carolina Community-Academic
    Partnership, 32
Novel Interventions in Children's Healthcare
    (NICH), 305
NRT. *See* nicotine replacement therapy
NSCH. *See* National Survey of Children's Health
NSDUH. *See* National Survey on Drug Use and
    Health
NTA. *See* Narcotic Treatment Administration
nudges, 12–13, 196–198, 203
nutrition, 365
    and built environment, 420, 429
    education, 122, 123
    labels, 10
    policy changes, 364
    worksite wellness interventions, 383–385
Nutrition Environment Measurement Survey
    (NEMS), 109

OARS. *See* open questions, affirmations,
    reflections, and summaries
obesity, 421
    acceptance-based behavioral treatment for,
        322–323
    barriers to treatment of, 323
    in children, 112, 316–317
    classification of, 317
    dietary modification, 317–318
    equity issues in behavioral treatment
        disparities in weight loss outcomes, 325–326
        social determinants of health and equity-
            minded frameworks, 326–328
    health equity-centered interventions, 332–333
    healthcare provider-directed and patient-
        centered interventions, 323–324
    metabolic and bariatric surgery, 330–331
    pharmacotherapy, 329–330
    physical activity, 318
    policy-level interventions, 333
    prevalence, comorbidities, and significance of,
        316–317
    relapse prevention/maintenance of change,
        331–332

self-monitoring, 319, 322
self-regulation, 322
standard behavioral treatment for, 318–321
weight stigma, 324
Obesity Society, 332
objective measures of health behaviors
community-level, 109–110, 112
individual-level (direct), 103–104, 106
individual-level (indirect), 104–105, 106–107
population-level, 110, 111, 112
Office of Disease Prevention and Health
Promotion, 374
older adults, 373
cancer screening of, 263
COVID-19 mitigation behaviors of, 89
fall prevention, 246–247
medication adherence of, 277
physical activity among, 144, 147, 149
representation in cancer screening research, 267
one-child policy (China), 216
open questions, affirmations, reflections, and
summaries (OARS), 198
opioid use disorder (OUD), 182
diagnosis of, 178
medications for, 178–179
opioids, 178–179
pharmacology of, 178
use
epidemiology of, 178
during pregnancy, 181–182
Opportunity Atlas, 5
oppression and privilege, systems of, 101–102, 266
organizational health promotion, 377
orlistat, 329
OSNAP Initiative, 365
OUD. *See* opioid use disorder
Our Voice initiative, 149
OurRelationship, 52
outcome expectations (social cognitive theory), 63
outpatient venography, 16
overdose prevention centers, 169, 170

PACV. *See* Parent Attitudes about Childhood
Vaccine
panic disorders, 342
Pap test, 258–259
parent and family factors framework, 45, 48–49
Parent Attitudes about Childhood Vaccine
(PACV), 205
parenting-focused interventions, 88
partnerships
and built environment interventions, 423–424
CBPR, 26, 29–32
motivational interviewing, 172
Pasteur, Louis, 22
patient adherence, 70. *See also* medication
adherence

and collaborative care model, 402
and CVD management, 276–277, 279, 280, 284
and diabetes management, 297
and mHealth, 128
and obesity management, 322
patient navigators, 261–262, 265
patient-centered interventions
for obesity management, 323–324
in schools, 361–362
patient-centered medical homes (PCMHs), 397,
398–399, 400
PBC. *See* perceived behavioral control
PCBH. *See* primary care behavioral health
model
PCMHs. *See* patient-centered medical homes
Pedestrian and Bicycle Information Center, 423
pedestrian crossings, 421, 426
pedestrian deaths, 420–421
pediatric weight management programs, 88–89
pedometers, 103
peer support interventions, 303
perceived barriers (health belief model), 62, 345
perceived behavioral control (PBC), 65, 66–67
perceived benefits (health belief model), 62, 345
perceived severity (health belief model), 62, 202,
345
perceived susceptibility (health belief model), 62,
202, 345, 346
performance accomplishments, and self-efficacy,
64
personalized medicine, 55
person-centered approach to behavior change,
405–407
pharmacy refill records, 107
phentermine-topiramate, 329
PHQ-9, 345
physical activity, 326
among Americans, prevalence of, 142–144
assessment, 101, 103, 106, 107, 112, 140–141
and built environment, 147–148, 419–420,
424–425, 427–428
citizen science, 149
definition of, 139
device-based measures, 103, 140, 141, 149
dissemination of interventions, 155
domains of, 140
ecological model of, 419
individual-level factors contributing to,
144–145
interventions, 150
behavioral and social approaches, 150
environmental and policy-based
approaches, 152–153
informational and technology-based
approaches, 150–152
multiple behavior change, 153–154
stealth, 153
targets/contexts of, 154

450 INDEX

physical activity (*cont'd*)
  leisure-time, 145, 147
  life-course perspective, 154
  monitors, 112
  for obesity management, 318
  physical and mental health-related outcomes
    of, 141–142
  promotion, future directions in, 153–154
  psychosocial and behavioral factors associated
    with, 145
  research, challenges and opportunities in, 154–155
  research, history and development of, 139–140
  in rural areas, 428
  self-report measures, 140, 141
  social ecological framework, 154
  social factors contributing to, 146–147, 150
  for weight loss maintenance, 332
  worksite wellness interventions, 381–383
Physical Activity Design Guidelines for School
  Architecture, 422
Physical Activity Guidelines for Americans, 141,
  143–144, 154
physical development, 84
physical education, 363, 364, 365
physical spaces for health promotion, 424–425
physiological state, and self-efficacy, 64
pill counting, 107
Pittsburgh Sleep Quality Index, 107
PLACES. *See* Population Level Analysis and
  Community Estimates
Planet Health, 364–365, 366
playgrounds, school, 424–425, 427
polysomnography, 106
population health, 21, 60. *See also* vaccines
  behavior measurement, 108–109, 110, 111, 112,
    113, 140
  definition of, 108
  outcomes, measurement of, 101
  surveys, 140
Population Level Analysis and Community
  Estimates (PLACES), 113
portion control (weight loss strategy), 321
poverty, 404
  and child marriage, 227
  impact on mental health, 343, 405
  and unintentional injuries, 240
precaution adoption process model, 131
pre-exposure prophylaxis (PrEP), 26, 27
pregnancy, 328. *See also* family planning and
  contraception
  substance use during, 174, 181–182
  unintended, 217
PrEP. *See* pre-exposure prophylaxis
present bias, 11
Prevention Research Centers Program (CDC), 29
preventive health screenings, 113–114
primary care behavioral health (PCBH) model,
  403–405

primary care settings, 392. *See also* healthcare
  system
  CMS reimbursement for, 323–324
  vs. specialty care, behavioral health standards
    of care in, 404
problem solving, 402
  behavioral family systems therapy, 50, 51,
    304
  diabetes management, 294, 299, 301–303, 308
  eating behavior change, 128–129
  as a weight loss strategy, 320
prohibitions, 9, 12
Project Toward No Tobacco Use, 366
Propeller Health devices, 106
protection motivation theory, 200, 201
psychological development
  and ADHD, 89
  in emerging adulthood, 82–83
psychological insulin resistance, 299

QALY. *See* quality adjusted life-years
quality adjusted life-years (QALY), 16, 17

RAA. *See* reasoned action approach
race/ethnicity, 87. *See also* Black Americans;
  Latinx people
  and AUD diagnosis, 174
  and breast cancer screening, 258
  and built environment, 421
  and cancer incidence and mortality rates, 253,
    254
  and childhood obesity, 112
  and CVD, 275
  disparities in mental health, 343, 344
  disparities in weight loss outcomes of
    behavioral treatment, 325–326
  and health disparities, 1
  and life expectancy, 2–3
  and lung cancer screening, 260
  and physical activity, 144, 318
  racialization of substance use, 184
  substance use in racial/ethnic minorities, 174,
    176, 178, 182
  and unintentional injuries, 239–240
racial and ethnic identity development, 87
racism, 87, 182, 253, 264, 266, 306
radionovelas, 221–222
REACH. *See* Reduction of Atherothrombosis for
  Continued Health Registry
readiness for change, 246, 302, 405–406
reasoned action approach (RAA), 73
reciprocal determinism, 27, 242
recreational cannabis, 176
recreational substance use, 168
Reduction of Atherothrombosis for Continued
  Health (REACH) Registry, 277

reflective listening, 198
reimbursement (health insurance), 323, 394
relapse prevention (RP) model, 68–69, 72–73, 321
relational hypothesis of motivational interviewing, 198
reliability (measurement), 102
reminders, 70, 261, 262, 268, 298, 406
remote food photography method (RFPM), 103
remote sensing, 416, 418, 430
remote work environment, 373–374, 375
reproductive health. *See* sexual and reproductive health (SRH)
resistance exercise training, 318
retatrutride, 329
RFPM. *See* remote food photography method
Royal College of Physicians and Surgeons of Canada, 396
RP. *See* relapse prevention model
rural areas, people in
  and built environment, 149, 428
  cancer screening of, 256
  telehealth for, 56

Safe Routes to School (SRTS), 428–429
Safer Choices, 365, 366
safer sex, promotion of, 224
safety culture, 244
Salud Con La Familia (Health with the Family) program, 53
sanitary statistics, 21–22
SASA!, 226
SASQ. *See* Single Alcohol Screening Question
SBIRT. *See* Screening Brief Intervention and Referral to Treatment
school feeding programs, 363
school-based health clinics, 361–362
school-based interventions, 357–358
  adaptability of, 365
  behavioral interventions, 362–363
  built environment interventions, 424–425, 427, 428
  challenges, 365–366
  community-engaged research principles, 366
  cost-effectiveness of strategies, 365–366
  eating behavior change, 132
  education, 358, 362
  future directions, 366–367
  guidelines for health behavior change, 359–360
  Hip Hop HEALS (Healthy Eating And Living in Schools), 64
  and infrastructure, 365
  multicomponent, 364–365
  patient-centered, 361–362
  physical activity, 152
  and policies, 364, 367
  promotion of equity in, 357, 358
  at system level, 363–364

types of, 360–365
vaccination programs, 222
Screening Brief Intervention and Referral to Treatment (SBIRT), 172, 175
SCRIP. *See* Stanford Coronary Risk Intervention Program
SCT. *See* social cognitive theory
SDGs. *See* Sustainable Development Goals
SDOH. *See* social determinants of health
second degree moral hazards, 9
sedentary behaviors, 140, 142–143, 375, 381–383, 424
SEL. *See* social-emotional learning
self- and family-management framework, 44, 45, 48
self-determinations theory, 125
self-care, 54, 284, 300, 342, 346–347, 350
self-efficacy, 48, 50–51, 63–64, 89, 127, 128, 153, 203, 224, 242, 319
self-efficacy theory, 200, 201
self-evaluation, 319
self-monitoring
  of eating behaviors, 121, 127–128, 131
  of physical activity, 143, 152
  for weight loss, 319, 322
self-regulation, 68, 245, 282
  of appetite, 121
  developmental model of, 47, 53–54
  and obesity management, 322
  and physical activity, 150
self-reinforcement, 319
self-report measures, 70, 107–108, 112–113, 140, 144, 152, 415, 416
semaglutide, 329, 330
SenseCam, 417
sensitivity (measurement), 102
SES. *See* socioeconomic status
sexual and gender-based violence (SGBV), 225
  child, early, and forced marriages and unions, 226–227
  ecological perspectives for understanding and preventing, 225–226
  SASA!, 226
sexual and reproductive health (SRH)
  contraception, 216
  contraception demand, 217–219
  defining, 212–213
  gender equality *vs.* equity, 215
  and gender inequality, 214
  history of global family planning programs, 215–216
  HIV/AIDS, 222–225
  human papillomavirus, 220–222
  rights-based perspective of, 213–214
  social-ecological perspective, 214–215
SFA. *See* smoke-free air policies
SG. *See* sleeve gastrectomy
SGBV. *See* sexual and gender-based violence

452 INDEX

shared-use agreements, 427–428
short message service (SMS). *See* text messaging
sin taxes, 10, 11–12
Single Alcohol Screening Question (SASQ), 174
single parents, 55, 377
skin cancer, 244–245
skip-stop elevator, 425
sleep behaviors, measurement of, 101, 106–108
sleeve gastrectomy (SG), 330
SlimFast, 318
Small Town and Rural Multimodal Networks guide, 428
smallpox vaccination, 194, 195
smallpox variolation, 192–193, 203
SMART (Specific, Measurable, Attainable, Realistic, Timely) goal model, 127
Smart Growth, 422, 426
smoke-free air (SFA) policies, 11
smoking. *See also* tobacco use
  bans, 10
  cessation
    individual-level theories of health behavior, 72–73
    interventions, 55, 67, 68
  in children/adolescents, 180
  e-cigarettes, 174, 180, 381
  and lung cancer deaths, 3, 4
  and lung cancer screening, 260
  sin taxes, 11–12
SMS. *See* short message service
Snow, John, 22
social assertion (weight loss strategy), 320
social breaks, 185
social cognitive theory (SCT), 63–64, 70, 71, 72–73, 125, 131, 150, 151, 202, 224, 245, 278, 318, 322, 363
social determinants of health (SDOH), 1–2, 4, 33, 34, 91, 92, 182, 239, 306, 333, 343. *See also* built environment
  assessment, 101
  and behavioral weight loss treatment, 326–327
  and cancer screening, 264, 266
  definition of, 326
  and individual-level theories of health behavior, 75
  and physical activity, 146–149
social determinants of substance use, 167–168
social distancing during COVID-19 pandemic, 102, 147
social drivers of health, 23
social ecological theory, 41, 44, 45
  parent and family factors framework, 45, 48–49
  self- and family-management framework, 44, 45, 48
  therapeutic triangle in healthcare, 46, 49–50
social marketing, 153
social media, 86, 151

benefits of, 86–87
  interventions, 53, 70
  misinformation about vaccines in, 204
social networks, 4, 32, 279
  for addressing vaccine hesitancy, 221
  for HIV/AIDS prevention, 26–27
  and physical activity, 146, 147, 150, 151
social norms, 13, 71, 203, 222, 224, 237, 244–245
social regulation, developmental model of, 47, 53–54
social support, 32, 279
  for diabetes management, 303
  dimensions of, 146
  for eating behavior change, 128
  and physical activity, 146–147, 150
  via companionship, 147
social workers, 93, 284, 304, 350, 352–353
social-emotional learning (SEL), 362–363
socialization, 88, 419
society-oriented drug care, 168
socioecological model(s), 23, 154
  characteristics of, 23–26
  complex nature of human environments, 25
  dynamic nature of behavior, 26
  elements of individual's environment, 25–26
  and health behavior measurement, 101–102
  and HPV interventions, 221–222
  influence of multiple factors on behavior, 24–25
  multilevel intervention for HIV prevention, 26–27
  sexual and reproductive health, 214–215
  study participants, 25
  variation in individual behavioral responses, 26
  for worksite wellness initiatives, 378
socioeconomic status (SES)
  and cancer screening, 255
  and injury risk, 239
  neighborhood, and childhood obesity disparities, 112
  and sin taxes, 12
socioemotional development, 84–85
South Carolina Department of Health and Environmental Control, 305
Special Turku Coronary Risk Factor Intervention Project (STRIP), 275
specialization (economics), 6
speech-language pathologists, school-based, 361
speeding behavior, 241–242
SRH. *See* sexual and reproductive health
SRTS. *See* Safe Routes to School
SSOs. *See* systematic social observations
stages of change model. *See* transtheoretical model
stair use, 425
stakeholder mapping, 377

Stanford Coronary Risk Intervention Program (SCRIP), 281
statins, 275, 276, 277
stealth interventions, 153
stigma, 109, 113–114
    and cancer screening, 259, 267
    and HIV/AIDS prevention/management, 25, 26, 27
    and substance use, 184–185
    weight, 324, 393
stimulus control (weight loss strategy), 320
stimulus narrowing, 318
stool DNA tests, 259
story immersion, 71
strengths-based approach, 50, 327
stress, 69, 324
    and obesity, 328
    prevention, 376
    worksite, 375
        wellness interventions, 385–387, 388
STRIP. *See* Special Turku Coronary Risk Factor Intervention Project
structural determinants of health, 21, 23, 33, 114, 155, 275, 327, 328
structural racism, 264, 266
    and cancer incidence and mortality rates, 253
    definition of, 327
    measures of, 109
structural stigma, 109, 113–114
structural support (social support), 146
subjective measures of health behaviors
    community-level, 111, 112–113
    individual-level, 105, 107–108
    population-level, 111, 113
subjective norms (theory of reasoned action), 65
substance use, 164, 166
    alcohol use/alcohol use disorder, 174–175
    barriers for treatment, 185
    cannabis use/cannabis use disorder, 176–177
    chaotic, 166
    in children and adolescents, 180–181
    cocaine use and cocaine use disorder, 179
    community-based prevention programs, 167
    deconstructing social stigma, 184–185
    functional, 166
    GOMER (Get Out of My Emergency Room), 184
    harm reduction, 166, 168–170, 182, 183, 185
    impact on brain development, 181
    individualist orientation of prevention programs, 167
    opioids/opioid use disorder, 178–179
    during pregnancy, 181–182
    prevention strategies, 166–167
    in racial and ethnic minorities, 182
    recreational, 168
    research, future directions for, 185–186
    risk reduction, 166
    social determinants of, 167–168
    tobacco use/tobacco use disorder, 171–174
    training, curriculum time of, 184
    xylazine, 179–180
substance use disorder (SUD), 164, 341, 342
    diagnostic criteria for, 165
    frequent flyers, 184
    general principles for preventative care, 182–183
    public policies that promote health equity, 183–184
    3Cs of, 165
substitute goods, 6–8, 15
SUD. *See* substance use disorder
sugary drinks/beverages, 123
    screening, EHR-based, 401–402
    taxes for, 12
SunSafe, 365
SunSmart, 244–245
Sustainable Development Goals (SDGs), 212, 226
Switzerland League Against Cancer, 256
syringe services programs, 26
systematic social observations (SSOs), 415, 416, 417
systems theory, 40, 42–43

T1D. *See* type 1 diabetes
Task Force on Community Preventive Services, 243
Task Force on Practice Guidelines, 332
TEAM UP. *See* Transforming and Expanding Access to Mental Health in Urban Practices model
team-based care, 281, 394, 397, 399–400, 405
technical hypothesis of motivational interviewing, 198
technology, 86, 224, 407. *See also* eHealth; mobile health (mHealth)
    -based physical activity interventions, 150–152
    for eating behavior change, 131–132
    -enabled interventions, application of health behavior theories to, 70–71
    and health behavior measurement, 109, 113
    impact of interactive media use on development, 86–87
    for injury prevention, 248
    role in diabetes management, 306–307
    use in family-based interventions, 55–56
telehealth, 56, 94, 150
telemedicine, 279–280, 284–285
tetanus, 193
text messaging, 54, 70, 71, 224, 280
theory of planned behavior (TPB), 23, 65–67, 70, 72–73, 151, 200, 202, 203
theory of reasoned action (TRA), 65, 200, 201, 245

454 INDEX

theory of self-regulation and self-control, 245
theory of subjective culture and interpersonal
relations, 245
therapeutic patient education (TPE), 278–279
therapeutic triangle in healthcare, 46, 49–50
thimerosal, 205
thinking traps, 346, 347
tirzepatide, 329, 330
tobacco taxes, 11
tobacco use, 171
and built environment, 420, 427
cessation, 55, 67, 68, 72–73, 379, 393, 394, 427
in children/adolescents, 180
epidemiology of, 171
neurobiology of addiction, 171
during pregnancy, 181
worksite wellness interventions, 379–381
tobacco use disorder (TUD)
diagnosis of, 171
medications for, 173
motivational interviewing for, 171–172
treatment, clinical evaluation to facilitate,
171–172
total demand for family planning, 217
TPB. See theory of planned behavior
TPE. See therapeutic patient education
TRA. See theory of reasoned action
traffic crashes/injuries, 239
traffic safety, 244, 420–421, 426
traffic-calming measures, 426, 427
Tranq. See xylazine
Transforming and Expanding Access to Mental
Health in Urban Practices (TEAM UP)
model, 404
transgender people
Appalachian Access Project, 32
HIV prevention in transgender women, 26–27
representation in cancer screening research, 267
transportation, 423–424, 430
bicycling, 421, 426–427, 428–429
and cancer screening, 264
public, 25, 377
and sexual and reproductive health, 214
transtheoretical model (TTM), 23, 67–68, 70,
72–73, 126, 131, 151, 198, 226, 246–247,
278–279, 352, 395
triangulation, 102
TTM. See transtheoretical model
TUD. See tobacco use disorder
21st Century Cures Act, 397
24-hour recall interviews, 107
2030 Agenda for Sustainable Development, 358
type 1 diabetes (T1D), 54, 295. See also diabetes
management
BFST intervention in families of adolescents
with, 50–51
coping skills training for youth with, 48
and hypoglycemia, 299–300

and nighttime hypoglycemia, 108
prevalence and incidence of, 296
type 2 diabetes, 54, 82, 295. See also diabetes
management
prevalence and incidence of, 296
psychological insulin resistance, 299

UKPDS. See United Kingdom Prospective
Diabetes Study
UNAIDS. See Joint United Nations Programme
on HIV/AIDS
UNFPA. See United Nations Population Fund
unintentional injuries, 236–237
and built environment, 420–421
disparities, 239–240
ecological models, 242–244
education for behavior change, 241–242
fatal injuries, 237, 238, 239
health communications for behavior change,
244–245
integrative models, 245–246
legislation for behavior change, 242–243
nonfatal injuries, 237, 238
prevention of, 240–247
challenges to, 247–248
public health burden of, 237–238
social norms, 244–245
United Kingdom National Screening Committee,
256
United Kingdom Prospective Diabetes Study
(UKPDS), 297
United Nations Population Fund (UNFPA), 222
United States Department of Agriculture
(USDA), 10, 364, 367
United States Preventive Services Task Force
(USPSTF), 174, 256, 257, 258–260, 262, 268,
323, 397
unmet need for family planning, 217
U.S. Centers for Disease Control and Prevention
(CDC), 1, 2, 3, 28, 29, 100, 113, 221, 237, 243,
246, 295, 305, 316, 342, 359–360, 394
Division of Diabetes Translation, 305
Workplace Health Promotion, 374–375
U.S. Department of Health and Human Services
(USDHHS), 374
U.S. Green Building Council, 422, 429
U.S. National Physical Activity Plan, 375
USDA. See United States Department of
Agriculture
USDHHS. See U.S. Department of Health and
Human Services
USPSTF. See United States Preventive Services
Task Force

vaccine confidence, 205
vaccines, 192

affordability, 222
and autism, beliefs about, 200
decision making of governments about, 193–195
exemptions to, 194
health behavior models, 200, 201–203
history of, 192–193
mandates, 194–195
motivational interviewing for conversations about, 196, 197, 198–200
nudges for promoting, 196–198, 203
post-marketing surveillance of adverse events, 194
reasons for getting, 200–203
and recommendations of healthcare providers, 195–196
uptake, factors associated with, 201
uptake, increasing, 195–196
vaccine hesitancy, 195–196, 203–205, 221
vaccines, COVID-19, 95
acceptance, 95
mandates, 11, 12, 194–195, 364
and politicization, 95
uptake, and community trust on providers, 195
vaccination incentivization campaign, 16
validity (measurement), 102, 155
vaping, 171, 174, 180
varenicline, 173, 177
variolation (smallpox), 192–193, 203
verbal persuasion, and self-efficacy, 64
vicarious experience, and self-efficacy, 64
virtual reality (VR), 71, 151
VMMC. *See* voluntary medical male circumcision
voluntary medical male circumcision (VMMC), 224–225
VR. *See* virtual reality

Wakefield, Andrew, 204
Walk Score, 418
walking
and built environment, 149, 152, 415, 426
Safe Routes to School (SRTS), 428–429
walkability, 149, 426
wearable sensing devices, 132, 307, 416, 417
web-based geospatial data, 417, 418
webcams, 416, 418
web-enabled applications, 416, 417
WebMAP2, 49, 55
weighed food inventory, 106
weight loss, 127, 279, 303, 305. *See also* obesity
maintenance, 331–332
programs, actor-partner interdependence model for, 51–52
standard behavioral treatment for, 318–321
TTM based interventions, 68
weight stigma, 324, 393

WHO. *See* World Health Organization
Whole School, Whole Community, Whole Child (WSCC) model, 359, 363
women. *See also* pregnancy; sexual and gender-based violence (SGBV); sexual and reproductive health (SRH)
in behavioral weight loss intervention studies, 325
Black, 149, 258, 318, 325–326, 328
breast cancer screening, 257, 258, 262
cervical cancer in, 220
cervical cancer screening, 257, 258–259, 263
common cancers in, 253
intimate partner violence experienced by, 225
physical activity of, 144, 147, 149
women-of-substance health hubs, 170
worksite wellness interventions
built environment, 425
creating feasible goals and objectives, 388
equitable opportunities, 377
focus on modifiable behaviors that can lead to chronic disease, 388–389
nutrition, 383–385
organizational health promotion, 377
physical activity, 381–383
planning and implementing, 376–377
shared responsibility and accountability, 388
socioecological model for, 378
stakeholder engagement, 377
strategies, 377–379
stress and mental health, 385–387, 388
tobacco, 379–381
upper management, 377
wellness committees, 376, 377, 378
worksites/workplace
health behaviors at, 375
inequities in, 376
physical activity interventions in, 152–153
prevention strategies, 376
as a priority for intervention setting, 374–375
promotion of eating behavior change in, 132
risk factors for chronic illnesses at, 375
working population in United States, 373–374
WorkWell KS, 381
World Café method, 145–146
World Health Organization (WHO), 1, 86, 175, 192, 221, 257, 275, 295, 358
cycle of social determinants and mental disorders, 344
definition of health, 92
definition of mental health, 341
definition of reproductive health, 213
Expanded Program on Immunization (EPI), 194
SAGE Working Group on Vaccine Hesitancy, 205
WSCC. *See* Whole School, Whole Community, Whole Child model

456 INDEX

xylazine, 179–180

YFS. *See* Cardiovascular Risk in Young Finns Study
YMCA. *See* Young Men's Christian Association
Young Men's Christian Association (YMCA), 304–305
YourWay, 307

Youth Risk Behavior Surveillance System (YRBSS), 113, 140
YRBSS. *See* Youth Risk Behavior Surveillance System

zolpidem, 177
zoning codes/policies, 326, 427, 430